"**Health professional, scientist or lay citizen, one cannot fail to grasp the explosive significance of this book** and its main thesis—that biological weapons programs developed and field tested immune-system-destroying agents now cannot be contained. . . . **A cogent and readable yet carefully documented book.**"

—GARTH L. NICOLSON, PH.D.
PROFESSOR AND CHAIR IN CANCER RESEARCH, UNIVERSITY OF TEXAS

"**Thoroughly researched** . . . Horowitz vividly portrays the inept, dishonest and secretive science found in our country's national laboratories and in international organizations such as the World Health Organization. . . . **I suggest you read this brilliantly idiosyncratic volume.**"

—ED GEHRMAN
BOOK REVIEW—SONOMA COUNTY BAY PRESS

"Dr. Horowitz **courageously exposes the inner workings of the military–medical–industrial complex**, the people, and their mind set. This book provides the unsettling truth, yet, sets us free, by releasing us from tyranny. . . . Amen!"

—DA VID, M.D.
DIRECTOR, SAN FRANCISCO MEDICAL RESEARCH FOUNDATION

"**Horowitz has performed the miracle of summarizing a century of intrigue, fraud and deceit in one cohesive story.** We move from the filthy labs where contaminated vaccines are produced, to the polished executive offices of biowarfare contractors. . . . **This book is the most breathtaking thriller of the last millennium.**"

—EVA LEE SNEAD, M.D.
AUTHOR OF *SOME CALL IT AIDS—I CALL IT MURDER!*

"**The most massive, well-documented assembly of evidence** ever published in support of the idea the AIDS virus could have been manufactured as a biological weapon and then accidentally or purposely released into the world. . . . If you scoff at the notion, you won't be so cocky once you see how much evidence exists. **I recommend it most highly. . . . You'll never think of AIDS the same way again.**"

—RUSS KICK
REVIEW IN *OUTPOSTS 2: CATALOG OF RARE AND DISTURBING ALTERNATIVE INFORMATION*

"**An explosive book exposing the madness of modern medicine and a powerhouse of evidence to show why AIDS is a man-made disease.**"

—ALAN CANTWELL, JR., M.D.
AUTHOR OF *AIDS & THE DOCTORS OF DEATH*

"A compelling, remarkable book, *Emerging Viruses: AIDS and Ebola* , at the very least, reminds us that few who have power do not misapply it, few who have knowledge do not misuse it, and few who have money do not misspend it. This is **a tale of powerful, knowledgeable, moneyed, men who squander their souls as they seek to acquire others'**."

—ROBERT HARTWELL FISKE
AUTHOR OF *DICTIONARY OF CONCISE WRITING*

"**Clearly written, carefully reasoned and researched . . .** As a modern gadfly, Horowitz awakens us to nightmarish challenges we must respond to today if we do not want to wake up dead tomorrow. *Emerging Viruses* is **a historic contribution to the human species.**"

—THOMAS ELLIS KATEN
ASSOCIATE PROFESSOR OF PHILOSOPHY AND AUTHOR OF *DOING PHILOSOPHY*

"*Emerging Viruses : AIDS & Ebola* is **one of the most fascinating books I have ever read.** Each chapter is a learning experience. **I have had goose bumps and chills repeatedly** as I continued to read this amazing work in which **the documentation is overwealming.**"

—ROBERT COHEN
MEDICAL JOURNALIST AND AUTHOR OF *THE POISON IN MILK*

"**Health professionals and those involved in infectious disease research will find *Emerging Viruses* startling** . . . Certain to spark controversy, this provides quite a different view of virus mutations and evolution. "

—*THE BOOKWATCH*
MIDWEST BOOK REVIEW

"**A well documented chronology of the AIDS virus research effort** supporting the author's hypothesis that AIDS was the result of a manufactured virus created for military/population control objectives. **Fascinating, well researched, referenced and written. Four stars out of five.** "

— BOOK REVIEW
JOURNAL OF THE AMERICAN ASSOCIATION OF FORENSIC DENTISTS

"**Presents alarming documents**, all for the first time in one compendium, that causes us to pause, ask questions, and **challenges the scientific community for a fair-minded critical reevaluation of the causes of AIDS and its origin.** These questions are long overdue."

— GARY NULL, PH.D.
AUTHOR AND NATIONALLY SYNDICATED TALK SHOW HOST

Emerging Viruses: AIDS and Ebola

Nature, Accident or Intentional?

Leonard G. Horowitz, D.M.D., M.A., M.P.H.

Foreword by W. John Martin, M.D., Ph.D.

Tetrahedron, Inc.
Rockport, MA

BY LEONARD G. HOROWITZ

Deadly Innocence

Deadly Exposures

Dentistry in the Age of AIDS

AIDS, Fear and Infection Control

Emerging Viruses: AIDS and Ebola—Nature, Accident or Intentional?

To do evil a human being must first of all believe that what he's doing is good. . . .

Ideology—that is what gives devildoing its long-sought justification and gives the evildoer the necessary steadfastness and determination. That is the social theory which helps to make his acts seem good instead of bad in his own and others' eyes, so that he won't hear reproaches and curses but will receive praise and honors.

—Russian dissident Alexander Solzhenitsyn

DEDICATED TO THE SEEKERS OF TRUTH
and to those who, regardless of risk, labor tirelessly to tell it

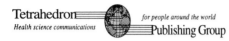

Tetrahedron
Health science communications

for people around the world
Publishing Group

Designed by Gary Kerr
Manufactured in the United States of America

10 9 8 7 6 5 4 3 2 1

Library of Congress Cataloging Requested
Horowitz, Leonard G.
   Emerging Viruses: AIDS & Ebola—Nature, Accident, or Intentional?
   p.   cm.
   Includes bibliographical references and index.
   1. Epidemiology—Popular works.   2. Communicable diseases—
   —Popular works.   3. Biological Weapons—CIA
   —NATO   4. Cancer—National Cancer Institute—Virus
   5. Ebola virus disease—Africa   I. Title.
Card Number: 95-61123
Additional cataloging data pending.

ISBN: 0-923550-12-7

Additional copies of this book are available for bulk purchases.
For more information, please contact:
Tetrahedron, Inc., 20 Drumlin Road, Rockport, Massachusetts 01966,
1-800-336-9266, Fax: 508-546-9226, E-mail: tetra@tetrahedron.org,
URL web site: http://www.tetrahedron.org

Expanded Reference Edition

Third printing

Contents

Part III. Covert Operations

Illustrations

Figures

Maps

To the Reader

THIS BOOK is painfully nonfiction—the story is true, the characters, scientific and political, are real. Secondary references have been checked and authenticated.

Since the importance of this information was clear, I labored to write for both critical health scientists and intelligent lay readers without losing either. Technical words are explained in lay terms for all to better understand.

Though many people—black, white, gay, straight, Jew and gentile—may wish to deny the implications of this work, the truth is the truth. As British statesman Edmund Burke said in the wake of the American revolution, "People never give up their liberties but under some delusion." Perhaps now, as AIDS consumes the lives, liberties, and pursuits of an estimated 30 million HIV-positive people worldwide, the time has come to vanquish our delusions about it and its origin.

Despite its social and scientific importance, the origin of HIV has been clouded in mystery. Based on the mass of circumstantial and scientific evidence presented herein, the theory that "emerging viruses" like HIV and Ebola spontaneously evolved and naturally jumped species from monkey to man must be seriously questioned.

There is an old saying in medicine, that diagnosis is required before treatment. The facts presented here, easily verified, may help diagnose the man-made origin of the world's most feared and deadly viruses. It is hoped this work will, therefore, help redirect AIDS science in search of a cure, free AIDS victims from the guilt and stigma attached to the disease, as well as prevent such "emerging viruses" from reemerging.

I offer this investigation into the orgin of AIDS and Ebola for critical review in the hope that it may also contribute to greater honesty in science, to political, military, and intelligence community reforms that are truly peace loving, and to self and social reflection as a preventative against inhumanity.

—LEONARD G. HOROWITZ

Foreword

All at once, it seems, new viruses and virus-related diseases have threatened the health of humans and many animal species. How did this situation arise? Could it be that scientific studies and the emergence of new pathogens are not totally unrelated events? In writing this text, Dr. Horowitz has bravely questioned the extent to which scientific research and lax government oversight may have contributed to the present and coming plagues.

Open debate on this issue has been soundly discouraged. Opponents to open dialogue on the apparent relationship between early viral research and the latest germ discoveries argue that little good, and considerable harm, would come from a full disclosure of the facts. Exposing the truth, many believed, would likely: 1) tarnish the reputations of certain scientists, 2) make it more difficult to maintain science funding, 3) promote antigovernment sentiment, and 4) likely leave many issues unresolved. Others argued that it was simply too late to undo past mistakes. The fact that a better understanding of the new viruses' origins could lead to new treatment approaches, and, more importantly, to ways of preventing future outbreaks, was disregarded.

In considering the recent genesis of HIV and the Ebola viruses, Dr. Horowitz's book has explored three areas of great general and scientific interest: 1) the history of intensive research into the viral causes of cancer wherein readers can become familiar with the many, now questionable, virus transmission experiments, 2) the CIA and Department of Defense efforts to develop and defend against biological weapons of germ warfare. Here Dr. Horowitz should be especially congratulated for presenting well-researched little known facts that, though highly disturbing, are an important piece of history that may also bear heavily on the emergence of new viruses, and 3) vaccine production. Clearly, as anyone who reads this book will conclude, there is a great need for more open dialogue concerning the past and present risks inherent in the production of live viral vaccines. It is this topic that I am pleased to address here.

In 1798, Edward Jenner, an English physician advanced the use of cowpox (vaccinia) virus for immunizing humans against smallpox. He recognized that pathogens can behave differently while infecting different species. Indeed, he theorized that the vaccinia infection, which caused mild problems for cows, caused more severe ailments in horses. Only after adapting to cows, did vaccinia acquire limited infectivity for humans. The open sores that humans developed were far less severe than those induced by smallpox (variola) virus and essentially remained localized to the site of inoculation. Moreover, contact with vaccinia virus caused individuals to become virtually immune to the widespread disease caused by the smallpox virus. The success of vaccination is reflected in today's total elimination of smallpox as a disease.

Jenner's vaccination approach was followed in the twentieth century by Pasteur's use of rabies virus grown in rabbit's brain, and by Theiler's finding that he could reduce the effect of yellow fever virus by growing it in chicken embryos.

These successes set the precedent for other scientists to attempt to reduce the pathogenicity of other human and animal viruses by inoculating them into foreign species. Although we now look back with some disdain at the crudeness of early immunization experiments—such as the 1938 injections of polio virus, grown in mouse brains, into humans, most people, including scientists, are unaware that we *still* use primary monkey kidney cells to produce live polio virus vaccine. Likewise, dog and duck kidney cells were used to make licensed rubella vaccines. Experimental vaccines, grown in animal tissues and intended for human use, were commonly tested in African monkeys, and it is likely that many of these monkeys were released back into the wild. This practice may have led to the emergence of primate diseases, some of which could have been transmitted back to humans.

Large numbers of rural Africans were also chosen as test recipients of experimental human vaccines.

In veterinary medicine, live viral vaccines have been widely used in domestic pets and in animals destined to become part of the food-chain. Undoubtedly, many cross-species transfer of viruses have occurred in the process. Even today, more than ten foreign species are used to produce currently licensed vaccines for cats and dogs.

The general acceptance of the safety of cross-species produced vaccines was supported in part by the generalization that there are inherent restrictions to the interspecies spread of disease. Thus, like vaccinia, most viruses are less harmful, but others can be far more dangerous after invading a foreign host. One dramatic example is that of the human infection caused by the herpes-type monkey B virus. This germ remains a rather harmless invader of monkeys, but place it in humans, and striking, severe, acute illness results which commonly ends in death. Likewise, a modified horse-measles-virus (morbillivirus) can be lethal to man. Other examples include the relatively mild dog distemper morbillivirus that was blamed for the death of some 3,000 lions in the Serengeti; the cat-adapted parvovirus that caused worldwide infection in dogs; and the mouse-derived lymphocytic choriomeningitis virus that caused severe hepatitis in monkeys.

It is the slow onset of disease that can be particularly baffling, especially when considering potential viral diseases transmitted through vaccines. Most acute diseases are relatively easy to recognize and amenable to further prevention. The delayed onset of chronic debilitating diseases that could be associated with animal viruses finding their way into a new species, e.g., man, are much more challenging. Here, the association between the germ and the symptoms it causes is obscured. Such an association would be especially hard to establish if the clinical features presented during the illness are poorly defined and mimic those of other known ailments. One example is the 1996 concern over the food-borne transmission of the prion disease scrapie. Initially carried by infected sheep, this protein caused bovine spongiform encepalopathy in "mad" cows. Then it was apparently passed on to humans resulting in juvenile Crutzfeldt-Jakob disease.

While in some cases disease transmission has been traced to certain vaccine lots, other times, even widely distributed licensed vaccines have been found to be contaminated. Yellow fever vaccine was known to contain avian leukosis virus.* During World War II, batches of yellow fever vaccines were inadvertently also contaminated with hepatitis B virus. Current measles, mumps, rubella (MMR) vaccines contain low levels of reverse transcriptase, an enzyme associated with retroviruses. Both Salk and Sabin polio vaccines made from rhesus monkeys contained live monkey viruses called SV40, short for the fortieth monkey virus discovered. As Dr. Horowitz documents, polio vaccines may also have contained numerous other monkey viruses, some of which may have provided some building blocks for the emergence of HIV-1 and human AIDS.

The finding of SV40 in rhesus monkey kidney cells, during the early 1960s, led to a rapid switch to African green monkeys for polio vaccine production. Kidney cells from African green monkeys, *still* being used to produce live polio vaccines today, may have been infected with monkey

---

* Editor's note: This is the retrovirus that causes leukemia in chickens.

viruses that were not easily detectable. The monkeys used before 1980, for example, were likely to have been infected with simian immunodeficiency virus (SIV)—a virus genetically related to HIV-1. The origin of this virus and whether it contaminated any experimental vaccines are issues that need addressing.

What makes vaccines so troublesome is that their production and administration allows viral contamination to breach the two natural barriers that often restrict cross-species infections:

First is the skin. Direct inoculation of vaccines breaches this natural barrier and has been shown to produce increased infections in animals and humans. Such was the case when SV40 was injected intramuscularly in contaminated Salk polio vaccine. Later it was learned that Sabin's orally administered polio vaccines were safer since the live simian viruses were digested in the stomach and thereby inactivated. Additionally risky, when it comes to breaking the skin barrier, is the chance of transmitting viruses from one person to another through the use of unsterilized needles.

Second is the unique and natural viral surface characteristics that reduce the chance that viruses might jump species. The mixing of vaccine viruses with others found in the cells and tissues used to develop the vaccine can potentially lead to the development of new recombinant mutants that are more adaptive and have wider host range than either of the original viruses. This can especially happen when a live viral vaccine produced in cells from one species is then given to another species.

Also of concern is the transmission of new genetic information along with the vaccine virus. For instance, early adenoviral vaccines, produced in rhesus monkeys' kidney cells, developed to protect people against respiratory infections, incorporated parts of the SV40 virus that remained as a vaccine contaminant even after production of the vaccine virus was switched to human cells. Numerous other vaccines, especially those that were used in early field trials in Africa, should be analyzed for those genetic components which characterize today's monkey and human pathogens.

Unfortunately, this new awareness of potential problems with live viral vaccines has had little impact on the viral vaccine approval process. Seemingly, U.S. government agencies, principally the FDA, have been reluctant to impose additional testing requirements on vaccines once they are approved for use. In effect, government officials are given a single opportunity to decide on a new vaccine's safety. Even then, government regulators themselves may be denied certain critical information belonging to the vaccine industry. Specifically, FDA regulations are written so as not to compel industry to reveal testing information not directly pertaining to the lots submitted for clinical use. The FDA is reluctant to admit its lack of knowledge about vaccines to the medical/scientific community. Yet, practicing physicians are expected to unquestionably endorse the safety of vaccines under all circumstances and to all individuals.

Aside from these bureaucratic barriers to viral vaccine safety assurance, there are additional major concerns. Since vaccine development information is considered proprietary—protected by nondisclosure policies—government officials and researchers must shield potential safety issues from public scrutiny. This censorship is rationalized by the all too persuasive argument that vaccines cannot be criticized lest the public become non-compliant in taking them. Finally, this silence is buttressed by the small number of people capable of critically evaluating vaccine manufacturing and safety testing procedures. In essence, health care professionals and the general public know little about the possible dangers of live viral vaccines.

As an illustration, the issue of possible simian cytomegalovirus (SCMV) contamination of live polio virus vaccines has been suppressed since 1972. On the eve of Nixon's war on cancer, a joint Lederle Corporation/FDA Bureau of Biologics study showed that eleven test monkeys, imported for polio vaccine production, tested positively for SCMV. The reluctance of the FDA to act on this matter was revealed in a corporate memo delivered the following year. Even in 1995, following a report to FDA officials concerning a patient infected with a SCMV-derived virus, no new in-house testing of polio vaccines for SCMV has occurred. Moreover, this author's specific requests for vaccine material to undertake specific testing, were denied on the basis of protecting "proprietary" interests.

This basic flaw in the regulatory process must be addressed—the FDA must be responsive to the medical–scientific community's need for accurate information regarding the potential hazards of products released for use in society. In the event that public health and safety concerns arise, industry should wave its right to maintain proprietary intelligence. This would enable the FDA to disclose more information concerning the safety of FDA regulated products to the medical–scientific community. Such a proposal should be included in the all pending and future FDA reforms.

It is against this background of possible risks of past viral vaccine studies, uncertain biological recombinants, bureaucratic censorship, a rising tide of medical consumerism in the information age, and an urgent need for legislative FDA reform, that Dr. Horowitz's work contributes. At minimum, what you are about to read exposes many important facts which, unfortunately, few people realize and all would be better off knowing. At best, this important text raises far greater hope that by knowing their origin, cures for the many complex emerging viruses, including AIDS, may be forthcoming.

—W. JOHN MARTIN, M.D., PH.D.*

* **Dr. W. John Martin**, a Professor of Pathology at the University of Southern California, is also the Director of the Center for Complex Infectious Diseases in Rosemead, California. Between 1976 and 1980, Dr. Martin served as the director of the Viral Oncology Branch of the FDA's Bureau of Biologics (now the Center for Biologics, Evaluation and Research), the government's principal agency in charge of human vaccines.

Prologue

"DAVID was an alcoholic, an active alcoholic," recalled Edward Parsons. "I say that—I have nothing to hide. I'm also a recovering alcoholic. When I met David, I spoke to him about sobriety and the possibility of becoming involved with AA, and I don't think that was at the time really an option for him."[1]

Robert Montgomery, the attorney for four of the six Florida dental AIDS victims, listened intently as the auburn-haired nurse and once closest homosexual friend of the infamous Dr. David Acer spoke under oath for the record.

"He would drink—start to drink and not be able to stop and become inebriated, sloppy, more aggressive, more assertive. He would come on to people a lot more easily."

"And you believe he may have intentionally infected his [dental] patients?" Montgomery questioned.

"Yes. What happened was David was angry. He was very angry. I guess he had a right to be. Kimberly Bergalis was very angry, so was the family. That's a natural reaction to a diagnosis like that [AIDS]. But I had a conversation with David that bothered me. It has bothered me for quite a while. Now, when ultimately these five patients came forward I was certainly surprised at that disclosure, and then heard that they were testing positive for the same strain of virus that David had apparently possessed. This is all based on media. This was not based on any conversation I had with him. But I was able to recall a conversation I had with him that bothered me."

Parsons paused to take a drink.

"Go on," prodded the counselor.

"He had been drinking," Parsons continued. "He—we discussed AIDS again. I think I mentioned a friend of mine had been diagnosed and he discussed with me—he verbalized some opinions and some feelings, and he said something to the effect that, well, our society does not want to address the issue because they perceive it to be a homosexual problem, and when it begins to affect younger people and grandparents, I think is the words he used, he said that maybe society will do something. I kind of just blew it away. I didn't think much of it.

"I asked him how his practice was going. He said fine, and that was the end of that conversation. I met with him again up at his home . . . , and we discussed it again. There was sort of an anger there about HIV and what our government was. We got into many, many political discussions where

HIV came from, the World Health Organization theory and all of these various conversations about it. . . . The perception within the gay community was that our government avoided the issue; neglected the issue. We discussed everything from the controversy surrounding Robert Gallo and the French researcher Luc Montagnier at the Pasteur Institute; Ronald Reagan. Just numerous conversations pertaining to AIDS."

"And this began in 1985?" Montgomery questioned.

"1985, that's correct."

"What did he say about Montagnier and Gallo?"

Parsons replied, "David believed that HIV was probably, if not created in a lab, he believed that HIV was introduced into the human population and various governments knowingly sat on this information for a period of years before they actually acknowledged [it]. . . ."

Montgomery looked puzzled. "Are you saying that you interpreted that . . . to mean that you felt Dr. Acer was potentially deliberately infecting his patients?"

"I think so," Parsons replied. "We had—as I said, we had numerous conversations about AIDS and politics and transmission. . . . He believed that there were solutions out there; that there were drugs and chemicals out there that could kill the virus and that there was a conspiracy. . . . Some sort of a conspiracy . . . .

"What he said was when HIV begins to affect mainstream—I think the word he used was mainstream America, when we start seeing people who are—I think the word he used was adolescents and grandparents, then maybe something will be done. . . ."[1]

• • •

The preceding legal testimony provided by Edward Parsons was passed on to authorities from the United States Centers of Disease Control and Prevention (CDC) and the Florida Department of Health and Rehabilitative Services (HRS). Investigators for these agencies then also interviewed Parsons. According to the U.S. General Accounting Office, HRS officials then delivered the incriminating testimony to the Florida attorney general's office. Both offices then failed to pursue a criminal investigation into the case "noting the absence of supporting evidence."[2]

Officially thwarted in his effort to relay his circumstantial evidence to the world, on October 1, 1993, Parsons's broadcast his claims with the help of Barbara Walters on ABC television's "20/20."[3] The authorities thereafter announced that Parsons's testimony was unreliable.

Dr. Robert Runnells, an expert witness hired by attorney Montgomery to argue Acer's negligence in infection control in the now famous Kimberly Bergalis case, openly discredited Edward Parsons in his book *AIDS in the Dental Office*.[1] Runnells wrote that Acer's close friend:

> consciously or subconsciously, may have begun championing the theory of Acer murdering his patients to keep the case before the public—to continue to emphasize to mainstream America that anyone can get AIDS—whether or not they are gay. In fact, it was [Parsons] who wanted desperately to carry the anti-homophobia message. Because Acer and Kimberly were constantly in the headlines, [Parsons] may have decided that the media would continue to carry a story that Acer may have intentionally injected his patients.[1]

Contrary to Dr. Runnells's and attorney Montgomery's claims, the mass of circumstantial and scientific evidence presented in my earlier book *Deadly Innocence: Solving the Greatest Murder Mystery in the History of American Medicine* [4] showed the most plausible way Dr. David Acer could have infected six patients with the AIDS virus between December, 1987 and July, 1989 was by intent, just as Edward Parsons alleged.

Deadly Innocence, along with three investigation reports I subsequently published in the scientific/health professional journals *AIDS Patient Care,*[6] *Clinical Pediatric Dentistry,*[7] and the *British Dental Journal,*[8] provided evidence that Dr. Acer was developmentally and behaviorally predisposed to become an organized serial killer. By reviewing Federal Bureau of Investigation (FBI) methods and materials, I learned that all serial killers kill for the sake of power, control, and revenge. The most important question in the *Deadly Innocence* investigation then became, "Against whom did Acer hold a vendetta?"

In light of Parsons's legal testimony and other evidence, it became evident that the dentist's primary vendetta was against the United States Public Health Service (USPHS) and the CDC whom he believed developed and intentionally deployed the AIDS virus. Indeed, he held the authorities accountable for his infection and the deaths of scores of others.

During a personal conversation with Parsons, he admitted to me that Acer was outraged by the notion that the American homosexual community had been specifically targeted to receive HIV-tainted hepatitis B vaccinations during the 1970s.

Though this theory, I later learned, was embraced by at least a half dozen health scientists and scholars throughout the world, in the United States, the "World Health Organization theory," as it is called, was principally advanced by Dr. Robert Strecker, a practicing internist and gastroenterologist with an additional doctorate in pharmacology. As a trained pathologist and insurance industry consultant, Dr. Strecker initially investigated the AIDS epidemic and virus under contract with a large insurance company. Following years of research, Strecker published a highly controversial videotape entitled *The Strecker Memorandum*.[9]

According to Edward Parsons, "David and I viewed *The Strecker Memorandum* at length and spent hours in heated discussion over its disturbing contents."[10] In *The Memorandum*, Strecker alleged that the AIDS virus was "requested," "created," and "deployed" and its effects were predicted long before the epidemic began. In short, Acer believed that he was one of millions of innocent victims of genocide.

The speculation that Dr. Acer was angry with "mainstream" America for not recognizing AIDS as everyone's problem was only part of the story that the authorities and media promoted. The fact is many people are similarly angry, yet they do not go around killing people. The explanation fell short of a plausible murder motive.

Acknowledging the possibility that Acer, a closet homosexual who never came to terms with being gay, may have held a vendetta against mainstream homophobes, I realized Acer's second plausible motive. As an intelligent, scientifically trained, solo practitioner, the terminally ill dentist would have realized he could never spread his virus throughout the entire U.S. population. What he could do, however, and what the evidence showed he intentionally accomplished, was to spread the fear of AIDS in health care throughout mainstream America.

In fact, the open letter Dr. Acer published, shortly before his death, spelled out his two principal vendettas against American public health authorities and mainstream homophobic society. Within eight brief paragraphs, published in Florida newspapers on September 6 and 7, 1990, Acer condemned the CDC six times for their alleged involvement in the viral transmissions and articulated his grave distrust of them. He ended by subtly expressing his fascination with the probability of initiating mass hysteria throughout the United States:

> It is important to be informed of this disease, so you are aware of the dangers and how it can and cannot be transmitted. As fear of the unknown is hard to deal with, but knowledge of what you fear can at least help you know what action to take, if any. . . . [5]

Following months of intensive investigation, HRS and CDC researchers failed to report Parsons's testimony, or give serious consideration to the murder theory. Rather, they speculated that this first and only documented cluster of doctor-to-patient HIV transmission cases was most likely "an accident." They published that injuries sustained by a fatigued and shaky Dr. Acer, who performed "invasive" procedures on his patients, were the most likely cause of the infections and not negligence (that is, the use of unsterilized instruments and equipment). In addition, after having the Florida Attorney General's Office review the facts, they rejected the "murder theory."

Later, following years of denial, the Barbara Walters interview of Edward Parsons, and the identification of Acer's sixth victim, Sherry Johnson, who received no invasive procedures aside from local anesthetic injections, the CDC exhumed the murder theory for plausible consideration. Dr. Harold Jaffe, Deputy Director for HIV/AIDS Science at the CDC, quickly concluded the case would likely remain "an unsolvable mystery."[11]

Adding to the confusion, in early June 1994, a CBS "60-MINUTES" report proposed that the victims themselves were to blame. The program accused Kimberly Bergalis, the elderly Barbara Webb, and the others of concealing sexual practices and other lifestyle risks, and said their infections came from random community exposures. Though this disinformation was quickly and easily debunked by official as well as independent investigators, for a grossly uninformed public, the cruel CBS hoax had left its mark.[12]

The Florida dental AIDS tragedy generated intense controversy, mass hysteria, needless concerns, political legislation, billions in financial costs, and even increased death and disease among those frightened away from health care. In light of the importance of the case, its toll on society, and the many questions it raised, I believed, prior to writing this book, that a final chapter in the case needed to be written. In a strange and unsettling way, this book at least shows that Acer's anger, though obviously not his actions, was justified. The mystery of his case, for many now, may be solved. Moreover, Acer may have fulfilled a remarkable destiny—creating one mystery to help solve a larger one—the origin of AIDS, Ebola and other "emerging viruses."

Abbreviations

AEC—Atomic Energy Commission
AEIPP—American Enterprise Institute for Public Policy
AIBS—American Institute of Biological Sciences
AIDS—Acquired immune deficiency syndrome
AIFLD—American Institute for Free Labor Development
AMI—Allan Memorial Institute
AMV—avian myeloblastosis virus
ARC—AIDS related complex
ARV—AIDS associated retrovirus
ASCC—American Society for the Control of Cancer
BSL—biological safety level (1–4)
BW—biological weapons
BPL—Boston Pubic Library
BPP—Black Panther Party
BLV—bovine leukemia virus
BL—Burkitt's lymphoma
BVV—bovine visna virus
CAIB—Covert Action Information Bulletin
CBW—chemical and biological warfare
CDC—Centers for Disease Control and Prevention
CFR—Council on Foreign Relations
CHINA—chronic infectious neuropathic agents
CIA—Central Intelligence Agency
CIC—Counter-Intelligence Corps
CNSS—Center for National Security Studies
COINTELPRO—Communist (Counter) Intelligence Program
CPUSA—Communist Party U.S.A.
CSH—Cold Spring Harbor
DCI—Director of Central Intelligence
DHEW—Department of Health, Education and Welfare
DNA—Deoxyribonucleic Acid
DOD—Department of Defense
DT—diptheria, tetanus
EBV—Epstein Barr Virus
ECT—electro-convulsive (shock) therapy
ELISA (test)—enzyme-linked immuosorbent assay
ERTS—Earth Resources Technology Satellite
FBI—Federal Bureau of Investigation
FELV—feline (cat) leukemia virus

FCRC—Frederick Cancer Research Center
FDA—Food and Drug Administration
FNLA—National Front for the Liberation of Angola
FOIA—Freedom of Information Act
FSA—Federal Security Agency
GAO—U.S. General Accounting Office
GRID—Gay related immune deficiency
HAV—human AIDS-related virus
HBsAg—hepatitis B surface antigen
HBV—hepatitis B virus
HELA—Henrietta Lack (cell line)
HIV—human immunodeficiency virus
HRS—Florida Department of Health and Rehabilitative Services
HSPH—Harvard School of Public Health
HTLV—human T-lymphocyte leukemia virus
IADB—Inter-American Defense Board
IARC—International Agency for Research on Cancer
IDA—International Development Association
ILC—idiopathic lymphocyteopaenia
INTELSAT—intelligence satellite
IPP—Institute Pasteur Production
JIC—Joint Intelligence Committee
JIOA—Joint Intelligence Objectives Agency
LAV—lymphadenopathy-associated virus
LBI—Litton Bionetics, Inc.
LSAF—Louisiana State Agriculture Farm
MIT—Massachusetts Institute of Technology
MKNAOMI—CIA code for secret biological weapons program
MKULTRA—CIA code for secret mind control program
MLV—mouse leukemia viruses
MMIC—military-medical-industrial complex
MMMV—maximally monstrous malignant virus
MPLA—Popular Movement for the Liberation of Angola
MSD—Merck, Sharp & Dohme
NAACP—National Assoc. for the Advancement of Colored People
NAS—National Academy of Sciences
NASA—National Aeronautics and Space Administration
NATO—North Atlantic Treaty Organization
NBC-New Bolton Center
NBRL—Navy's Biomedical Research Laboratory
NCAC—National Cancer Advisory Council
NCDC—National Communicable Disease Center
NCI—National Cancer Institute
NFF—Nicaraguan Freedom Fund

NGO—Nongovernmental Organization
NIAID—National Institute for Allergies and Infectious Diseases
NIH—National Institutes of Health
NRC—National Research Council
NSC—National Security Council
NSF—National Science Foundation
NYCBB—New York City Blood Bank
NYCBC—New York City Blood Center
NYUMC—New York University Medical Center
OPC—Office of Policy Coordination
OSRD—Office of Scientific Research and Development
OSS—Office of Strategic Services
OTRAG—Orbital Transport and Missiles, Ltd.
PAHO—Pan American Health Organization
PUSH—People to Save Humanity
RAPID—Resources for the Awareness of Population and
    International Development
RNA—Ribonucleic Acid
SCF—Save the Children Fund
SCMV—simian cytomegalovirus
SFV—simian foamy virus
SMOM—Sovereign Military Order of Malta
SOD—Special Operations Division of the Army
SVCP—Special Virus Cancer Program
SVLP—Special Virus Leukemia Program
SV(40)—simian virus (40)
TEREC—Tactical Electronic Reconnaissance
UNDP—U.N. Development Program
UNFAO—U.N. Food and Agriculture Organization
UNFPA—U.N. Fund for Population Activities
UNICEF—U.N. Children's Fund
UNITA—National Union for the Complete Independence of
    Angola
USAID—U.S. Agency for International Development
USIA—U.S. Information Agency
USPHS—U.S. Public Health Service
USDHEW—U.S. Dept. of Health, Education and Welfare
VEE—Venezuelan equine encephalitis
VVE—Venezuelan equine encephalomyelitis
VFHP—Voluntary Fund for Health Promotion
WRS—War Research Service
WBC—white blood cells
WHO—World Health Organization
WPPA—World Population Plan of Action

Part I
Introduction and
Scientific Background

Chapter 1
The "World Health Organization Theory of AIDS"

The World Health Organization (WHO) theory[1] festered in my mind like a disease. That the AIDS virus was cultured as a biological weapon and then deliberately deployed was unfathomable. How could WHO scientists and others in the United States Public Health Service (USPHS) consciously or even unwittingly create such a hideous germ? More inconceivable was the alleged targeting of American homosexuals and black Africans for genocide. The entire subject was beyond my wildest nightmares.

Frightened by the ramifications of such alleged atrocities, I spent months living in denial. As a behavioral scientist, I was no stranger to the subject of man's inhumanity toward man. I just feared what further research might reveal.

Eventually, curiosity wore down my defenses, and I attempted, on several occasions, to contact Dr. Robert Strecker for an explanation. For months, then, the telephone number I had for him rang continuously unanswered. Secretly, I was thankful. The secondary sources of information I had about *The Strecker Memorandum* were adequate for my needs, I rationalized.

The few documents I had on the WHO theory of AIDS came from a wholistic physician I met at a National Wellness Association conference. For years, the doctor documented, the word on the street in the gay community and among the black intelligentsia was that HIV was created as a bioweapon—a man-made virus bearing stark similarities to the bovine lymphotrophic virus (BLV) cultured in cows.[2] Although American authorities quickly moved to dispel the assertion, claiming African monkeys were the source of the scourge, Dr. Strecker insisted the germ came from cow and sheep sources.

Research showed a similarity between HIV and BLV. One report appeared in *Nature* in 1987.[2] Strecker heralded this and argued it was virologically absurd to believe HIV came from the monkey. Especially "since there are no genetic markers in the AIDS virus typical of the primate, and the AIDS virus cannot thrive in the monkey."[3] Still, the majority subscribed to the African green monkey theory.

According to Strecker, whose work was reviewed by medical physician Jonathan Collin in a 1988 issue of *Townsend Letter for Doctors*, the AIDS virus:

> . . . can and apparently does thrive in the cow, having essentially identical characteristics with the bovine virus and this, further, gives a hint of the role vaccinations have played in either accidentally or purposefully inducing the AIDS epidemic.[3]

Collin reported that Strecker's research made sense, particularly considering the virology and evolution of the AIDS epidemic.

Strecker's first point was that AIDS was nonexistent in Africa prior to 1975, and had it been the result of monkey bites occurring in the 1940s, as some alleged, the epidemic should have occurred in the 1960s and not late 1970s owing to the twenty-year timetable for case incidence doubling.[3]

More telling, Strecker obtained documents through the Freedom of Information Act (FOIA) that showed that the United States Department of Defense (DOD) secured funding from Congress in 1969 to perform studies on immune-system-destroying agents for germ warfare.[4] Strecker alleged that soon thereafter, the WHO, funded by the DOD, began experimenting with a lymphotrophic virus that was produced in cows, but could also infect humans. The WHO, Strecker noted, also launched a major African campaign against smallpox in 1977, which involved the urban population, not the rural Pygmies. Had the "green monkey" been responsible for AIDS, Strecker professed, the Pygmies of rural Africa would have had a higher incidence of AIDS than the country's urban populations. The opposite is true.[3]

Strecker reportedly examined WHO research that revealed their scientists, in the early 1970s, had studied viruses that were capable of altering the immunologic response capacity of T-lymphocytes. He noted that such viruses were found in 1970, but only in some animals including sheep and cows, and that the latter species is used to produce the smallpox vaccine.

Literature provided by The Strecker Group[5] urged readers to:

PLEASE WAKE UP!

> In 1969 . . . [the] United States Defense Department requested and got $10 million to make the AIDS virus in labs as a political/ethnic weapon to be used mainly against Blacks. The feasibility program and labs were to have been completed by 1974-1975; the virus between 1974-1979. The World Health Organization started to inject AIDS-laced smallpox vaccine into over 100

million Africans (population reduction) in 1977. And over 2000 young white male homosexuals (Trojan horse) in 1978 with the hepatitis B vaccine through the Centers for Disease Control/New York Blood Center. . . .

Collin, in his review, added:

Strecker remarks that it would be relatively easy to implant such viruses in the cow carcasses used to produce the smallpox vaccine. When the smallpox vaccine sera was recovered from the animal carcasses, animal lymphotrophic viruses could be carried or mutated or incorporated in the vaccine. . . . [T]he epidemiology of multiple "contaminated" smallpox vaccines given in the early 1970s would provide exactly the right timetable for such a widespread AIDS epidemic in Africa today.[3]

Strecker vigorously promoted his theory that the AIDS virus was transmitted to the American homosexual community during the course of the experimental hepatitis B vaccination program sponsored by the USPHS between 1978 and 1979.[1,3,6]

I recalled reviewing this research as a post-doctoral student at Harvard.[6]

At that time, Collin wrote:

The USPHS notes the recipients were sexually active, having more than one sexual partner, and at particular risk for developing hepatitis. The homosexual populations given the vaccination were in six major cities, including New York, San Francisco, Los Angeles, St. Louis, Houston and Chicago. Epidemiologically, these cities now have the highest incidence of AIDS and ARC, as well as the highest death rates from AIDS.[3]

After reading this, I began to question more of what I learned about the origin of AIDS. My curiosity, piqued by the DOD appropriations request for 1970 (see fig. 1.1) beckoned me to investigate further.

Fig. 1.1. Department of Defense Appropriations Hearings for 1970 on the Development of Immune-System Destroying Agents for Biological Warfare

SOVIET CHEMICAL AND BIOLOGICAL WEAPONS

Mr. SIKES. The statements indicate that the Soviets have made extensive progress in chemical and biological weapons. I would like you to provide for the record a statement which shows what they are doing in this area and with some indication of their capabilities in this area.

Mr. POOR. We will be happy to provide that.

(The information follows:)

The Soviet Union is better equipped defensively, offensively, militarily, and psychologically for chemical and biological warfare than any other nation in the world. She has placed a great deal of emphasis on these systems in her military machine. Utilizing a wide spectrum of chemical munitions, the Soviets consider that chemical tactical weapons would be used in conjunction with nuclear weapons or separately, as the case may dictate. The Soviet agent stockpiles include a variety of agents and munitions capable of creating a wide range of effects on the battlefield. The Soviet soldier is well equipped defensively. He trains vigorously and for long periods of time utilizing his equipment. He looks upon chemical as a real possibility in any future conflict, and respects his protective equipment. The research program in the Soviet Union for chemical warfare and biological agents has encompassed every facet from incapacitating to lethal effects, both offensively and defensively.

(Additional classified information was supplied to the committee [including the testimony below].)

SYNTHETIC BIOLOGICAL AGENTS

There are two things about the biological agent field I would like to mention. One is the possibility of technological surprise. Molecular biology is a field that is advancing very rapidly and eminent biologists believe that within a period of 5 to 10 years it would be possible to produce a synthetic biological agent, an agent that does not naturally exist and for which no natural immunity could have been acquired.

Mr. SIKES. Are we doing any work in that field?

Dr. MACARTHUR. We are not.

Mr. SIKES. Why not? Lack of money or lack of interest?

Dr. MACARTHUR. Certainly not lack of interest.

Mr. SIKES. Would you provide for our records information on what would be required, what the advantages of such a program would be, the time and the cost involved?

Dr. MACARTHUR. We will be very happy to.

(The information follows:)

The dramatic progress being made in the field of molecular biology led us to investigate the relevance of this field of science to biological warfare. A small group of experts considered this matter and provided the following observations:

1. All biological agents up to the present time are representatives of naturally occurring disease, and are thus known by scientists throughout the world. They are easily available to qualified scientists for research, either for offensive or defensive purposes.

2. Within the next 5 to 10 years, it would probably be possible to make a new infective microorganism which could differ in certain important aspects from any known disease-causing organisms. Most important of these is that it might be refractory to the immunological and therapeutic processes upon which we depend to maintain our relative freedom from infectious disease.

3. A research program to explore the feasibility of this could be completed in approximately 5 years at a total cost of $10 million.

4. It would be very difficult to establish such a program. Molecular biology is a relatively new science. There are not many highly competent scientists in the field, almost all are in university laboratories, and they are generally adequately supported from sources other than DOD. However, it was considered possible to initiate an adequate program through the National Academy of Sciences-National Research Council (NAS-NRC).

5. The matter was discussed with the NAS-NRC and tentative plans were made to initiate the program. However, decreasing funds in CB, growing criticism of the CB program, and our reluctance to involve the NAS-NRC in such a controversial endeavor have led us to postpone it for the past 2 years.

It is a highly controversial issue and there are many who believe such research should not be undertaken lest it lead to yet another method of massive killing of large populations. On the other hand, without the sure scientific knowledge that such a weapon is possible, and an understanding of the ways it could be done, there is little that can be done to devise defensive measures. Should an enemy develop it there is little doubt that this is an important area of potential military technological inferiority in which there is no adequate research program.

The above testimony of Acting Assistant Secretary of the Army for Research and Development, Charles L. Poor, was printed on page 79 of the public record cited below. However, Dr. MacArthur's above statements were deleted. Dr. MacArthur was, at the time, the deputy director of the Department of Defense. The complete testimony was found initially by military investigator Zears Miles and subsequently by attorney Theodore Strecker, J.D., through the Freedom of Information Act (on page 129 of the supplemental record). A copy of the original classified document was later published on page 124 of *Deadly Innocence* by this author in 1994. Source: Department of Defense Appropriations for 1970. Hearings Before a Subcommittee of the Committee on Appropriations House of Representatives, Ninety-First Congress, Part 5 Research, Development, Test, and Evaluation, Dept. of the Army. Tuesday, July 1, 1969, page 79. Washington: U.S. Government Printing Office, 1969.

Chapter 2
WHO Plays in the Big Leagues

JACKIE, my wife and co-investigator had been instrumental in helping me research the Florida dental AIDS tragedy for *Deadly Innocence*.[1]

The loving mother of our now two children, Jackie began her working career as a dental assistant for the Saskatchewan Dental Plan in Canada. We met in Cancun, Mexico, waiting in line at Carlos and Charlie's Bar and Grill. At the time, she was looking for a job and I needed an assistant. The rest is history.

Besides her big blue eyes, long silky auburn hair, slight build, and innocent appearance, what attracted me most about my future wife was her survival instinct. She had spent almost two months touring the back roads of Mexico virtually unchaperoned. This girl's a survivor, I respectfully considered.

Over the years, I found this trait increasingly comforting, particularly while confronting the many frightening realities we encountered during our research.

"The WHO Does What?"

"The only thing I know about the World Health Organization," I said to Jackie after learning of Strecker's theory, "is that it's a prestigious internationally supported organization that develops health and vaccination programs for developing countries."

It suddenly seemed odd to me that over the course of my training—more than four years of college, three years of dental school, ten years of postdoctoral research and teaching, and sixteen years of clinical dental practice—I had learned very little about the WHO.

"I don't even know what's involved in becoming a WHO member," I admitted. "The name sure imparts an air of scientific aristocracy."

Eventually, as the novelty of Strecker's theory wore off, and further attempts at contacting Strecker by phone failed, I decided to venture into the dungeons of Harvard's Countway Medical Library to prove "the null hypothesis"—that nothing was true about Strecker's memorandum.[2] What I unearthed, however, in back issues of the *WHO Chronicle* was engaging.

Dozens of *WHO Chronicle* articles that I photocopied and brought home revealed that by 1968 the WHO had been solely in control of the world's experimental "biologicals" for almost two decades.[3]

> WHO has exerted a powerful influence on the quality control of biological substances since its very inception in 1948. . . . Since 1952, when WHO interest in the establishment of international requirements for such biological products began, various possible measures have been examined for attempting to achieve a greater degree of uniformity in the quality, safety, and potency of vaccines, antisera, etc. . . . for the control of substances of particular interest to WHO in relation to its mass immunization and mass prophylaxis schemes in developing countries. . . . The main purpose served by these international standards, reference preparations, and reference reagents is to provide a means of ensuring worldwide uniformity in expressing the potency of preparations used in the prophylaxis, therapy, or diagnosis of human and animal disease.[3]

The coordinating body for all this work I learned was "the WHO secretariat." The Geneva-based organization maintained several full-time officers and part-time consultants who worked in collaboration with several other laboratories in other countries:

> The laboratories most deeply involved are the WHO International Laboratories for Biological Standards within the departments of biological standards of the Statens Seruminstitut, Copenhagen, the National Institute for Medical Research, London, and the Central Veterinary Laboratory, Weybridge, England. Between them, these laboratories undertake the detailed work of organizing international collaborative assays and of holding and distributing the international biological standards and many of the international biological reference preparations and international biological reference reagents. The initiative for setting up standards and reference preparations usually comes from a WHO Expert Committee on Biological Standardization, which is convened annually in Geneva. It comprises recognized experts in the field, who serve without remuneration in their personal capacity and not as representatives of governments or other bodies, together with members of the WHO secretariat. This Expert Committee also establishes the international standards and reference preparations on the basis of the results of the international collaborative assays.

> For pharmaceuticals generally, still including some biologicals, the drawing up of standards is in the hands of the Expert Committee on Specifications for Pharmaceutical Preparations, in collaboration with the WHO secretariat and with the help of the Expert Advisory Panel on the International Pharmacopoeia and Pharmaceutical Preparations. Needless to say, close liaison is needed between the secretariat, the Expert Committee on Biological

Standardization, the Expert Committee on Specifications for Pharmaceutical Preparations, and various other expert committees on, for example, antibiotics, tuberculosis, yellow fever, and cholera.[3]

Another article[4] discussed the WHO's "National control activities" which provided advice and encouragement when countries became "conscious of the need for controlling biologicals." WHO helped them establish and develop their "national control laboratories."[3]

It was quickly apparent that the WHO set the standards for the development, manufacture, distribution, and administration of essentially all pharmaceuticals used throughout the world (see fig. 2.1).[3,4]

As seen in figure 2.2, they were also intimately involved in determining which drugs should be made or remain illegal.[4]

Besides assembling teams of scientists to develop, test, and standardize new (and ancient) drugs, the WHO applied similar administrative leadership to develop plans for attacking all the woes of humanity. Polio, yellow fever, cholera, smallpox, whooping cough, diphtheria, tetanus, measles, anthrax, typhoid, tuberculosis, influenza, and even the common cold were all targeted. The WHO's approach to controlling communicable diseases was spelled out by their Assistant Director-General, Dr. A. M. Payne:

> Mass campaigns against certain communicable diseases require an initial attack sustained uninterruptedly over a relatively large area within a short period of time. . . . In smallpox, for instance, the buildup of new susceptibles in the absence of routine vaccination creates an explosive situation resulting in the familiar pattern of epidemics of smallpox followed by epidemics of vaccination. . . .[5]

WHO's Developing Viral Network

Applauding WHO's support for pioneering work in viral research, Dr. D. A. Tyrrell reported the common cold (rhino) virus provided valuable insights into the burgeoning field of virology. In the early 1960s, WHO designated Tyrrell's research unit in the United Kingdom and the National Institutes of Health (NIH) in Bethesda, Maryland, as "two International Reference Centres . . . in order to promote their [respiratory virus] study."

From here, newly developed techniques for virus cultivation, Tyrrell wrote, were widely applied:

Hundreds of strains of rhinoviruses have been isolated and shown to be anti-genically distinct from at least some other strains. They have been reported in the scientific literature under a confusing variety of designations, and it was accordingly decided at a meeting of the Directors of the WHO Virus Reference Centers to undertake collaborative study in which sera and strains were distributed to a number of laboratories so that cross neutralization tests could be performed of all well-characterized and apparently new strains. *This work was supported by the US Vaccine Development Board* [emphasis added] and coordinated by the two WHO International Reference Centres. . . .

"Work on these viruses," Tyrrell continued, demanded "a supply of cells" that were "sensitive to such organisms." It required considerable work to find such cells. Often cell lines would "change their sensitivity after prolonged cultivation." The Reference Centres, thus, maintained stocks of cells, "stored in liquid nitrogen," which they distributed to labs conducting viral research throughout the world.

Some viruses that failed to grow in the usual tissue cultures, Tyrrell revealed, "were propagated in cultures of the human trachea and nose," that is, "in the organs and tissues in which they multiply in nature." These viruses, some "new rhinoviruses," and other new types "never before detected in man were "disseminated through the WHO network of Virus Reference Centres."[6]

"So, let me get this straight," Jackie said. "World renowned scientists developed WHO policies and practices, studied and distributed viruses, with financial support from groups like the 'U.S. Vaccine Development Board.' Was the board, like the WHO connected to any pharmaceutical companies?"

"I'm not sure," I replied, "but most likely. There was obviously lots of money to be made with vaccines, and only a few companies made them."

"Which ones?"

"Well Merck, Sharp and Dohme (MSD) is one of the largest, and they did fund the hepatitis B vaccine research Strecker alleged spread HIV to homosexuals in America."

Another report four months later showed Israeli scientists were supported by the WHO to study the genetic determinants of the human immune response.[7]

A few others stated that the WHO was funding several programs designed to evaluate the specific disease vulnerabilities of minority groups—from American Indians[8] to African natives[9]—through the collection and analysis of "gene pools" and "blood supplies."[10]

"That's just what the Nazis did," Jackie recalled.

"Here are a couple more articles noting the WHO and the U.S. Vaccine Development Board also funded 'large-scale human trials' of newly developed vaccines made from both bacteria[11] and viruses."[12,13,14]

"Let me see."

I passed the reports over to my co-investigator.

"Just as Strecker reported," Jackie said after reading the articles carefully.

"Yeah. I hate to say it, but maybe there's something to his theory. Their 'smallpox eradication program' used vaccines made from antisera made largely in the United States and given for free to African countries, including Kenya, Ethiopia, Guinea, The Democratic Republic of the Congo, and Rwanda.

"The Democratic Republic of the Congo, which eventually became Zaire, they said would 'have a sufficient production capacity to supply the needs of all the African countries south of the Sahara.'"[13,14]

"That's interesting, and very noble," Jackie retorted somewhat cynically. "Zaire—the center of the African AIDS belt—supplying neighboring countries with the technology and expertise they needed to become healthier and more self-sufficient is great. I only wonder who paid for it and why?"

"I just read that their vaccine development committee endorsed a 1970 African campaign budget of $14 million," I answered.[15]

"That was a lot of money for those days."

"About how much in present dollars?" I asked my more mathematically gifted partner.

"Say about five times that, around $70 million."

"Much of it apparently came from the United States and other world governments interested in Africa. And periodic infusions of more cash for revaccination campaigns were needed and supplied."[16]

The Lausanne Laboratories

In 1964, shortly after President Kennedy's assassination, the WHO created the International Reference Centre for Immunoglobulins at the University of Lausanne, Switzerland. Three years later, the WHO Regional Reference Centre for Immunology (Research and Training) was designated at the same site. Its director, Dr. Rowe, reported that the center was established to broaden the WHO's "range of activities" in-so-far-as the "study of antibodies and immunoglobulins," the naturally produced proteins that defend the body against attack by toxins and germs. Rowe noted the WHO's special interest in cell-mediated immunity, that is, the cells that recognize antigen (foreign proteins associated with germs and toxic substances), secrete antibody, and are themselves able to attack foreign cells. Primary defense cells, called lymphoid cells, Rowe noted, were under intensive investigation to determine how they initiated and maintained the immune system, "paramount . . . in determining the pathogenic effects of infectious agents ranging from viruses to parasites."[17]

"Apparently their experiments went well," I remarked. "In December 1969, the WHO issued its second five-year research report on viral experiments it had funded or conducted since 1959."

The report stated,

> In the years 1964-68 the principal advances in virology were in knowledge of the fundamental structure of viruses and cells and of their interrelationships and interactions. A much greater understanding was gained of the natural behavior of viruses as infectious agents, of the pathogenesis of virus diseases, and of the means of controlling many of the common virus diseases—generally by improving existing vaccines or by developing new ones.
>
> Though direct proof of a causal relationship between viruses and human cancer still escapes the numerous investigators working on this subject, the quest continues to be energetically pursued. The hypothesis that at least some malignant neoplastic diseases such as leukemia are associated with virus infection is perhaps even more strongly expressed now than in the past.[18]

The article went on to state that Russian and American researchers were privy to the same vaccines, viral samples, and information about how the human immune system could be bolstered or destroyed by old and newly developed germs, including those produced from monkey viruses.[17,18]

"All this during the cold war," Jackie noted.

Green Monkeys, "Slow" Viruses, and $10 Million

"Strecker's material said that the DOD provided one contract in 1970 for $10 million for the development of a synthetic biological agent with no natural immunity. Which WHO reference center got that?" Jackie asked.

"It had to have been one in the U.S."

"For sure, but where?"

14

"There were only two possibilities," I said, "Atlanta, Georgia, and Bethesda, Maryland."[17-19]

The Atlanta lab, was run by the CDC's predecessor—the National Communicable Disease Center (NCDC). The Bethesda lab was run by the NIH. The later was cited in the *WHO Chronicle* as one of the initial two International [virus] Reference Centers. Yet, it was reported to be inadequately equipped to handle dangerous smallpox viruses. These were allegedly handled in Atlanta.

"If that's the case, it's not likely they would have handled deadly viruses like HIV either," Jackie reasoned.

"Not necessarily," I responded. "The smallpox virus and the DOD requisition may have posed different risks."

Shortly after our conversation, an article by Charles Siebert in *The New York Times Magazine* clarified the biological safety level (BSL) risk rating system used by the CDC and the NIH:

> In the hierarchy of precaution taken against biological threats at the CDC, BSL 1 and 2 are the lowest level of safety. Work is done there only with non- or moderate-risk organisms—viruses that cause colds, for example, or bacteria that cause diarrhea. At BSL 3, known as "the hot zone" or the "blue suit lab," workers visit with highly transmissible viruses or with those viruses or bacteria for which there is no known cure. There are only two BSL 4 labs in the country, one at the United States Army Medical Research Institute for Infectious Diseases [USAMRIID] at Fort Detrick in Frederick, Md., and the one in Atlanta.[20]

Our road atlas showed us Frederick was very close to Bethesda. I picked up the telephone to learn more.

An administrator at the NCI's Tumor Cell Biology Lab in Bethesda confirmed Siebert's report. Additionally, the woman told me, "The AIDS virus is considered a BSL 3 hazard. It's being studied in Bethesda as well as numerous labs across the nation."

We also learned that, once developed, the most dangerous viruses planned for use as biological weapons were shipped to the Pine Bluff Arsenal for storage.[21]

Among the tens of thousands of viral strains cultured, developed, and transported for study by WHO reference centers, we learned that two received special attention and an inordinate share of research dollars: monkey viruses, including the simian pox virus, and the "slow" viruses, particularly visna and scrapie.[17-19, 22] We read these reports carefully since Strecker noted the AIDS virus bears the greatest likeness to the human-bovine (cow) lymphotrophic (lymph-cell-targeting and cancer-causing) virus combined with sheep visna virus.[2]

Monkeypox was of great interest to researchers, the *WHO Chronicle* said, for two reasons. First, the monkeypox virus was found closely related to the variola-vaccinia virus group, which causes and immunizes against human smallpox. Second, the monkey is man's closest relative in the animal kingdom, and experimental results using monkeys were expected to provide the best indication of what might occur in humans exposed to the same elements.[17-22]

Alternatively, "slow" viruses were of the greatest interest to WHO, CDC, NIH, and NCI scientists between 1968 and 1974. The reasons for this were not as obvious. The *WHO Chronicle* reported:

> Recent interest in the "slow" viruses, in particular those causing chronic degenerative disease of the nervous system—the CHINA (chronic infectious neuropathic agents) viruses—has come from painstaking work with visna and scrapie, degenerative diseases of the central nervous system of sheep, and kuru, a degenerative disease of the central nervous system of man restricted to the Fore people of New Guinea and their immediate neighbours.[18]

"Why so much interest in two sheep viruses that cause nerve disorders and don't infect humans?" Jackie asked.

"I'm not sure."

"And what about kuru? Who are the 'Fore people of New Guinea'? What makes them so important that viral centers around the world took up their cause?"

"Well, let's look it up." I walked over to our library and pulled out a copy of *Steadman's Medical Dictionary.*

"Kuru, it says is":

> A highly localized, fatal disease found in New Guinea, resembling paralysis agitans [a nervous disorder with frequent bouts of shaking]; found among certain cannibalistic people who ingest raw brain of recently deceased victims of the disease. Also called a laughing sickness.[23]

"When in history has helping cannibals been a world priority?" I wondered.

"Never," Jackie responded. "The notion seems utterly *harebrained.*"

"Oh. That was awful."

"Sorry, I couldn't help myself."

We read on:

CHINA viruses are distinguished by the languishing character of the infection process they initiate. The incubation period in the host may be months or years, and the disease itself may progress laggardly towards an irreversible deterioration of the victim. Cells infected with "slow" viruses are in general neither impaired nor stimulated to proliferate. Their functions are impaired but the nature of the dysfunction has not as yet been clarified.[18]

"It's remarkable how closely this matches several of the most prominent features of AIDS," I said. "And there's more":

The resistance of the scrapie agent to heat, ether, formalin, and other enzymatic and chemical agents, as well as its very small particle size, poses the question whether it is a conventional virus, an incomplete virus, or some other agent. . . . The findings of different [research] groups are at variance and in several instances are totally inexplicable within our present concept of infectious agents. . . .[18]

"That reads just like the DOD order for a 'new infective microorganism' that couldn't be defended against," I remarked.

The article went on to state that additional experiments had been conducted in order to prompt the human immune response "by the injection of double-stranded RNA."[18]

"HIV is a single-stranded RNA 'slow' virus," I explained. "And gene cutting and splicing techniques were well developed at that time."[24]

"Could they have cut double-stranded RNA to make single stranded RNA?"

"I'm not sure, but what I don't understand is, here, the *WHO Chronicle* stated the primary objective of their viral research program was "to acquire a thorough knowledge of the virus diseases so that prophylactic and other public health measures can be introduced as soon as possible."[18]

"What's the matter with that?"

"Look at *what* they were studying to accomplish it. Two rare diseases that only affect sheep and one totally remote virus that makes brain eaters laugh themselves to death."

"Do you think they might've been looking at these things for use as biological weapons?" Jackie asked and then added, "Think about it— scrapie—a totally unconventional germ that they're not even sure what it is. You can't kill it with heat or chemicals, and there are 'still no tissue culture systems or antibody systems' by which enemy defenses could be prepared."

"And 'at variance' and 'totally inexplicable' with the current knowledge at that time," I added, "the enemy would not only be surprised, but baffled and helpless."

We reflected again on the DOD document that detailed their desire to acquire:

> a new infective microorganism which could differ in certain important aspects from any known disease-causing organisms. Most important of these is that it might be refractory to the immunological and therapeutic processes upon which we depend to maintain our relative freedom from infectious disease.

> It is a highly controversial issue and there are many who believe such research should not be undertaken lest it lead to yet another method of massive killing of large populations. . . .[25]

The following week we learned that despite heavy opposition by the public and House of Representatives, the United States Congress gave the Army $23.2 million for biological warfare research. About half of that, at least $10 million of taxpayer money, went directly toward funding the manufacture of immunosuppressive agents allegedly for defense.[26]

"In essence, this one 1970 DOD biological weapons appropriation cost more than half of all the money the WHO spent in Africa that year for all of their health care and vaccination programs." Jackie calculated.

Fig. 2.1. WHO Requirements for Biological Substances

Year	Subject
1958	General Requirements for Manufacturing Establishing and Control Laboratories (revised in 1965)
1958	Poliomyelitis Vaccine (Inactivated) (revised in 1965)
1958	Yellow Fever Vaccine
1958	Cholera Vaccine (revised in 1968)
1958	Smallox Vaccine (revised in 1965)
1959	General Requirements for Sterility of Biological Substances
1961	Poliomyelitis Vaccine (Oral) (revised in 1965)
1963	Pertussis Vaccine
1963	Procaine Benzylpenicillin in Oil with Aluminium Monostearate (revised in 1965)
1963	Diphtheria Toxoid and Tetanus Toxoid
1965	Dried BCG Vaccine
1965	Measles Vaccine (Live) and Measles Vaccine (Inactivated)
1966	Anthrax Spore Vaccine (Live—for Veterinary Use)
1966	Human Immunoglobulin
1966	Typhoid Vaccine
1967	Tuberculins
1967	Inactivated Influenza Vaccine
1969	Immune Sera of Animal Origin (to be published)

Source: Mathews AG. WHO's influence on the control of biologicals. *WHO Chronicle* 1969;23;1:3-15.

WHO'S INFLUENCE ON THE CONTROL OF BIOLOGICALS

by A. G. Mathews *

This seems to be a most appropriate time to review the work of WHO in relation to the quality of biological products, for in 1968 the Organization completed its twentieth year of existence. It is during its second decade that WHO has exerted a particularly direct influence in this field, by virtue of the establishment of a series of Requirements for Biological Substances (see Table 1).

International biological standards

However, in a somewhat less direct fashion, WHO has exerted a powerful influence on the quality control of biological substances since its very inception in 1948. The work of setting up and distributing international biological standards was not started by WHO but was taken over, already in an advanced stage of development, from the Health Committee of the League of Nations. Indeed the first few international standards for biological substances were established by a national body, the Statens Seruminstitut, Copenhagen, a few years before the creation of the Health Committee. The very first such standard—the International Standard for Diphtheria Antitoxin, which consists of a dried hyperimmune horse serum—was established in 1922 and it is still in use today. It says much for the forethought and wise choice of the early authorities, as well as for the stability of at least some biological products, that a single preparation has served world requirements for a period of 46 years. The supply of this particular

standard is expected to last for at least another 46 years.

From this small start in 1922, and up until 1948, when WHO was established, the number of international standards distributed by the League of Nations grew to 32, in the categories enumerated in Table 2. The total number of international biological standards issued by WHO is now 79, and in addition there are 56 international biological reference preparations. Also, in recent years, 96 international biological reference reagents have been established by WHO. Generally, these are intended as reference materials for substances used in the diagnosis of disease and in the identification of micro-organisms. Many leptospiral typing antisera are included among these reagents, and a recently established set of viral typing antisera is being rapidly expanded. Table 2 gives a classification of the current international preparations, with comparative figures for 1948.

In general, the main purpose served by these international standards, reference preparations, and reference reagents is to provide a means of ensuring world-wide uniformity in expressing the potency of preparations used in the prophylaxis, therapy, or diagnosis of human and animal disease. Most of the substances for which these international standards, etc. have been established could not, at least at the time of their establishment, be characterized fully by chemical and physical means. The activity of an ill-characterized substance may be measured by biological assay, and the results may be best expressed as a ratio of its activity to the activity of a closely similar physical specimen, designated the international standard. In many cases, the defining of an international

* Chief of Quality Control, Commonwealth Serum Laboratories, Melbourne, Australia. The article is based on a paper presented to the Australian Pharmaceutical Science Association at a seminar on drug control, University of Otago, Dunedin, New Zealand, February 1968.

3

Chapter 3
Cold War, Biological Weapons, and World Health

THE Francis Countway Memorial Library is a stone's throw from Harvard's School of Dental Medicine where I had served on the faculty. A modern structure of glass and concrete, the building looks somewhat misplaced amid the grandeur of its centuries old Gothic marble neighbors.

What seemed ironically amusing about the building is that this tribute to health science learning would be diagnosed as a "sick building." After a couple of hours in the Countway, people commonly became ill. Headaches and dizzyness were the most frequent symptoms. The graduate students next door at the School of Public Health always joked that the library was contraindicated for women in their third trimester of pregnancy. Nevertheless, here's where I conducted most of my post-doctoral research.

Access to Countway from Boston's Northshore was relatively painless. An hour's train-ride dropped me off at the old Boston Garden. Two transfers and a half-hour later I disembarked the Huntington Avenue street car on Harvard medical turf. A brief trek through two concrete corridors, a pair of glass doors, and a guarded gate, and I was at work.

The first floor of Countway is mostly administrative offices, reference books, and on-line services. Computer literature searches are easily conducted here. The *Index Medicus* and current stacks are located down an open stairway on the first lower level. Current periodicals are neatly arranged on display shelves filling the south side of the gymnasium-size floor. Work desks line the walls and are in greatest demand on the same sunny side of the room.

The older stacks and copy machines are all in the basement. There is no natural light here and barely any oxygen. At the heart of this floor are eight high-speed copiers. All are almost always in use filling the room with heat and noise. Faculty and students alike await their turns seated uncomfortably at the center of the room on cracked black vinyl love seats. The lights flicker like a strobe. This is Countway's dungeon—where I accessed the scientific literature dating to the late 1960s. Sweat and time quickly disappeared here.

Prelude to a Protocol

After our cursory review of early *WHO Chronicle* reports, my search was on for articles about biological warfare (BW). There were many.

In February 1967, as international protests resounded against the Vietnam War, more than 5,000 domestic scientists petitioned President Lyndon Johnson (and soon thereafter Richard Nixon) to "reexamine and publicly state" the government's research and deployment policies on chemical and biological weapons. Their request was met with stoic silence. Notes from White House science adviser Donald Hornig to correspondents simply said, "thank you for your interest in national security."[1]

The official government position on chemical and biological warfare (CBW) had been articulated by Deputy Defense Secretary Cyrus Vance a year earlier:

> I have indicated that we seek international understandings to limit chemical and biological warfare and that we have not used weapons of the sort condemned by the Geneva protocol. [Though "agent orange," the powerful defoliant, was being used heavily in Vietnam at that time, only later was it acknowledged to be highly toxic to humans as well.] I should also point out that we have at the same time maintained an active chemical and biological program. In the last few years we have placed increasing emphasis on defensive concepts and material. As long as other nations, such as the Soviet Union, maintain large programs, we believe we must maintain our defensive and retaliatory capability. It is believed by many that President Roosevelt's statement in 1943 which promised "to any perpetrators full and swift retaliation in kind" played a significant role in preventing gas warfare in World War II. Until we achieve effective agreement to eliminate all stockpiles of these weapons, it may be necessary in the future to be in a position to make such a statement again.[1]

Worldwide Protests

Between 1967 and 1972, debate raged over whether America's CBW industry should be scrubbed[2-5] or bolstered.[6,7] Dr. Joshua Lederberg relayed the consensus of protesters in a 1971 *Science* article.[8] Germ warfare he wrote:

> . . . has been universally condemned as a vile perversion of scientific insight. This emotional reaction is buttressed by a rational consideration of the strategic and political instabilities that would follow from threatened uses of biological weapons and of the possibilities of worldwide spread of infectious

disease. In the interest of world order and to reduce the possibilities of igniting world conflict, the development, stockpiling, and general accommodation of biological weaponry must be controlled by international agreement.

Lederberg, a professor of genetics at Stanford University's School of Medicine described work in synthetic small gene assembly. He warned that very soon through "chemical operations on DNA components," researchers would be able to synthesize small viruses and engineer their design "to exquisite detail." He argued that biological weapons stand "apart from all other devices in the actual threat that it poses to the health and life expectancy of every human being whether or not he is politically involved in belligerent actions."[8]

> In a word, the intentional release of an infectious particle, be it a virus or bacterium, from the confines of the laboratory or of medical practice must be condemned as an irresponsible threat against the whole human community. . . .

> We have learned in recent years that viruses undergo constant evolution in their own natural history, not only by mutations within a given strain, but also by the natural cross-hybridization of viruses that superficially appear to be only remotely related to one another. Furthermore, many of us carry viruses in our body cells of which we are unaware for years and which may be harmless—though they may eventually cause the formation of a tumor, or of brain degeneration, or of other diseases. At least in the laboratory, we can show that such latent viruses can still cross-breed with other viruses to give rise to new forms. . . .

> We are all familiar with the process of mutual escalation in which the defensive efforts of one side inevitably contribute to further technical development on the other, and vice versa. . . . And the potential undoubtedly exists for the design and development of infective agents against which no credible defense is possible, through the genetic and chemical manipulation of these agents.[8]

Nature, Science, and *Lancet* published dozens of articles expressing grave concerns over the fate of humanity should biological weapons research continue. One such article entitled "The Biological Bomb," written by an anonymous author, discussed the ethical implications of biological weapons research—an industry that lay "at the heart of the cellular nucleus, ticking us to destruction."[9]

Dr. V. W. Sidel, a Boston physician, declared that not only should medical personnel refuse to participate in such activities, but physicians "must actively protest against the development, production, and use of biological weapons." Failure to do so, he argued, represented an insult to the medical profession, complicity, and one of the greatest dangers to society.[9]

Scientists could not "retain public esteem if they did nothing about the present state of the world," declared another protestor. The delicate balance between good and evil was "changing rapidly" and the "present juncture" was seen as crucial.[9]

In Britain, several groups frustrated by the secrecy surrounding experiments conducted at Porton, England's CBW research facility, lobbied their government too. Protestors included Nobel Prize winners Professor Sir Cyril Powell, Professor H. F. Wilkins, and Dr. F. Sanger. All desired to have the Ministry of Health assume responsibility for Porton from the Ministry of Defense to assure that all CBW research would be strictly defensive.[10]

Another English notable, Lord Ritchie-Calder, summoned support for an international biological weapons accord and haled one group of scientists who were devoted to preventing diseases over another who was busy "devising man-made epidemics."[9]

Likewise, another anonymous author published in *Lancet*:

> The whole field [of biological warfare] bristles with difficulties. Organisms for biological warfare can be produced quickly, cheaply, and easily; many are required in ordinary and perfectly legitimate ways for production of vaccines; clandestine research could easily be conducted; storage is scarcely necessary, for chemical plants and even breweries could be quickly switched to producing harmful microorganisms in enormous quantities; and delivery systems are multiple. . . .

> The Government could give a sound basis to its Geneva proposal by declaring all future work carried out at Porton declassified. . . . This would carry especial conviction if . . . it were linked to participation with WHO. . . . In 1963 Prof. Roger M. Herriott[11] of the Johns Hopkins School of Public Health, suggested that the United States should offer to place its biological laboratories under WHO if Russia and other countries agreed to do the same. The risks to national security in this procedure are a good deal less than might be thought, for despite all the secrecy, it seems to be difficult for any country to steal a march on another in this sphere where the essential basic knowledge is so readily obtainable.

> These large and frankly political questions may hardly seem of pressing concern to the medical profession. But biological warfare implies a misuse of medical science for which doctors cannot evade responsibility. Medical knowledge and medical participation are inherent in most of its projects, and the profession's silence on this issue is liable to be interpreted as consent. The secrecy demanded is also contrary to the principles of medical ethics and is totally rejected in every other medical activity. If the fetters of secrecy were

discarded and an international orientation adopted, more immediate and constructive thought could be given to feeding the world's 1000 million undernourished citizens.[12]

Though this author's heart was in the right place, I thought it naive to think that placing all "biological laboratories under the WHO's control," would have made any difference. Americans were sharing secrets with the Russians through the WHO network anyway.

Moreover, the WHO made it clear that security wasn't an issue. They expressed their objections to safeguarding DNA research this way:

> The requirements for high security laboratories may be an inordinate burden (who, in fact will pay for them?) in relation to the prospective gains. The best strategy here seems to be the development of safe vectors: plasmids and bacteria engineered to have little chance of survival outside the laboratory. In fact, in the long run this is a safer procedure than relying upon uncertain human compliance with fixed rules and regulations.[13]

Discussing the "remaining controversies" in the field of genetic splicing and hazardous germ development—techniques that require "rather complicated analyses of the remotest kinds of risks," WHO reported:

> Those who regard themselves as guardians of the public safety must count not only the speculative hazards of these marginal situations, but also the costs to the public health of impeding their investigation.
>
> This partly voluntaristic [recommended] approach will not satisfy a demand for absolute assurance that no foolish experiment is ever attempted. But the history of human institutions should suffice to show that no system of sanctions can have such a perfect outcome.[11]

These were the WHO's reservations to safeguarding hazardous gene research despite the fact that the one who brought the issue of increasing security to the floor of WHO debate was Professor Lederberg. The world renowned geneticist, Lederberg, at the time, was serving as a member of the WHO's Advisory Committee on Medical Research.[13]

The Proponents of CBW Research

My computer search also revealed that though opponents of CBW research appeared to outnumber proponents by at least three to one, the typical BW advocacy position was expressed in numerous publications. Donald McCrary in *Science,* for instance, wrote:

What is apparently overlooked and totally ignored by these petitioners is that [the war in Vietnam] . . . is not an academic exercise divorced from life and death. It is a very real exercise in how to achieve a goal, however distasteful, with a minimum of casualties among our own combat personnel. I believe that any technique, weapon, tactic, or strategy that will minimize casualties among our combat personnel is right, and any technique, tactic, or strategy that preserves the combat effectiveness of our opponent is wrong.[14]

But in March 1970, even WHO consultants noted that all biological agents permit the danger that if a disease capable of spreading widely is produced, it may get out of control and become "a source of disaster to the attacker as well as the attacked."

The viral infections suitable for use in warfare include yellow fever, tick-borne encephalitis, Japanese encephalitis, dengue, Venezuelan equine encephalitis (VEE), chikungunya, O'nyong-nyong, Rift Valley fever, influenza, and small-pox. Tick-borne encephalitis may be taken as an example of the agents belonging to this group. Susceptibility is almost universal, and the ease with which the Far Eastern virus can be grown in the laboratory and its high infectivity and lethality by the aerosol route make it likely that a case fatality rate of 25% would be achieved. . . .

The attacking country could, of course, attempt to protect itself, e.g., by immunization, but . . . more virulent forms of the organism concerned might develop or the massive doses used might be such that ordinary levels of immunity would be useless. *Thus it is possible that biological agents may be used tactically, rather than strategically, to achieve the simultaneous infection of key groups of people, and the military consequences might well be of major importance.* . . . A decision to develop chemical and biological weapons implies that they will ultimately be used.[emphasis added]

The consultants even predicted "a virulent mutant" that could "spread rapidly to produce an uncontrollable epidemic on a large scale." In addition, they warned, if mutants were deliberately produced, there was the "ever-present risk of an accidental escape."[15]

Psychosocial Consequences

WHO consultants additionally predicted grave psychosocial consequences of such an escape, including mass hysteria:

They thus present a real danger that is conducive to both anxiety and fear. Anxiety in particular may result from the fact that many chemical and all biological agents are undetectable by the senses, so that there are no warning signs to enable people to defend themselves. In addition, with biological agents, there is the latent period between infection and illness and the fact that the extent to which an infection may spread through a community is unpredictable. As a result, an exposed person cannot be sure whether he has been infected or know how ill he will be or when the danger has passed. A further confusing factor is that many of the symptoms of illness are also symptoms of emotional stress.[15]

That sounded remarkably similar to the "fear of AIDS epidemic" I had frequently written and talked about.[16-18]

In the event of an attack, the researchers added:

Panic . . . may be so great that . . . those who have not been affected will view those who have as potential agents of disease. The response to a chemical or biological attack may require precautionary or other measures on such a scale that extraordinary means of social control will have to be introduced and these may remain in force long after the need for them has passed. Thus, an attack may lead to social changes out of all proportion to the actual damage done.

Isn't that interesting, I thought. They even predicted social changes like the need to legislate AIDS as a disability rather than a disease, and requiring infection control measures that have yet to prove their value in saving costs or lives.

WHO consultants further predicted that the masses would try to avoid anything that would bring them in contact with deadly germs. Much of this avoidance was expected to be disproportionate to the actual risk.

In my role as a health professional AIDS educator, I recalled several similar experiences. One had occurred a few weeks earlier following a television interview in Rockford, Illinois. A viewer called me at the station to express her concern about leaving her house. The last time she went shopping, she said a storekeeper handed her a box of laundry detergent. She noticed a few cuts on his hands and refused to touch him or the box. She just panicked, left the store, and hadn't gone shopping since.

"Even though casual contact can't transmit HIV," I said to the station receptionist, "people are still afraid—especially of shaking hands with AIDS patients or HIV carriers." *Exactly what was predicted*, I reflected.

Besides this, the consultants even envisioned extensive health and medical emergencies as a consequence of a biological attack, "including mass illnesses, deaths, and epidemics." They expected that "WHO might be called upon to furnish technical assistance in dealing with allegations that chemical or biological weapons had been used . . . and in achieving disarmament."[15]

The authors concluded:

27

As long as research on the military use of chemical and biological agents is continued . . . new agents of even greater destructive power [may be discovered]. . . . It is clear, therefore, that the best interests of all Member States, to say nothing of mankind in general, require that the development and use of chemical and biological agents as weapons of war be outlawed in all circumstances. The nations of the world must renounce the use of such weapons, in accordance with the resolutions on chemical and biological warfare adopted by the United Nations General Assembly and the World Health Assembly.[15]

Sadly, I realized, their notice fell before blind eyes. Army medical scientists allegedly wanted vaccines and diagnostic methods developed quickly in the event of a viral attack.[19]

Between 1967 and 1968, the Johnson administration lanquished amid cries for America's withdrawal from Vietnam. Richard Nixon was then propelled to the White House and soon thereafter, toward détente. Superficially, under Nixon, the world seemed safer. But in the viral research laboratories of the NIH, the "cold war" raged.

During this time, the NCI, under NIH administrative direction, provided the CDC with prototype "reagents"—viruses, vaccines, antibodies, and cell lines—as the American and international viral research program advanced.[21-23]

Who Bit First, the Texan or the Simian?

Once we considered the cold war climate in which bioweapons research advanced, we reviewed the WHO's written accounts of the NIH's and NCI's primary role in manufacturing human "prototype" viruses, including new strains of simian viruses, for world distribution and testing.[21,23]

In 1969, the *WHO Chronicle* reported:

Representative working stocks and . . . [vaccines] for the various viruses are being prepared and tested. The distribution of these reagents will be through WHO or the National Institutes of Health, or on their instructions. Obviously certain limitations must be imposed on distribution, as it will be impossible to produce sufficient amounts of the reagents to send them out indiscriminately. Reference reagents also have been prepared in the centre [the WHO immunology laboratories at Lausanne], as well as in other cooperating laboratories *under the auspices of the Research Reference Reagents Branch and National Cancer Institute, U.S. National Institutes of Health*, [emphasis added] for many of the prototype human viruses and, to a more limited extent, for simian viruses. Reagents prepared against newly recognized simian viruses will be distributed only to recognized investigators in primate research.[21]

Another WHO report added:

> As additional means of providing advanced training, three meetings on the joint activities of WHO virus reference centres and national virus laboratories have been held, one in Atlanta in 1967, one in Prague in 1968, and one in Dakar in 1968. At these meetings most of the time was devoted to laboratory bench work. They were designed not only to disseminate information on recent advances and on new techniques but also to foster closer relations between regional reference centres and national laboratories.[23]

"Isn't that nice," Jackie observed, "'closer relations' and germ warfare method and material exchanges between NATO allies and communist bloc countries at the height of the cold war."

After another hour of reading, Jackie said "I'm going to bed. Are you coming?"

"Wait till you read this," I replied.

"Haven't you had enough for one day?"

"You know the theory that a simian monkey bite caused an African to get AIDS," I said. Well here's a report by two doctors from San Antonio that suggests that the simian may have first been bitten by a Texan."

"What?"

I showed her the article and pointed to the section that explained that in 1969, WHO encouraged researchers to use simian monkeys as "animals phylogenetically close to man."[21] They recommended establishing "biomedical systems that will permit the evaluation of different zoonoses [infections or infestations shared in nature by man and lower animals to] . . . yield information on human disease."[21]

"WHO scientists were concerned about the potential risks of introducing 'a new group or species' of such animals into research since this might be 'potentially dangerous' for both the animals and the investigators," I explained. "They noted that an 'exchange of organisms' might occur from the laboratory into nature affecting both animals and man that, 'in most instances, result in inapparent and latent infections rather than in overt illness.' Here, read this."

"No, I'm tired. Read it to me in bed."

We marched off to the bedroom, got settled, and then I began to read.

"It says here that 'overt human and non-human illness is possible,' as it apparently occurred with 'Herpesvirus simiae disease, Yaba-like disease, and haemorrhagic disease, the outbreak in Germany associated with African green monkeys, and the spread of a number of bacterial infections.'"[21]

"This is nightmare material," Jackie protested.

"Wait," I continued to read:

The importance of such occurrences is enhanced by the fact that simians come from diverse geographical areas. A possibility exists, therefore, that new and exotic agents may be transported internationally, introducing an unrecognized clinical syndrome into the animal colonies and perhaps into the human population as well. Thus, while the use of non-human primates in certain experimental studies is to be commended, disregard for the potential problems would be foolhardy indeed.[21]

"The report goes on to say that despite their concerns, the authors reported working with various governmental agencies as well as commercial firms to obtain 'reference seed virus and specific antisera' for dozens of monkey types and related diseases. With funding from the NIH and methods and materials from the NCI, the doctors continued to grow their simian monkey viruses until the WHO ordained them the 'WHO Collaborating Laboratory on Comparative Medicine: Simian Viruses.' They're located at the Southwest Foundation for Research and Education [currently called the Southwest Foundation for Biomedical Research]."

"Listen to their 'specific aims:'"

(1) the development of a working repository for simian viruses;

(2) the provision of a source of reagents such as certified reference seed virus strains and specific antisera;

(3) the provision of consultation services, including serum survey data, on the existence of antibody to various viruses of human and simian origin in various genera and species of primates;

(4) the provision of diagnostic services, including the identification and characterization of viruses for primate research workers unable to identify isolates obtained from their primates (this would also include screening for human viruses);

(5) the provision of information and the organization of exchanges of organisms between primate centres and other health organizations; and

(6) the training of interested students in virological laboratory procedures associated with primate investigations.[21]

"And here again, they stated they received their 'working stocks' of viruses and antisera from the NIH's Research Reference Reagents Branch as well as from the NCI, and that they were now creating their own new forms of viruses and vaccines."

"Sounds like a 'clearinghouse' for simian viruses," Jackie responded with one eye open. "Just what the world needed. Now can we go to sleep."

"Not yet. Consider the financial payoff. They already acknowledged working with private companies. In the late 1960s and early 1970s they stockpiled everything that might be needed, and undoubtedly lucrative, in the event of a future simian virus outbreak. They clearly acknowledged the Marburg virus outbreak in Europe and Africa as a sign of times to come. It also says they would continue their 'present cooperation with investigators using primates in cancer studies.'

"What's interesting," I continued, "is that they blamed the monkeys for transmitting these newly discovered viruses which they most plausibly isolated, cultured, and then inoculated into the animals. Here's how they closed:"

> Perhaps it should be reemphasized that there is a very practical, important side to this programme. Recent outbreaks of human and simian disease in several centres handling simians indicate that these animals are responsible for the transmission of the etiological agents.[21]

"How treasonous," Jackie chuckled. "The monkeys asked to be jailed so they could later be held responsible for their crimes against humanity. How dare they transmit deadly viruses back to the humans who were infecting them."

I joined in the comic relief. "Yeah. Maybe instead of three monkeys symbolizing denial, it should be three NCI virologists with their eyes, ears, and mouths covered.

"The last thing it says is that:"

> It is highly probable that more such incidents can be expected. The work to be done at the centre will do much to evaluate and elucidate the situation, and the centre may be called upon for assistance.[21]

"That's the best example I think I've ever heard of successful entrepreneurs creating their own niche market," Jackie chided.

Early Cancer Research Under WHO

The next morning after getting Alena, now three, off to day care, Jackie and I reviewed the last of the WHO's viral research reports.

We immediately learned that the WHO's intensified interest in viruses dated from around 1950 with the initiation of their "smallpox eradication programme."

Initially, a number of countries "generously donated smallpox vaccine to the WHO Special Account for Smallpox Eradication," and by 1971, more than 37 million doses had been distributed with Russian contributions outpacing America's by more than two-to-one.[29]

Yet, despite such international investments, the mammoth undertaking, we learned, returned only mixed results since many vaccinated countries experienced repeated outbreaks of deadly smallpox.[25-29]

Besides smallpox, the *WHO Chronicle* stated the importance of viral infections on cancer as early as 1965. The WHO's Scientific Group on Viruses and Cancer met in Geneva that year to plan a common research agenda. The Group, comprised of international representatives, including three from the United States and one from Russia, cited the need to study viruses since cancer cells maintained altered genetic material.[30,31] Consequently, they recommended attempts be made "to determine the structural alterations in cellular nucleic acids," that is, the basic chemical building blocks of all life. They desired to search for all parts of the virus genome, the genetic makeup or reproductive blueprint of the viruses, their chemical reaction triggers, or enzymes, or other "virus-associated intracellular substances." They ordered study of the "specific changes in the metabolism" of virus infected cells, and wrote:

> Any genetic structure peculiar to viruses suspected of causing cancer should be identified and mapped out. Immunological methods might prove of value, since virus-transformed cells carry antigenic [that is, foreign chemical] markers. . . . A first step in such research would be to induce transformation [cancers] in various experimental animals with viruses that commonly infect man. . . .[30]

> The Group also suggested that, although there is no reason at present to suspect transmission of animal cancer viruses to man, any possible relationship that might exist between bovine [cow] lymphosarcoma [cancer of the lymphatic cells and tissues] or other mammalian leukemias and human leukemia should be explored, both by epidemiological studies and by laboratory research on suspected etiological agents.[31]

"That's exactly what Strecker alleged brought on the AIDS epidemic," I said. Could this research have really created HIV and AIDS-related diseases like lymphomas and sarcomas?

Hot Viruses During the Cold War

It soon became obvious that by the late 1960s, the WHO's viral research program shifted into hyperdrive.[32-35] After reading several papers about their major advances, my attention focused on additional written confirmation of the USPHS's and the NCI's leading role in the WHO's viral and cancer research program.

Perhaps not coincidentally, at the exact time the DOD petitioned Congress to fund their AIDS-like virus project, the WHO announced its center for viral research and development was the NCI.[36-39]

By 1968—ten years into their viral research program—the NCI and WHO reference centers in Copenhagen, Denmark, and Lausanne, Switzerland, had served as authorized technical advisers and suppliers of "prototype virus strains, diagnostic and reference reagents [e.g., antibodies], antigens, and cell cultures"[22] for more than "120 laboratories in 35 different countries."[23]

Within a year of this announcement, this number increased to "592 virus laboratories. . . . [O]nly 137 were outside Europe and North America."[24] Over these twelve months, four of the most active centers, including the CDC and NCI, distributed "2,514 strains of viruses, 1,888 ampoules of antisera mainly for reference purposes, 1,274 ampoules of antigens, and about 100 samples of cell cultures."[22] More than 70,000 individual reports of virus isolations or related serological tests had been transmitted through the WHO network.[23]

"This sounds like something out of a James Bond novel." Jackie responded. "I expect to read the word *SPECTRE* any minute now."

Instead, we read that the NIH in Bethesda and the National Communicable Disease Center in Atlanta, the predecessor of the CDC, had made great progress in testing vaccines produced in large quantities in horses. We soon learned that the horses were actually stabled and tested in Frederick, MD at Fort Detrick, America's premier biological weapons testing center.

Chapter 4
The Road to Fort Detrick
Runs Through Bethesda

ONCE again, from the bowels of Countway's dusty basement came a wealth of information about Fort Detrick. As the WHO and NCI viral research quietly expanded, a growing wave of world opposition to biological weapons (BW) came crashing down on Detrick's gate.

The scene was set in 1968 as these Army biowarfare labs were operating at full tilt on numerous assignments, including the testing of synthetic viruses designed to attack the very nature of human immunity.

At the same time, medical experts and political leaders from around the world shamed America for its continued BW program and its use of chemical weapons in Vietnam.

As a calculated public relations ploy designed to bolster sagging public opinion and counter threatened congressional funding, Detrick's public relations department announced the Fort's plan to celebrate its silver anniversary. In response, protests erupted on Detrick's perimeter.[1-8]

Detrick's Silver Anniversary

Fort Detrick was the nation's, and likely the world's, "largest and most sophisticated" BW testing center. The facility employed some 300 scientists, including 140 microbiologists, 40 of whom had PhDs, 150 specialists "in other disciplines ranging from plant pathology to mathematical statistics," and between 700 and 1,000 supporting staff. The operation occupied "some 1,230 acres of federally owned land" upon which 450 structures were maintained. It produced annually "some 900,000 mice, 50,000 guinea pigs, 2,500 rabbits . . . and 4,000 monkeys." There was also a large "corral" area for holding larger animals such as horses, cattle, and sheep. The cost of running Detrick's BW research alone was reported as $21.9 million in 1969.[1-3]

Among the academic festivities planned for Detrick's twenty-fifth anniversary was an international symposium dealing with the "entry and control of foreign nucleic acid" into cells during the process of human and animal immunosuppression. The frank threat of manipulating nature's own genetic blueprint for life, and celebrating its possibilities, brought sharp protests from leading scientists. Despite their harshest warnings, on April 4 and 5, 1969, Detrick played host to the American Institute of Biological Sciences (AIBS)–sponsored event.

The AIBS involvement additionally outraged conscientious objectors. A boycott ensued that was believed to be unparalleled in the "stormy history of relationships between the military and the scientific community."[4]

Science news reported:

> At least 16 scientists refused to give papers at a Detrick-sponsored symposium on nucleic acids as part of a half-spontaneous, half organized protest against the use of science for destructive military purposes. Some scientists rejected Detrick's invitation shortly after it was received; others accepted the invitation, but then, after receiving letters and calls from their colleagues, decided to withdraw. Four scientists even withdrew after the final program had been printed, thus forcing Detrick to rearrange the program at the last minute.

> Pickets marched outside Detrick's main gate carrying signs that proclaimed "Fort Detrick IS NOT a Respectable Scientific Institution" and "Fort Detrick Scientists are Prostitutes." One sign asked "Want to Get Sick? Consult Your Local Physician at Fort Detrick"; and several signs were decorated with drawings of skulls.[4]

Mark Ptashne, a Harvard graduate researcher, declined on the grounds that he found Detrick's work "highly repellant" and did "not want my name associated with Fort Detrick." Dean Fraser, a professor of microbiology at Indiana University, balked at celebrating research conducted in an effort to develop BW. He wrote in declining his invitation, "It seems at best a little like commemorating the creation of the electric chair and at worst like celebrating the establishment of Dachau."[4]

Even some AIBS officials appealed the event. Dr. John Allen and a group of AIBS board members published a clarification notice in *Science* citing their principal concerns:

> It is not appropriate nor proper for an organization representing a large segment of the biological community to actively participate in a celebration honoring 25 years of biological and chemical warfare research. . . . It is not proper for AIBS to lend its name and prestige to this celebration indirectly conveying the impression that AIBS actively favors this aspect of Defense Department activity. . . . The essential issue is a moral one. . . .[5]

World consensus among physicians and scientists was much the same.

Calling Fort Detrick

Considering that the symposium papers on the *"entry and control of foreign nucleic acid"* might hold important information, I decided to call the library at Fort Detrick. By this time, I realized the NCI had been the Fort's chief tenant for over two decades. After phoning directory assistance for their number, I soon contacted one of the NCI's chief librarians.

It took her several hours to field my request for the papers generated during the beleaguered symposium. "I'm sorry, I wasn't able to find any publications relating to that conference, but it's possible the library at the Army's Cancer Research Facility may have them. Would you like their number?"

"Sure."

Unfortunately, the Army's Cancer Research Facility librarian reached a similar dead end. She called me back and said, "You know, you might try calling the public relations office to see if they can dig up the information for you."

Within minutes, I was speaking with Mr. Norman M. Covert, the chief public relations officer for the United States Army Garrison at Fort Detrick.

What a great name for a secret military facility's public relations officer, I mused.

I found Mr. Covert exceptionally knowledgeable about the history of The Fort, and very kind as well. He recalled the late 1960s being a period of widespread dissent but could not recall the symposium.

"Protestors held a twenty-four-hour vigil outside the gates for a full year," he lamented. "I documented it in my new book about our fifty-year history. Would you like to receive a copy?"

"Well, sure, but how much is it?"

"Oh, there's no charge. I'll be happy to send you one."

Two days later, *Cutting Edge*[9] arrived in the mail, and I devoured the eighty-seven page hardcover in a few hours.

Merck: On the "Cutting Edge" of Biological Warfare

According to Covert's version of Detrick's anthology, The Fort celebrated its "Birth of Science" in 1943 for two purposes defined by President Roosevelt and the War Department. They were to "develop defensive mechanisms against biological attack; and they were to develop weapons with which the United States could respond 'in kind' if attacked by an enemy which deployed biological weapons." Covert wrote:

> From the moment of its birth in the highest levels of government, the fledgling biological warfare effort was kept to an inner circle of knowledgeable persons. George W. Merck was a key member of the panel advising President Franklin D. Roosevelt and was charged with putting such an effort together. Merck owned the pharmaceutical firm that still bears his name.

"Merck! If that don't beat all," I wailed.

My surprise was based on the knowledge that the hepatitis B vaccine Strecker alleged infected the American gay community was almost certainly manufactured by Merck's company. To confirm my suspicions, I dug out the *New England Journal of Medicine* report that I had studied years earlier. The paper reported that, indeed, the homosexual hepatitis B vaccine study had been supported "by a grant from the Department of Virus and Cell Biology of Merck, Sharp and Dohme Research Laboratories, West Point, PA." The "National Heart, Lung, and Blood Institute, of the U.S. Public Health Services's National Institutes of Health" also provided grant money for the project.[10]

Then I recalled another interesting fact from the *Deadly Innocence* investigation. Robert Gallo's Cell Tumor Biology Department at the NCI, that had been credited for having discovered the AIDS virus in 1984, bore a resemblance to Merck's "Department of Virus and Cell Biology."

I leafed to the page that discussed the Merck vaccine and read:

> The vaccine was prepared in the laboratories of the Department of Virus and Cell Biology Research, Merck Institute for Therapeutic Research, West Point, PA. . . . The vaccine, made from the plasma of HBsAg [hepatitis B surface antigen] carriers . . . was treated. . . . A large number and variety of tests were carried out by the manufacturer on the initial plasma pools, the antigen concentrates, and the vaccine to insure microbial sterility and the absence of extraneous viruses. The vaccine was also tested for live hepatitis A virus (HAV) in marmosets [South and Central American monkeys] and live HBV [hepatitis B virus] in susceptible chimpanzees. The placebo, also prepared in the Merck Laboratories, consisted of alum alone in the vaccine diluent.[10]

So, they produced the experimental and placebo vaccines. They allegedly tested them both for "extraneous viruses." But wait, I thought. It's not clear whether they tested the placebo vaccines. Perhaps there was no need to test the placebo, but could there have been a potential for sabotage?

A Mysterious French Connection

In fact, a few days later, alone again in Countway's dungeon, I discovered a 1983 *Nature* article[11] that said that France's Institut Pasteur—credited along with Luc Montagnier for having isolated LAV, the first AIDS virus (identical to Robert Gallo's HTLV-III)—was under suspicion for allegedly importing tainted hepatitis B vaccine serum from the United States. The news report said:

> [Their] independent commercial offshoot, Institut Pasteur Production (IPP). . . was accused of clandestine importation of American blood plasma (automatically suspected of AIDS contamination) to help with manufacture of hepatitis B vaccine. A chimpanzee was also said to have died in testing the first batch of such vaccine: it was an apparent scandal.

The report noted the IPP was up against:

> . . . fierce competition with its American rival, Merck, Sharp and Dohme. Both companies are seeking lucrative contracts in Asia, and particularly in China where IPP had foreseen a market of "dozens of millions of doses of vaccine," an order of magnitude larger than its previous sales. . . .[11]

With so many millions of doses worth billions of dollars in revenue, I realized, there was certainly potential motive for industrial espionage.

The article did not cite, however, the source of the American plasma, an omission possibly due to liability concerns. But it could have been Merck or one of its subsidiaries, I reckoned.

It was certainly plausible that the imported plasma had been as tainted as our domestic blood supply had been until screening procedures began in 1986. If tainted though, I reasoned, it could have just as easily been sabotage—an intentional targeting of a competitor. It would have been easy to hide and hard to trace the source of HIV in contaminated vaccines months or even years after they were administered.

> As for some of *Libértion*'s accusations, the truth now seems a little difficult to establish since French Health officials who earlier were said to have been "furious" about not having been informed by IPP about the use of American plasma now have to accept a Ministry of Health statement that the ministry was, in fact, informed, and had granted authorization from the first date of importation in March 1982. . . .[11]

That was two years before Gallo announced the discovery of HIV, I reflected.

... In this particular chimpanzee, treated with the first lot of vaccine to be based in part on American plasma (3 per cent of the total), there was a small lesion of the liver. Two French and one American expert concluded it was "nonspecific" and the vaccine was marketed with approval.... However, there had been "some disagreement" (says Dr. Netter) among the experts about the nature of the lesion. When a kit for detecting human T-cell leukaemia virus (HTLV)—a suspected AIDS agent—arrived from the United States [by way of Dr. Robert Gallo's NCI research lab no doubt], the ministry requested a new test. Marketing was stopped for a while but the [second] test proved negative and sales were resumed.[11]

That meant Montagnier and the French had used Gallo-supplied antibodies for AIDS-like virus testing two years before they announced the discovery of HTLV-III or LAV—the AIDS virus. How could that be? I recalled that Margaret Heckler, Secretary of Health and Human Services, announced in 1984 that they would not have such a test kit available for at least six months. How bizarre, I thought.

The article concluded:

Libértion is left with one substantial point: that confusion over the origin of IPP's plasma, and an early lack of information about the chimpanzee, which resulted in the facts being "discovered" by journalists, indicate a lack of "clarity" in IPP's affairs; and that it would have been much better for the company if the confusion had not been allowed to arise. IPP might heartily agree.[11]

In any case, I considered, the fact that the press discovered the confusion meant they were tipped off, and who stood the best chance of capitalizing on IPP's negative publicity more than their foremost competitor—Merck, Sharp and Dohme.

More Merck Nostalgia

According to Covert's *Cutting Edge*, the United States biowarfare effort began "in the fall of 1941 when Secretary of War Henry Stimson wrote to Dr. Frank B. Jewett, then president of the National Academy of Sciences (NAS):

Because of the dangers that might confront this country from potential enemies employing what may be broadly described as biological warfare, it seems advisable that investigations be initiated to survey the present situation and the future possibilities. I am therefore, asking if you will undertake the appointment of an appropriate committee to survey all phases of this matter. Your organization already has before it a request from The Surgeon General for the appointment of a committee by the Division of Medical Sciences of the National Research Council to examine one phase of the matter. I trust that appropriate integration of these efforts can be arranged.[9]

I noted the reference to the NAS's National Research Council (NAS–NRC), recalling its part in the DOD appropriations request for funding AIDS-like virus research and development (see fig. 1.1).

A year later, Secretary of War Stimson added:

The value of biological warfare will be a debatable question until it has been clearly proven or disproven by experiences. The wide assumption is that any method which appears to offer advantages to a nation at war will be vigorously employed by that nation. There is but one logical course to pursue, namely, to study the possibilities of such warfare from every angle, make every preparation for reducing its effectiveness, and thereby reduce the likelihood of its use.[9]

A couple months after this report to President Roosevelt, Stimson was authorized to develop a civilian agency to "take the lead on all aspects of biological warfare." It was assigned to the Federal Security Agency (FSA) to obscure its existence, and George Merck was named director of the new War Research Service (WRS).[9]

As a result of this covert effort, according to Detrick's public relations director, "recombinant DNA research techniques" were being employed "through which certain organisms . . . [were] cloned to produce weaker, stronger or mutations of the original." These experiments, Covert wrote, became the "legacies of Fort Detrick, but it was not done in the Fort Detrick laboratories."

In other words, I thought, the road to Fort Detrick leads through Bethesda. If Covert printed the truth, the AIDS-like virus prototypes were developed outside the Fort and brought in for testing. The only other regional facilities with the means and organisms needed to produce immune-system-destroying viruses, in 1969-1970, was right down the road in Bethesda at the NCI's labs,[12] or in West Point, Pennsylvania at MSD's.[10]

The NAS on CBW

On October 13, 1969, following the onslaught of opposition to Fort Detrick's silver anniversary festivities and the international CBW race in general, the NAS responded—not by disclosing its clandestine efforts to support the development and testing of BW and antidotes, but by addressing the controversy at a "Symposium on Chemical and Biological Warfare."[13] The meeting was chaired by Dr. Matthew S. Meselson, Director of the Biological Laboratories, Harvard University, and included three presentations from American CBW notables.

Attorney George Bunn, a former General Counsel for the United States Arms Control and Disarmament Agency presented a session dealing with "Gas and Germ Warfare: International Legal History and Present Status," during which he heralded the "success" of "the Geneva Protocol of 1925 which prohibits the use of gasses and bacteriological methods of warfare. More than 80 countries have ratified this treaty. . . . Many in recent years. The United States, the one country most responsible for the drafting of the treaty, has still not become a party to it," he noted.[13]

The chairman, commenting on Bunn's presentation, wrote:

> This winter a group of 21 nonaligned states at the United National General Assembly introduced a resolution declaring as contrary to international law as embodied in the Geneva Protocol the use in war of all toxic chemical agents directed at men, animals, or plants. Its sponsors made clear that the resolution applied to irritant gases and anti-plant chemicals such as those used by the United States in Vietnam. Just this month, the resolution was passed by a vote of 80 to 3, with only Portugal, Australia, and the United States in opposition.[13]

Next, Han Swyter, formerly with the DOD, addressed the NAS assembly with the "Political Considerations and Analysis of Military Requirements for Chemical and Biological Weapons." He commented:

> We are talking about a dollar magnitude of only hundreds of millions of dollars annually. This is insignificant in an $80 billion Defense budget. On the other hand, these funds could instead be spent on other scientific or medical research, on welfare, or on housing. . . .

The entire chemical and biological warfare research budget for 1969, Covert reported, was $300 million. Research for herbicides, such as the ones used in Vietnam that were "designed to kill food crops or strip trees of foliage to deprive enemy forces of ground cover," was granted $5 million.[9] I found it interesting that twice this amount—$10 million—was requested and received by DOD for developing an AIDS-like virus that same year.[14]

After reading this, I reflected on Covert's admission in *Cutting Edge* that despite preparations for President Nixon to ratify the 1925 Geneva Accord, "Nixon assured Fort Detrick its research would continue."

Lt. Col. Lucien Winegar, Covert wrote, said it would "be fair to assume" that the Frederick, MD labs:

. . . would continue to work with dangerous organisms used in offensive BW since any defense required knowledge of those agents. Continuation of the defensive research program was authorized in the biological warfare convention.[9]

The "Grisly Business" of CBW

Within months of Winegar's announcement, Swyter said before the NAS:

Chemical and biological war is grisly business. I am going to approach it unemotionally, much as an economist analyzes the need for mythical widgets, rather than like a Dr. Strangelove, gleefully plotting the destruction of millions by plague or anthrax. My general approach—that is, identifying objectives, breaking the problem into smaller manageable parts, and examine each part in terms of objectives—is being used at the Pentagon. *Secretary Laird has a group, known as his Systems Analysis Office, which examines the need for each kind of military capability* much as I will examine for you the need for chemical and biological capability. Unemotional analysis of the need for war-fighting capability goes on every day. [emphasis added]

The first kind of capability I will analyze is lethal biologicals. . . . These are population-killing weapons. In situations in which our national objective would be to kill other countries' populations, lethal biologicals could be used.

If we want to kill population, we can now do that with our strategic nuclear weapons—our B-52's, Minutemen, and Polaris. We keep the nuclear capability whether or not we have a lethal biological capability. A lethal biological capability would be in addition to our nuclear capability rather than a substitute for it.

Therefore, we do not need a lethal biological capability.[13]

Failing to describe the benefits of biological versus nuclear weapons for population control, the former Defense Department analyst rhetorically concluded that since a ". . . crude biological capability is economically available to very many nations."

. . . a decision to have capability, to have an option for that rare situation, requires weighing the uncertainties of nonproliferation with the value of human life, perhaps of tens of thousands of Americans. If we decide today that we would be willing to sacrifice our soldiers in the situation I described, we do not need a capability. However, if we want the option to decide later, perhaps we need an incapacitating [as opposed to lethal] biological capability.[13]

Ivan L. Bennett, Jr., a former Deputy Director of the United States Office of Science and Technology, was the last one to address the NAS general session. The topic of his presentation was "The Significance of Chemical and Biological Warfare for the People." He began by defining biological weapons as "organisms, whatever their nature, or infective material derived from them which are intended to cause disease or death in man, animals, or plants, and which depend for their effects on their ability to multiply in the person, animal or plant attacked."[13]

"Both chemical and biological agents lend themselves to covert use in sabotage," he noted, against which it would be exceedingly difficult to develop any really effective defense.

> As one pursues the possibilities of such covert uses, one discovers that the scenarios resemble that in which the components of a nuclear weapon are smuggled into New York City and assembled in the basement of the Empire State Building. In other words, once the possibility is recognized to exist, about all that one can do is worry about it.[13]

General military philosophy according to Bennett:

> says that our national security demands that we "keep all options open" no matter how limited the need for or the utility of a given option may be. Similarly, arguments of cost-effectiveness or maintaining an option because it is "cheap" should be countered by asking, "Relative to what?"

> Indeed, insofar as lethal chemical and biological weapons are concerned, all arguments for possessing them finally come down to the basic assertion that if the Soviets or some other potential aggressor possesses them, then we must have them too. . . . In essence, then, the real military effectiveness of lethal CBW, in terms of inflicting casualties, will accrue to the force that initiates use against an unwarned enemy. . . .[13]

Kissinger and Nixon Respond

The following month, as a calculated diplomatic measure, Dr. Henry Kissinger, Nixon's National Security Counsel director and foreign policy chief, advised the president to sign the Geneva accord. History proved the act was a public relations ploy intended to silence American BW critics, bolster sagging public opinion regarding American military efforts, and respond to threatened congressional funding for additional BW research.

President Nixon—pressured on the one hand to respond to growing public criticism of America's involvement in Vietnam, and on the other by DOD militarists citing their unwillingness to "sacrifice our soldiers" should Russia deploy their biological weapons—renounced the "first use of lethal chemical weapons . . . incapacitating chemical[s], . . . and biological weapons" of any kind in support of the objectives of the Geneva Protocol of 1925.

Covert wrote:

President Nixon, scoring a major international diplomatic victory on November 25, 1969, signed an executive order outlawing offensive biological research in the United States. . . . Nixon said the Nation would destroy its stockpile of bacteriological weapons and limit its research to defensive measures.[9]

The President articulated his BW concerns this way:

"Biological weapons have massive, unpredictable, and potentially uncontrollable consequences. They may produce global epidemics and impair the health of future generations. I have therefore decided that:

• The U.S. shall renounce the use of lethal biological agents and weapons, and all other methods of biological warfare.

• The U.S. will confine its biological research to defensive measures such as immunization and safety measures, and

• The Department of Defense has been asked to make recommendations as to the disposal of existing stocks of bacteriological weapons."[13,15]

Nixon's recommendation to Congress went further than the position of many other countries that had earlier ratified the protocol in suggesting that "bacteriological weapons will never be used, whatever other countries may do."[15]

In an accompanying document, Nixon's Secretary of State William P. Rogers made it clear that "the United States Government considers that toxins, however manufactured, will be considered as biological weapons and not chemical weapons." In this and other ways, *Nature* observed, "the position of the United States on chemical and biological weapons" had been "transformed within the short space of a year." (see fig. 4.1)

The Ruse

By November 1970, a year after Nixon ratified the Geneva Protocol, nothing had changed except the public's perception of CBW risk.[16] Rather than receive the promised annual cut in biological warfare research funding, the DOD's BW budget increased from $21.9 to $23.2 million. The stockpiled bioweapons Nixon pledged would be rapidly destroyed remained intact in Pine Bluff, Arkansas, and the announced transition of Fort Detrick from a

BW testing facility to a solely defensive NIH run health research lab had not occurred.

Nature carefully followed the events from Washington, Bethesda, and Fort Detrick, and reported:

> The general absence of forward movement in the direction pointed by President Nixon is ascribed by some to skillful delaying tactics by the Army, which is held to be determined not to drop its biological weapons until its hand is forced. . . . Nixon seems not to have been properly briefed on the extent of the likely opposition [to the cuts].[16]

I later learned that, indeed, Nixon may not have been properly advised, but the ruse was by no means an accident.

The BPL Exercise

"Would this library have the Rockefeller Commission's report on CIA Wrongdoing?" I asked Mike, one of several Countway librarians stationed at the on-line services center. I was interested in following up a hunch that the CIA, reportedly involved in LSD and other drug experiments, might have also been involved in viral research. A Canadian colleague had mentioned the Rockefeller report might be available through a local library.[17,18]

"Let me check," Mike replied; then he quickly keyed in a few words on his PC. "That's over in the BPL, The Boston Pubic Library. They have a copy available in the government documents office."

"All right. Thanks."

That afternoon I visited the BPL's government documents office and asked one of the librarians for assistance in tracking down the CIA wrongdoing report.

"That'll be a few minutes," the librarian responded after I handed him my completed request form. "Have a seat and we'll bring it right to you."

I made myself comfortable in a seat adjacent a functioning PC. The screen displayed a search menu that beckoned my curiosity. Just for the hell of it I thought, I typed the words, "biological weapons" and "CIA" in the subject field. Then I pressed the Enter key. To my surprise, the screen filled with data—references regarding the CIA and biological weapons. Somewhat astonished, I suddenly realized how easy it was to access information I assumed would be classified. I selected and then output the information to the printer.

The hardcopy included Soviet, Caribbean, and Cuban *International Affairs* references. "Belitskiy on How, Where AIDS Virus Originated," read one title. It documented a Moscow World Service broadcast in English. Another, "Commentary Accuses U.S. of Developing AIDS Virus," was broadcast by the Havana International Service. A third in the Caribbean press was tagged "German Claims AIDS Created by Pentagon."[19-21]

Moments later, the BPL librarian returned with the Rockefeller Commission report about the CIA. Before he left, I asked how I might locate the documents I had just learned about. He told me they were on microfilm two floors up. Within a couple of hours, I had retrieved and read them all. Apparently, several researchers throughout the world—Dr. John Seale from London, Dr. Maneul Servin in Mexico, and Dr. Jacobo Segal from Berlin—had alleged what Strecker had. The Russian report even cited a West German company named OTRAG for having conducted green monkey virus experiments in Zaire that had allegedly led to the development of "a mutant virus that would be a human killer."[19]

I filed these documents neatly away for later reference.

The Rockefeller Commission Report on CIA Wrongdoing

In the spring of 1970, after Congress granted DOD funds for the development of AIDS-like viruses, the CIA illegally "forwarded two checks totaling $33,655.68 to the White House. . . ." This money, the report said, was used to help fund Richard Nixon's upcoming reelection campaign, and was allegedly spent for direct-mail expenses.[18]

So as Nixon administration officials were stalling the announced biological weapons cutback, the president was being rewarded by America's espionage establishment, I realized, though the two may not have been related.

In April 1970, E. Howard Hunt, most famous for orchestrating the Watergate break-in which led to President Nixon's resignation, allegedly "retired from the CIA after having served in it for over twenty years."

With the help of the CIA's External Employment Affairs Branch, The Rockefeller Commission reported that Hunt then obtained a job with Robert R. Mullen and Company, a Washington, D.C., public relations firm, a CIA "front".[18]

> The Mullen Company itself had for years cooperated with the Agency by providing cover abroad for Agency officers, carrying them as ostensible employees of its offices overseas.

Hunt, while employed by Mullen, orchestrated and led the [Dr. Lewis] Fielding and Watergate break-ins and participated in other questionable activities. . . .

During 1971, the CIA, at the request of members of the White House staff, provided alias documents and disguise materials, a tape recorder, camera, film and film processing to E. Howard Hunt. . . .

Some of these materials were used by Hunt and [G. Gordon] Liddy in preparing for and carrying out the entry into the office of Dr. Fielding, Daniel Ellsberg's psychiatrist. In particular, the CIA at Hunt's request developed pictures taken by him of that office in the course of his reconnaissance for the break-in.[18]

It took till 1974 before a stunned public learned that at least four CIA operatives had engineered "Watergate" allegedly to discredit Senator Edward (Ted) Kennedy who was viewed as Nixon's only formidable Democratic rival.

Nostalgic Foreshadowing

In retrospect, Ted Kennedy's brother Bobby had been considered a "shoe-in" for defeating Nixon in the 1968 presidential election. He was assassinated not long after Dr. Martin Luther King was shot and killed. Besides embodying the Kennedy mystique, Bobby was gaining in the polls for being sharply critical of America's increasingly unpopular involvement in Vietnam. In particular, both John and Bobby Kennedy had found the use of chemical and biological weapons abhorrent. [18,22]

These horrors, Bobby said, were the responsibility of all American citizens, not just the administration's policymakers. "It is we," he said, "who live in abundance and send our young men out to die. It is our chemicals that scorch the children and our bombs that level the villages. We are all participants."[22]

Unlike his brothers, Ted Kennedy's position on CBW and related "defense" research was one of moderate tolerance. He alleged that "society must give its informed consent to technological innovation." On the other hand, he argued that the "prospects of significant medical advances" surely outweigh the "hazards of saying no" to such exploration. "The particular field of DNA-splicing research," he commented not long after Bobby's assassination is "far from being an idle scientific toy."[23]

Ted Kennedy, I also learned that afternoon in the government documents library, had been appointed to serve as vice president of NATO during the Nixon and Ford administrations.[24]

Onward and Upward

With Jack and Bobby out of the way, the King-led civil rights movement in disarray, and Ted on board and politically neutralized, the manufacturers of war and biological weapons got on with their business.

Researchers at the NCI were now hard at work filling the DOD's order for AIDS-like viruses. Because of the adverse political climate, and Nixon's superficial endorsement of the Geneva accord, funding needed to be secured covertly through an "amendment to the appropriation bill for the Departments of Labor and of Health, Education and Welfare."[25]

This was how it came to pass that Fort Detrick—the world's largest and most active biological weapons facility—was virtually overtaken by the NIH and NCI for allegedly "peaceful uses." The cost of the conversion (approved by the U.S. Senate) was $15 million.[25]

> The proposals by the National Institutes of Health were judged the most meritorious and seem to have had the agreement in principle of Mr. Robert Finch, previous Secretary of the Department of Health, Education and Welfare, and Dr. Lee Dubridge, former science adviser to the President. . . .[25]

All of Fort Detrick's staff were, as *Nature* reported, "looking forward with great expectation to taking on the health research projects the National Institutes of Health would assign the laboratories. . . ." Since many scientists at Fort Detrick were "in any case involved in basic research and some are already cooperating in projects with the National Cancer Institute, there would not be much of a shift."[25]

Not surprisingly then, among the projects heralded for immediate action at the new NIH-run facility, was "research on hazardous viruses." The NCI, it was reported, would "use Fort Detrick for the containment and large scale production of suspected viral tumor agents."[25]

The following year, 1971, in the heat of his reelection campaign, Nixon launched the "war on cancer" and soon thereafter, hailed Dr. Robert Gallo, the head of the NIH and NCI's Section on Cellular Control Mechanisms, for having discovered leukemia's alleged cause—an "RNA-retrovirus." It was then announced that the NCI would have a vaccine for cancer available by 1976.[26]

This knowledge brought me back to Countway for the final hour of my day. In a mad rush to find anything Gallo had published, my search led me to a fascinating and disturbing discovery: As this history-making announcement was being made, Gallo was drafting a review article describing his group's methods of injecting ribonucleic acids from one strain of virus into other strains in an effort to create mutants that functioned just like the AIDS virus. In essence, they developed AIDS-like viruses by the early 1970s. Their stated purpose was to alter a host's genetic immunity allegedly to control cancer. Experiments were designed to produce an assortment of lymphocytic leukemias, sarcomas, and opportunistic infections in chickens, mice, rats, sheep, cats, monkeys, and humans.[27]

Thirteen years later, President Reagan's Secretary of Health and Human Services, Margaret Heckler, hailed Dr. Gallo for having "discovered the virus which causes AIDS."[28]

The train ride home that night was one I will always remember. It's amazing what you can dig up in libraries, I thought as I solemnly contemplated the lessons of the day.

Fig. 4.1. President Nixon Visits Fort Detrick in 1972

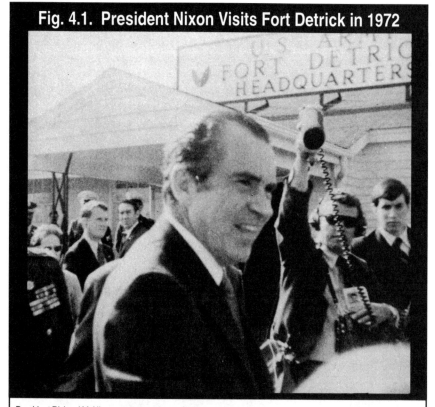

President Richard M. Nixon greets members of the press outside former Fort Detrick Headquarters in November 1972. Nixon, under advisement of Henry Kissinger, established Frederick Cancer Research and Development Center in former Army laboratory buildings. This change he heralded by saying the U.S. was "beating its swords into plowshares." Source: Covert NM. Cutting Edge: A history of Fort Detrick, Maryland 1943–1993. U.S. Army Garrison Headquarters, Fort Detrick, Maryland 21702-5000, p. 83.

Chapter 5
The Emperor's New Virus

"You discovered WHAT!?" Jackie shrieked.

"I found out that Robert Gallo may have created the AIDS virus about a decade before he allegedly discovered it."

"Come on."

"Well, I'll know more tomorrow. I'm going back to the dungeon to search his early work."

"You think there's a paper trail? But why would he have published something so incriminating?"

"Because he couldn't have possibly predicted that his creations might have caused an epidemic a decade later. Besides, Randy Shilts characterized Gallo as having a huge ego in *And The Band Played On*,[1] and those types like to see their names in print."

I had quickly read Shilts's highly regarded work about two years earlier. Though I skimmed through much of it, my most vivid memory was that Gallo erected barriers for colleagues racing against time in search of the deadly AIDS virus.

"You know the old saying 'publish or perish.' Today I discovered that Gallo's lab at the NCI put AIDS-like viruses together by the mid-1970s. They proudly published it."

"Really?"

"I might be wrong, but my intuition is telling me to thoroughly check it out; especially now that I know that the NCI, and most likely Gallo's lab, was the principal beneficiary of the $10 million DOD AIDS-like virus contract.[2]

"How do you know that?"

"By putting the pieces together," I replied. "The NCI was the WHO's chief virus distributor and they took over Fort Detrick. And Gallo was their top retrovirologist, that is, immune-system-destroying germ expert. Anyway, I'll find out more in the morning. I'm leaving for Boston again early."

That night I couldn't sleep. Questions darted through my mind at lightening speed: Had WHO officials known that their viral "reagents" and laboratory instructions were being used by biological weapons developers? How could they not have? Immune system destroying "slow" cancer viruses were the rage back then. Were WHO officials connected to NAS-NRC members who worked for the DOD? Was Gallo a member of the NAS-NRC, and if so, was he directly involved in their negotiations with the DOD? Had he participated in the controversial Fort Detrick symposium on "entry and control of foreign nucleic acid?" Could he have been injecting RNA into cells to create cancers and analyzing white blood cell control mechanisms as early as the 1960s? This would have drawn DOD attention to his work for potential application in BW research.

It struck me odd that soon after the WHO published its report on chemical and biological warfare, the *WHO Chronicle* ceased publishing its "Current Research Projects" column that had appeared almost monthly until 1969. Had the military contractors hushed the *WHO Chronicle* up? Had the CIA—the counterintelligence arm of the Defense Department—protested the practice of giving CBW secrets away?

"I can't sleep," I said to Jackie who was dozing soundly.

"I'm getting up to read."

Gallo Sounded Dreadful in "The Band"

Driven to satisfy my wakeful curiosity Gallo, I walked to the den, flicked on the reading lamp, and thumbed to the index of *And The Band Played On*. I then settled back into the recliner and began to read the sections Shilts had written about him.

Robert Gallo, I immediately learned, was the son of a hard-working president of a Connecticut metal company. His mother, Shilts simply described as charismatic, extroverted, and clannish.[3]

In 1949, at the age of thirteen, young Robert suffered a "turning point" in his life. His younger sister struggled unsuccessfully to fight leukemia. While she was at the hospital, Gallo met the famous Harvard University cancer expert, Sydney Faber, and other researchers who worked to save his sister from death. This experience sparked Gallo's desire to become a research biologist.[3]

An uncle who taught zoology at the University of Connecticut encouraged young Robert to study at a local Catholic hospital with a grossly cynical research pathologist. Here, as a teen, Gallo performed numerous autopsies.[3]

Later, above his mother's garage, while attending Providence College, he slew scores of mice and studied diligently.[3]

He graduated from Jefferson Medical College in 1963 and then went on to a two-year postdoctoral residency program at the University of Chicago. Next he became a clinical associate in the Medical Branch of the NIH's National Cancer Institute. Here, assigned to work in the children's leukemia ward at the NIH Hospital, he swore he would "never work with patients again."[3]

Later he was appointed to head the NCI's Cellular Control Mechanisms Section of the Human Tumor Cell Biology Branch, and then in 1972, he became the Chief of Lab Tumor Cell Biology at the NCI.

From 1966 to 1970 Gallo earned fame investigating the theory that viruses played a role in leukemia and other forms of cancer. His efforts examined the role of retroviruses and focused on the unique enzyme reverse transcriptase—the chemical that retroviruses used to reproduce themselves in victim cells. Identifying reverse transcriptase aided scientists in detecting retrovirus infections, and represented a significant advance. Yet, few scientists appeared particularly impressed by Gallo's work. At that time, retroviruses were seen to infect chickens, mice, and cats, but not humans.[4]

Following his discovery of interleukin-II, a natural substance that kept cultured T-cells alive and multiplying, Gallo's "career advanced smoothly—until the false alarm of 1976. It appeared that he had discovered a new virus, and proudly, Gallo announced it to the world. When it turned out that an animal virus had contaminated his cell line, and there was no new virus, Gallo's reputation plummeted."[4]

"For all his accolades," Shilts recorded, "Bob Gallo remained a controversial figure in science." Critics saw him as pompous and arrogant. In scientific politics, "he could be ruthless" and "not always reliable." Gallo himself recognized this criticism reflected "the shadowy side of his character." In his mind however, this pride and arrogance, was required "from the few brave scientists who challenged nature to yield its secrets."[4]

Among his most valuable contributions to the AIDS research effort, Shilts acknowledged, was Gallo's cell culturing and virus typing techniques.

> . . . By easily being able to grow lymphocytes, Gallo had already overcome a formidable research barrier. Some viruses eluded decent study simply because scientists couldn't figure out how to propagate their host cells.[5]

... Experiments to detect antibodies [blood markers that are used to indicate exposure to a foreign substance or an active infection] to the Human T-cell Leukemia virus, HTLV, were performed easily with reagents sent from Dr. Bob Gallo's lab. . . .[6]

What troubled me after reading these sections was the realization that he had the cell lines to culture the AIDS virus and the antibodies to detect it *before* anyone in the world knew what *it* was.

My selected review of *The Band* quickly drew my attention to another interesting oddity. Gallo, credited with having identified HTLV—the first isolated retrovirus known to cause leukemia in humans, in 1980, had apparently shown his retrovirus was linked to a Japanese outbreak of leukemia. Apparently, Gallo had first discovered this unique retrovirus; then "searched worldwide for a disease that it might cause."[7]

"That's kind of like playing pin the donkey on the tail," I muttered to myself. "A very unusual approach to medical science."

Allegedly by chance, Gallo stumbled upon Japanese researchers who were searching for T-cell leukemia's viral culprit. Identifying HTLV, forged a major scientific breakthrough in virology. It also disturbed scientists who recognized that such a killer, due to its long incubation period, could spread widely before it caused disease or was even suspected.[7] Something which Gallo was undoubtedly aware with the NCI's charter membership in the WHO "lentivirus" or "slow" virus research network.

Still, scientists remained doubtful about the importance of Gallo's work and the future of retrovirus research altogether. Many stuck to the belief that such germs preyed mainly upon chickens, pigs, and cats.[7]

So I suspected Gallo's early work probably involved chickens, pigs, and cats. That's interesting, I thought as I remembered reading in Shilts's anthology that AIDS patients suffered complications very similar to cats infected with feline leukemia virus:

> Both feline leukemia and this new gay disease were marked by a trail of opportunistic infections that seemed to take advantage of an immune system weakened by a primary infection. In cats, the infection was a leukemia virus that knocked out the cats' immune systems and left them open to a number of cancers. Clearly, some similar virus was doing the same thing to these homosexual men, and they were getting cancer too. Secondly, feline leukemia has a long incubation period; this new disease must have long latency too, which is the only way it was killing people in three cities on both coasts before anybody even knew it existed.[7]

Dr. Don Francis, one of the CDC's chief virologists, Shilts noted, quickly realized this association. Next, he examined the unique affinity the mystery disease had to gays and intravenous drug users, and how similar this was to the distribution of hepatitis B cases. He rapidly concluded, "Combine these two diseases—feline leukemia and hepatitis—and you have the immune deficiency."[8]

Slow Start Against a "Hot" New Virus

"More than a year into the epidemic," Shilts reported, "the Nationai Institutes of Health had no coordinated AIDS plan. Everything was done on the basis of temporary assignments. . . . At Bob Gallo's lab at the NCI's Division of Tumor Cell Biology," things could have been different, but they were much the same. Only "about 10 percent of the staff effort went into poking around the devastated lymphocytes of AIDS patients." This, despite the availability of generous NIH funding.[9]

Even more suspicious was the fact that nearly a year after the NCI acknowledged the need to channel its resources to fight the oncoming epidemic, the institute withheld its request for funding proposals, and failed to free available funds for AIDS researchers outside Bethesda.[9]

With all the financial resources at its disposal, and the earnest need, why had they held up everyone's search for the AIDS virus?

Furthermore, Shilts wrote that by the end of 1982, "Gallo had had it up to here with this goddamn disease."[9]

But that was only about eighteen months after the CDC announced there may be an epidemic brewing. I recalled that it was in June 1981 that the CDC reported in *Morbidity and Mortality Weekly Report* (*MMWR*) the first cases of what would soon be called GRID—Gay-Related Immune Deficiency disease—the first acronym given AIDS.

It also struck me as odd that Gallo suspected a retrovirus—his career's passion—and then he decided to quit. Shilts wrote that "AIDS had always created some discomfort for Gallo, who hailed from traditional Italian-Catholic stock in New Jersey. There was all this dirty talk of 1,100 partners, fist-fucking, and other exotic sexuality; frankly, Gallo found it embarrassing to talk about."[10]

Again, my mind flashed back to Strecker's hypothesis and then questioned—If the NCI began taking over Fort Detrick in 1970 for the expressed purpose of developing defenses against retrovirus attacks and immune deficiency epidemics, then why did they not respond to this suspected retrovirus crisis over a decade later? Was it because the disease was principally striking Africans and homosexuals?

Brilliance, Treachery, or Both

Between 1978 and 1983, Gallo's lab continued to pay little attention to AIDS at the "lethargic NCI." In those days, the NCI's chief retrovirologist allegedly perceived the cause to be more frustrating and distracting than legitimate.[11]

During this period of AIDS research, Gallo's behavior appeared at best erratic and at worst contemptuous. Shilts recorded a series of suspicious interactions in which Gallo all but sabotaged international research efforts to isolate the AIDS retrovirus.

One episode involved Dr. Max Essex, a Harvard researcher who had flown in to Atlanta to discuss with Gallo the results of a test he conducted on behalf of the CDC. The CDC had sent a cell line teeming with viruses to Essex to determine if HTLV-I or HTLV-II—the viruses Gallo's lab initially discovered and then reported as AIDS suspects—was involved. To find out, Essex used "monoclonal antibodies" that had come from samples Gallo had previously supplied. But when Gallo learned the group was still using his materials, he blew up.

"How can you collaborate with me and you're doing stuff behind my back?" Gallo exploded. "If you're using my materials on anything, I need to know about it in advance. You need my approval."

Gallo spent the better part of an hour berating Essex and embarrassing CDC doctors. "This was the ugly side of the National Cancer Institute that the CDC researchers sometimes talked to each other about," Shilts wrote. The NCI appeared to be "a repository for researchers concerned with little more than personal glory." Gallo's outburst confirmed the "darkest suspicions about the NCI."[12]

Another bizarre tale involved Dr. V. S. Kalyanaraman. Kaly, as he was called, had been recruited by Dr. Don Francis at the CDC to develop a "top-rate retrovirus lab" in late 1983. Kaly had gained fame for his HTLV-II discovery while working under Gallo.

> When cajoling did not persuade Kaly to stay in Bethesda, Gallo resorted to threats: He would not let his researcher take any reagents to any retrovirus from his NCI lab to the CDC. He'd have to culture his own viruses and antibodies, Gallo said. Meanwhile, Don Francis heard in early August that Gallo

had asked top officials at the National Cancer Institute to stop the CDC from hiring the younger researcher. . . . [When] Gallo knew these efforts would not succeed . . . he phoned Don Francis directly.

Gallo said there was no need for two government agencies to replicate retrovirus research efforts. When this approach failed, Gallo warned, "There's no way we will collaborate with you." He saw "no evidence of CDC goodwill" toward the NCI.

Allegedly, for that reason, he withheld experimental reagents including the antibodies needed to identify AIDS-like viruses.[13]

Later, Gallo voiced his concern to colleagues that the CDC was conspiring to determine the cause of AIDS and then "run without me," fearing he would get no credit.

At various times, Gallo warned Francis not to work with other researchers, especially the French. "Don't form tertiary relationships," Francis was told. "Keep me in a prime relationship with AIDS and cherish the goodwill."[13]

Shilts also reported that Gallo's collaboration with Luc Montagnier was altogether shameless. When Montagnier had allegedly discovered what later turned out to be the AIDS virus, he asked Gallo to supply the antibody needed to examine the retrovirus's dissimilarity to Gallo's HTLV-I. "Oddly," wrote Shilts, "his antibody had been almost inactivated when it arrived from Dr. Robert Gallo's lab." Montagnier labored to run the analysis anyway.

But that also seemed odd. The report I had read in *Nature* revealed that Montagnier already had Gallo's HTLV antibody test kit as early as 1982.[14]

Shilts also reported that after writing up the results and submitting his paper to *Science* for publication, Montagnier learned that Gallo was sent the manuscript as "part of the review process." Gallo criticized the work and informed Montagnier that the acronym he had used to initially name his retrovirus, "RUB," was offensive. The NCI chief retrovirologist then persuaded the French researcher to claim his find was from the HTLV family of viruses that he had discovered.[15]

Collusion at the Top

Jim Goedert was one of many AIDS researchers at the NIH who was foundering for lack of staff and money. In April 1983, he approached the NCI for assistance and was met with a response far less than was expected given Gallo's widely recognized work with reverse transcriptase. Shilts wrote:

> [T]he NCI lab where he sent his blood samples . . . [allegedly] did not have the capabilities to look for reverse transcriptase, the sure marker of retroviral infection. The tests were never run. Life as an AIDS researcher at the National Cancer Institute, he later remarked, meant "chronic frustration."[16]

Later:

> On Capitol Hill, Representative Ted Weiss experienced similar frustrations when he attempted to review unclassified NCI and CDC documents. Weiss, assigned by the House Subcommittee on Federal AIDS Funding to review CDC budget records, obtained through less-than-formal channels a National Cancer Institute memo, ordering that before any interviews with congressional investigators, NCI researchers should advise agency officials and "invite" a top administrator to attend.

So much for an independent review, Weiss thought.

Another memo, sent by CDC Director William Foege, instructed federal agency chiefs that, "All material submitted to the Congress must evidence the Department's support of the administration's stated policies."[17]

Change of Heart

Despite his "distaste for the whole subject of AIDS," by April 1983, Gallo could see that "the stakes were being redefined."[4]

The French were about to publish their findings as was Max Essex at Harvard. "So on April 11, 1983, the NCI's Deputy Director Peter Fishinger called a meeting for 4:30 P.M. in the director's conference room. This marked the first gathering of the NCI Task Force on AIDS." Here, Gallo forcefully acknowledged his concern about the French who had delivered a lymph node for him to study.[4]

"I believe a retrovirus is involved, and we're going to prove it or disprove it within a year," declared Gallo. "We're going to spend a year and nail this down one way or another."

Allegedly then, Fishinger promised Gallo that he could have the full resources of the NCI's elite laboratory in Frederick (Fort Detrick), Maryland.[4]

Montagnier's Alleged Discovery

Once Montagnier learned that the new retrovirus he had isolated was not a leukemia virus, but something completely unique, he chose to rename it LAV, or lymphadenopathy-associated virus, rather than RUB or HTLV. . . . Shilts chronicled:

> Montagnier was surprised that there wasn't more enthusiasm about the Pasteur Institute's announcement of a new retrovirus. Most scientists wanted to defer final judgment until more research came from Robert Gallo's lab. . . . Gallo was, after all, a far more famed retrovirologist, and he was talking HTLV. . . . Montagnier was gaining more confidence that the Pasteur Institute had indeed discovered the virus that caused AIDS. Still, he was stumped as to which family of viruses LAV belonged. If not HTLV, then what?

> The chance encounter with another virologist on the Pasteur campus gave Montagnier the final piece to the puzzle. The associate mentioned a family of viruses, primarily found in animals, called lentiviruses. Lenti means slow. These viruses go into the cells, lie dormant for a while, and then burst into frenzied activity. Montagnier had never heard of the family before. . . .[18]

"What!" I exclaimed, breaking the night's silence. I couldn't believe my eyes. He had never heard of the family of slow viruses before? "That's absolutely ludicrous." How could he not have heard about the hottest rage in virology during the late 1960s and early 1970s?

What I had just read in Shilts's book didn't jibe with my knowledge of the scientific reality. Something was up with the French connection that Shilts completely overlooked. Something deeply troubling.

Montagnier allegedly spent the night reading about cattle viruses and was amazed to find LAV had the same morphology, the same proteins, and even the same look under the electron microscope.[18]

The French Francis Fracas

Prior to hailing the discovery of HTLV-III as the AIDS virus, Gallo, representing the NCI, met with Don Francis from the CDC and Dr. Jean-Claude Chermann from the Pasteur Institute to negotiate the claims that would be made to the international press. The discussions, wrote Shilts, "quickly acquired the mood of delicate arms negotiations among parties who shared only mutual distrust."[19]

Gallo absolutely refused to discuss specifics about his upcoming HTLV-III publication in Francis's presence. Francis was frequently required to leave the room while Chermann and Gallo conferred privately. "The Pasteur scientists were astonished that one branch of the U.S. government should hold another in such low regard."[19]

Ultimately, Don Francis determined from electron micrographs he had obtained from Europe that Montagnier's and Gallo's retroviruses were the same. In light of the germ's dissimilarity to the HTLV family of retroviruses, he argued in favor of the French naming the virus. Following intense negotiations, however, the naming issue remained unresolved, though the three researchers worked out an agreement to jointly announce the discovery of the AIDS virus by the CDC, NCI and Pasteur.

Shilts then chronicled Gallo's efforts to sabotage this agreement and claim the lion's share of credit for himself. Standing alongside Chermann in the pissoir, he offered, "We can do this together—just the Pasteur Institute and the NCI," he said. "We don't need the CDC." Chermann dismissed the proposal. The next morning, during breakfast with Don Francis, Gallo remarked that he would probably get the most credit during the announcement because he maintained the most HTLV-III isolates. Then he offered Francis the proposal Chermann refused the night before. "We don't need the Pasteur Institute," he argued. "The CDC and the NCI can announce this ourselves."[19]

On April 23, 1984, the announcement was made by Margaret Heckler, Secretary of the Office of Health and Human Services, that Robert Gallo, essentially unaided by the French and CDC, had discovered the AIDS virus.

"The doctors who accompanied Heckler to the podium blanched visibly," Shilts noted, "when she proclaimed that a blood test would be available within six months and a vaccine would be ready for testing within two years." The blood test had already been available for over two years, I reflected, but I understood why they blanched with the announcement of a vaccine.[20]

The Emperor's New Virus

Ten months later at a prestigious AIDS meeting in New York, Dr. Joseph Sonnabend revealed that Gallo's HTLV-III and Montagnier's LAV were "identical . . . to a degree that would not be anticipated with two independent isolates from the same family."

"Would you be brave enough to voice explicitly the implications of what you're saying here?" Sonnabend was asked by an attending physician.

"No, I wouldn't," Sonnabend replied. "I'm not the right person to be saying that."

"Neither am I," said the other doctor.

"What are you talking about here?" asked an Associated Press reporter. "Do you know something that you are not saying?"

"They appear to be the same actual isolate," Sonnabend finally admitted. "Or some strange coincidence."

"What are you suggesting?" another person asked.

Dr. Mathilde Krim, the conference organizer, chimed in, "Dr. Montagnier felt very appropriately that he was not the person to point this out."

"Nobody's pointed it out quite exactly yet," voiced a frustrated reporter.

"It's perhaps a complicated notion for you to understand," said Krim, "but I think you are coming close."

Donald Drake, a veteran science writer for the *Philadelphia Inquirer* was one of few journalists present who understood the meaning of Sonnabend's remarks.

"Are you suggesting that Gallo swiped his virus from the French?" Drake queried.

"Or Montagnier swiped Gallo's virus, or we are dealing with a very strange coincidence," replied Sonnabend diplomatically.

"A light bulb goes off," blurted the *San Francisco Chronicle* panelist.

It was now understood by all in attendance. In virology, it is inconceivable that a genetic variation between two different viruses could be less than 1 percent as was the case with Gallo's HTLV-III and Montagnier's LAV. As Shilts put it, "That would be like finding two identical snowflakes. It simply didn't happen."[21]

Sonnabend was pointing out the scientific fact that Gallo had simply cloned the virus Montagnier had sent him, then claimed it was his discovery, or Gallo had supplied Montagnier with his virus, and now both were claiming credit for the discovery.

Disharmony in "The Band"

Even more disturbing than the French–American AIDS fracas, however, was the possibility that Gallo may have indeed discovered the virus, not in 1984, but at least a decade earlier, and the French most likely knew about it.

Support for this frightening theory existed, I realized, not only in the suspicious and offensive actions Gallo and the NCI took in trying to prevent others from discovering the AIDS virus.

Apparently, Gallo resisted and resented the challenge of identifying the suspected retrovirus as late as December 1982. Shilts reported with masterful clarity:

> Because the genetic material of retroviruses is made of RNA that must be transcribed to DNA for the construction of viral duplicates, retroviruses need a special enzyme to reproduce—the reverse transcriptase enzyme. By November [1982], Gallo's lab had found evidence of reverse transcriptase in the infected lymphocytes of AIDS patients. This enzyme, in effect, had left the footprints of a retrovirus all over the lymphocytes. *But it was impossible to find the damned retrovirus itself.* [emphasis added] That was the rub.
>
> In addition, *Gallo's staff couldn't keep the lymphocytes alive.* They died. Any leukemia virus, Gallo knew, caused the proliferation of cells, not their death. People with leukemia have too many white blood cells. When Gallo's staff added lymphocytes from the blood from AIDS patients, however, to lymphocytes in culture, the lymphocytes would die without any proliferation. The frustration was galling and, by November, Gallo had made what would prove to be among the most important decisions of his career. He gave up.[10]

This doesn't make any sense, I thought. Gallo discovered interleuken-II. Six months earlier, "an associate of Gallo said that he had started culturing lymphocytes from a GRID patient in a special culture medium Gallo had developed that contained interleukin-II." The IL-II, Don Francis recognized was a perfect addition to a growth medium for lymphocytes. "By easily being able to grow lymphocytes, Gallo had already overcome a formidable research barrier," Shilts reported.[11]

Now, I considered, Gallo was quitting because he allegedly couldn't keep infected lymphocytes alive long enough to study them or isolate their attackers. I found both hard to believe. First of all, the French discovered how to keep their lymphocytes alive quite rapidly. Why couldn't Gallo who had far more experience in the field? Second, Shilts noted earlier Margaret Heckler's correct comment that Gallo alone had discovered how to reproduce the virus in large enough quantities to develop a blood test—a test used by the French as early as 1982.[20] Third, to reproduce the virus, he needed the cell lines in which to grow them—lymphocytes which he had apparently kept alive long before the French. Fourth, if the French had isolated AIDS viruses using Gallo's largely inactivated antibodies to tag them, then how come Gallo couldn't find them with his superior-quality reagents? And finally, seasoned researchers just don't give up so easily.

But that was not the worst of it. Following the official United States government announcement that Gallo had discovered the AIDS virus, Shilts wrote:

> How timely was the discovery of the long-sought AIDS virus? . . . *As it turned out, the AIDS virus was not a particularly difficult virus to find. The French took all of three weeks to discover LAV* [emphasis added] and had published their first paper on it within four months. This early publication lacked the certainty of a definitive discovery, but the French had enough evidence to assert they had found the cause of AIDS by the summer of 1983, seven or eight months into the research process.[22]

And their efforts had been allegedly delayed by Gallo's inactivated antibodies, I reflected.

> Nor was the NCI research marked by great longevity. Gallo's announcement of forty-eight isolates of HTLV-III came just twelve days past the first anniversary of the April 11, 1983, NCI meeting in which the researcher swore he would "nail down" the cause of AIDS. Meanwhile, at the University of California in San Francisco, it took Dr. Jay Levy about eight months to gather twenty isolates of a virus he called AIDS-associated retrovirus, or ARV, which he too believed to be identical to LAV. Levy's research was hampered by lack of resources and did not begin in earnest until after the arrival of his long-sought flow hood and the release of UC research funds impounded the previous autumn.[22]

And all the discoveries used methods and materials developed, perfected, and supplied by Dr. Gallo, I realized.

The next day, I learned that the testing methods and reagents for identifying RNA reverse transcriptase in virus-infected cells as well as antibodies to detect retroviruses, Gallo and coworkers developed more than ten years earlier than had been publicized.[22-27]

Gallo was among the world's champions at quickly identifying reverse transcriptase enzyme and RNA retroviruses. Long before identifying the growth hormone interleuken-II,[26,27,29] Gallo and coworkers identified more than a dozen human lymphocyte and RNA tumor virus growth stimulants.[30] His primary business was allegedly trying to determine the cause of leukemia, a cancer associated with the rapid proliferation of white blood cells. Thus, methods and materials used to increase the reproductive rate of RNA retroviruses and the white blood cells they infected, Gallo and company researched in depth in the early 1970s. It was highly suspicious then that following a decade of successfully doing so, he was suddenly unable to keep RNA retrovirus-infected lymphocytes alive.

So, I considered, if this was a lame excuse to quit searching for the easily isolated AIDS virus, then what was his real motivation?

As "most CDC researchers privately believed,"[22] Shilts wrote, it is inconceivable that Gallo would not have readily isolated the "true" AIDS virus well before 1982 given his formidable background and resources.

"What delayed the NCI, therefore, was not the difficulty in finding the virus but their reluctance to even look."[22]

With all the glory attached to the earliest discovery of the AIDS virus, what powerful force could have moved the world's citadel of retrovirus research—Gallo and the NCI—away from the challenge that could have been met so handily?

There were few plausible explanations—only more horrifying questions. Had Gallo been ashamed of creating the virus years earlier, so he tried to block its discovery, terrified it might be traced to BW research?

I never did get any sleep that night.

Chapter 6
Gallo's Research Anthology:
The AIDS Buck and Virus Stops Here

EARLY the next morning, I made my way to Countway's *Cumulated Index Medicus* to look up all of Gallo's early work. I started my search in 1965, figuring it would have taken him at least five years to establish himself as an expert in the field of retrovirology by 1970. The 1965 and 1966 year-books cited nothing of Gallo's efforts, but 1967 held two such references in what became a long list of Gallo publications. By days end, I held a stack of nearly forty research reports published by Gallo and coworkers before 1975.

It took me about two weeks of reading, with frequent referencing of medical texts for explanations to technical information that I found diffi-cult to understand. My earlier lessons in biochemistry, cell physiology, ge-netics, and virology all needed refreshing. With my head buried in scientific literature, I saw very little of my family those weeks.

I began my review of Gallo's papers by organizing them chronologi-cally. I read each paper, highlighted important details in yellow, then noted the purpose, conclusions, and potential relevance to the development of AIDS-like viruses. In the end, I held six pages of tables summarizing the data (see fig. 6.8).

Introduction to Retrovirology

A fundamental understanding of what HIV is and how it works is required before discussing the development of AIDS-like viruses by Gallo and his coworkers.

The AIDS virus is an extremely unique germ. Most astonishing is that it incorporates elements that cause normal white blood cells (WBCs) to produce more viruses through a somewhat unnatural and uniquely back-ward process.

One of HIV's main components is a single chain of genetic material. This single strand is called RNA, short for ribonucleic acid. It comprises sugars combined with chemical (molecular) rings called purines and pyrimidines (see fig. 6.2).

After the virus gets into a T4 lymphocyte or CD4 helper cell (a type of WBC), its RNA genetic code directs the blood cell to produce a similar nucleic acid chain called DNA, short for deoxyribonucleic acid. DNA is the genetic blueprint all cells use to reproduce normally.

DNA directs the manufacture of all new proteins and other cell parts, including RNA. In the case of an RNA retrovirus infection, however, this natural direction is commandeered to run in reverse. In this case, the viral RNA directs the manufacture of deadly foreign DNA, which then commands the cell's reproductive machinery to produce more viruses rather than healthy new cells.

This switch in reproductive control is accomplished partly because RNA and DNA are very much alike. The only difference between them is the substitution of one sugar-linked molecule, called uracil in RNA, for another one, called thymine, in the DNA (see figs. 6.1 and 6.2).

As shown in fig. 6.3, AIDS viruses have a special attraction for T4 lymphocytes. These blood cells possess special magnetlike CD4 receptors. These attachments normally serve to detect and help destroy foreign invaders, called antigens, via a complex immunological defense system. These CD4 receptors bind to a portion of HIV's outer envelope known as the gp 120 antigen. The CD4-gp 120 interaction allows the AIDS virus to be transported across the lymphocyte's protective outer membrane, and once inside the cell, the viral envelope opens releasing the unique RNA and special enzymes into the human cell.[1]

Then, by means of the special reverse transcriptase enzyme—so named because it prompts the "reverse" process of copying DNA to RNA—the RNA code is copied to produce a new "proviral DNA" strand. This enzyme is technically called RNA-dependent DNA polymerase. It directs the cell to produce a DNA gene sequence from the viral RNA template, the exact opposite of what normally occurs in the non-infected cell.

This DNA provirus then enters the cell's nucleus where genetic materials are stored. Here the provirus is inserted into the host's normal gene sequence through the work of another unique enzyme known as viral endonuclease. The endonuclease enzyme functions like a pair of scissors. It cuts open the cell's normal DNA strand allowing the newly formed provirus to be inserted.

Fig. 6.1. The Molecular Structures Comprising Nucleic Acids RNA and DNA—Life's Building Blocks

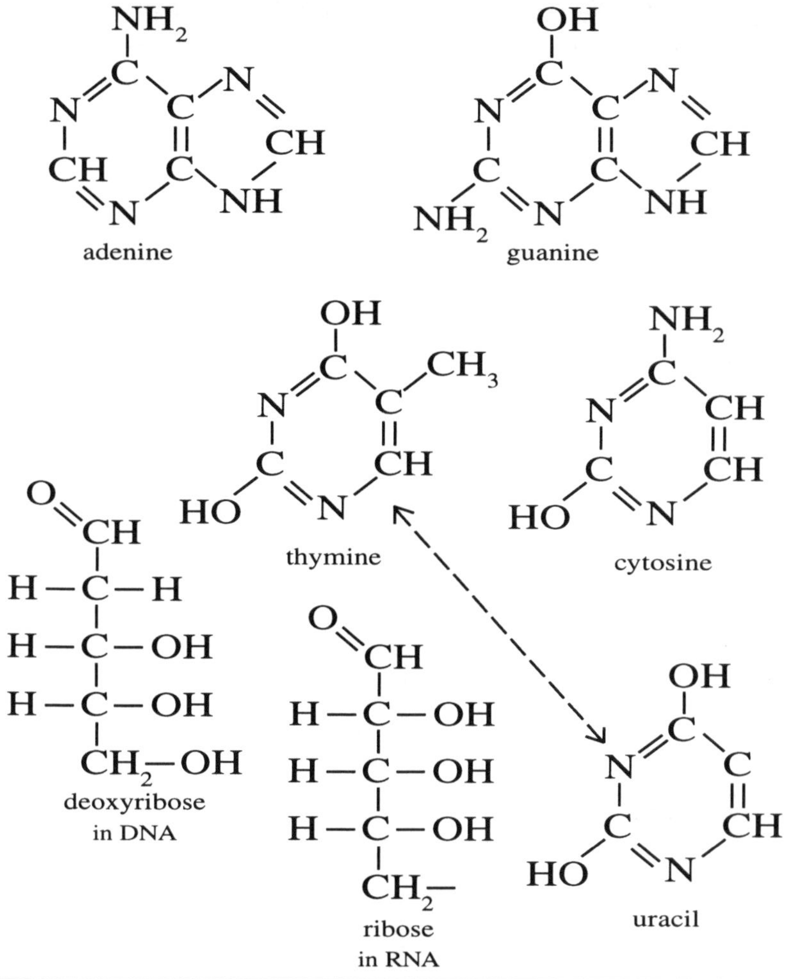

Source: Asimov, I. *The Intelligent Man's Guide to Science. Volume II. The Biological Sciences.* New York: Basic Books, Inc. 1960, pp. 526-527.

Later, during normal cell operation, the provirus directs new viral proteins to be produced, which eventually bud off the cell forming new viruses.[1]

This is the theory Gallo advanced first in 1972 during the "war on cancer" in order to explain retrovirus related cancers such as lymphoma,

Fig. 6.2. A Model of the Nucleic-Acid Molecule

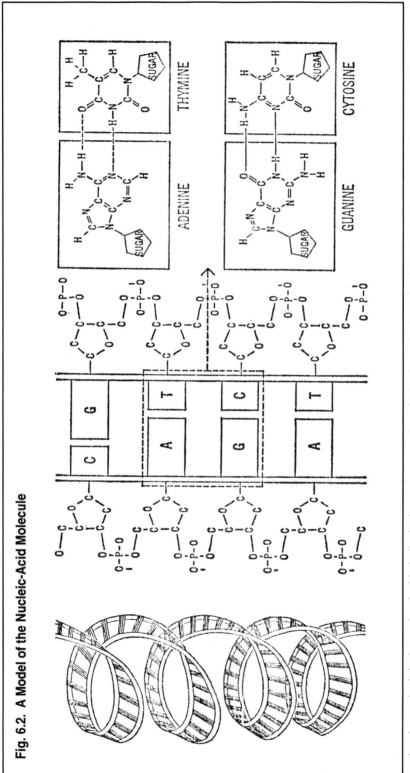

The drawing at the left shows the double helix; in the center a portion of it is shown in detail (omitting the hydrogen atoms); at the right is a detail of the nucleotide combinations. Source: Asimov I. *The Intelligent Man's Guide to Science.* Volume II, The Biological Sciences. Basic Books, 1960. p. 532. Reprinted with permission.

Fig. 6.3. Replication of the AIDS Virus—HIV/CD4 Cell Interaction

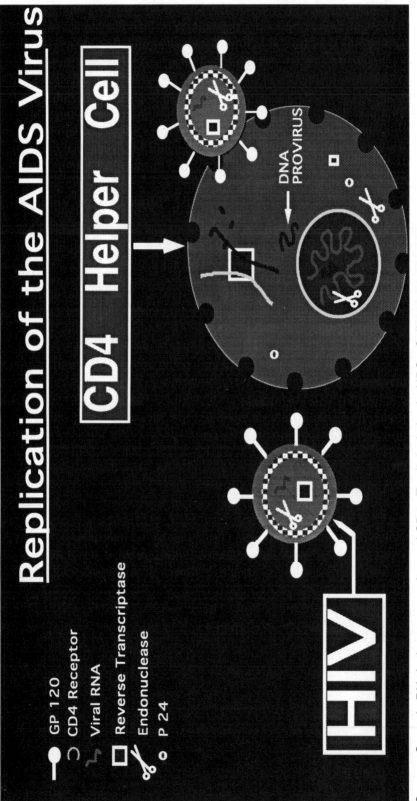

Source: Germain RN. Antigen processing and CD4+ T cell depletion in AIDS. *Cell* 1988;54:441-414.

leukaemia, and sarcoma. Twelve years later, he advanced the same theory to explain AIDS.

Gallo's Cancerous Creations

In 1971, the year following the $10 million DOD appropriation for the development of AIDS-like viruses,[8] the NCI acquired the lion's share of the Fort Detrick facilities, and the Cell Tumor Biology Laboratory's output increased as measured by the publication of eight scientific articles by Gallo and his coworkers compared to at most four in previous years.

Among Gallo's earliest reports was the discovery that by adding a synthetic RNA and cat leukaemia virus "template" to "human type C" viruses—those associated with cancers of the lymph nodes—the rate of DNA production (and subsequent provirus and virus reproduction) increased as much as thirty times. Gallo and company reported that such a virus may cause many cancers besides leukaemias and lymphomas, including sarcomas.[10]

Regarding Gallo's widely accepted 1983 speculation that the AIDS virus arose from an African monkey virus that naturally jumped species and then was carried by Portugese seamen to Japan (see fig. 6.4), in 1971 he and his team published a seemingly conflicting statement. "Only one virus [of 27 then known RNA retroviruses] which contains reverse transcriptase," they wrote, "does not seem to be oncogenic [cancer causing]"— the simian foamy virus.[10]

At the time, simian foamy viruses were known to be common, humanly benign, vaccine contaminants. Had the simian virus simply jumped species then, I considered, it is doubtful it would have gained the cancer-causing capabilities seen in AIDS. Additional mutations would have been needed to make it so carcinogenic.

Then, suddenly, there it was. "Mama Mia!" I exclaimed. "I can't believe he published this." Gallo and company, including frequent coauthor Robert Ting from Litton Bionetics, reported modifying simian monkey* viruses by infusing them with cat leukaemia RNA to make them cause cancers as seen in people with AIDS (see fig. 6.5).[9,10]

Furthermore, Gallo and his coworker Seitoku Fujioka concluded from studies conducted in late 1969 or early 1970 that they would need to further "evaluate the functional significance of tRNA changes in tumor cells." To do this, they designed an experiment in which "specific tumor cell tRNAs" were "added directly to normal cells." They explained that one way of doing this was to use viruses to deliver the foreign cancer producing

---

* The word "simian" before monkey, introduced by the mass media, is actually redundant. Since most people now associate the two, however, particularly in connection with the origin of the AIDS virus, the phrase "simian monkey" will be used in this book to mean just "monkey."

Fig. 6.4. Possible Origin of HTLV

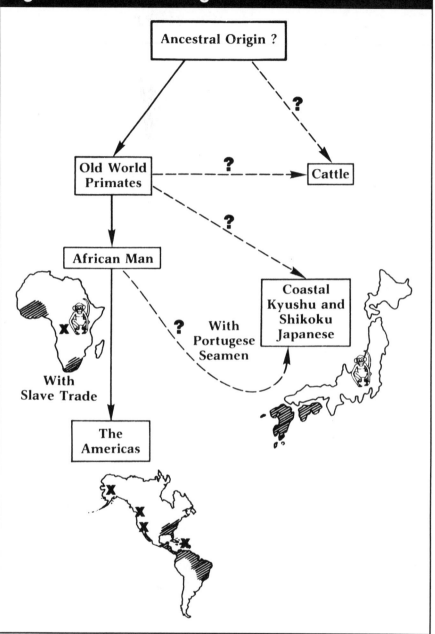

This diagram was presented by Dr. Robert Gallo of the National Cancer Institute during his introductory speech before a meeting on "Human T-Cell Leukemia Viruses" at the Cold Spring Harbor Laboratory in New York. Source: Essex M and Gallo R. *Human T-Cell Leukemia Viruses: Abstracts of papers* presented at the Cold Spring Harbor Laboratory Meeting, Sept. 14-15, 1983. New York: Cold Spring Harbor Laboratory, 1983, p. iv.

tRNA to the normal cells. The viruses that they used for this purpose, were the simian monkey virus (SV40) and the mouse parotid tumor (polyoma) virus.[11]

These experiments, I realized, could have easily established the technology for the development of HIV—allegedly of simian virus descent—which similarly delivers reverse transcriptase and a foreign cat leukemia/sarcoma-like RNA to normal human white blood cells.

Obvious Link to NATO

That same year, Gallo and his coworkers presented research describing the experimental entry of bacterial RNA into human WBCs before a special symposium sponsored by the North Atlantic Treaty Organization (NATO).[2] The paper published in the *Proceedings of the National Academy of Sciences* discussed several possible mechanisms prompting the "entry of foreign nucleic acids" into lymphocytes.

I flashed back to my knowledge of the controversial symposium on the *entry and control of foreign nucleic acids*, held on April 4 and 5, 1969, at Fort Detrick, and noted Gallo's link to this work.

Here was documented evidence that senior investigator Robert Gallo presented the methods and materials used to produce AIDS-like viruses before NATO military scientists at "the NATO International Symposium on Uptake of Informative Molecules by Living Cells" in Mol, Belgium, in 1970.[2]

I sat stunned while reading that Gallo and his coworkers had also published studies identifying (1) the mechanisms responsible for reduced amino acid and protein synthesis by T-lymphocytes required for immune system failure;[3] (2) the specific enzymes required to produce such effects along with a "base pair switch mutation" in the genes of WBCs to produce the small DNA changes needed to create extreme immune system failure;[4] and (3) the methods by which human WBC "DNA degradation" and immune system decay may be prompted by the "pooling" of nucleic acids, purine bases, or the addition of specific chemical reagents.[5]

A subsequent study published in 1970 by Gallo and his colleagues identified RNA-dependent DNA polymerase. Gallo's team noted that this enzyme was responsible for gene amplification and biochemical cytodifferentiation (the development of unique WBC characteristics including cancer cell production) and leukaemogenesis (the production of leukemia).[6] Another of their studies identified L-Asparaginase synthetase—an

Fig. 6.5. Development of AIDS-like Viruses by Robert Gallo and Associates at the NCI and Litton Bionetics

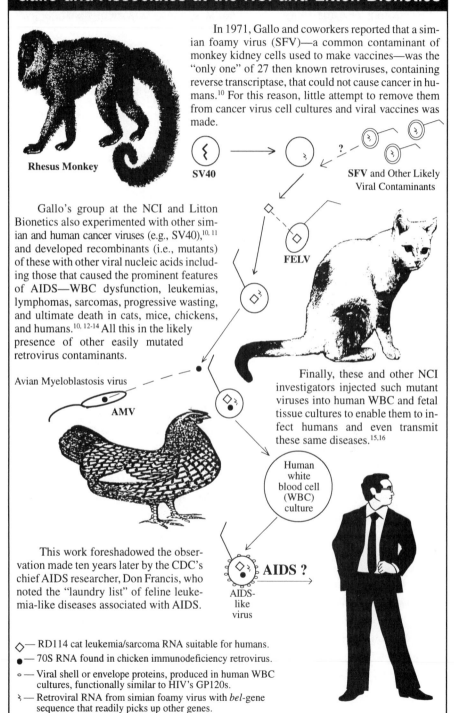

In 1971, Gallo and coworkers reported that a simian foamy virus (SFV)—a common contaminant of monkey kidney cells used to make vaccines—was the "only one" of 27 then known retroviruses, containing reverse transcriptase, that could not cause cancer in humans.[10] For this reason, little attempt to remove them from cancer virus cell cultures and viral vaccines was made.

Rhesus Monkey

SV40

?

SFV and Other Likely Viral Contaminants

Gallo's group at the NCI and Litton Bionetics also experimented with other simian and human cancer viruses (e.g., SV40),[10, 11] and developed recombinants (i.e., mutants) of these with other viral nucleic acids including those that caused the prominent features of AIDS—WBC dysfunction, leukemias, lymphomas, sarcomas, progressive wasting, and ultimate death in cats, mice, chickens, and humans.[10, 12-14] All this in the likely presence of other easily mutated retrovirus contaminants.

FELV

Avian Myeloblastosis virus

AMV

Finally, these and other NCI investigators injected such mutant viruses into human WBC and fetal tissue cultures to enable them to infect humans and even transmit these same diseases.[15,16]

Human white blood cell (WBC) culture

This work foreshadowed the observation made ten years later by the CDC's chief AIDS researcher, Don Francis, who noted the "laundry list" of feline leukemia-like diseases associated with AIDS.

AIDS ?

AIDS-like virus

◇ — RD114 cat leukemia/sarcoma RNA suitable for humans.

● — 70S RNA found in chicken immunodeficiency retrovirus.

○ — Viral shell or envelope proteins, produced in human WBC cultures, functionally similar to HIV's GP120s.

⟩ — Retroviral RNA from simian foamy virus with *bel*-gene sequence that readily picks up other genes.

important enzyme that, if blocked, will cause treatment-resistant leukemias and other cancers.[7]

Just what the DOD ordered, I recalled,

> [M]ake a new infective microorganism . . . most important . . . that it might be refractory to the immunological and therapeutic processes upon which we depend to maintain our relative freedom from infectious disease.[8]

Creating More AIDS-Like Viruses

By 1972, Gallo and coworkers studied portions of simian monkey and mouse salivary gland tumor viruses to determine differences in RNA activity between infected versus uninfected cancer cells.[9] They wrote:

> [B]y studying viral or cellular mutants or cell segregants . . . which have conditional variations in virus-specific cellular alterations, it should be possible to more precisely determine the biological significance of the . . . RNA variation reported here.[9]

The group was trying to determine the importance of various viral genes on the development of human cancers and immune system collapse. They reported their desire to use this information to find a cure for cancer, but at this time their activity was more focused on creating various cancers and carcinogenic viruses that could infect humans.[9-11]

From this work, I also realized, Gallo was actually cloning simian monkey viruses as early as 1970. So allegations that he had cloned Montagnier's virus were buffeted by the fact that he had over a decade of practice in the procedure.

Another example of Gallo's work in creating new viruses to cause cancer in humans was published for the benefit of the NAS. Here Gallo and company examined the activity of the special AIDS-linked DNA polymerase enzyme in normal versus acute immature leukaemic lymph cells, that is, lymphoblasts. To do so, they evaluated the single stranded "70S RNA retrovirus" found in chickens, which caused prominent features of AIDS, including WBC dysfunction, sarcomas, progressive wasting, and death (see fig. 6.5).[12]

Gallo and his team injected this chicken virus RNA into human WBCs to determine if the cells were prompted to produce proteins and new viruses called for by the viral RNA.[13] Another Gallo team evaluated the human cancer-causing effects of the single-stranded 70S RNA reverse transcriptase enzyme—a genetic catalyst essentially identical to the one found in HIV. They used cat leukemia viruses (FELV) and Mason-Pfizer monkey viruses to deliver these carcinogens to normal human lymphocytes.[14]

I instantly realized that this work foreshadowed the observation made ten years later by the CDC's chief AIDS researcher, Don Francis, who noted the "laundry list" of feline leukemia-like diseases associated with AIDS.[15] Had Francis known about this early work? I considered it most conceivable that he would have.

Other Gallo publications detailed the steps involved in creating immune-system-destroying-cancer-causing viruses by adapting monkey, rat, and bird leukemia and tumor viruses for experimental use in a human (NC-37) cell line.[16] One Gallo team discussed the synthesis of new RNA tumor viruses induced by 5-iodo-2'-deoxyuridine (IdU), a constituent of RNA in rodent cell cultures, and noted that chemical treatment might be used to halt the reverse transcriptase-linked viral reproduction cycle.[17]

They were apparently looking for a cure for AIDS-like symptoms as early as 1972.

Then I read a Gallo team discussion in 1973, which concerned the origin of the RD114 cat-human virus. "It can always be argued," they wrote, that a virus that jumped species would be expected to have foreign protein markers, that is, antigens, that differ "from the antigen found on the viruses of known" origin.[18]

So if Gallo and his coworkers had synthesized HIV for military or medical purposes from various animal virus components, I realized, it would be difficult if not impossible to prove.

Finally, in another report published in the *Proceedings of the National Academy of Sciences*, Gallo and associates proclaimed they had isolated a virus-like particle from human acute, that is, quick-acting, leukemic WBCs. This particle, they noted, has a specific density of 1.16—1.17g/ml, which allowed it to be repeatedly recovered without being destroyed by physical handling. Moreover, it was capable of producing the principal rapidly growing cancers seen in AIDS, including leukemias, sarcomas, and carcinomas.[19]

In conclusion, I learned that Gallo and his group of researchers created numerous AIDS-like viruses for more than a decade before Luc Montagnier announced the discovery of LAV.

Links to the DOD

Throughout my review of Gallo's research, besides citing the NCI as his chief source of support, the names Bionetics, Bionetics Research Laboratories, and Litton Bionetics, Inc., repeatedly appeared (see fig. 6.6).

For days, I wondered who or what Bionetics was? This mystery ended when I retraced Ted Strecker's steps through the Ninety-first Congress's House hearings on DOD appropriations for 1970. The *Congressional Record* contained several sections dealing with chemical and biological weapons funding. One contained the list of major Army contractors shown in fig. 6.7.

Bionetics Research Laboratories, a subsidiary of Litton Industries, Inc. was sixth on the list of acknowledged biological weapons contractors.[20]

Later congressional records showed that Bionetics's affiliate— Litton Systems, Inc., a subsidiary of Litton Industries, Inc.—was among the most frequently contracted companies involved in BW research and development between 1960 and 1970.[20] Additional BW contractors with whom Dr. Gallo or his coworkers associated during the late 1960s and early 1970s included the Universities of Chicago, Texas, Virginia, California, Yale, and New York.[21]

Breaking the News

I emerged from my two weeks of laborious isolation noticeably pale. My mind raced with questions about the risk of continuing the investigation. I also wondered how I would break the whole truth about my findings to Jackie. The pragmatist in our family, she would immediately consider the sensitivity of the information and its potential affect on our lives.

Following a brief summation of my findings aided by the six pages of tables I had developed (see fig. 6.8), Jackie shattered a long and anxious silence. "What are you going to do now?"

"I don't know. What do you think I should do with this kind of information?"

"Bury it! Or else we'd better get the hell out of this country. Do you know what the risk is in getting this information out?"

"I don't even want to think about it."

"Well you'd better think about it," she ordered. "Look what happened to Strecker's brother and that congressman from Illinois.

"And what about Strecker? Have you been able to reach him?"

NATURE VOL. 228 DECEMBER 5 1970   927

RNA Dependent DNA Polymerase of Human Acute Leukaemic Cells

by
ROBERT C. GALLO

Section on Cellular Control Mechanisms,
Human Tumor Cell Biology Branch,
National Cancer Institute,
National Institutes of Health,
Bethesda, Maryland 20014

STRINGNER S. YANG
ROBERT C. TING

Bionetics Research Laboratories,
Bethesda, Maryland 20014

An RNA dependent DNA polymerase analogous to that of RNA tumour viruses has been found in lymphoblasts of leukaemic patients but not of normal donors. The enzyme can use an RNA template from mammalian cells to synthesize DNA.

RECENT reports by Temin[1] and Baltimore[2] that an RNA dependent DNA polymerase activity is present in oncogenic RNA viruses, now confirmed and extended in other laboratories[3-5], provide a mechanism by which an RNA virus may insert stable genetic information into a host cell genome.

The aetiology of human acute leukaemia is not known, but a role for RNA oncogenic viruses in human neoplasia has been proposed for several reasons[6]. Although RNA virus particles have not been clearly associated with human leukaemia, we have examined human leukaemic cells for the presence of an RNA dependent DNA polymerase because: (1) it is possible that RNA virus particles are regularly present in human leukaemic cells but cannot be detected by ordinary means. The presence of a unique enzyme might be a more sensitive index. (2) The virus particles may never be formed but the viral genome would be integrated and undetected, yet functional in the host cell. The enzyme could be required for subsequent formation of additional viral DNA used in infection of other host cells. (3) Information flow from RNA to DNA raises interesting questions regarding gene amplification during biochemical cytodifferentiation. This mechanism could have considerable implications for cell growth and differentiation[7], and because human leukaemia has been considered a disorder of cell differentiation, it may also have implications for leukaemogenesis[8,9].

Choice and Preparation of Cells

Several considerations influenced our choice of cells. First, acute leukaemia was selected rather than the chronic form because the characteristics of the former cell type are more malignant and less often contaminated with other types of leucocytes. In leukaemia of an acute "blastic" type, a population of almost 100 per cent blasts can be obtained directly from a patient. Second, the lymphoblastic type was chosen rather than the myeloblastic (granulocytic type) because the latter are more likely to be associated with other more differentiated cells of the myeloid (granulocytic) series. These cells contain abundant lysosomes with high nuclease activities, making any RNA analysis or polymerase assay extremely difficult[9]. Third, proliferative lymphoblasts can also be obtained from normal human volunteers. This is achieved by transformation of normal peripheral blood lymphocytes to lymphoblasts with a mitogenic agent. Fourth, the polymerase activities of tumour cells are generally higher than those of normal adult organs. A much greater content of various polymerases would be more likely to lead to a spurious interpretation of a unique polymerase in such cell types. For this reason, we would expect a better controlled comparison between normal and neoplastic cells of comparable DNA and RNA polymerase activities.

The simple use of peripheral blood leucocytes, which consist primarily of fully mature non-proliferating granulocytes and lymphocytes, cannot be considered as controls for leukaemic blast cells, particularly in view of the fact that these cells have minimal or no detectable DNA dependent DNA polymerase activity[9]. On the other hand, after 72 h of stimulation of normal human lymphocytes with phytohaemagglutinin (PHA), DNA synthesis is maximal[10]. In addition, Loeb et al.[11] have reported a 30 to 100-fold induction of DNA polymerase at this time, so that activities reach levels comparable with neoplastic cells, and Hausen et al.[12] have reported an induction of RNA polymerase in lymphocytes stimulated with PHA. We have confirmed both these findings (unpublished results). Fifth, human cells obtained directly from peripheral blood instead of human tissue culture cell lines were chosen for these initial investigations because they obviously are a more true reflexion of the disease. Furthermore, there is much less chance of contamination with microorganisms or of developing mutations not relevant to leukaemogenesis.

The leukaemic cells utilized in this study, therefore, were peripheral blood lymphoblasts obtained from three patients with acute lymphoblastic leukaemia (ALL). In each, the number of lymphoblasts was more than 100,000/mm³ of blood. Two patients were untreated and the third received hydroxyurea for one day. Normal lymphocytes were obtained from the peripheral blood lymphocytes of forty-eight normal donors.

The lymphocytes were separated from other blood cells, as previously described[13], except that an additional nylon column chromatographic step was carried out to obtain more pure cell populations (more than 98 per cent lymphocytes). These cells were incubated with the mitogenic agent and harvested after 72 h as previously described[13]. In our conditions, at 72 h the number of cells transformed to lymphoblasts and the rate of DNA synthesis are maximum[10]. After terminating the incubation, the cells were extensively washed with 0·15 M NaCl and used for polymerase assays.

RNA dependent DNA Polymerase Activity

Nucleic acid "free" preparations were made by gentle manual homogenization (Ten-Broeck) of purified lymphoblast pellets in 3 volumes of 25 mM Tris-sulphate buffer, pH 8·3; 1 mM $MgSO_4$: 6 mM NaCl; 4 mM dithiothreitol; and 0·1 mM EDTA. The samples were centrifuged at 15,000 r.p.m., and the supernatants and pellets separated. The pellets of membranes and nuclei were washed with the same buffer with gentle homogenization. After centrifugation the wash (second supernatants) was combined with the first supernatants and the nuclei-membrane pellets removed.

Nucleic acids were removed from the supernatant fractions by successive precipitations with $MnCl_2$ and

Fig. 6.7. Major United States Army Biological Weapons Contractors for Fiscal Year 1969

Mr. Mahon. List for the record the major contractors and the sums allocated to them in this program in fiscal year 1969.
(The information follows:)

The following list contains the major contractors and amounts of each contract.

Contractor	Fiscal year 1969
Miami, University. of Coral Gables Fla	$645, 000
Herner and Co., Bethesda, Md	518, 000
Missouri, University of, Columbia, Mo	250, 000
Chicago, University, of Chicago, Ill	216, 000
Aerojet-General Corp., Sacramento. Calif	210, 000
Bionetics Research Laboratories, Inc., Falls Church, Va	180, 000
West Virginia University, Morgantown, W. Va	177, 000
Maryland. University of, College Park, Md	170, 000
Dow Chemical Co., Midland, Mich	158, 000
Hazelton Laboratories, Inc., Falls Church, Reston, Va	145, 000
New York University Medical Center. New York, N.Y	142, 000
Midwest Research Institute. Kansas City, Mo	134, 000
Stanford University, Palo Alto, Calif	125, 000
Stanford Research Institute, Menlo Park, Calif	124, 000
Pfizer and Co., Inc., New York, N.Y	120, 000
Aldrich Chemical Co., Inc., Milwaukee, Wis	117, 000
Computer Usage Development Corp., Washington, D.C	110, 000
New England Nuclear Corp., Boston, Mass	104, 000

Source: Department of Defense Appropriations For 1970: Hearings Before A Subcommittee of the Committee on Appropriations House of Representatives, Ninety-first Congress, First Session, H.B. 15090, Part 5, Research, Development, Test and Evaluation of Biological Weapons, Dept. of the Army. U.S. Government Printing Office, Washington, D.C., 1969, p. 689.

"No. Every time I call, the phone just rings and rings. And that other doctor from Georgia who wrote that article about Strecker, William Douglass, I've left a half-dozen messages for him on his answering machine, but he's never returned one."

"Well you better find out if Strecker's still alive before you do anything else," Jackie said.

That night before bed, after her initial shock lessened, I said, "You know, this thing is bigger than just us. This is about the world. The kind of world we'll leave behind for our children."

"I know it," Jackie replied. "That's what scares me most."

Fig. 6.8. The Early Research of Dr. Robert Gallo at the National Cancer Institute and Its Implications in Relation to the Theory of Synthetic HIV Development

Year and Subject of Investigation	Study Conclusions	Possible Relationship to HIV Synthesis
1967		
Gallo RC. The Inhibitory Effect of Heme on Heme Formation *In Vivo*. Possible Mechanism for the Regulation of Hemoglobin Synthesis. *Journal of Clinical Investigation* 1967;46;1:124-132.	Red blood cell 'heme' synthesis depends upon a feedback system that is self-limiting. The "possible site of negative feedback control" in red blood cell production is considered.	None.
Gallo RC, Perry S and Breitman TR. The Enzymatic Mechanisms for Deoxythymidine Synthesis in Human Leukocytes. *Journal of Biological Chemistry* 1967;242;21:5059-5068.	Amino acid synthesis in white blood cells, and subsequent cell reproduction is regulated by special enzymes. These control factors can be modified by inorganic substances (e.g. arsenate or phosphate).	Mechanisms for inhibiting white blood cell production. In AIDS there is a reduction in the number of white blood cells from the thymus (i.e., T-lymphocytes) and resulting immunosuppression.
1968		
Gallo RC and Perry S. Enzymatic Abnormality in Human Leukaemia. *Nature* 1968;218:465-466.	Special enzymes are altered in white blood cells of leukemia patients. Study shows which enzyme (i.e. pyrimidine deoxynucleoside) is associated with chronic leukemia and what will likely cause a reduction of this enzyme to prompt leukemia.	Specific enzymes associated with (chronic myelogenous) leukemia found, and apparent requirement to create a "base pair switch mutation" in the protein (genes) of white blood cells to create immune system dysfunction.
Gallo RC and Breitman TR. The Enzymatic Mechanisms for Deoxythymidine Synthesis in Human Leukocytes: Comparison of Deoxyribosyl Donors. *Journal of Biological Chemistry* 1968;243;19:4936-4942.	Human white blood cell reproduction is largely regulated by independent enzyme-linked mechanisms. Both activities are the function of one protein.	The production of one of four major building blocks of DNA (i.e., deoxythymidine) in human white blood cells (leukocytes) can be stimulated or inhibited by manipulating "the function of one protein" within the cells.
Gallo RC and Breitman TR. The Enzymatic Mechanisms for Deoxythymidine Synthesis in Human Leukocytes: Inhibition of Deoxythymidine Phosphorylase by Purines. *Journal of Biological Chemistry* 1968;243;19:4943-4951.	Further evidence that human white blood cell reproduction is largely regulated by independent enzyme-linked mechanisms associated with the addition of the base components of nucleic acids which can affect the synthesis of DNA and cell replication.	DNA in human leukocytes can be inhibited by the addition of various reagents (including the "pooling" of purine bases within the cell). This may cause "DNA degradation" and immune system dysfunction…
Gallo RC, Perry S and Breitman TR. Inhibition of Human Leukocyte Pyrimidine Deoxynucleoside Synthesis by Allopurinal and 6-Mercaptopurine. *Biochemical Pharmacology* 1968;17:2185-2191.	The nucleic acid base purine plays a role in the regulation of human white blood cell reproduction (which is largely regulated by independent enzyme-linked mechanisms), but not as much as the pyrimidine bases studied previously (and cited above).	Though related to the treatment of childhood leukemia, this study provides evidence that human leukocytes can be inhibited to a larger degree by the building blocks of RNA and DNA.
1969		
Gallo RC and Perry S. The Enzymatic Mechanisms for Deoxythymidine Synthesis in Human Leukocytes: Comparison Between Normal and Leukemic Leukocytes.	Same findings as cited above	Same findings as cited above
Gallo RC, Whang-Peng J and Perry S. Isopentenyladenosine Stimulates and Inhibits Mitosis in Human Lymphocytes Treated with Phytohemagglutinin. *Science,* 1969: 165:400-402.	Transfer RNA (tRNA) components from plants affects human lymph cells. Stimulation or inhibition ofcell division depends on the concentrations of reagents used. tRNA components may be useful in treating cancers and "has potential immunosuppressive properties."	Relates to human lymphocytes (immune cell division control mechanisms as well as immunosuppressive influence of tRNA. AIDS virus is RNA virus which causes immunosuppression.
1970		
Herrera F, Adamson RH and Gallo RC. Uptake of Transfer Ribonucleic Acid by Normal and Leukemic Cells. *Proceedings of the National Academy of Sciences* 1970;67;4:1943-1950. "Presented at the NATO International Symposium on Uptake of Informative Molecules by Living Cells, Mol, Belgium, 1970.	Uptake of foreign (bacterial) tRNA by mammalian leukemia and normal immature human white blood cells is determined by "an energy independent, carrier-mediated, mechanism." Paper offers several possibilities of what this mechanism might be.	Paper links Gallo not only to National Academy of Sciences at the time DOD contracted with them to develop immune deficiency causing biological weapons, but also to Senior NCI research position in "entry" of foreign nucleic acids into cells" to effect immunosuppression—This at the time of controversial Fort Detrick symposium. Paper also implies Gallo's link to NATO's applied "defense" research.
Gallo RC and Longmore JL. Asparaginyl-tRNA and Resistance of Murine Leukaemias to L-Asparaginase. *Nature* 1970;227:1134-1136.	L-Asparaginase synthetase (a unique enzyme) plays a key role in controlling the growth of tumors. By blocking this enzyme's activity, tumors can be "derepressed"—that is, made resistant to chemotherapies—and stimulated to grow.	Study focuses on key enzyme in white blood cells which if repressed will induce leukemia and other cancers as well as make the exposed animal cells treatment resistant. This work lays the foundation for discovery and work on reverse transcriptase enzyme in RNA retroviruses.
Gallo RC, Yang SS and Ting RC. RNA Dependent DNA Polymerase of Human Acute Leukaemic Cells. *Nature* 1970;228:927-929.	An RNA dependent DNA polymerase analogous to that of RNA tumour viruses has been found in lymphoblasts (immature white blood cells) of leukaemic patients but not or normal donors. The enzyme can use an RNA template from mammalian cells to synthesize DNA.	Reverse transcriptaseenzyme identified responsible for "gene amplification," "biochemical cytodifferentiation," (i.e. development of unique cell characteristics including cancer cell production) and "leukaemogenesis. "With HIV, this enzyme causes infected T-4 Lymphocyte to produce additional viruses as well as lose their own competence.

Acknowledged Funding Source/Biological Weapons Contractor: † Litton Bionetics; √ Bionetics Research Labs: § Univ. of Calif.; ∞ Univ. of Texas: ◊ Univ. of Chicago: ⊥ Yale U.

	Year and Subject of Investigation	Study Conclusions	Possible Relationship to HIV Synthesis
	1970 continued		
	Gallo RC and Pestka S. Transfer RNA Species in Normal and Leukemic Human Lymphoblasts. *Journal of Molecular Biology.* 1970;52:195-219.	This study identified the transfer RNA responsible for the production of every amino acid in human tissues. It found at least 56 species of tRNA from both normal and leukemic cells. Most species were very similar except for tyrosyl-tRNA and glutaminyl-tRNA where the differences were "most pronounced."	Report focused on defining specific alterations in tRNA responsible for "abnormal cellular regulatory mechanisms in neoplastic cells." Such findings would provide knowledge as to where a tRNA molecule might need to be modified (by a virus) to produce leukemia and perhaps other cancers.
	1971		
√ 8	Gallo RC, Sarin PS, Allen, PT, Newton WA, Priori ES, Bowen JM and Dmochowski L. Reverse Transcriptase in Type C Virus Particles of Human Origin. *Nature New Biology* 1971;232:140-142.	Discovery of reverse transcriptase activity in human type C virus associated with lymphoma. By adding a synthetic RNA and Feline (i.e.,cat) leukaemia virus "template" to the human virus, the rate of DNA production (and subsequent provirus synsthesis) increased two and thirty times respectively. This human "type C virus" possesses a DNA polymerase (reverse transcriptase) which can utilize both endogenous (i.e., its own natural) RNA, or "exogenous RNA" as a template, (i.e.,foreign RNA extracted from other cells or viruses) to produce the effects on the human cells coded for by the new genetic material.	Report stated this type of virus may cause many types of cancers besides leukaemia and lymphoma including sarcomas. HIV causes sarcoma development. "Only one virus [of 27 known RNA retroviruses] which contains reverse transcriptase," article said, "does not seem to be oncogenic (cancer causing),"—the "simian" (monkey) virus. This contradicts the claim that a monkey virus was a natural precursor to HIV. Evidence presented here that this humanly benign retrovirus was being modified by the addition of cat leukaemia RNA, and other synthetic products to increase its DNA output and protein synthesis, that is, its disease causing capacity.
	Gallo RC, Whang-Peng J and Adamson RH. Studies on the Antitumor Activity, Mechanism of Action, and Cell Cycle Effects of Camptothecin. *Journal of the National Cancer Institute.* 1971;46:789-795.	At lower concentrations, dibutyryl adenosine cyclic 3',5'-monophosphate increased DNA synthesis and the rate of cell division of normal human lymphocytes responding to the stimulant phytohemagglutin (PHA)—a foreign plant derived substance. At higher concentrations of reagent, the opposite response was found. Cyclic 3',5'AMP "may be useful in immunotherapy."	None apparent at present time.
	Gallo RC, Whang-Peng J. Enhanced Transformation of Human Immunocompetent Cells by Dibutyryl Adenosine Cyclic 3':5'-Monophosphate. *Journal of the National Cancer Institute.* 1971;47;1:91-94.	Camptothecin, a naturally occurring antitumor drug extended survival time for mice bearing various experimental leukemias; the plasma cell tumor, but less effective against a mast cell tumor and a reticulum cell sarcoma.The alkaloid also killed cells in three cell lines. DNA synthesis was strongly inhibited but not RNA or protein synthesis. The drug may be useful for specific tumors.	None apparent at present time.
◊	Riddick DH and Gallo RC. The Transfer RNA Methylases of Human Lymphocytes: Induction by PHA in Normal Lymphocytes. *Blood*1971;37;3:282-292.	Phytohemagglutinin (PHA) treated human leukaemic lymphocytes contain increased tRNA enzymes (methylases) different from normal lymphocytes which was "dependent on the synthesis of new RNA" which has been methylated consistent with some tumors and cancer viruses.	Human lymphocytes (immune cell) control mechanisms is influence bytRNA. AIDS virus influences this control mechanism to ultimately cause immunosuppression. Later research found unique cellular proteins which specifically bind to HIV including those of a "PHA stimulated human CD4+ lymphoblast cell line.
◊	Riddick DH and Gallo RC. The Transfer RNA Methylases of Human Lymphocytes: II. Delayed Induction by PHA in Lymphocytes From Patients With Chronic Lymphocytic Leukemia. *Blood*1971;37;3:293-298.	Phytohemagglutinin (PHA) treated human leukaemic lymphocytes induces quantitative and qualitative changes in tRNA methylase enzymes similar to those seen in normal lymphocytes, but the sequence of events of PHA interaction with chronic lymphocytic leukemia (CLL) lymphocytes leading to enzyme induction is delayed.	Same as above plus additional finding that chronic lymphocytic leukaemia cells contain fewer Phytohemagglutinin, PHA, receptors than normal lymphocyte cell membranes. This factor may be somehow related to the specific binding of HIV to CD4+ lymphocytes as seen in AIDS patients.
	Levine L, Vunakis HV and Gallo RC. Serologic Specificities of Methylated Base Immune Systems. *Biochemistry*1971; 10;11:2009-2013.	Protein synthesis in cells is dependent on nucleic acids—the basic building blocks of DNA and RNA.The two major categories of these "bases" purines and pyrimidines can be biochemically methylated and are then easily identified by specific antibodies.This can be helpful in diagnosing tRNA changes in some tumors and leukaemias	Study provides the first published evidence of Gallo's work in developing antibodies which can detect problems with tRNA in white blood cells. This represents the basic research upon which he advanced the technology to produce the only antibodies available to detect the human T-lymphocyte viruses (HTLV-I, II, and III),and were required in identifying HIV. Currently, the HIV antibodies developed from this early work, were patented and sold by Gallo and the NCI to produce the blood tests used to detect HIV infection.
	Fujioka S and Gallo RC. Aminoacyl Transfer RNA Profiles in Human Myeloma Cells. *Blood*1971; 38;246-252.	Between human normal lymphoblasts (immature lymphocytes) and human myeloma cells (cancerous antibody-forming plasma cells manufactured in bone marrow) minor differences were noted in only 2 of 20 amino acid tRNA complexes—aspartyl-tRNA and larger differences in tyrosyl-tRNA—were observed.Consequently, this apparent defect in white blood cell differentiation in humans may be due to an abnormality in the "translational control" of these two amino acid—tRNA complexes. Additional analysis of the tyrosyl-tRNA found the presence of "more hydrophobic groups such as methyl groups in the tRNA of the neoplastic (cancerous) cells." This tied in with evidence cited above of the importance of tRNA methylase enzymes in the induction of leukaemia from viruses.	Gallo and Fujioka concluded from this study conducted in late 1969 or early 1970 that they would need to further "evaluate the functional significance of tRNA changes in tumor cells," by designing an experiment in which "specific tumor cell tRNAs" would be "added directly to normal cells." It was explained that one way of doing this was to use viruses to deliver the foreign cancer producing tRNA to normal cells. The viruses which were then being employed to do this, the report noted, was the simian monkey virus (SV40) and the mouse parotid tumor (polyoma) virus. Such experiments could have established the technology and provided a model for the development of HIV—allegedly of simian virus descent—which similarly delivers foreign RNA to normal white blood cells.

Acknowledged Funding Source/Biological Weapons Contractor: † Litton Bionetics; √ Bionetics Research Labs; § Univ. of Calif.; ∞ Univ. of Texas; ◊ Univ. of Chicago; ∆ Yale U.

	Year and Subject of Investigation	Study Conclusions	Possible Relationship to HIV Synthesis
	1971 continued		
√	Gallo RC. Transfer RNA and Transfer RNA Methylation in Growing and "Resting" Adult and Embryonic Tissues and in Various Oncogenic Systems. *Cancer Research* 1971;31:621-629.	Human acute leukemia likely involves a block in leukocyte maturation due to a "disorder of protein synthesis." This is indicated by reduced DNA synthesis in cancerous cells and a build-up of heavy weight tRNA—time changes in specific amino acids within the white blood cells. At this time changes in specific amino acids into proteins—in young leukemic cells. (The amino acids are delivered by tRNA to the RNA, the ribosomal 'assembly station.') In this report, Gallo questioned whether acute lymphocytic leukemia was associated with a specific change in tyrosyl-tRNA, and whether lymphosarcoma was related to a specific change in seryl-tRNA. "Similar to the results with RNA virus-transformed cells, the tumor derived from the polyoma (mouse parotid tumor) cells showed higher tRNA methylase activity.	In this study, Gallo used several virus-transformed cells including the simian (monkey) virus (SV40) the murine (rat or mouse) sarcoma virus, and the polyoma (mouse parotid tumor) virus infected cells. At this time changes in specific amino acids within the white blood cells' RNA and DNA were being manufactured in the lab and studied to determine the related effects on the immune cell structure and function. Combine this research, and the available technology to isolate and inject genes from different viruses to produce a unique RNA retrovirus, and Gallo et. al., had all the requirements needed to produce HIV. The next questions are: 1) Did he attempt to combine different viruses to induce specific cancerous and immune system alterations, and 2) if so, which specific viral species and components might he have used to create an AIDS virus?
	Gallo RC. Reverse Transcriptase, the DNA Polymerase of Oncogenic RNA Viruses. *Nature* 1971;39:1:194-198.	Article reviews and updates knowledge regarding the importance of reverse transcriptase enzyme in cancer causing RNA tumor viruses. Important questions which Gallo proposed be researched including: "What are the detailed biochemical mechanisms for this enzyme?" and "Does the enzyme in viruses from higher forms differ from that of lower animals?"	None obvious in this summary report.
	1972		
†	Gallagher RE. Ting RC and Gallo RC. A Common Change of Aspartyl-tRNA in Polyoma- and SV Transformed Cells. *Biochimica Et Biophysica Acta* 1972;272:568-582.	A major difference in aspartyl-tRNA (Asp-t-RNA) was demonstrated in polyoma (mouse parotid tumor) cells and SV40 (simian monkey tumor) cells. The "pattern of Asp-t-RNA is due to selective cellular gene expression," which "may be related to the function of the DNA oncogenic (cancer causing) virus genome (gene structure)" in infected cells. In addition, "a potential advantage of selecting virus-transformed tumor cells for study is that tRNA differences discovered may be correlated with the virus genome function," with the ability to produce virus-related antigens and their effects.	In this study, Gallo and coworkers studied portions of different viruses to determine if "the tRNA difference (in cancer cells) may be related to the properties of neoplasia (cancer development) in general, or, more specifically, to the function of the DNA oncogenic (cancer causing) virus genome (genetic code) inserted in the infected cells? They stated that "by studying viral or cellular mutants or cell segregants...which have conditional variations in virus-specific cellular alterations, it should be possible to more precisely determine the biological significance of the aspartyl-tRNA variation reported here." This work shows the analysis of different viral genes was underway to determine what effects each might have on developing cancer. They reported their desire to use this information on cancer causing viruses to find a cure for cancer, but at this time they applied their knowledge more towards creating various cancers and new viral species, than towards eradicating them.
	Smith RG and Gallo RC. DNA-Dependent DNA Polymerases I and II from Normal Human-Blood Lymphocytes. *Proceedings of the National Academy of Sciences* 1972; 69;10:2879-2884.	"A DNA polymerase has been found in blood lymphoblasts [immature white blood cells] from individuals with acute leukemia that, unlike lymphocyte DNA polymerases from normal individuals, transcribes 70S viral RNA."	The 70S RNA virus is single stranded RNA retrovirus found in chickens which causes some prominent features of AIDS, including white blood cell dysfunction, sarcomas, progressive wasting, and death.
√	Robert MS, Smith RG and Gallo RC. Viral and Cellular DNA Polymerase: Comparison of Activities with Synthetic and Natural RNA Templates. *Science* 1972;176:798-800.	"Two DNA polymerases purified from normal human lymphocytes (NHL) are distinguishable from the viral reverse transcriptases of avian [chicken] myeloblastosis virus and mason-Pfizer monkey virus by their relative affinity for select templates....Criteria for distinguishing the activity of viral reverse transcriptases are discussed," including "...the ability of viral reverse transcriptases, but not the cellular DNA polymerases, to react with purified single-stranded 70S RNA templates." Also: "The importance of using rigorously purified 70S RNA cannot be overemphasized. In early experiments, NHL DNA polymerases I and II showed reactivity with feline (cat) leukemia virus (FELV) 70S RNA," however this was an artifact of contamination. "All of these distinguishing criteria will enable more critical determination to be made as to whether a viral-like reverse transcriptase is associated with neoplastic disease. The RNA-dependent DNA polymerase from human acute leukemic cells satisfies all these criteria for a reverse transcriptase.	This report also indicates Gallo and co-workers were evaluating single stranded RNA reverse transcriptase activity in cat leukemias as well as chickens. In 1982, Dr. Don Francis, a chief virologist at the CDC noted the "laundry list" of feline leukemia-like diseases and the sexual transmissability of AIDS, and remarked, "Combine these two diseases—feline leukemia and hepatitis—and you have the immune deficiency." The possibilities in relation to HIV synthesis and the implications of this study speak for themselves.

Acknowledged Funding Source/Biological Weapons Contractor: † Litton Bionetics; √ Bionetics Research Labs; § Univ. of Calif.; ∞ Univ. of Texas; ◊ Univ. of Chicago; ∆ Yale U.

Year and Subject of Investigation	Study Conclusions	Possible Relationship to HIV Synthesis
1972 continued		
∞ Talal N and Gallo RC. Antibodies to DNA-RNA Hybrid in Systemic Lupus Erythematosus measured by a Cellulose Ester Filter Radioimmunoassay. *Nature New Biology* 1972; 240:240-242.	"The RNA tumour viruses apparently replicate by means of an RNA-dependent DNA polymerase (reverse transcriptase) that produces virus specific DNA which presumably is integrated into the host genome. The first product of this process is a DNA:RNA hybrid…Antibodies to such hybrids might strengthen the role for viruses in this disease."	Gallo and Talal concluded that—"A continued search for antibodies to natural hybrids seems warranted." The importance, specificity and difficult task of isolating antibodies to reverse transcriptase RNA tumor viruses described in this report, provided the incentive to develop the antibody isolation techniques and antibodies which AIDS researchers throughout the world sought from Gallo alone.
† △ Borrow SN, Smith RG, Reitz MS and Gallo RC. Stimulated Normal Human Lymphocytes Contain a Ribonuclease-Sensitive DNA Polymerase Distinct from Viral RNA-Directed DNA Polymerase. *Proceedings National Academy of Sciences* 1972;69;11:3228-3232.	Ribonuclease-sensitive DNA synthesis was found in normal human blood lymphocytes stimulated with the foreign plant derived antigenic substance called phytohemagglutinin (PHA),but not in the unstimulated lymphocytes. DNA polymerase purified from this fraction does not transcribe specific regions of "naturally occurring, exogenously supplied single-stranded RNA," that is the "70S RNA from RNA tumor viruses." This distinguishes this enzyme from the RNA-directed DNA polymerase (reverse transcriptase) found in cancer causing RNA viruses and human leukemic cells.	In this study, Gallo and co-workers experimented with the single stranded RNA from chicken viruses which were known to cause leukemia in the birds. They essentially injected the single strands of RNA into the human white blood cells to see if the normal DNA enzymes present in the lymphocytes would be able to work with the viral RNA to produce a radioactively labeled protein.This study shows that by the early 1970s Gallo was injecting foreign single stranded RNA from animal viruses to determine their effects on human white blood cell structure and functioning. The AIDS virus, as you may now know, is a single stranded RNA retrovirus which as shown in this study, provides an enzyme mechanism foreign to the cell's natural protein synthesis mechanism in order to produce protein, that is, reproduce itself.
√ Gallo RC, Abrell JW, Robert MS, Yang SS and Smith RG.Reverse Transcriptase From Mason-Pfizer Monkey Tumor Virus, Avian Myeloblastosis Virus, and Rauscher Leukemia Virus and Its Response to Rifamycin Derivatives. *Journal of the National Cancer Institute* 1972;48;4:1185-1189.	The partially purified polymerases from RNA tumor viruses exhibited similar characteristics which enabled the virus' "reverse transcriptases" to be distinguished from the purified cellular enzymes. "Since the existence of RNA-dependent DNA polymerase (RDDP) was first reported, RDDP has been found in all RNA tumor viruses. Included in this class are the following 3 viruses: Mason-Pfizer monkey tumor virus (M-PMTV), avian myeloblastosis virus (AMV), and Rauscher Murine (rat/mouse) leukemia virus (RLV). M-PMTV is of interest, since it is a primate RNA virus adapted to a human cell line, NC-37. This cell line was initially derived from the peripheral blood of normal human lymphocytes. This system has been used in our laboratory as a model for the detection of the RDDP in human neoplastic cells. The data also demonstrated the ability of the viral and not naturally occurring enzymes to utilize single-stranded RNA for protein synthesis which may be increased dramatically by the incorporation of thymidylic acid and adenylic acid.	Here, Gallo and coworkers publish experiments using monkey leukemia viruses as well as chicken and mouse viruses to test for their effects on normal human DNA-directed protein synthesis in white blood cells. Many authorities believe the AIDS virus bears great similarities to the simian monkey virus with which Gallo's lab was also working (See Fujioka and Gallo, 1971; and,Gallo, Miller, Saxinger and Gillespie, 1973). In addition, the researchers acquired additional evidence that as previously noted some amino acids, in this case, thymidylic and adenylic, can greatly increase the rate of RNA reverse transcriptase directed DNA synthesis when added to the "synthetic DNA-RNA hybrid." This aspect of the study reflects the minute detail which went into influencing the expression of foreign (in this case monkey virus) RNA on human white blood cells.
† Wu AM, Ting FC, Paran M and Gallo RC. Cordycepin Inhibits Induction of Murine Leukovirus Production By 5-iodo-2'-deoxyuridine. *Proceedings of the National Academy of Sciences* 1972; 69;12:3820-3824.	"RNA tumor viruses replicate via a transcription of proviral DNA… The discovery of RNA-dependent DNA polymerase…supports the idea that the genetic information of RNA tumor viruses can exist in an infected cell (or transformed cell) in a form of DNA termed a "provirus." In this study, "the production of RNAviruses induced by 5-iodo-2'-deoxyuridine, IdU," (a constituent of RNA) in [mouse/rat] cell lines" was blocked by a chemical (Cordycepin 3'-deoxyadenosine), a known inhibitor of poly (A) (this term refers to a chemical polymer of adenylic acid which is a condensation product of adenosine and phosphoric acid; a nucleotide found within all nucleic acids). N^6(△²-Isopentenyl) Adenosine, a plant hormone (among a class of hormones called cytokinins known to be a "causative agent in certain plant pathogens or cancers and component of the tRNAs of numerous forms of plant and animal life") was found within the tRNA of	In the above study, Gallo et al found that adenylic acid a basic (nucleotide)component of RNA and DNA can "greatly increase the rate of RNA directed protein synthesis from DNA through the reverse transcription mechanism. In this study they concluded that chemicals which can block the adenylic acid portion of viral RNA can inhibit this protein synthesis/viral reproduction mechanism, though not without side effects. In regard to HIV synthesis, in this study new forms of RNA retroviruses were being synthesized by the addition of 5-iodo-2'-deoxyuridine , that is IdU, a foreign RNA component introduced into normal rodent white blood cells. Clearly, the researchers were manufacturing a new strain of virus here and checking to see if chemotherapy could stop it from reproducing itself through the reverse protein synthesis mechanism typical of RNA retroviruses.
† Gallo RC, Hecht SM, Whang-Peng J and O'Hopp S. N^6-(△²-Isopentenyl) Adenosine: The Regulatory Effects of a Cytokinin and Modified Nucleoside From tRNA on Human Lymphocytes. *Biochimica Et Biophysica Acta* 1972; 281:488-500.	lymphosarcoma cells from cancer patients at levels "four times as great as that in normal lymphocytes" from healthy humans. This synthesis cannot be the primary site of action" of this drug which causes "remarkably similar effects " as phytohemagglutinin on "stimulated lymphocytes at comparable concentrations).	Gallo's group is clearly considering the possibility of using N^6-(△²-Isopentenyl) Adenosine or related plant hormones to both inhibit and stimulate cancer cell division, they appear at this point to have narrowed their attention on to the tRNA segments composed of adenosine or adenylic acids.

Acknowledged Funding Source/Biological Weapons Contractor: † Litton Bionetics; √ Bionetics Research Labs; § Univ. of Calif.; ∞ Univ. of Texas; ◊ Univ. of Chicago; △ Yale U.

	Year and Subject of Investigation	Study Conclusions	Possible Relationship to HIV Synthesis
	1972 continued		
√	Ting RC, Yang SS and Gallo RC. Reverse Transcriptase, RNA Tumour Virus Transformation and Derivatives of Rifamycin SV. *Nature New Biology* 1972;236:163-165.	Derivatives of the antibiotic rifamycin derived from bacteria were used to inhibit the effects of rat and mouse leukaemia-sarcoma viruses preventing the formation of cancer cells. "This suggests that reverse transcriptase is necessary for transformation by RNA tumour viruses."	Reverse transcriptase, the unique enzyme found in HIV is here shown to be required for leukaemia and sarcoma viruses to produce their cancer causing effects. HIV attacks white blood cells, that is leukocytes, and causes a rare skin cancer known as Kaposi's sarcoma.
√	Smith RG, Whang-Peng J, Gallo RC, Levine P and Ting RC. Selective Toxicity of Rifamycin Derivatives for Leukaemic Human Leucocytes. *Nature New Biology* 1972;236:166-171.	Certain rifamycin derivatives have been found to be more toxic for fresh human leukaemic blood cells than for normal blood cells. These particular antibiotics also inhibit the reverse transcriptases of both human and viral origin.	This work advanced the use of certain antibiotics in an effort to fight human leukemia. Though it bears no relationship to the development of HIV or other AIDS-like viruses, it might be interpreted as having contributed to the development of chemotherapies for cancer as well as possibly AIDS patients. The authors did indicate that normal cells would also be harmed along with cancer cells.
	Gallo RC. RNA-Dependent DNA Polymerase in Viruses and Cells: Views on the Current State. *Blood* 1972;39:1:117-137.	The presence of an RNA-dependent DNA polymerase or reverse transcriptase has been found in every RNA oncogenic virus...It is assumed that the role of the enzyme is to convert viral 70S RNA to a DNA copy, allowing the viral genome to be inserted into the host cell.	Though this summary and update report on reverse transcriptase and its link to cancer bears no relationship to the development of HIV or other AIDS-like viruses, Gallo did discuss beginning to develop antibodies which could help detect this enzyme which is currently used to identify HIV infections.
	1973 Gallo RC. Reverse Transcriptase and Neoplasia. *Biomedicine* 1973;18:446-452.	"Reverse transcriptase, the DNA polymerase of type-C RNA tumor viruses, can be distinguished from the DNA polymerases of normal cells by biochemical and immunological approaches. The enzyme is required for formation of the provirus, the RNA tumor viruses, and hence, for infection of cells by these viruses...A reverse transcriptase related to the reverse transcriptase of type-C RNA tumor viruses (leukaemia-lymphoma-sarcoma complex) has been unequivocally demonstrated in some human acute leukemic cells and its presence has been suggested...in other human cancers...Work on reverse transcriptase has contributed to major progress in tumor virology and to molecular biology in general in a very short period."	This review article summarizes Gallo's research on the unique reverse transcriptase enzyme associated with HIV and other RNA tumor viruses. Here the theory of how HIV and other such viruses replicate is explained—ten years before Luc Montagnier at the Pasteur Research Institute isolated HIV from the white blood cells of AIDS patients. The biochemical and immunological detection techniques which would later be used to detect HIV infection were also discussed here. It is remarkable that the type-C RNA tumor viruses Gallo studied and discussed here produced a similar complex of diseases associated with AIDS including a "leukemia-lymphoma-sarcoma complex."
†	Wu AM, Ting RCY and Gallo RC. RNA-Directed DNA Polymerase and Virus-Induced Leukemia in Mice. *Proceedings of the National Academy of Sciences* 1973;70:5:1298-1302.	"The results of this study suggest that RNA-directed DNA polymerase is essential for induction of leukemia by exogenous virus and correlate with the previous observation that the same [Rifamycin antibiotic] derivatives block viral transformation [in cell cultures].	Besides Litton Bionetics, a documented U.S. D.O.D. biological weapons contractor, being cited as the major funding source for these experiments, The Special Virus Cancer Program from Hazleton Laboratory in Vienna, Va. was mentioned as the supplier of Rausher leukemia viruses used in this study. This is noteworthy as Hazleton's Reston Va, monkey facility was the site of the frightening Ebola-like virus outbreak in December, 1989. Nowhere in Richard Preson's best seller *The Hot Zone* was Hazleton mentioned as an actual supplier of RNA tumor viruses. In fact, Preston alleged the deadly viruses came from either the Phillipines or Africa.
§	Paran M, Gallo RC, Richardson LS and Wu AM. Adrenal Corticosteroids Enhance Production of Type-C Virus Induced by 5-Iodo-2'-Deoxyuridine from Cultured Mouse Fibroblasts. *Proceedings of the National Academy of Sciences* 1973;70;8:2391-2395.	RNA tumor viruses can be stimulated to reproduce in mouse cells by the addition of adrenal corticosteroids and many other hormones. Cordycepin (a crystalline antibiotic obtained from the bacteria *Cordyceps militaris*) was shown to be an inhibitor of RNA synthesis in RNA tumor viruses.	No apparent relation to the development of AIDS-like viruses or of identification or treatment methods for AIDS. Paper does provide interesting acknowledgment: The cordycepin antibiotic used in the experiment had been obtained from the "Drug Development Branch of the National Cancer Institute." The NCI, the authors wrote received the drug from "Merck and Co., Incorp." Document provides evidence of link between Gallo, the NCI, and the documented biological weapons contractor Merck and Co. Also, apparent is connection of Merck and Co. to a special branch of the NCI responsible for the development of new pharmaceuticals, developed apparently with federal and taxpayer assistance.

Acknowledged Funding Source/Biological Weapons Contractor: † Litton Bionetics; √ Bionetics Research Labs; § Univ. of Calif.; ◇ Univ. of Chicago; ∆ Yale U.; ∞ Merck and Co.;

Year and Subject of Investigation	Study Conclusions	Possible Relationship to HIV Synthesis
1973 continued Gillespie D, Gillespie S, Gallo RC, East JL and Dmochowski L. Genetic Origin of RD114 and Other RNA Tumour Viruses assayed by Molecular Hybridization. *Nature New Biology* 1973;224:52-54.	The group tested "RNA from RD 114 virus, potentially an RNA tumour virus of human origin," to see if reverse transcription occurred to give rise to additional RD 114 virus. This study concluded that "the reverse transcriptase of RD114 is not closely related to any tested viral reverse transcriptase. It is believed that the gs1 antigen of tumour viruses is species specific...Unless it is shown that one species can produce only one type of gs1 antigen, however, it can always be argued that RD114 is a new cat virus with a gs1 antigen that differs from the antigen found on the viruses of known feline origin. Also, it was noted that "only viruses which had been grown in the original tumour cell and had never been purified as a cell free extract before the final collection hybridized [that is joined] strongly and specifically to cell DNA.	Many researchers believe that the RD114 virus evolved from a cat virus to later infect humans. This report stated that: "Some experiments have been reported which have led to the belief that RD114 is not a cat origin or is likely to be of human origin." Just as Gallo's research team argued in this paper, "it can always be argued that the" HIV evolved as a simian virus with antigens [foreign proteins which prompt an immune response] that differ "from the antigen found on the viruses of known" monkey origin. Also, the group concluded that "RNA tumour virus maintained in tissue culture [as opposed to a cell line in culture] often do not produce the pathology of the original virus and give cause for questioning the indiscriminate use of the viruses transferred from one type of cell to another." Apparently, the group was not concerned about creating new viruses; rather that the new viruses they created would not mutate to other less deadly forms before they could capture and study them thoroughly.
Gallo RC, Miller NR, Saxinger WC and Gillespie D. Primate RNA Tumor Virus-Like DNA Synthesized Endogenously by RNA-Dependent DNA Polymerase in Virus-like Particles from Fresh Human Acute Leukemic Blood Cells. *Proceedings National Academy of Sciences* 1973;70;11:3219-3224.	"DNA polymerase activity in human acute leukemia is recovered from a cytoplasmic subcellular fraction having a density [1.16-1.17g/ml] characteristic of RNA tumor virus particles of animals...the purified enzyme uses synthetic template-primers with a specificity like RNA-dependent DNA polymerase [reverse transcriptase] of viruses and different from the major DNA polymerases of normal proliferating leukocytes; and ...the DNA synthesized [within the cells] by RNA-dependent DNA polymerase contained among its sequences a high proportion (50%) capable of hybridizing to RNA isolated from a primate type-C sarcoma virus and/or a murine sarcoma virus [that is, a Kirsten (rat) sarcoma-leukemia virus complex]...The DNA-synthesizing activity was recovered in a particle not disaggregated [that is, not broken apart or destroyed] by physical manipulation unlike the vast majority of cytoplasmic particulate material, which had a density of 1.16-1.17g/ml...The present results stress the importance of purification of the cytoplasmic particle to obtain a suitable DNA probe, [that is, a particle which can initiate the invasion of normal DNA by foreign viral RNA].	Here in the *Proceedings of the National Academy of Sciences*, Gallo and co-workers proclaim they have isolated a virus-like particle from human acute (that is, quick acting) leukemic (white) blood cells. This particle they state has a specific density of 1.16-1.17 g/ml, can be repeatedly recovered without being destroyed by physical handling, and has the capability of producing the principal rapidly progressing cancers associated with AIDS including leukemias, sarcomas, and carcinomas. In essence, Gallo and company announced isolating AIDS-like virus particles more than a decade before Luc Montagnier announced the discovery of LAV [HIV]. It is also interesting to note that to accomplish this result, Gallo and co-workers reported here using several types of RNA tumor viruses including:"SiSV (NRK)—simian [monkey] sarcoma virus grown in normal rat kidney (NRK) cells; MuSV (Kirsten [type])—a [rat/mouse] sarcoma-leukemia virus complex grown in NRK cells which originated by repeated infection of rats with a Gross-type murine leukemia virus;...AvLV (ANV), avian [bird] leukosis [leukemia] virus, strain avian myeloblastosis [bone marrow cancer];...FeSV (Gardner), feline [cat] sarcoma-leukemia virus,... and several other RNA animal viruses.
1974 Wu AM and Gallo RC. Interaction between Murine Type-C Virus RNA-Directed DNA Polymerases and Rifamycin Derivatives. *Biochimica et Biophysica Acta* 1974;340;419-436	Similar to those reported previously	None more apparent than above
1985 Fisher AG, Collatti E, Ratner L, Gallo RC, Wong-Staal F. A molecular clone of HTLV-III with biological activity. *Nature* 1985;316:262-265.	"A clone containing the full-length HTLV-III proviral DNA was inserted into a plasmid [a extrachromosomal hereditary determining replicating unit other than a gene from the cell nucleus] and used to transfect cord blood T cells from normal newborn humans...this molecular clone is infectious...and causes marked cytopathic [cell death] on T-cell cultures..."	This paper along with Gallo's earlier publication (see Gallagher, Ting and Gallo, 1972) shows that the methods and materials needed to clone Luc Montagnier's LAV, but also the capacity to develop a foreign germ capable of infecting normal newborn human cells with the genetic material needed to cause marked T-cell death; identical to the AIDS virus.
Ratner L, Haseltine W, Patarca R, Livak KJ, Starcich R, and Gallo RC et al. Complete nucleotide sequence of the AIDS virus, HTLV-III. *Nature* 1985;313:277-284.	The complete genetic building block sequence of two human T-cell leukemia type III (HTLV-III) proviral DNAs are identified and described.	As Strecker reported in 1986, this large group of researchers including Gallo found the HTLV family of retroviruses similar but not identical to the bovine leukaemia virus (BLV).

Acknowledged Funding Source/Biological Weapons Contractor: † Litton Bionetics; √ Bionetics Research Labs; § Univ. of Calif.; ∞ Merck and Co.; ◊ Univ. of Chicago; Δ Yale U.

Chapter 7
An Interview with
Dr. Robert Strecker

THE next morning, I tried contacting Strecker again. First I dialed what I thought was his published telephone number. Again, it rang continuously unanswered. Then I called the number directory assistance had given me for Dr. William Campbell Douglass, a physician from Clayton, Georgia, who had published an article entitled "WHO Murdered Africa," which supported Strecker's theory. As in past attempts, a machine instructed me to leave a message.

"Is there anyone there!? This is about the sixth time I've called. I've been trying to reach you for months. I'm trying to reach Dr. William Douglass. I need to get in touch with Dr. Robert Strecker. My name is Dr. Len Horowitz, and this is an emergency. If anyone can answer, would you please return my call?" I then left my 800 number and hung up.

Two days later I received a call from a Mr. William Douglass. I was delighted. He immediately informed me, however, that he was not the person I sought.

"I've been getting a couple of calls a month for Dr. Strecker, so I finally decided to get his number. If you like, I can give it to you."

"Please. I would really appreciate it."

Finally! I thought as I quickly dialed the magic numbers, feeling the end of my frustration might be near.

"Hello, this is Dr. Strecker's office," a woman's kindly voice answered.

Following a lengthy introduction, the woman informed me that Dr. Strecker was indeed alive, well, and practicing internal medicine in Needles, California. He was busy seeing patients, I was told, but I was assured he would return my call that evening.

"All right!" I affirmed as I hung up the phone. Then I quickly relayed the good news to Jackie.

The information on Strecker's whereabouts immediately helped to ease her concerns.

On the Line

That night, Robert Strecker returned my call with news about his ongoing crusade to bring the "truth to light." We spoke at length about our independent investigations, immediately developing the warm rapport that two black sheep isolated from the establishment's scientific flock might.

Pondering safety, I asked, "Has anyone from the government ever bothered you over all these years?"

"Not really," he replied. "Since the suspicious deaths of my brother and Representative Huff,[1] I've just gone about my business. There was one incident though that occurred shortly after I sent reports of my findings to all the health and intelligence agencies."

"What happened?"

"Well, first, the CIA warned all agencies that I was a communist and told them not to take anything I said seriously. My brother Ted obtained a copy of the release they sent out through the Freedom of Information Act. Their counterintelligence efforts apparently worked."

"Do you still have a copy of the release?"

"I wish I did," Strecker replied. "It disappeared along with a lot of other records Ted and I had collected. Shortly after Ted's death, my office was burglarized."

"Interesting," I said. "Who do you think did it?"

"I believe it was the CIA, but I obviously can't prove it."

Following an illuminating conversation, Robert—as he preferred to be called—and I agreed to mail each other copies of our previous publications. He would send me a copy of *The Strecker Memorandum,* which I still had not viewed, and I would send him *Deadly Innocence,* which he had not heard about.

Then we also agreed to exchange interviews. I set up a time to be a guest on "He Said/She Said," a radio program Strecker co-hosted with Betsy Prior on KGER-AM, Los Angeles, and he agreed to be interviewed for this book.

The Strecker Interview

Several weeks went by before we could coordinate our schedules for my telephone interview with Strecker. By this time, I had watched *The Strecker Memorandum*, and considered, as Acer had, Strecker's position that AIDS had been "predicted, requested, created, and deployed."

Strecker, I now knew, was a stocky, earnest-looking man in his late 40s or early 50s. His dark blond hair glistened as he spoke. His wire-rimmed glasses and slightly graying temples portrayed a more mature, intelligent, demeanor than what his boyish face disguised. He spoke quickly and easily, accompanied by an unmistakable Midwestern drawl. He appeared to me to be a once all American, football hero type, whose athleticism and idealism was quickly dashed by the nature of medical education and academic politics.

I began the interview by reading from a list of questions I had prepared for Robert to answer:

LEN: Robert, first off, what convinced you that the AIDS virus was synthetically manufactured?

ROBERT: What convinced us [The Strecker Group] was the fact that this new agent had suddenly appeared out of nowhere. That the virus had characteristics of animal viruses more so than human viruses, and that the genetic structure of the AIDS virus actually looked like the viruses that appeared in animals that would not normally adapt themselves in humans. . . .

That could have occurred spontaneously, but not by the process that scientists have normally talked about. For instance, not by the virus running in primates [the highest order of mammals, including man, monkeys, and lemurs] because if you look at the genetic structure of the AIDS virus, what you find is that the codon choices [the specific sequence of three (purine and pyrimidine) bases in the viral RNA that codes for the production of a specific amino acid by the infected cell] included in the AIDS virus are not existent in primate genes.

Therefore, to assume that they simply mutated in order to adapt themselves into primates in the case of AIDS is vanishingly small although still possible.

What happened is that the virus either mutated in cattle and sheep, and then was artificially adapted to humans by growing in human tissue cultures, which they [virologists] do and in which they are easily manipulated in that manner—or the virus was actually constructed in a laboratory by gene manipulation, which was available to scientists in the early '70s although many of the techniques were not talked about until the mid '70s, because the biowarfare laboratories throughout the world have always been about five to ten years ahead of other laboratories working on all kinds of projects.

In addition, a clearer reason is, if you look at the appearance of the 'human retroviruses,' the fact is that there were a host of these things that appeared all at the same time. So, you have to explain not only the appearance of HIV-I, but also HIV-II, HTLV-I, HTLV-II, HTLV-IV, HTLV-V, HTLV-VI, ad nauseam.

And so, to say that these things all spontaneously mutated at the same time in nature, and in the same direction, to infect human beings spontaneously and spread disease in worldwide epidemic proportions, in my opinion, is absurd compared to the known fact that scientists were working with exact progenitors of these viruses in their laboratories, which we can document.

The Green Monkey Theory

LEN: But what about the green monkey theory—the theory that a green monkey bit an African or someone had sex with an ape?

ROBERT: That's just nonsense. . . . Green monkeys are about the size of chickens. So the idea of a human having sex with a female monkey the size of a chicken is, of course, absurd.

In addition, the theory that a transmission occurred through biting, of course, is always said to be close to impossible. If you look at the CDC and everybody else, they say that biting is not an easy way to spread these diseases except in the case of the purported green monkey which is suddenly the way it was spread.[2]

We don't believe that the viruses came from primates or from green monkeys. In addition, if you look at the whole theory that was published in *Rolling Stone* . . . which accused Wistar Institute of spreading AIDS to Africa in the polio vaccines of the early 1960s; Wistar, of course, says that they have now reviewed all their stocks [without finding any incriminating evidence for the allegation]. . . . Wistar Institute is one of the world's biological leaders in 'retrovirus, virus, and cancer causation, cancer research,' [and is] located in Philadelphia.[3]

And these viruses were originally known by their Philadelphia names. They were called 'NBC' for New Bolton Center, which is also in Philadelphia. And if you look up the original AIDS virus, in our opinion, that goes back to cattle viruses that were called NBC, New Bolton Center I through about XIV or XVI.[4]

And we identified HTLV-I and HTLV-II and HTLV-III in those first cultures that were adapted to human beings by growing them in human tissue culture. . . .

For many years actually, you could simply call up New Bolton and say, "Give me some NBC-XIII." And they would send it to you. And then when AIDS appeared around 1978 or so, all of a sudden the NBC line all disappeared. You could no longer order them.

LEN: How interesting.

The Cow Theory

ROBERT: Yeah. It is interesting. And so we tracked NBC, I think it's [NBC-] XIII . . . back to Louisiana State Agriculture Farm (LSAF) cow BFC-44. And what happens was you see, they were looking a lot at HTLV-I, which is like bovine leukemia virus (BLV),[5] and this cow at the LSAF got they thought a BLV infection. She got huge lymph nodes in the neck just like HTLV-I/BLV in cattle. And then she apparently conquered it because the lymph nodes went down; she got better after a mononucleosis-like disease, and she made lots and lots and lots of antibodies against this virus.

Then about five or six years later, she started losing weight rapidly, developed diarrhea, and died with pneumonia. And they autopsied her and of course she had no immune system left.

And as far as we can tell, that was the original bovine visna virus isolate.

LEN: What year was that?

ROBERT: 1969. And that virus was capable of wiping out T-cells selectively, it produced syncytium [a mass of cell fluids containing many cell nuclei formed by the joining of originally separate cells as a result of infection or disease][6] in tissue culture, and it does everything that AIDS does.

LEN: Now, who was studying that?

ROBERT: That was isolated from the LSAF outside of New Orleans.

LEN: So Gallo wasn't the only one studying that virus?

ROBERT: No, everybody was. These [cultures] were [widely distributed]. If you go back and look at the veterinary literature, they were looking at all the BLV, bovine leukemia virus lines, bovine syncytium viruses, and bovine visna viruses. And all these things were being studied. . . .

Well, at this point, they were still essentially noninvasive because they were restricted to animals. But, then what happened was in the late '60s and early '70s they started growing these in human tissue.

Early Researchers

LEN: Now when you say 'they,' can you be more specific in terms of the labs that you're familiar with that were doing this work?

ROBERT: Yeah, well virtually every lab in the world that was doing sophisticated lymphocyte studies. But particularly Gallo and company at the NIH, ahh . . . ahh . . . actually there were only a few guys you know—Gallo, Montagnier, a couple of guys that are dead, Baltimore,[7] Teman,[8] and a few others and a few veterinarians. . . .

Dmochowski was interesting because he was the first one to show that you could basically adapt retroviruses to different mammalian species by growing them in the tissue cultures that you wanted them to go to. Now he's down in Texas.[9]

Miller, in 1969, took bovine leukemia virus and injected it into chimpanzees, and the chimpanzees formed antibodies against the virus.[10] So they concluded that these chimpanzees were immune. And so that was the decision for telling everybody that bovine viruses in human beings posed no threat; which is relatively true, there is a species barrier.

Since the 1950s and even the 1940s Burny,[11] Bobrow,[12] and all these guys from Europe said these [bovine] viruses posed a threat to humans, so they began a whole program of mass extermination of cattle in Europe that carried BLV and other viruses.[13]

In this country, half of our herds are infected with BLV, BFC, or BVV, and the only thing that has prevented, in my opinion, everyone from dying of T-cell leukemia is the fact that pasteurization of the milk kills viruses.

Now if you look at the distribution of T-cell leukemia across the upper United States, from like Minnesota to Wisconsin, there's a huge incidence of T-cell leukemia in dairy farmers.

And if you actually look at some of the studies done in France, they found that guys working in meat-packing plants had a greater incidence of T-cell leukemia too.[13]

So there's all this evidence that T-cell leukemia is related to BLV, which it certainly is, [and] for sure, if you culture the virus in human tissue and adapt it, what you get [is an HTLV-I-like virus that thrives in humans]. . . .

If you look at BVV, bovine visna virus,[13] . . . it's very closely related [to HIV], but it's still not there; it's not the same as AIDS because what you have is bovine visna virus—a virus growing in cattle—and that's not adapted to humans yet. To adapt it to humans, you've got to grow it in human tissue, as they were doing in those early '70s. And what they discovered was that it was a selective T-cell destroyer [just as the AIDS virus is].

French/American "Bull"

ROBERT: Do you know what the true conflict [was] that occurred between Gallo and Montagnier?

LEN: The one that I'm aware of was that Montagnier allegedly gave him what he thought was the virus, and Gallo supposedly cloned it.

ROBERT: That was all bull. . . . Because they both had the viruses growing in their labs in the early 1970s.

The real problem was, and what happens is—suppose you take a culture of lymphocytes, you take T-cell lymphocytes and you dump in HTLV-I or II. What happens to the T-lymphocyte culture?

LEN: It gets infected, and it proliferates.

ROBERT: That's exactly what happens. The tissue grows and grows and grows in human beings. That's what results in leukemia. You have to take the cells out; they get so packed that the tissue culture dies.

Now what happens when you dump bovine visna or AIDS virus into the same tissue cultures?

LEN: The cells don't grow.

ROBERT: Exactly! They're lysed. They die. So when you come back in a day or two and look, there's nothing left except debris. And so Gallo couldn't figure out how to make enough virus for the antibody tests. They needed virus in quantities to get everything going. And they couldn't get them to reproduce long enough to get large quantities of virus.

I felt the urge to interrupt Strecker at this point since I had questioned this same allegation before when Randy Shilts advanced it in *The Band*. Instead, I remained silent, heeding my father's recommendation that I could, "learn more from listening than speaking."

ROBERT: So that's the real argument. And what Montagnier figured out was if you dump in Epstein-Barr virus on to the T-lymphocytes, you immortalize them. . . . They will just sit there and make virus for you, which is why if you have an Epstein-Barr virus infection on top of an AIDS virus infection you're in sorry, sorry shape. . . . The immortalized Epstein-Barr-virus-infected T-cells will just churn out AIDS viruses day after day after day. . . . And so that was the real thing that Montagnier discovered. . . .[14]

LEN: And that's not published anywhere?

ROBERT: Oh sure it's published. But it's the true argument versus the suspicious argument that, "You stole my virus." That's all a lot of bull because they both had the virus, and they both knew what they were doing from day one in my opinion.

If that was true, I considered, then Gallo would have also known about the Epstein-Barr virus effects, which I recalled he also published.[14] So I questioned Strecker:

LEN: Now when I look back at the research literature, at least in the *Index Medicus*, Montagnier did not have too many publications in this field [in the early 1970s], whereas Gallo had been churning out the publications.

ROBERT: Except that Montagnier had worked with Gallo![15]

LEN: They did?

ROBERT: Yeah, they were in the same [building] or on the same hallway.

LEN: At the NCI?

ROBERT: Yes! . . . Montagnier was over here . . . around 1965 or so; he and Gallo were working together. . . . They're all connected.

LEN: Interesting.

I had not considered the possibility that Gallo and Montagnier had known about each other's work prior to 1978 as Shilts documented.

ROBERT: And then when . . . Donald Francis and what's his name? When they published that cat house experiment, and questioned, "Is it possible that there's a human retrovirus similar to this one." Of course [there was]! Gallo had already isolated HTLV-III. . . . And his office was only twenty-five feet away.

I sat up on the edge of my seat taken by the allegation. *The Band* presented Francis as somewhat of a hero during his alleged conflict with Gallo and other NCI administrators over withholding support for AIDS research. I suspected he knew about Gallo's early research, and Strecker was now alleging the same.

LEN: You mean Don Francis from the CDC? Francis was originally at the NCI before he went to the CDC?

ROBERT: Yes. . . . He was working there right next to Gallo. And that's when they did their famous cat house experiments showing that the cats were transferring the viruses back and forth amongst themselves. And then they wrote this article that said, "Is it possible. . . ."[16]

I mean, they knew or else they didn't talk for the whole time. They knew that there was a similar virus out there growing in human beings. . . . Gallo had already isolated it, and their labs were twenty-five feet apart.

LEN: Now what I seem to have dug up in the *WHO Chronicle,* is that the first American laboratory to be sent any of the viral strains from which they began was the NCI.[17]

ROBERT: Yeah. Well, I think that's a lie. I mean, I think the viruses were growing in the basement of the NCI all along. . . . Do you know about the meeting between Gallo, Montagnier, and Salk?

LEN: No.

ROBERT: Oh my God! Anyway, a year or two ago, and this is documented in *Science* or somewhere, Gallo, Montagnier, and Salk met in San Diego to write up the history—the official history—of their discoveries.[18]

LEN: Salk? The polio virus Salk?

ROBERT: Yeah, they met down there and made up a story. . . . And I personally believe that virtually everything they wrote was bull. . . . We [referring again to his brother and other colleagues in The Strecker Group] understood that they used to meet like two or three times a week and decide what to tell next—how to package it, how to discuss it. In other words, they already knew everything because they'd been working on it since the early 1970s. They basically knew they had the same stuff [retroviruses and reagents] because if you look at what happened, their discoveries were too quick. . . .

LEN: OK. Explain this now. Why did Gallo in 1980 become so frustrated that he couldn't keep the [T-lymph] cells alive, so allegedly he quit.

ROBERT: What?

LEN: According to Shilts, Gallo dropped out of the AIDS race for about two years.

ROBERT: I don't believe that either. I don't know what he was doing in that time frame, but he was still working on AIDS; there's no doubt about that.

LEN: According to Shilts, Gallo had only about 10 percent of his lab going on the AIDS problem. He said that Gallo stonewalled researchers throughout the world [by] not providing the antibodies, not providing the cell lines that were required to identify and cultivate the virus.

ROBERT: Yeah. . . . Why would they want to give things away when they knew what was going on already, and it was a matter of Gallo and Montagnier deciding who was going to tell what when. . . . Do you know the story about the patent?[19]

LEN: Gallo ripped Montagnier off.

ROBERT: Yeah. That's what brought the split. You see we [the United States] tried to take all the money.

LEN: Well, that's what they've done.

ROBERT: Yes. Yes. Yes. So that's what got the French so angry. And what was Montagnier going to do? Come out and say, "Well, we lied. We've been doing this work all along. We're all crooks."

So that's, in my opinion, what happened. Anybody with any scientific credibility knew that Gallo stole the virus if that's what they were talking about because they [HTLV-III and LAV] were identical. . . . But I think that the big war was really a war over money.

LEN: Oh, for sure.

ROBERT: Yeah. Anybody with any sense knew; I mean retrovirologists laugh about it because they knew that Gallo stole it. It was only the press that was blind.

LEN: But how do you reconcile the first comment that they all had these things and then later that he [Gallo] cloned it [Montagnier's LAV]?

ROBERT: They had them, and you can grow the virus in perpetuity if you keep constantly changing their cell line as it kills it. That doesn't mean you can grow it in any quantity. In other words, every lab in the world—and these were all over the world, they weren't just here and in France; they were in Germany and Russia and everywhere—[and] a lot of people had the [human] cell lines, and they had the cattle cell lines [in the early 1970s]. . . . And we know they had, in 1976, BVV, bovine visna virus, growing in brain tissue in Brussels because we have papers on that. One paper said that the AIDS[-like] virus would infect [human] brain tissue. And the guy even wrote, "Is it possible that this is a cause of slow virus disease of man?"[20] So, I mean, they were everywhere.

The "Conspiracy of Cells"

ROBERT: Plus, they were growing in cattle naturally, and we were using fetal calf serum as growth medium for every cell culture in the world. . . . The theory was that since these were extracted from fetuses, they were sterile, but in fact, they weren't.

Because the AIDS virus and BLV-I and II were being transferred in the gene lines. And so they were potentially transferring these viruses into every tissue culture throughout the world. . . .

So it gets very mixed up. You've got to read a book called *Conspiracy of Cells*, by Michael Gold.[21] This is a story about Walter Nelson Reese who worked in the highest containment laboratory in the NIH—the BSL 4 lab. That's where they keep their tissue cultures, and they had like 300 to 400 of them. And in 1981, Walter Nelson Reese published a paper [in *Science*] saying that over a third of them were Henrietta-Lack-cell-contaminated cell lines.

Henrietta Lack was a black lady who worked at Hopkins in the late 1950s. She died around 1965 or so while she was still working there . . . [from] a tumor of the uterus that literally ate her alive. And that tissue was the first human tissue that was grown in perpetuity in tissue cultures. Because up till then, they would only grow one or two divisions and then die, and her tissue called HELA—that's where HELA comes from, Henrietta Lack—was the first [cancer cells] that would grow in tissue cultures.

Now those cell lines were sent all over the world, and what happened was that scientists were contaminating their tissue culture cells with HELA accidentally. And in the early 1970s, I think '72 under Nixon, the Russians sent us six cell lines that they thought contained human cancer-causing viruses. And those were sent to Walter Nelson Reese who was the keeper of the cell lines in the United States. He was in San Francisco, and it was his job to keep the cell lines straight and not contaminate them.

That was [during] the great "war on cancer," that's where all this stuff came from. The NIH was funded in '72 with billions of dollars to find the cancer virus. . . .

Nixon was trying to steal the show from [Teddy] Kennedy by coming up with a virus and vaccine against cancer. They said, "Let's find a virus." So that's where the big cancer virus hypothesis came from.

Now when we got these six cell lines from the Russians . . . Reese started looking at them and discovered that they were all female; then he discovered that they were all black. And so he questioned, 'How many black females are there in Moscow who have cancer?' And, of course, what he discovered was that these were all Henrietta Lack cell contaminants that contained monkey viruses. And so all that stuff the Russians sent us was in fact a fraud. But . . . it was a very embarrassing thing because they thought they had got there first, and what we proved was that they were awful scientists.

So then what Walter Nelson Reese did is that he started looking at all the cell lines of the United States, and closely. And [then he] discovered that at the NIH, over a third of them were HELA contaminated.

What happened was that when they would open their tissue culture lids, they would aerosolize small particles into the air. They would float around and drop into another cell line, and HELA's so aggressive that it will literally take over. And so it just takes one cell to drop into another cell line and it takes over, and it amalgamates, and those were called HELA contaminated.

And so what the NIH did to him [Dr. Reese] was, of course, de-funded him and put him out of business. Because he proved they were all a bunch of idiots.

LEN: Oh—I see.

ROBERT: So then the problem was you had a whole bunch of HELA-contaminated cell lines floating around and being sent out as clean cell lines and they weren't; they were actually human cancer malignant cell lines, and some of them contained viruses that were from other species.

And so it represented a big problem. Plus, they were throwing in fetal calf serum which was contaminated with these bovine viruses.

So you had a mixture for a natural [disaster]. I mean, the thing is, like they said in the '72 conferences, it's a wonder that we don't have worse disasters. You just wonder why we haven't been annihilated by these idiots.

If, for instance, you look at the tissue cell culture that was used to determine x-ray tolerance of human tissue, it turns out it's a HELA-contaminated cell line. Which means the most radiation-resistant cell line in the world is used as the standard to determine how much radiation a human should be exposed to!

LEN: Unreal.

ROBERT: Well, that's all documented in *Conspiracy of Cells* by Michael Gold. . . . Walter Nelson Reese now runs an art gallery. They put him out of business. . . .

The "Patient Zero" Theory

LEN: All right, let's get back . . . to the situation with AIDS. What about the "patient zero theory?"

ROBERT: That's nonsense. First off, this guy lived in Canada and flew primarily in Canadian cities, yet you must propose that he only had sex in American cities because the disease broke out in specific American cities where he allegedly had sex.

In addition, it doesn't make any sense if you look at the time frame. AIDS broke out in '78 in Manhattan and then in '80 in San Francisco. It didn't break out in Montreal in '79, or in Toronto, in Quebec, or Ontario in '80, whatever. It broke out in select cities in the United States in a select time frame which corresponds exactly to the hepatitis B study.[22]

LEN: OK. Let's talk about that study for a minute. If you could conceive of a way that vaccine could have been contaminated, how could it have happened?

ROBERT: Two ways. One way accidentally and one way intentionally.

LEN: All right then, elaborate. . . .

ROBERT: Well the vaccine was prepared from gays first off, and then it had plasma expanders that came from cattle added to it.

LEN: So the hepatitis B vaccine is produced through the bovine serum.

ROBERT: Yes. . . . It had expanders put into it as a mechanism of production.

LEN: Like serum?

ROBERT: Yeah, serum. . . . Because they needed to expand the volume.

LEN: Now is the vaccine produced in cow carcases?

ROBERT: No, it's made from humans.

LEN: The hepatitis B vaccine [is made] from the gay men's serum?

ROBERT: And also from straight men's serum.

LEN: OK.

ROBERT: And . . . that's the most interesting thing. Why did they make two separate vaccines?

LEN: Yeah. Why?

ROBERT: Because the epitopes[23] [surface molecules] of hepatitis B [antigens] in gays was different than in straights. . . . So what does that tell you?

LEN: I'm not quite sure.

ROBERT: Well it tells you there's not a lot of exchange going on between the two pools. Because if there were, the hepatitis B would not have separated into two epitopes. So if there was a lot of exchange, the information would have been heterogeneous in the pools, not homogeneous and not different [between homosexual and heterosexual men].

Now suppose you introduce a virus which is transferred like hepatitis B into the gay pool or population. When will it show up in the heterosexual pool?

LEN: I don't know. When?

ROBERT: Well it will take it a long time to show up there, because what you know is that the exchange of information going on between homosexuals and heterosexuals is limited.

So Szmuness was the guy who conducted that study.[22] Szmuness came from Poland, and was educated in Moscow. He somehow managed to escape [from Poland] to the United States with his family in tow, and ended up in New York City . . . as the head of the New York City Blood Bank.

That is interesting, I thought as I reflected on my recent tour of the National Holocaust Museum in Washington. The Nazis, I learned, had done extensive blood and genetics research in an effort to discriminate and exterminate mixed breeds from their racist and white supremacist world. A Russian-educated Polish researcher with Szmuness's credentials could have best survived Nazi-occupied Poland by joining the Nazi's research effort, or post–Nazi Poland by serving Russia. How did he end up in the United States? I wondered if there was a link between the Nazi effort to exterminate homosexuals and Szmuness's study that targeted gays with allegedly tainted hepatitis B vaccines? The German-owned Merck Company, after all, funded the study and produced the experimental and control vaccines.[22]

LEN: So [still somewhat perplexed, I asked,] that's the theory of unintentional infection?

ROBERT: Well, the fact is that the vaccine could have been prepared in a way that unintentionally infected them. Yes. [But] it might have been intentionally contaminated by somebody [also]. . . . They may have been testing gays trying to develop an immunity against something they knew was already ripping through Africa. . . . It could be that they were testing it just to test it, or it could be that somebody intentionally was trying to exterminate gays, or in our opinion, it could be that their actual goal was to exterminate the United States.

Strecker's latter remark took me by surprise. It was the first thing he said which to me made no sense.

LEN: The actual goal was to try to exterminate the United States? And that's one of your most plausible explanations?

ROBERT: Yes.

LEN: And who would have been behind that?

ROBERT: Some foreign party. The Russians or someone who didn't like us. Because the Russians have talked about that for fifty years. There have been KGB biological warfare experts that have been trying to do that to us for fifty years.

I felt intuitively uncomfortable with Strecker's explanation. I recalled his comments about Walter Nelson Reese which proved the Soviets knew far less about viral biotechnology than American researchers. Moreover, it seemed farfetched to believe the Russians had somehow managed to infiltrate the New York City Blood Center which appeared to be the starting point for the AIDS epidemic in America. This part of Strecker's theory would have required Szmuness, or one of his associates, to have been a secret agent working for Russia.

LEN: OK, but why would they have started with gays?

ROBERT: For a very obvious reason. And that is because nothing would be done. Just think about this. Suppose you put this virus in the heterosexuals or kids. What kind of response would have occurred compared to the response that did occur?

LEN: Right. That's for sure. Quite different. I appreciate that, but still, even to this day, the heterosexual spread is limited compared to the spread in the gay population.

ROBERT: Only in this country.

LEN: Right.

ROBERT: If you look in the world, what percentage of the world's AIDS cases are heterosexuals?

LEN: Ninety percent.

ROBERT: Over 90 percent. Right. Exactly . . . It's only in this country that you have this strange, unexplained predominance of homosexuals. Now, that's why you have to remember what I just told you. What happens when you put a virus that is transferred like hepatitis B into the homosexuals? When does it appear in heterosexuals?

LEN: Not for a long time.

ROBERT: Exactly . . . [That's why] I think it was pure genius.

Now people say, "Well nobody would think of that." And my answer to that is: "Well, I thought of it. So why couldn't they think of it?"

LEN: I still like my theory better.

Problems with the 'communist theory' flooded my head. Strecker noted the Russians were way behind us in viral research. How would the Russians have gained access to the viruses in Gallo's or Merck's labs in the first place. Even if Szmuness had been a Russian agent, he would have needed to gain access to the viruses first in order to contaminate the vaccines. Also, had the Russians created AIDS-like viruses shortly after Gallo surely did, then why had Gallo become the world's preeminent retrovirologist and not some Russian? Also the patents are worth millions. Why would the United States and not Russia hold the patents on the AIDS virus antibodies and cell lines?

ROBERT: Yeah. I mean I don't have the answer. I'm just telling you my theory.

African Vaccine Trials

LEN: OK. So that's the intentional theory.

ROBERT: Yeah. It could've been an experiment. It could've been intentional to get rid of gays. It could've been intentional to infect all of us.

LEN: OK.

ROBERT: And you see what happened. In our opinion, IARC, the International Agency for Research on Cancer, took these viruses to Africa in the early 1970s and tested them. Because we think they were trying to get the virus/cancer hypothesis proved; they wanted to develop a vaccine, and they wanted to find out which of those [viruses] were actually causing cancer because they weren't sure.[24]

So how do you prove it. How do you prove Koch's postulates[25] in the case of virus and cancer?

LEN: Difficult.

ROBERT: Yeah. You've got to test them.

LEN: Right.

ROBERT: It's like saying because you have lung cancer in women; it's because they wear hose. That doesn't prove anything. You've got to have causation. So they were stuck.

Now that's what was said in our references. They said, "let's test it; let's test it in humans with the same degree of sophisticated experiments that we use in animals." What does that mean?

And then they published their test sites. And the test sites are exactly where AIDS is. We had these huge laboratories over there.[24]

LEN: And what year was that?

ROBERT: 1972, I think. . . . It says that epidemiological studies are of no use per se. So what do you conclude?

LEN: That they're going to have to test it in a population.

ROBERT: Exactly. And then it says we're going to test these things in sibships—brothers and sisters from the same family. And they were going to study the time course of the infection. And then we said, well, what do you mean by that?

And they said, well, we're gonna study the antibody response. And I said, well you already knew the antibody response. How could there be any time course to that. The only thing that a time course could refer to is an infection. Which means you had to have active particles. That's all in the references.[26] Anyway in 1972 they said, let's make a T-cell destroyer. That's out of the bulletin of the WHO.

LEN: That I know.

ROBERT: The same year, they said let's test it, and then let's inject it. And then they published their test sites which is a map of Africa where they have all their test sites, and that corresponds exactly to the outbreak of AIDS.

LEN: Do you have those maps anywhere?

ROBERT: They're in the references [we published].[26] They're also in the Federal Register. . . .

So we think that they went over there and tested it. . . . Then somebody put it back into us or simply used it in us.

Again, I thought, it makes more sense to place the source of the experimental AIDS viruses in Bethesda and not Russia given that the WHO had made the NCI, and not a Russian institution, the initial distributor of viral testing reagents.[27-29] And since the initial homosexual outbreak of AIDS was in New York, Szmuness and his New York colleagues along with Merck researchers seemed to be the prime suspects. Then I wondered whether there were any documented links between Gallo's group and Szmuness?

Manufacturing AIDS-Like Viruses

LEN: OK. Now let's get a little bit more specific about the virus itself. With regard to the AIDS virus, had it been specifically manufactured, what might have been the first steps? What do you think the researchers began with?

ROBERT: I think they began with bovine visna virus, which they knew was a T-cell destroyer. And they made that by crossing bovine and visna [viruses] in cattle. . . .

Visna is the virus in sheep. Its characteristic is a destroyer, and they wanted a T-cell destroyer. So they took a T-cell attacker—the bovine leukemia virus and crossed it with a visna to make a T-cell destroyer, which is exactly what they got.

But then all they had was a T-cell destroyer in cattle which wasn't very good for humans. So then they grew it in human tissue, and when you do that it adapts to human beings (see fig. 7.1). And there are a host of ways to get these things to grow in tissue even if the receptors won't take [the virus]. . . .

LEN: They could have delivered the viral RNA a number of ways.

ROBERT: Yes. One of the ways is by pseudovirus formation. . . . Pseudovirus formation is where you put in a simultaneous mixture of cells and viruses, and what happens is, for instance, if you put bovine and visna viruses in with herpes virus; in the packaging process, you'll get BVV genome inside a herpes coat and visa versa.

So then you separate out all the herpes ones, and it just infects any cells which are sensitive to herpes. And you can artificially introduce BVV into a herpes-sensitive cell, because it has BVV on the inside and herpes on the outside.

LEN: I remember reading through studies about that technique being used.

ROBERT: Yeah. Another way is you treat 'em with heat, and they open up. Or you can use some detergents that will open them up, or there's a host of different things; even some viruses will tend to open them up. It makes the cells permeable even though they normally wouldn't be, so you can introduce the one you want to get in even though there's no real receptor for it.

LEN: OK. So it could've been bovine visna virus, BVV, but also there was some speculation it could have been scrapie, another sheep virus, right?

ROBERT: Yeah, well. . . . Scrapie's a little bit different than visna, but basically I don't think scrapie's a retrovirus. It's like it, but it's not the culprit.

LEN: During our first conversation, you also mentioned, like other researchers, you could actually take a look at the AIDS virus, and it looks like it's been spliced in particular regions.

ROBERT: Oh yes. Actually, looking at it was one of the first things that told us what it was because BVV and AIDS, of course, look identical, and there weren't that many 'D-type' retroviruses. There were only a few.

The 'D-type' are cylindrical-shaped retroviruses which of course BVV and AIDS are identical. Besides the fact that they were both magnesium dependent and were T-cell attackers that would produce syncytium and could wipe out cells.

And then what you do is look at the genome. Actually, a paper by Gallo published in *Science* I think about '83, or '86, said he took the restriction endonucleases [scissor-like enzymes] and treated the virus, and showed that when the virus falls apart, that where it falls apart are exactly at the gene lines.

In other words, it manages to fall apart just at the places where they could have constructed it.

LEN: Is that right? Just where the foreign pieces might have come together?

ROBERT: Yes, it falls apart in ten or twelve places . . . because those endonucleases cut at specific points.

But, what's interesting is . . . if it occurred spontaneously [in nature], why would it fall apart exactly where the genes occurred—the gag, pol, envelope, the tat genes?[30] Everything sort of cuts apart just the way you would put it together if you were constructing it. . . . [This] we thought [was] the strongest piece of evidence that would have said they actually put it together entirely in a lab.

LEN: And how might they have done that then? Let's say they started with BVV.

ROBERT: Well, in this case if you start with BVV, you just manipulate it to grow it in human tissue to adapt it to humans.

If you started with BLV and visna, you would . . . take the viruses, cut them up [with enzymes], then chromatograph them so that they're homologous. That is, the ten different parts [separate], then you take each different part that you want uniquely and put it together with other parts and zip 'em up.

LEN: And how do they 'zip 'em up' or combine them?

ROBERT: They have enzymes that sow them back up just like they've got ones which cut 'em apart. These are repair enzymes.

LEN: Then they separate those particular viruses, and they put them into cells?

ROBERT: They put them into serum . . . [add] your enzymes and [other] parts and wait for awhile. And then throw [everything] . . . into a culture and see what happens."

I was still a bit fuzzy.

ROBERT: But you see that's work. You don't have to do that. Nature does it all for you. All you do is take a cow and simultaneously inject bovine in one hip and visna in the other, and the cow is your mixer. And it will do it for you automatically. Because what happens is the viruses are so unstable that they will recombine and produce every thermodynamically stable recombinant possible.

LEN: Interesting. It's unbelievable.

ROBERT: Yeah. You see that's why everybody says, "We didn't make these viruses! We didn't have the techniques."

LEN: That's nonsense.

Fig. 7.1. Theoretic Manufacture of AIDS-Like Viruses From Bovine Leukemia and Sheep Visna Viruses

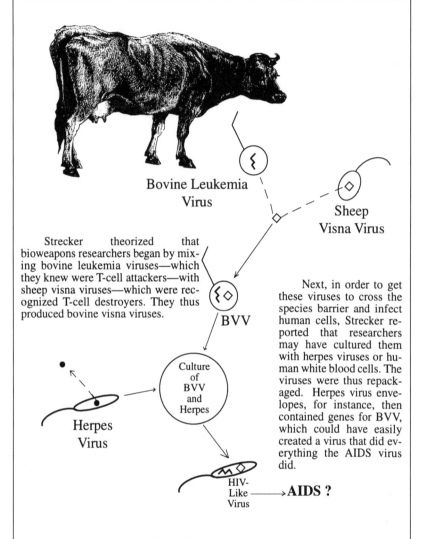

Bovine Leukemia Virus

Sheep Visna Virus

Strecker theorized that bioweapons researchers began by mixing bovine leukemia viruses—which they knew were T-cell attackers—with sheep visna viruses—which were recognized T-cell destroyers. They thus produced bovine visna viruses.

BVV

Next, in order to get these viruses to cross the species barrier and infect human cells, Strecker reported that researchers may have cultured them with herpes viruses or human white blood cells. The viruses were thus repackaged. Herpes virus envelopes, for instance, then contained genes for BVV, which could have easily created a virus that did everything the AIDS virus did.

Culture of BVV and Herpes

Herpes Virus

HIV-Like Virus ——→ AIDS ?

ᴍ — Bovine leukemia virus RNA with reverse transcriptase
◇ — Sheep visna virus RNA with reverse transcriptase
● — Herpes virus DNA found in infected humans

Diagram depicts the theoretic manufacture of AIDS-like viruses according to Robert Strecker, M.D., Ph.D., beginning with the bovine leukemia virus and sheep visna virus. Support for this theory was presented by Fort Detrick, NCI researchers Gonda MA, Braun MJ, Carter SG, Kost TA, Bess Jr JW, Arthur LO, and VanDer Maaten MJ. Characterization and molecular cloning of a bovine lentivirus related to human immunodeficiency virus. *Nature* 1987;330, 388-391.

ROBERT: Right. That's bull too, but, of course, our answer is: "Well . . . the virus makes itself." So you don't even have to implicate them for the genetic [engineering] viewpoint, if you don't want to.

Strecker then provided a unique, common sense, metaphor for the emergence of HIV.

ROBERT: It's like saying you've got a baby with no arms and legs and somebody dressed it up and took it to a party in Beverly Hills. Well, it sure couldn't do that and get there by itself!

Evidence Against Simians

LEN: What about simian monkey viruses? Why do they have scientists throughout the world claiming HIV is a simian monkey type of virus?

ROBERT: Because they get money for that. You know. . . . Here . . . send more money. Let me tell you about the simian AIDS virus.

First off, how does simian AIDS virus work? It produces a protein that causes AIDS in simians, and it's very easy to make a vaccine against a protein. And that's actually a derivative of the Mason Phizer monkey virus, which is another laboratory creation . . . another man-made virus made in the lab which was a simian virus that was being used for various things. It will cause AIDS in apes, but it doesn't do it [like HIV]; it does it by making a protein that wipes out their immune system.

LEN: Is it also a specific T-cell destroyer?

ROBERT: No. . . . The virus produces a protein, and the protein messes up the immune system. And it's very easy to make a vaccine against a protein.

But AIDS works entirely differently. It wipes out the T-cells and works inside of macrophages. . . . It inhibits the processing plant. AIDS is really a problem of macrophages, not of lymphocytes. . . . The virus makes the macrophage dysfunction.

What really is supposed to happen is that the macrophage is supposed to chop up the virus and present it to the T4 cell [thymus-derived cells] for the production of delayed immunity, and then to the B [bone-marrow-derived] cell for antibodies. But what happens is that the macrophage can't process it.

LEN: OK. So what happens then?

ROBERT: They run around the body and inject it into other cells. That's how the virus gets into other cells. That's how the virus gets into cells that don't have receptors for it.

LEN: So the macrophage actually reproduces the virus and then distributes it?

ROBERT: Yes. That's exactly what happens. That's how it gets into the brain. It's carried across the blood–brain barrier by macrophages that then inject it into brain cells.

LEN: Because T4 lymphocytes don't cross the barrier?

ROBERT: Yeah, they do, but they don't inject it. . . . They don't have sex with cells, whereas the macrophages do. And also the viruses are bigger than the pores of the membranes, so they can't get across directly. So something has to carry it.

Strecker's Colleagues

LEN: Now let's discuss some of your colleagues. Others have reported similar findings to yours. During our first conversation, we talked briefly about John Seale.[31] What do you know about his work?

ROBERT: Seale started writing about AIDS in '81 or so, even before us, and he was the first guy to say AIDS was not a venereal disease, and that it appeared to be artificial and spreading in an unusual manner, which was really just looking at the fact that the virus appeared in different areas of the world at the same time.

ROBERT: By the way, do you know the story of Parvo II?

LEN: No.

ROBERT: Parvo-II virus is a dog virus that appeared simultaneously around the world at the same time and proceeded to kill hundreds of millions of dogs.

How does a virus appear in Australia, Europe, and Asia all at the same time?"

LEN: American Airlines.

ROBERT: Right. American Airlines.

We both laughed.

ROBERT: OK. And then instead of spreading contiguously [from one dog to another], the viruses were spreading and popped up [in different areas around the world] as if directed mutations had occurred [and been delivered by humans].

And Parvo II was eventually proven by genetic techniques to be feline panleukopenic virus which had contaminated dog vaccines.[32]

So Seale was observing the same thing with AIDS. How was this virus appearing at different spots in the world at the same time in a sense without any contiguous spread? I mean, even if you look at the gay [transmission] theory [if AIDS started in Africa, Haiti, Paris, and then New York], why wasn't there AIDS in Miami, or New Orleans, or Dallas. I mean those guys were going to Haiti [New York, Africa, and Paris] far more than the gays from San Francisco. I mean none of this theory makes any sense!

Then Segal began to write the same thing.

LEN: Jacabo Segal, from Humboldt University in Berlin?[33]

ROBERT: Yes. He was at the Institute of Biology in East Berlin. He was writing the same stuff, but again, he thought that the virus was constructed from HTLV-I and visna. And that's correct except he didn't go far enough because really HTLV-I is just bovine leukemia virus in man.

So both [Seale and Segal] were saying the same sort of stuff, but neither one could exactly figure out how it was done. And so that's basically what we figured out, how it occurred. And we believe it occurred at Fort Detrick. . . . And Segal was probably supplied information by the KGB.

This sudden reference to the KGB threw me again. Somehow I needed to reconcile why Strecker, who believed the Russians may have brought AIDS to America, also recognized Fort Detrick as the source of the scourge.

ROBERT: The Russians wrote in over 400 public places that the virus was constructed over here. And if you remember our good surgeon *genital* went over there and made a deal with them. I don't know if you know anything about that?

LEN: Which surgeon general was that?

ROBERT: Koop.

LEN: No. I didn't know that.

ROBERT: Yeah. Koop went to Russia—to Moscow—and basically made a deal with them to stop talking about it and we'd give them our money.

That doesn't surprise me, I thought, reflecting on the alleged apology Gorbachev offered Reagan according to Covert's *Cutting Edge*.[34]

LEN: That's what I figured cause something like that is talked about vaguely in the book that I got from Fort Detrick. By the way, have you seen that book?

ROBERT: No.

LEN: You've got to get a copy of it. It came out in 1993. It's the fifty year history of Fort Detrick. It's free. They'll send it to you.

ROBERT: Well they won't send me one.

Strecker seemed to relish that possibility and his notoriety.

LEN: Oh they will. It's by a very nice guy. He's the public relations director for the fort. His name is Norman Covert. Imagine that?

ROBERT: Norman Covert? [Strecker laughed heartily] Is that a code name?

LEN: That's his real name. It's perfect, huh?

ROBERT: Well, do you know anything about what's going on there, the anthrax building?

LEN: Yes. I read about that.

ROBERT: Do you know about the Ebola building?

LEN: Vaguely.

ROBERT: Well they've got another building that's contaminated now; that they can't get into because of Ebola. You know they've got a whole bunch of problems. There's a bunch of people in Frederick [Maryland] that believe everything we talk about. We've quite a few supporters there, because they've had a lot of problems with strange illnesses. And so they're not entirely unsuspicious.

I shuttered for a moment considering the fact that I was scheduled to visit Frederick on my way to present an AIDS education seminar in Western Pennsylvania later in the year.

LEN: Robert, here's another one—Dr. Manuel Servin of the National Autonomous University of Mexico said that research conducted at Columbia by the U.S. Army was starting to point to the deadly disease in Haiti. He said that an unexplained accident caused the virus to spread to an employee of Haitian origin, and this person he believed, brought it back to Haiti. What do you think of that theory?[35]

ROBERT: No. There were like 47,000 Haitians working in Zaire at the time of these experiments. . . . So we think they either got it from the vaccine project or from the gays that were infected.

LEN: OK. So there were tens of thousands of Haitians working on health and welfare activities in Zaire during the 1970s?

ROBERT: Yes.

LEN: OK. So here's another one. There was a European physician who told a Russian journalist that he believed he was working for a DOD subcontractor with orders to mutate simian monkey viruses to produce fast-killing human viruses.[31] Had you heard that?

ROBERT: No, but that's entirely possible.

LEN: And this report went on to say that the experiment was considered a partial failure because they got a slow-acting virus rather than a fast one. They were allegedly looking for fast acting killers.

ROBERT: Except that quick viruses are, of course, worthless because they're too easy to defend against. I mean a very fast-acting virus is not any good.

LEN: What do you mean?

ROBERT: Frank Fenner talks about all the characteristics. . . . Ahh. . . . It's out of . . . . Cold Springs Harbor, that's the other great biowarfare palace. It's the Eugenics Institute. . . . Cold Springs is in upstate New York. . . . That was the place started by Margaret Thanger and others. Now they're, of course, the big biological warfare place under the guise of just research.

Anyway, Cold Springs Harbor put out a big thing on MMMV, that is, the 'maximally monstrous malignant virus,' and then they gave all the characteristics. And they talked about what it would take to produce this kind of virus. And, of course, all the characteristics are exactly those of the AIDS virus except for one thing, and that is, aerosolized transmission—which we believe is potentially possible.

Oh, God forbid, I thought. I hadn't heard that theory before. Given Strecker's obvious intelligence and formidable knowledge, his assertion startled me.

ROBERT: But they produced papers about what makes viruses malignant and monstrous. And one of the things is that they work slowly, and not fast. And that they are constantly mutating. Exactly the characteristics of AIDS.

LEN: Interesting. It's unbelievable.

ROBERT: Yes it is.

Final Recommendations

LEN: Now, the first time we spoke, you mentioned something about . . . a forthcoming cure for AIDS. How might it work?

ROBERT: Well, it's very simple in theory; complicated in practice. Basically, just as viruses are little crystals, you might hit them with electromagnetic frequencies and destroy them. Just as you can shakedown a crystal and destroy it without disrupting the surrounding house, you can [theoretically] disrupt viruses without destroying the surrounding cell structure.

LEN: Are there laboratories working on that?

ROBERT: Not that I know of.

LEN: OK. Now there was something in the news the other day that the French had allegedly discovered a cure. Have you heard anything new?

ROBERT: Nah. I haven't heard or seen anything. . . . I can't believe the word would not be all over everywhere if they thought [they had a cure] . . . particularly the French.

Now you see also what is Pasteur? The Pasteur Institute is their biowarfare institute, the same as Porton Down [in England], the same as Ivanofsky Institute [in Russia], the same as the Tokyo Institute. These are all the biowarfare centers for these countries; they're also the great AIDS research centers for these countries.

LEN: Right. It figures.

Now my last question. If you could tell people one thing about AIDS or your theories, what would it be?

ROBERT: The whole story. Everything. How the virus was made; that it was manmade, and we think it represents a threat to the human species.

LEN: And if there's some positive thing that people can do you might recommend, what would it be?

ROBERT: Other than no IV drugs, reduce their [sexual] promiscuity, and no blood products, start by questioning some of the things that they hear which may or may not be true.

Chapter 8
HIV-1, 2 and the "Big Bang"

THE morning after the Strecker interview, I handed Jackie the tape of our conversation. "Here, listen to this," I said. I then walked off to my office to do some more reading.

A few hours later, Jackie, who had slain much of her fear following word of Strecker's whereabouts, walked in holding the cassette. "This is completely unbelievable," she protested. "The part about the HELA cells, aerosolized in labs, ending up all over the world, is absolutely horrifying."

"The whole thing is horrifying, if you ask me," I responded. "I have a few problems with what he alleged, particularly the Russian theory, but most of what he said seems plausible. I'm going to check on his references tomorrow."

"You're going back to Harvard?"

"Yeah. I want to read some of the articles he mentioned, and see if they have *Conspiracy of Cells.*"

Early the next morning, I made my now routine excursion to Countway to investigate Strecker's allegations. Unfortunately for humanity, I found scientific evidence to support the vast majority of his claims.

His BLV/BVV theory of AIDS virus engineering was indeed sound. The methods Strecker cited as those used by cancer researchers to establish new strains of deadly viruses were generally accepted and widely practiced.[1,2]

In addition, evolutionary trees had been developed showing the close relationship between HTLV-I and II and BLV, as well as between HIV and VISNA (see fig. 8.1).[3]

One conflicting report, however, emerged from the NCI. The report alleged the risk of BLV or BVV transmission to humans was nil. In a Cold Springs Harbor Laboratory publication, Dr. S. G. Devare wrote:

> There is evidence that BLV can be transmitted to sheep through unpasteurized milk. . . . In one instance leukemia has been reported to have developed in a chimpanzee fed milk from a leukemic cow. . . . However, sera from patients with various forms of cancer, as well as from individuals in contact with cattle, lacked detectable levels of antibodies to BLV proteins. . . . These observations confirm those of others . . . and suggest that BLV is not likely to pose a serious natural hazard to humans.[4]

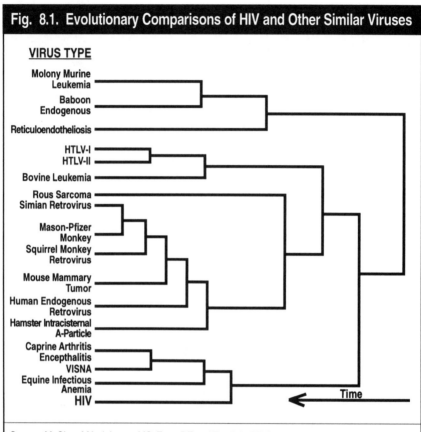

Fig. 8.1. Evolutionary Comparisons of HIV and Other Similar Viruses

VIRUS TYPE

Molony Murine Leukemia
Baboon Endogenous
Reticuloendotheliosis
HTLV-I
HTLV-II
Bovine Leukemia
Rous Sarcoma
Simian Retrovirus
Mason-Pfizer Monkey
Squirrel Monkey Retrovirus
Mouse Mammary Tumor
Human Endogenous Retrovirus
Hamster Intracisternal A-Particle
Caprine Arthritis Encepthalitis
VISNA
Equine Infectious Anemia
HIV

Time

Source: McClure MA, Johnson MS, Feng DF and Doolittle RF. Sequence comparisons of retroviral proteins: Relative rates of change and general phylogeny. *Proceedings of the National Academy of Sciences* 1988;85:2469-73.

My internal dialogue questioned again, "What about unnatural hazards like intentional mutations and tainted vaccine injections?" If chimpanzees were susceptible to cow milk transmitted leukemia, then humans might be also; particularly if the inoculated BLV or BVV was experimentally cultured in human WBCs, as researchers had routinely done.[5]

Additionally disturbing was an article I found about human breast milk in *Nature New Biology*—a journal in which Gallo published much of his work.[6,7] This report, by other members of the NCI staff, found "type C particles"—simian sarcoma virus type structures—in mother's milk that resembled "known oncogenic RNA viruses" isolated from monkey breast tumors. As in Gallo's NAS report,[8] in which he manipulated simian sarcoma virus RNA to synthesize a "DNA probe" for human cancer research, the particles found by this group of researchers had an identical density of 1.16–1.19g/ml[-1].

What left me cold was the fact that Gallo and others at the NCI were manipulating simian monkey viruses to create human killers, screening American women for these agents, and then oddly enough, locating these same "particles" in their lactates.[6-8] I couldn't help wondering—Might at least some of the world's childhood leukemia cases be linked to nursing infants exposed to NCI simian monkey cancer viruses? Could such experiments have gone awry exposing American women to breast-cancer-causing viruses too?

I made note of the fact that the authors acknowledged their NCI coordinators—Drs. Bryan, Manaker, and Clausen—for their efforts.[6]

Shilts vs. Strecker on Montagnier and Gallo

Strecker indicated The Wistar Institute was alleged to have spread AIDS through tainted polio vaccines. In researching background on Wistar, I learned that Hilary Koprowski served as a chief virologist at the facility during the late 1960s and early 1970s.[9]

I found it interesting to read that Koprowski also served as co-chair for the "Second International Symposium on Tumor Viruses" held at Royaumont, France, on June 3–5, 1969. During Koprowski's session—titled "Persistence and transcription of the viral genome in virus-transformed cells mechanism of induction," he presented the "Presence of SV_{40} [Simian virus 40] genome in transformed cells and mechanism of rescue operation"—Luc Montagnier, then with the Institut du Radium, Orsay, France, attended.

Montagnier also presented a paper at this symposium ("Alterations de la surface des cellules BHK21 en rapport avec leur transformation par des virus ongogenes") in which he discussed the nature of changes occurring at cell surfaces following exposure to cancer-causing viruses.[10]

In addition, Montagnier was apparently present at the general session in which Drs. Huebner, Todar, and Sarma from the NCI presented "'Switched off' vertically transmitted C-type RNA tumor viruses as determinants of spontaneous and induced cancer: A new hypothesis of viral carcinogenesis."[11]

During their presentation, this NCI-affiliated group acknowledged, as Gallo did shortly after, that their search for cancer-causing viruses was only marginally fruitful. They said:

[O]nly Burkitt's African lymphoma survives as a cancerous entity, the natural occurrence of which could be regarded as consistent with [a foreign virus] such as the herpes-like Epstein Barr virus (EBV). . . . Although EBV infections have also been associated with nasopharyngeal cancers, racial (genetic) factors and perhaps religious practices appear to be important contributing factors.

Despite extensive sero-epidemiologic [blood surveys] and experimental tumor induction studies of the "oncogenic" DNA viruses . . . none have been established as significant causes of spontaneous cancers in their natural hosts. . . .

These various convincing arguments against DNA and other horizontally [species to species] spread viruses as possible significant causes of natural cancer led us to ask this very pertinent question: Do any of the known oncogenic viruses have properties and/or behavior patterns consistent with the well known . . . [naturally occurring] . . . cancers? We concluded that the only candidates were the RNA tumor viruses of the C and B types, the prototypes of which are the sarcoma and leukemia viruses. . . . Except for the B-type mammary tumor virus . . . the C-type virus we believe represents the only well established oncogenic group of viruses that can be considered seriously in the etiology of . . . naturally occurring cancer.[11]

Meaning? Shilts was mistaken and Strecker was undoubtedly correct. Montagnier apparently knew as much as Gallo not only about "slow" C-type viruses, and simian monkey viruses including SV_{40}, but also about the suspected relationship between EBV and Burkitt's African lymphoma—a WBC cancer affecting genetically and behaviorally predisposed black people.

Moreover, it was obvious and highly suspicious that Montagnier, Koprowski, as well as Gallo knew that the "only candidates" for cancer causing viruses potentially useful as human bioweapons, were the "RNA tumor viruses . . . the prototypes" that caused the rare AIDS-related cancers—sarcoma, lymphoma, and leukemia.

More troubling, these researchers acknowledged cancer studies conducted in New York City that provided evidence of the probable association "of virtually all human cancer occurring in different age groups and in different ethnic groups in each of many different years."[12]

As Jackie had noted the similarity of the NCI's blood studies to those conducted by the Nazis, here was evidence that New York researchers confirmed as early as 1960, exactly which ethnic groups would be most susceptible to lymphoma, leukemia, and sarcoma virus attacks.

The IARC and African AIDS

Strecker's theory that IARC brought AIDS to Africa is based on the knowledge that the organization, along with the Cancer Division of the WHO, worked with the International Union Against Cancer (IUAC)—a nongovernmental, voluntary agency "devoted solely to promoting the campaign against cancer in its research, therapeutic, and preventive aspects."[13]

The NCI reported that IARC was established in 1965 under the auspices of the WHO. Initially sponsored by the five most active NATO countries—the Federal Republic of Germany, France, Italy, the United Kingdom, and the United States—and based in Lyon, France, IARC began work with a budget of $750,000 per year. The budget for 1973 was $3.5 million as ten other countries joined the organization, including the Soviet Union.[14]

Indeed, when attention began to focus on the apparent link between virus infections and cancers, IARC focused its research efforts principally on Africa. The reasons for this are also suspicious. Despite the existence of cancers in most parts of the world, IARC targeted esophageal cancer and liver cancer both in black African populations.[14]

The NCI reported:

The incidence of cancer of the esophagus shows very wide geographic variations. It has also increased significantly in recent years in certain population groups, notably the black community in the United States, for as yet undetermined reasons.[14]

In an effort to determine the reasons:

... the Agency is investigating a "hot spot" for rumenal cancer in cattle (the equivalent of esophageal cancer in man) in Kenya which affects 10% of all beasts in a very limited area and which may provide clues to the possible etiology of esophageal cancer in those human situations were alcohol is not important.[14]

Liver cancer was second on the list of IARC priorities. To determine the relationship between aflatoxin, a toxic chemical produced by the fungus *Aspergillus flavus*, and liver cancer, IARC studied individuals in Kenya and elsewhere in Africa.[14]

The problem has been further compounded by recent work on hepatitis virus and liver cancer. Serologic studies show that the hepatitis B antigen (HBag) is associated with $\leq$ 50% of liver cancers in Africa and Asia [two areas of the world wherein AIDS prevalence rates are highest], being found in about 6%

Fig. 8.2. Geographic Distribution of Some NCI and IARC "Collaborative Agency" Programs

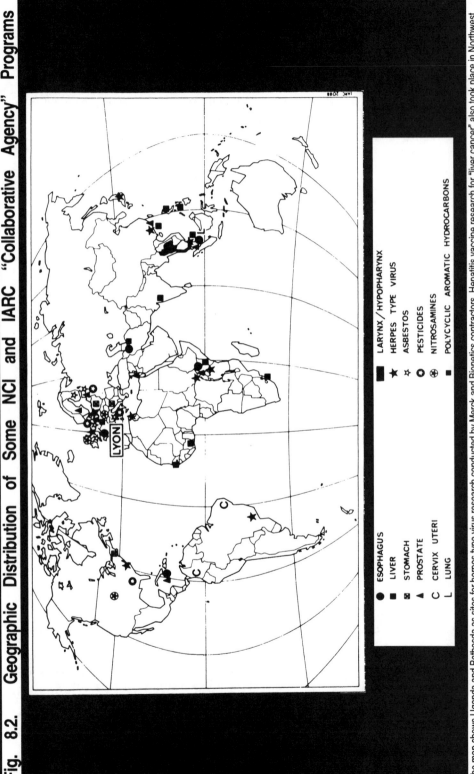

The map shows Uganda and Bethesda as sites for herpes type virus research conducted by Merck and Bionetics contractors. Hepatitis vaccine research for "liver cancer" also took place in Northwest Uganda, where experts believe the Marburg, Ebola, Reston, and AIDS viruses originated. Source: Higginson J and Muir CS. Epidemiologic program of the International Agency for Research on Cancer (IARC). In: *The National Cancer Program and International Cancer Research. National Cancer Institute Monograph* 1974: 40-65.

of controls. Much lower frequencies were obtained in North America and in Europe. While much remains to be discovered about HBag, there now exist 2 putative etiologic agents, one chemical and the other viral. Intensive study is needed to show whether they are both in fact responsible for liver cancer, and if so, whether they operate independently or together. A survey of 5,000 individuals has been carried out over 2 years in West Africa to determine the natural history of HBag.[14]

Besides IARC's interest in hepatitis B:

Even more important perhaps are the sero-epidemiologic studies being carried out with the support of the U.S. National Cancer Institute, Bethesda, Maryland, and the East African Virus Research Institute, Entebbe, Uganda. The Agency has been studying nasopharyngeal carcinoma in Asia and Burkitt's lymphoma in Africa, neoplasms associated serologically with a herpesvirus [a C-type RNA retrovirus]. A mass survey has been organized which will follow a population of approximately 35,000 children in Africa over a sufficient period of time to see whether the development of Burkitt's lymphoma in that population is in fact linked with infection by the virus. The logistic problems are considerable, but no other possible approach has been suggested to date.[14]

A map (see fig. 8.2) depicting the nature of IARC-sponsored programs in Africa and elsewhere was also published in their report.[14]

Recognizing that hepatitis-B-virus related cancer research was a concern for IARC as well as Merck, Inc., I searched to understand why. The answer was apparent in a chapter of *Prospects for Vaccines Against Cancer* written in the early 1970s by Maurice R. Hilleman—Chief of the Division of Virus and Cell Biology Research at Merck Institute for Therapeutic Research—Gallo's counterpart at the Merck labs in West Point, Pennsylvania.[15] Hilleman explained the company's interest in viral vaccines this way:

It is well established that a great many factors have something to do with cancer: ionizing radiation, environmental carcinogens, age of host, hormones, genetic factors, and the like. It is also well established that a great variety of tumors of animals are caused by viruses, and one needs only to point to the role of viruses in the malignant neoplasia of rodents, cats, fowl, frogs, and bovines with ancillary information obtained in studies of cancer in monkeys and man. This leads to the concept that the one indispensable element in cancer may be a virus or its genetic material, and all other factors may only be secondary. In taking this position, we are reinforced by the fact that cancer cells seem to have a new genetic input that allows them to make new and unique antigens that are present in the cells and on their surfaces. Carcinogenic chemicals and physical agents, such as ionizing radiation, do not provide such input—they only rearrange the output. If it is true that virus infection is indispensable in cancer, then the prevention of viral infection or the negation of the viral effect might permit the breaking of an essential link in the neoplastic chain and so make the prevention of cancer possible.

This then has provided the motivation for seeking the virus or viruses that cause cancer in man. Current research in viral etiology of human cancer has been focused on the C and B type RNA viruses that are being linked with leukemia, sarcoma, and breast cancer mainly by the demonstration of viruses or viruslike particles in human neoplastic tissues and secretions. To date, however, no reliably propagable RNA virus has been recovered from human neoplasia that can be considered to be a serious candidate for an etiologic role in man; this in spite of the intense competitive effort given to it and in spite of the private and public proclamations to the contrary.

The DNA viruses have fared somewhat better, and the herpesviruses can be seriously considered as candidates for several neoplasias in man including Burkitt's lymphoma and nasopharyngeal carcinoma and possibly also cervical and prostatic neoplasia and Hodgkin's disease. As with the RNA viruses, however, proof of etiologic role remains elusive and is frustrated by the inability to carry out direct etiologic studies in the human species.[15]

Regarding the use of the "Feline Leukemia-Sarcoma Model" for vaccine production and cancer research, Hilleman noted:

In judging the probability for developing vaccines against cancer, it is necessary to consider the means for spread of the virus, whether it be horizontal as in infectious disease [like animal to animal or cross species transmission] or vertical as in transmission from mother to offspring either through transplacental infection or through integration in the germ plasm [genes]. . . .

The feline leukemia-sarcoma complex presents an excellent model in comparative oncology for testing vertical versus horizontal spread of cancer and for evaluating the effectiveness of vaccines. It is the prime model for RNA oncogenic viruses that is being pursued in our laboratories. The cat might be considered an especially meaningful model for such studies, since the cat, like man, is outbred, and it is subject to many, if not most, of the same environmental carcinogens to which man is subject and which might play a role in the induction of cancer. The rates for spontaneous leukemia and sarcoma in cats are low and roughly in the same range as in man, considering the difference in life span. Most important, while cats do harbor covert indigenous leukemia viruses, horizontal transmission of the oncogenic virus does occur [whereas] the role of the vertically transmitted . . . cancer . . . is in serous doubt.[16] Significantly, adult immunologically competent cats can be infected artificially or naturally with the virus and this can result in the induction of leukemia. *With further study, it may be hoped that this model will present the means whereby live, killed, and subunit vaccines can be evaluated for prophylactic and therapeutic efficacy and whereby information can be obtained that can be applied eventually to the development of vaccines for use in man* [emphasis added].[15]

Finally, Hilleman acknowledged the use of simian cancer viruses, two of which were herpesviruses—herpesvirus saimiri "recovered from kidneys of squirrel monkeys (*Saimiri sciureus*) and herpesvirus ateles isolated from kidney culture of a black spider monkey (*Ateles geoffroyi*)"—known to "cause lymphoma or reticulum cell tumor and leukemia" when injected into other monkey species. "These viruses," Hilleman wrote, "present excellent models for studies for immunologic interruption of cancer in primate species using live, killed, or subunit viral vaccines. They are of special importance because of their possible use in elucidating the interactions among Epstein-Barr virus, Burkitt's lymphoma, and nasopharyngeal carcinoma in man."[15]

Now I better understood what Nixon's "war on cancer," and the "cancer virus hypothesis" was really about—the search for *the* virus and vaccine. I also realized why the generals on the battlefield—Gallo at the NCI, Hilleman at Merck, and Don Francis at the CDC—were fooling around with leukemic cats and simian monkeys. These models they claimed might provide the most powerful weapons against human immune-system-destroying germs.

Tribute to Don Francis

Attempting to investigate Strecker's claim that Drs. Gallo, Francis, and Montagnier were long-time workmates at the NCI, I sought Francis's biography in *American Men & Women of Science*.[17] In a nutshell, here's what I learned:

Donald Pinkston Francis was born in Los Angeles, California, on October 24, 1942. He married in 1976 and had two children. Educated at Northwestern University, he received his M. D. degree in 1968, and then an honorary Doctor of Science degree from Harvard in 1979. His specialty was noted as "medical epidemiology and virology." From 1978 to the time of this writing he served as chief of the epidemiology branch at the Hepatitis Labs Division of the CDC.

Francis's professional experience included service as an International Fellow in the Children's Bureau of the U.S. Department of Health, Education, and Welfare in Punjab, India, in 1968; internship and residency in pediatrics at the Los Angeles County, University of Southern California Medical Center, 1969–1971; USAID service as a state epidemiologist in infectious disease in Rivers State, Nigeria, in 1971; American epidemiologic intelligence service officer for the CDC, 1971–1973; and medical officer for the World Health Organization's smallpox vaccine program in the Sudan—which abuts the northern border of Zaire and Uganda—the "Hot Zone" wherein the AIDS, Ebola Zaire, and Ebola Sudan viruses allegedly jumped species three years after Francis's tour of the Sudan ended.[18] He then went to India from 1973 to 1975. And, finally, he received an infectious disease fellowship at the Channing Lab at Harvard Medical School from 1975 to 1977.

He currently holds a position at my alma mater, Harvard School of Public Health (HSPH), which he began as Fellow in Microbiology in 1976. His mailing address was listed as the Division of Oral Diseases, CDC, Atlanta, GA 30333.[17]

I found nothing to indicate Francis and Gallo shared common workplaces in the early 1970s although Francis received several grants from the NCI during that time. He also shared with Gallo several acquaintances, including Max Essex at the HSPH Department of Microbiology, with whom he co-authored many feline leukemia virus reports.[19] Consistent with Strecker's allegation of collusion, however, it's hard to imagine this most esteemed group of American type-C RNA retrovirologists were unaware of each other's studies and findings during this important time in cancer virus research.

Given his unique early 1970s cat leukemia virus research, hepatitis B virus studies, medical intelligence background, and Third World service record, the fact that Francis noted the laundry list of cat leukemia/sarcoma virus symptoms among gay men and intravenous drug users in the early days of the AIDS epidemic made me question his knowledge and service record even more.

"Combine these two diseases," Francis said to a gathering of colleagues, "feline leukemia and hepatitis, and you have the immune deficiency."[20]

Surely Francis knew what Hilleman had clearly explained. He would have known that Gallo had taken monkey viruses, extracted their humanly benign DNA, infused their empty viral shells with cat leukemia/sarcoma RNA, and then cultured the genetically engineered mutants in human WBCs to allow them to cross the species barrier.[21] The CDC's hepatitis chief might have had an inkling that this new retrovirus he suspected of causing GRID might have come from Gallo's or Hilleman's labs, or another NCI research group that manipulated viruses in this way, particularly since he, Gallo, and Essex presented their cat retrovirus research at the same session of a 1980 Cold Spring Harbor conference in which cat leukemia and sarcoma virus mutations, cloning, and cross-species transmissions were discussed.[22]

If Shiltz were alive, he might now realize an alternative reason why Francis was particularly "incredulous" that the NCI had successfully stalled the AIDS research effort.[20] Could their stalling have provided time to organize and administer an effective disinformation campaign? Surely, Francis knew more than he was saying.

Francis in Ebola Territory

I also found it interesting that Francis directed the emergency response team sent by the WHO to control the outbreak of the dreaded Ebola virus. Shilts chronicled this activity well:

> The horrible fever had swept seemingly from nowhere into the border region between Zaire and Sudan, on the fetid banks of the Ebola River. The disease was a blood-borne virus, wickedly spreading both through sexual intercourse, because infected lymphocytes were in victims' semen, and through the sharing of needles in local bush hospitals. The absence of modern precautions to protect doctors also spread the blood-borne disease among medical personnel through routes unimaginable in more civilized countries.

> During this 1976 outbreak, local Danish doctors in the remote hospitals in Zaire, people like Ib Bygbjerg and Grethe Rask, were impressed with the vigor with which the team from the World Health Organization (WHO) had moved to stamp out this deadly disease that became known as Ebola Fever. When it became obvious that the disease was spreading through autopsies and ritual contact with corpses during the funerary process, Dr. Don Francis, on loan to the World Health Organization from the CDC, had simply banned local rituals and unceremoniously burned the corpses. Infected survivors were removed from the community and quarantined until it was clear that they could no longer spread the fever. Within weeks, the disease disappeared as mysteriously as it had come. . . .[23]

Six years later, on January 6, 1982, Francis "could not escape the memories of the horrible Ebola Fever outbreak," wrote Shilts. His recollections became more acute when he received "a phone call from Dr. Guy de The in Paris, another veteran of African epidemics."[23]

Dr. de The had studied the latest data from Africa. The common cases of benign Kaposi's sarcoma were not in question. Typically, Kaposi's sarcoma in African males responded to treatment. Francis, however:

> had already heard of the *new, more virulent KS that had been reported first in Uganda in 1972*. But there was more, de The said. In the western Nile district of Uganda, young men living together were getting not only the typical, easygoing Kaposi's sarcoma, but the nasty kind, like that tearing through the bodies of American homosexuals. These Africans also suffered from the lymphadenopathy that marked the early stages of the American disease, de The said. There had to be some connection. [emphasis added]

Of course, Francis thought. A new virus from Africa. It was where Bob Gallo at the National Cancer Institute figured his new retrovirus for Human T-cell Leukemia came from too. After all, HTLV only struck in the portions of Japan settled by Portuguese traders, who apparently had brought the microbe with them from Africa some 500 years ago. The African links reinforced Francis's hypothesis about a transmissible agent . . . [but] The National Cancer Institute didn't seem terribly interested in the disease.[23]

Come on Shilts, I respectfully implored the deceased journalist, you were a lot smarter than that. Why would it have taken 500 years for an African virus to express itself in Japan while everywhere else in the world it reared its ugly head in less than a decade 90 percent of the time? Had Gallo figured his new retrovirus came from Africa because that's where the experiments were taking place in the race to create special cancer viruses and vaccines? A race in which he, Francis, and Hilleman were major contestants; a race to create dozens of leukemia/sarcoma RNA retroviruses for vaccine tests in black Africans in the "Nile district" of Northwest Uganda, and American homosexuals in New York City?

Finally, I found it interesting that following a successful stint in Nigeria as a USAID infectious disease researcher and a couple of years in Sudan on behalf of the CDC and WHO as a smallpox vaccination program officer, Francis was assigned a principal role in the gay male hepatitis B vaccine study funded by the CDC and Merck, Sharp & Dohme.[24]

Notes on Duesberg

As I was searching the literature, another prominent name in AIDS research circles kept appearing—Peter Duesberg. As detailed in *Deadly Innocence* [25] and elsewhere,[26] Duesberg is regarded as an esteemed American scientist, a member of the NAS, and is credited for having initially mapped the genetic structure of retroviruses. Unlike most AIDS scientists, however, Duesberg has, since the mid-1980s, argued that AIDS is completely atypical of an infectious disease and not likely caused by the retrovirus Gallo and Montagnier identified.

How is this possible? I questioned during the *Deadly Innocence* investigation.

To be an infectious disease, traditionally, scientists had to prove a cause–effect relationship between the suspected germ and the symptoms it is alleged to cause when the germ spreads to other hosts. As Strecker alluded, these standards, known as "Koch's postulates," are based on three tests.

First, the suspected germ must be found in everyone with the disease. Not all people with AIDS test positive for HIV infection. These patients would now likely be diagnosed as having Idiopathic Lymphocyteopaenia (ILC)—a disease in which WBCs spontaneously disappear for no apparent reason.

Second, the germ should not be present in individuals without the illness. Yet, of the estimated 1 million Americans who are believed to be HIV carriers, three-quarters have not developed AIDS. Furthermore, in a recent *CBS News* report, scientists noted that 8 percent of those who carry HIV antibodies have remained symptomless for more than a decade, suggesting that they may be carrying a weaker strain, or doing something special to prolong their health. Positive thinking, exercise, and good nutrition may be part of that special something.[26]

Third, researchers should be able to reproduce the illness in laboratory animals using isolated germ cultures. Duesberg argued that, with AIDS, this has proved difficult.

In the August 5, 1992, issue of *In These Times*, health writer Benjamin Goldman and AIDS journalist Michael Chappelle reported that defenders of the HIV hypothesis simply rejected Koch's postulates as being outdated. They stated that Harold Jaffe, the senior AIDS/HIV investigator at the CDC, and Robin Weiss, a British AIDS researcher, argued:

> What seems bizarre is that anyone should demand strict adherence to these unreconstructed postulates 100 years after their proposition.[26]

Reporters Goldman and Chappelle, however, noted the advice of Nobel Laureate Walter Gilbert of Harvard University:

> "Someone scientifically trained would not make that statement. Koch's postulates are an attempt at rigorous proof. If you cannot fulfill Koch's postulates, you've got a problem. You can deal with that either with hard thinking or with soft thinking. If you can block the virus and thus block the disease, that would constitute hard evidence that you were right." But in the absence of a successful treatment, Gilbert characterizes the attempt to dismiss Koch's postulates and fall back on incomplete epidemiological statistics as "soft-minded."[26]

I questioned, might Koch's postulates—the scientific test to prove etiology of naturally occurring infectious diseases—be outdated and dismissed only because they don't hold for *unnatural* man-made infectious diseases?

In any case, Duesberg has argued for more than a decade that you can find HIV in any burned-out, drugged-out, and sexed-out individual. He has consistently "blamed the victims" of AIDS for living unhealthy lives. His

Fig. 8.3. NIH Progress Report On Testing Mutant RNA Sarcoma and Leukemia Tumor Viruses at the Univ. of Calif. By Duesberg and Others, 1971

CALIFORNIA, UNIVERSITY OF (NIH 71-2173)

Title: Studies on the Structure and Replication of Viruses and Mechanism of Regulation

Contractor's Project Directors: Dr. Howard K. Schachman
                                 Dr. Peter Duesberg

Project Officers (NCI): Dr. Robert J. Huebner
                         Dr. James T. Duff

Objectives: Research on the structure of viruses includes studies on the type specific antigens, nucleoid structure and viral subunits of RNA tumor viruses, and the nucleic acids of various mutant viruses such as the radiation or chemically induced variants of Rous virus. Research on the replication of RNA tumor viruses includes studies on the RNA-dependent DNA polymerase and other enzymes of these viruses, and the analysis of temperature sensitive mutants of Rous sarcoma virus. Research on the mechanisms of regulation include transcriptional control by a satellite virus and factors controlling the growth of mammalian cells in culture.

Major Findings: This is a new contract and major findings have not been reported.

Significance to Biomedical Research and the Program of the Institute: These studies may provide important insight into the mechanism by which RNA tumor viruses bring about malignant transformation, and perhaps will lead to significant advances in the understanding of the causation and control of human neoplastic disease.

Date Contract Initiated: June 1971

NIH progress report shows Dr. Peter Duesberg, at the University of California (UC), in 1971, directed studies which paralleled Dr. Gallo's at the NCI. Duesberg intended to explain "the mechanism by which RNA tumor viruses bring about malignant" changes in humans. Mutant sarcoma viruses were used for this purpose following studies inoculating cows and monkeys with simian sarcoma and leukemia viruses by Leo Bustad and Robert Huebner at UC and the NCI. This evidence, along with a conference discussion, raises serious questions regarding Dr. Duesberg's more recent publications asserting HIV cannot cause AIDS. Source: NCI staff. *The Special Virus Cancer Program: Progress Reports #8 and #9.* Office of the Associate Scientific Director for Viral Oncology (OASDVO). J. B. Moloney, Ed., Washington, D. C.: U. S. Government Printing Office, 1971, p. 233.

arguments are difficult to dispute since physicians and scientists have known for years that strong host resistance is a key factor in determining whether or not an infectious germ can take root, grow, and ultimately overwhelm the immune system. Moreover, he has claimed that HIV is very difficult to spread—which it is. With rare exception, it generally requires larger doses of viruses in more healthy individuals to claim lives. So nothing Duesberg has said is new.

In fact, Duesberg's position is exactly that held by prominent NCI and NIH researchers from the beginning of the epidemic. As Shilts wrote, it is "incredulous" that "the National Cancer Institute [in 1982] was still fiddling around with half-baked theories that GRID was caused by poppers or sperm. But those were the presentations the NIH researchers made at the conferences. None of them was talking about what Francis thought was the most obvious cause, a new viral agent."[24]

The fact is that Duesberg—like Gallo, Montagnier, Francis, Hilleman, and a few others—had been part of a core group of investigators funded by the NCI to study "special" viruses and their links to cancer.[27]

In 1971, for instance, Duesberg became a "project director" for the University of California's contract (NIH 71-2173; see fig. 8.3) to study the mechanisms regulating mutant RNA tumor virus reproduction and sarcoma development; the RNA-dependent DNA polymerase related effects Gallo and his teams studied. This work followed sarcoma and leukemia virus studies on monkeys and cows, also conducted at the University of California with NCI funding.[27]

The same year, during a meeting in Paris attended by Gallo and Montagnier, Duesberg presented evidence that RNA leukemia and sarcoma viruses can be manipulated and observed to produce the "provirus DNA" needed to successfully reproduce in nature and cell cultures.[28] Earlier, Duesberg evaluated the effects of chemotherapy (using the antibiotic Actinomycin-D) on mouse leukemia viruses (MLV).[29] Later, he examined leukemia and sarcoma viruses to show how mutants of varying oncogenicity are formed.[30]

Most pertinent to Duesberg's main argument—HTLV-III does not cause the immune deficiency and cancers seen in AIDS, Duesberg and Gallo, in 1973, debated essentially the same question: Can "special" type C-RNA tumor viruses, such as those captured from monkeys and modified for human experiments, cause cancers? Duesberg answered affirmatively, "That is absolutely right."[31]

The discussion occurred following Gallo's presentation, "On the Origin of Human Acute Myeloblastic Leukemia: The Virus-'Hot Spot' Hypothesis." Gallo was joined by Dr. Wu, who presented two related papers as an emissary of Litton Bionetics.[32]

During the session's open discussion, Gallo questioned whether the genetic "Hot Spot" that caused cells to become cancerous was responding to an external or internal virus-like particle:

GALLO: Are there viral (type-C RNA tumor virus) genes in some normal cells? Everyone by now must believe that there are some virogenes in at least some normal cells. I would like to know where they came from—or which came first—are these virogenes in fact really cell genes which the virus utilizes? Duesberg should speculate on this.

DUESBERG: That's too much for me. That's like all theories on the origin of life: Where do whales come from, where does God come from, where does a 'clean chicken' come from? But I would like to return a question to you, maybe somewhat related to that. I think we can at least divide those viruses which cause cancer and those which are subvirus-like things which may be a consequence of cancer. I think that those which are causing cancer may be like the men and the other more or less like the boys. So I think that shouldn't be confused too much. I think these subviral particles or endogenous viruses or incomplete endogenous viruses or enzymes might in fact well be a consequence of cancer rather than its cause. But I think there is little doubt that Rous SV [mouse sarcoma virus] or AMV [bird virus] can be the cause of cancer."

GALLO: I kind of agree with that, at least they cause chicken cancer, *I think the information for carcinogenesis may be packaged into only very special type-C RNA tumor viruses.* But I wouldn't even make those viruses that you call boys any less important because boys can become men. Moreover, we have now demonstrated that the reverse transcriptase in human leukemic cells and the viral related nucleic acid is related not to endogenous non-oncogenic type-C viruses, but specifically to type C viruses which in fact *are* oncogenic such as the woolly monkey simian sarcoma virus.

DUESBERG: *That is absolutely right. . . .*[Emphasis added][31]

In essence, Gallo stated, and Duesberg acknowledged, that only "very special" retroviruses could be expected to produce AIDS-like immunosuppression and cancers, as this had already been proven in monkeys and other animals. In fact, AIDS-like viruses, they agreed, caused cancers in chickens and monkeys before they were clearly modified to infect humans.

In contrast, since the publication of his objections to the HIV=AIDS paradigm in 1988, Duesberg has diverted public attention from the facts by arguing that HIV is insufficient to cause AIDS.[33] Like counterintelligence propaganda that presents mostly truth, what he doesn't tell is most revealing.

Duesberg argues correctly that unhealthy lifestyles and abused drugs—including the commonly used AIDS drugs AZT, ddi, ddc, 3TC, and protease inhibitors—cause toxic side effects that reduce immune system strength. What he and his followers fail to discuss, however, is their knowledge that the so called "neutralizing antibody" response to HIV infection, allegedly protective, may in fact be part of an autoimmune response to virus/host protein-complex formation.[33] In other words, as the virus contacts, then attaches to, host proteins (antibodies included) these antigenic complexes can trigger additional antibody responses, autoimmune diseases, and infectious disease susceptibilities.[33]

Thus, in light of Duesberg's documented ties to the NAS and NCI, at the exact time the NAS informed the DOD that AIDS-like viruses could be developed in five years for $10 million, his earlier admission, and his incomplete message, I wondered whether the professor intended to provide a disinformation smokescreen for these organizations? Consistent with Hegel's approach to counterintelligence propaganda, Gallo's HIV=AIDS thesis, coupled with Duesberg's HIV≠AIDS antithesis, caused "synthesis"—mass confusion.

Earliest AIDS Cases

One important consideration remained before the basic premise of man-made HIV development could be reconciled. The literature held several accounts of alleged AIDS cases and HIV discoveries predating the work of Gallo, Hilleman, Duesberg, et al., that is, prior to the 1960s or early 1970s.

A literature search conducted to investigate such claims revealed several interesting discoveries.

I first read a series of reports published in *The Lancet* regarding the earliest alleged AIDS case—a "25-year-old former naval seaman" who died of cytomegalovirus and pneumocystis infections in 1959.[34] The claim was made by University of Manchester researcher Gerald Corbitt and co-workers. Having meticulously extracted the seaman's tissues from paraffin blocks initially developed to make autopsy slides, DNA amplification methods were used to "search for very small quantities of HIV proviral DNA in target cells." The group found the suspected particles in several of the recaptured tissues, and the news media broadly heralded the event.

Several years later, Drs. David Ho and Tuofu Zhu of the Aaron Diamond Research Center in New York reexamined Corbitt's tissues in an effort to investigate the theory that HIV evolved somehow from tainted poliovaccines during the 1950s. Ho and Zhu determined that the DNA sequences found by Corbitt and his colleagues were essentially identical to a strain of HIV circulating in the United States during the late 1980s. This raised "the spectre of specimen contamination."[35]

This contamination, the evidence showed, "was more likely to be [caused] by another clinical specimen" than by improper DNA probing techniques. And when additional methods were used to learn more, the New York researchers concluded that the tissues examined were "derived from at least two individuals."

Thus, the Corbitt group's finding was invalidated.

Corbitt, allegedly mystified by what Steve Connor of London's daily *The Independent* called a calculated hoax or mammoth error, later requested the material be reexamined by a third party.[36, 37]

HIV in Zaire in 1959?

Another study supported by grants obtained by Robert Gallo's and Don Francis's colleague Max Essex and his Harvard associate P. Kanki, alleged to have found one HTLV-III (HIV)-positive plasma specimen among 1213 from central Africa dating back to 1959.[38] Much ado accompanied this find especially since it was said to have come from Zaire. Essex's group also reported that the presence of HIV in the sample had been confirmed by three other laboratories using "different techniques." According to the scientific consensus, however, an independent confirmatory test was never done.[39]

The "three other laboratories" that Essex alleged checked his group's work, may not have been impartial. These included: Gallo's lab in Bethesda, Dr. C. Schable's lab at the CDC, and Abbott Laboratories.[38]

Abbott Labs are best known for having licensed and produced: the ELISA screening test for HIV. This test had also been used by Saxinger, Gallo, and others who claimed 60 percent of Ugandan children were infected with HIV by the early 1970s.[40] This report was later debunked by several research groups that noted the esteemed NCI researchers had failed to use HIV specific testing methods or materials.[41-44]

Abbott also licensed and marketed the hepatitis core antigen test purchased by New York City Blood Center officials, following years of delay, and before the ELISA test was available, to help identify blood units suspected of HIV infection. The company had also supplied expertise and the radioactive experimental reagents Szmuness required for his New York homosexual hepatitis B vaccine trial. Furthermore, Abbott Labs ended up commercially marketing MSDs hepatitis B vaccine.[45, 46, 47]

Moreover, the hepatitis B vaccines suspected of having transmitted HIV to American homosexuals, was researched by Abbott's L. R. Overby who was intimately connected to NYUMC hepatitis B chief Saul Krugman. Together, they evaluated hepatitis B susceptibility and vaccination methods in the New York subjects during the mid-1970s.[48]

As it turned out, additional confirmatory studies could not be carried out by independent investigators as the specimens containing the "Leopoldville strain" HIV had been lost by the Essex team.[39]

AIDS Case in 1968?

In 1984, researchers published evidence that "Robert R.," a fifteen-year-old, black, male, heterosexual, born and reared in St. Louis, had died of AIDS-like illnesses.[49] Later, in 1987, scientists provided evidence that the boy's blood contained antibodies to HIV.[50]

"If a virus related to HIV," they concluded, "has been present in the United States, Africa, or elsewhere for several decades, its failure to spread in an epidemic fashion earlier may reflect a recent genetic change in the virus and/or sociocultural factors involving sexual practices or numbers of sexual partners."[50]

By 1990, advanced gene analysis techniques allowed scientists to re-examine this case, at which time they determined that "Robert R." had not died of AIDS. His blood never contained HIV.[39]

This evidence and more led the consensus of international AIDS researchers to conclude that some radical event between 1970 and 1975 had changed the HIV-1 progenitor from a virtually harmless germ, essentially noninfectious to humans, to a silent killer.

Dr. Gerald Myers, chief of the special HIV Sequence Database AIDS Project of the U.S. Government's Los Alamos National Laboratory, may have articulated this position best when he said "the preponderance of evidence still argues for an explosive event in the mid-1970s." Furthermore, regarding the origin of AIDS, he insisted HIV-1 was a fairly new virus, surely only a few decades young.[39]

Alternatively, Ho and other virologists proposed that HIV-1 may have been ancient, but the mass of epidemiological evidence indicates a dramatic change occurred in the 1970s, most likely due to human events more than biological ones in the natural evolution of the virus.[39]

What might those human events have been?

Obviously, they would have needed to take place simultaneously in North America and Africa. An iatrogenic event, involving vaccines being tested on both continents on monkeys and people offers the most plausible, and in fact only, explanation being advanced.[39]

Polio Vaccine Theory of AIDS

Chief among these theories, I learned, is the polio vaccine theory. A fascinating article entitled "Simian retroviruses, polio vaccine, and origins of AIDS" by Walter Kyle sparked a flurry of debate in *The Lancet*.[51] Kyle, a New Hampshire attorney who represented a client who had become paralyzed, apparently from contacting someone who had received the poliovaccine, raised a number of concerns. Chief among them was the fact that live SV40, the simian virus that Gallo, Koprowski, and many others had manipulated for "cancer research," had been known by government officials and vaccine manufacturers to contaminate "all Salk inactivated vaccine" as well as "Sabin's original seed strains." Max Essex and his colleagues, Kyle noted, "reported that the African green monkey, the species used in the production of most live poliovaccine in the U.S., was a reservoir of SIV."[52]

> Presumably the regulatory authorities concluded that the presence of any such monkey virus would not affect man because there would be no transfer from the digestive tract to the lymph and blood systems and because there was no reason to suspect inter-species transfer. At that time this must have seemed correct, otherwise there would surely have been an outbreak in the child recipients of the vaccine.

Thus, government and industry standards overlooked SV40 and SIV vaccine contaminants in the range of 100 viruses per dose.

Kyle then explained that during the mid-1970s, homosexual men in the U.S. were prescribed SIV tainted poliovaccines in efforts to treat their herpes infections. Indeed Kyle's theory was so plausible that researchers around the world, including some ordered by the Food and Drug Administration (FDA), began testing suspected vaccine lots for type-C RNA tumor viruses.

Kyle concluded:

> My hypothesis that the virus particles found in those vaccine lots were HIV (or some variant) can be tested by analyzing stored samples by the polymerase chain reaction (PCR). Reverse transcriptase analyses of released vaccine have shown up positive for such simian viruses up to 1985, and a critical look should now be taken at all such vaccines. If US government laboratories have already done PCR tests on stored samples of the incriminated lots of poliovaccine which remain, the results should be made public.[51]

Several rebuttals to Kyle's controversial report were subsequently published. Some investigators expressed the opinion that "the origin of AIDS is unimportant," and that research time and money might be better spent finding a cure. This led Raphael Stricker and Blaine Elswood, two California scientists, to respond that Kyle's work, though "hardly surprising," was very important for three reasons:

> the sociological reason is that victims of the disease should not be blamed for starting it; the scientific reason is that new therapies for AIDS could be developed from an understanding of its origin; and the ethical reason is that the sequence of events culminating in AIDS should never be allowed to happen again.[53]

Kyle's theory also brought praise and criticism from Thomas F. Schulz of London's Institute of Cancer Research. It was "legitimate to ask whether one advance in medicine, such as the highly successful vaccines against poliomyelitis, might not inadvertently have given rise to another catastrophe, AIDS," he wrote. However, there were reasons why Kyle's theory was questionable. Foremost among these was Schultz's concern that African green monkey immunodeficiency viruses (SIV_{agm}) are "not C-type viruses." They differ significantly from HIV. So much so, Schultz argued, that they would not be suspected of causing human AIDS even though they had contaminated the poliovaccine lots.[54]

What Schultz and *The Lancet* omitted, however, was the fact that "initial reports of the discovery of HIV and SIV classified them as type-C viruses," Kyle relayed during a telephone interview.[55] "Although now called lentiviruses, they go through a stage of type-C morphogenesis during replication and look similar to the type-C viruses."

Additional support for Kyle's theory came in the *Journal of Virology*. "RNA viruses in general, and lentiviruses, in particular, undergo extensive genetic variation as a result of error-prone replication and recombination such that they are considered to exist as 'quasispecies,'" that is, a population of relatives with similar genes.[56] One researcher noted "the exceptional ability of HIV-1 to mutate results in rapid development of quasispecies which evade host defenses and become resistant to various antiviral" agents.[57]

Further supporting Kyle, and relating to Gallo's early work in the development of AIDS-like viruses, researchers later observed that HIV undergoes "type-C morphogenesis. . . . Although not classified as type-C viruses, lentiviruses follow a similar assembly strategy, by which capsid [shell] formation and budding [of the virus from the infected cell] occur simultaneously."[58] SV40's shell, likewise, is called a "capsid," I recalled. Perhaps not coincidentally, then, during the metamorphosis of HIV, researchers found "a reproducible peak of viral protein in the fraction corresponding to a density of approximately 1.15 to 1.16g/ml . . . in gradients of *gag* HIV," that is, the gene that codes for the inner shell, capsid-like structure, of the AIDS virus.[58]

The number "1.16" jogged my memory. Gallo reported it also, but in 1973, after *repeatedly* recovering the same density "virus-like particle" from human leukemic cells that was capable of producing the principal rapidly growing cancers seen in AIDS including sarcomas, leukemias, and carcinomas (see page 75).[59] The FDA's Bureau of Biologics, as Kyle noted in *The Lancet*, also found a similar characteristic in the "adventitious virus" found in some live polio vaccine approved by the FDA and released in 1977.[51]

Could the SV40 capsid have become the "inner shell" of a more complex retrovirus following recombination with SFV, FELV, chicken leukemia and perhaps other viruses? The scientific evidence was mounting.

Furthermore, Shultz explained the differences between HIV-1, HIV-2, and SIV$_{agm}$ and made a very important observation—HIV-2 is virtually identical to a monkey virus found only in *captive* macaques.

> The closest primate relative of HIV-1 is a lentivirus isolated from chimpanzees (SIV$_{cpz}$) and the closest relative of HIV-2 found in free living monkeys is SIV$_{sm}$ from sootey mangabeys. Both HIV-2 and SIV$_{sm}$ are closely related to SIV$_{mac}$ from macaques (a virus found only in captive macaques and *one which may have been transmitted to this species in captivity*). . . . All this means that . . . it is uncertain whether the viral particles observed by electronmicroscopy and reverse transcriptase assays [as Kyle reported in certain poliovaccine lots] were indeed SIV$_{agm}$. They may have represented endogenous retroviruses (*retroviral genomes carried in germline for millions of years and activated and packaged into virion particles under the conditions of tissue culture*).[54] [emphasis added]

In other words, the vaccines may have been tainted with monkey virus genes that for millions of years posed no threat to humans, but had acquired HIV-like capabilities, including the capacity to produce AIDS in humans, while being accidentally or intentionally altered in laboratories during human tissue culture processing.

Therefore, Schulz agreed, that it was important to "take up Kyle's suggestion and examine any remaining vaccine lots by the polymerase chain reaction" that might identify HIV or related lentiviruses.

Significantly, Kyle observes a more recent Ho et al. report that HIV-2 primarily appears in the wild in sexually active adult sooty mangabeys, not in immature monkeys, a fact which additionally discredits the evolutionary origin of AIDS theory.[55,60]

Finally, Schulz commented on the Elswood–Stricker theory that "certain live poliovirus vaccine lots dispensed in Zaire in 1957 to 1960 and prepared on African green monkey kidney cell cultures could have been inadvertently infected with a monkey lentivirus hypothesized to represent the ancestor of HIV-1." While this theory was compatible with the idea that the AIDS epidemic began in Africa, Schulz reiterated his belief that the AIDS agent *could not have been SIV$_{agm}$*. Suspecting, however, a related hybrid or intermediary might have given rise to HIV-1 during vaccine manufacture, he wrote, "it would be of scientific and practical interest to identify the retroviral particles present in some of the poliovirus vaccine lots."[54]

The same might be said for the hepatitis B vaccine lots used on New York's gay men I realized.

Max Essex, HIV-2, and the Origin of HIV-1

Perhaps not coincidentally, then, the discovery of monkey AIDS viruses dated back to the earliest days of the recognized human epidemic. According to Laurie Garrett's text, *The Coming Plague*, in 1969, researchers at the California Primate Research Center in Davis witnessed the first outbreak of AIDS-like symptoms among forty-two macaques. The monkeys suffered severe T-cell immune system depression, lymphomas, Kaposi's-like skin patches, and a host of opportunistic infections. Two similar outbreaks occurred in 1976 and 1978 in the same facility.[39]

Next, Garrett chronicled another French–American AIDS fracas, this time between Luc Montagnier and Max Essex regarding HIV-2 (initially dubbed HTLV-IV by Essex's group and LAV-II by the French).[39]

Essex and colleagues alleged discovering this virus among healthy Senegalese female prostitutes.[61] They reported the women's immune response to HTLV-IV and SIV_{agm} were equally strong. Essex claimed this find was "the missing link" to HIV-1 since it was very similar to the monkey virus, and humanly benign.[62]

Eventually, Gallo published a detailed genetic analysis of SIV_{mac} and HTLV-IV that indicated these viruses were *identical*. Presumably, Gallo's group argued, Essex's laboratory had been contaminated. Monkey and human tissues were somehow mixed.[63]

Yet, how could SIV_{mac} and HTLV-IV/HIV-2—identical new retroviruses, determined to be laboratory contaminants by Schulz, Gallo, and others, with roots in the monkey virus kingdom—be infecting Senegalese women and not macaques in the wild? The laboratory was the only common denominator, I realized. For HIV-2 to infect Senegalese women and *only humans in the wild, not monkeys*, the carriers would have needed to be exposed iatrogenically, that is, by the hand of man. Vaccines were the most plausible way. Particularly since SIV_{agm}, a documented vaccine contaminant, was also present in these women.[51,54]

Later, during the 1996 National AIDS Update Conference, held in San Francisco, I had the opportunity to ask Max Essex, during his press conference, how, other than through vaccines, could HIV-2, a laboratory monkey virus contaminant not found in monkeys in the wild, have gotten into his Senegalese subjects?

After beating around the bush for several minutes unwilling to answer the question directly, he defended, "I can tell you how my monkeys got infected. . . . Researchers had inoculated the monkeys with human tissues during experiments [unrelated to HIV] prior to them coming to my lab."

Though Essex's comment failed to explain just how HIV-1 and HIV-2 got into black Africans and gay Americans in the first place, it did provide an insider's view of human error commonly associated with laboratory contamination, including the threat of viral contaminants being spread from humans to monkeys and back again.

Indeed, the laboratory was the only common denominator, I realized, and experimental vaccines were the most likely transmitter.

The "Big Bang" Theory

Various researchers determined that HIV-2 preceded HIV-1's evolution. As family trees were constructed for these and related viruses based on archeoepidemiology, or what others called molecular epidemiology, scientists concluded the two HIVs shared a recent common ancestor—SIV (or SIV$_{agm}$).[39]

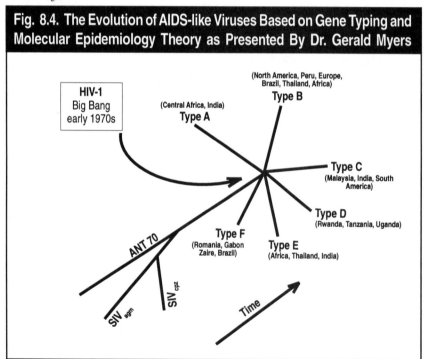

Fig. 8.4. The Evolution of AIDS-like Viruses Based on Gene Typing and Molecular Epidemiology Theory as Presented By Dr. Gerald Myers

Chief of the special HIV Sequence Database AIDS Project at the Los Alamos National Laboratory, Myers stated "the preponderance of evidence still argues for an explosive event in the mid-1970s." Regarding the origin of AIDS, he insisted, HIV-1 evolved fairly recently from SIV$_{agm}$. SV40, the monkey virus Gallo and Bionetics researchers genetically altered in a series of steps and then cultured in human WBCs to alter its outer membrane characteristics, may have been a building block for HIV-2 and HIV-1. Additional evidence suggests that SIV$_{agm}$ may have been man-made as well. Source: See chapter 6, and Myers. G, MacInnes K, and Myers L. "Phenogenetic Moments in the AIDS Epidemic," Chapter 12 in S. S. Morse, ed., *Emerging Viruses* (Oxford, Eng.: Oxford University Press, 1993).

During the 1990s it was discovered that: (1) HIV-1 and HIV-2 were about 43 percent homologous or similar; (2) SIV$_{agm}$ and HIV-1 were also about 43 percent alike; (3) SIV$_{agm}$ and HIV-2/SIV$_{mac}$ were genetically 72 percent alike; and (4) SIV$_{agm}$ and SIV$_{mac}$ envelopes were 91.4 percent homologous.[39]

I considered this information along with the phylogenetic tree developed by Gerald Myers (see fig. 8.4),[64] and realized that Myers's mid-1970s "Big Bang" theory coincided with: (1) the completion of efforts on behalf of the DOD to create AIDS-like viruses for biological warfare; and (2), the work of Gallo and Litton Bionetics researchers as diagramed in figure 6.5.

I wondered whether a similar series of SIV$_{agm}$ cancer virus vaccine experiments might have resulted in the mutations and phylogenetic variations consis-

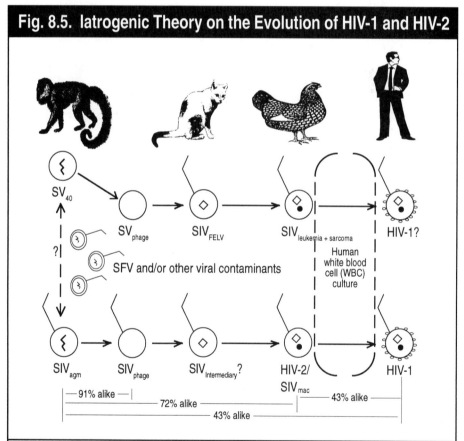

Fig. 8.5. Iatrogenic Theory on the Evolution of HIV-1 and HIV-2

A new theory on the origin of the HIVs from simian virus progenitors modified through laboratory experiments. Diagram shows the HIVs and SIVs most likely evolved from the "type-C" cancer viruses that were genetically altered and then cultured or inoculated into human tissues during cancer virus and vaccine studies conducted by NCI researchers during the late 1960s and early 1970s. These studies were not limited to monkeys, cats, and chickens. Cow, sheep, horse, rodent, and human viruses were also hybridized and likely contaminated laboratory cell cultures and experimental vaccines. This theory best explains how HIV-2/SIV$_{mac}$, a simian virus found only in laboratory and not wild monkeys, was found by Max Essex in Senegalese female prostitutes.

tent with all the findings above, including those reported by Schulz and Kyle regarding the possible iatrogenic origin of HIV-2/SIV$_{mac}$, HIV-1, and AIDS.

I realized that by genetically altering monkey viruses, and monkey virus vaccine contaminants, as many researchers, including Gallo and those at Bionetics, had done *prior* to culturing them in human tissues, they might have created AIDS virus progenitors like SIV, HIV-2, and others to which Schulz and Kyle were referring.

Putting all the facts together, I now understood how humanly benign DNA monkey viruses, like SV40, SIV$_{agm}$, and other common retrovirus vaccine contaminants like SFV, could have, over the period of a few decades, become RNA retroviruses that, through contaminated vaccines, spread to millions of people around the world.

SV40 may have been a building block for SIV$_{agm}$, which was 72 percent identical to HIV-2, and 43 percent like HIV-1. The highly unstable monkey retrovirus SFV, or other possible contaminants, including the leukemia, sarcoma, and immunodeficiency mutants Gallo and others put together, could have easily recombined with SV40, SIV$_{agm}$, or SFV. Together, they might have undergone the laboratory transformations, and vaccine transmissions, resulting in the AIDS pandemic today.

In late 1995, Bill Narayan, a Kansas Medical Center virologist reported a similar transformation in reverse—making SIV, that can cause monkey AIDS, from HIV-1. He used a hybrid of SIV and HIV-1 that contained "the core of the monkey virus and the outer coating of the human virus. This hybrid was supplied by Max Essex's group at Harvard. Narayan's study, funded by "the philanthropic foundation of Hoechst Marian Roussel, Inc., formerly known as Marian Merrell Dow Inc.," was heralded as important for developing a new vaccine against AIDS. The study was later awarded a $1.6 million grant from the NIH.[65]

Indeed, the iatrogenic origin theory of AIDS, the synthetic development of HIV-1, HIV-2, and a host of other killer viruses, seemed most plausible (see fig. 8.5 and discussion in Chapter 6).

After digesting all the facts, I concluded that claims of HIV's existence prior to the 1970s had to be seriously questioned, and those who made them, particularly Gallo and Essex, appeared to have on several occasions incriminated themselves.

Up to my neck in this world of cancer research, scientific misconduct, and counterintelligence, it seemed very hard to distinguish incompetence from duplicity.

Part II
The Political Terrain

Chapter 9
Early Targeting
of Minority America

I returned home from Boston later that evening and gave Jackie an overview of my findings. After digesting the recap, including the scoop on Francis and Duesberg, she asked a question that seemed to come from left field.

"Let's think about this for a minute," she adjured. "What was happening politically around the time cancer viruses first came in vogue? Who was in power?" Jackie, reared in Canada knew little about the politically volatile 1960s and early 1970s.

After a few seconds of considering the question, I replied "The '60s and early '70s were a political nightmare. President Kennedy was assassinated in 1963. The cold war and Vietnam was heating up, and the use of nuclear weapons was on everyone's minds, particularly those at the Defense Department."

"Do you think Kennedy's assassination had something to do with the CIA?" she asked.

"A lot of conspiracy buffs think so. Why? What are you getting at?"

"Military science doesn't evolve in a vacuum. Nor do global epidemics. You remember the famous French microbiologist René Dubos? He considered the powerful influence social and environmental factors wielded on every epidemic. He concluded, "The germ is nothing; the terrain is everything."[1] The world's greatest epidemics have always been preceded by great social/political upheaval. I just want to know who was behind the orders to develop AIDS-like viruses, why, and what was happening politically at the time."

With those questions in mind, the next day, we went to our local library and borrowed several books that provided additional insights into the dark forces at work during Camelot's demise. Soon thereafter, Jackie questioned whether the CIA's alleged involvement in the Kennedy and King assassinations might be linked to the targeting of blacks, or even homosexuals, by those with genocidal motives. Initially, the consideration seemed farfetched. Though now I considered the epidemic iatrogenic, I still had difficulty with the notion of intent. But the more I thought about it, the greater the urge I felt to investigate the possibility. At worst, it would be a great history lesson.

Concluding Camelot

So we began to study the political 'terrain' upon which the Kennedy and King assassinations took place. By the end of this seemingly unrelated investigation, Jackie's proposed link between the politics of Camelot lost and the development of AIDS-like viruses seemed frighteningly plausible.

It was during this bleak period of American history that biological weapons contractors began to realize the possibility of genetically engineered virus delivery systems for untraceable genocide.

Moreover, by the mid-1960s, the checks and balances between the legislative and executive branches of government ceased to function. J. Edgar Hoover's position as "the effigy of anti-Communistic, crime-fighting vigilance" had grown to such an extent that legislative oversight of the FBI and CIA was essentially non-existent.[2]

It was during this period that shadow governors like Hoover began to grossly abuse their freedom with the press. According to New Jersey Congressman Neil Gallagher, ousted as a result of a smear campaign waged by Hoover and his media liaison Roy Cohn, information was "controlled" and "the bastards" were in charge of a multitude of disinformation channels.[2]

The American political system, infected by the most evil forces imaginable—under Hoover, Lansky, and the military/industrial complex—functioned metaphorically like the retroviruses Gallo and his coworkers were about to create. Both macroscopic and microscopic menaces transmitted disinformation and created the many pathological life forms needed to control, grow, kill, and remain undetected.

The military/industrial complex in association with organized crime had overrun the nation's natural immune system—the checks and balances for truth and justice established under the United States Constitution. American government became a cancerous growth that consumed rather than abetted the public's health and welfare.

By the time we finished reading *Citizen Cohn*[2] by von Hoffman, and *Secrecy and Power* by Powers,[3] it was clear the FBI and CIA officials who administered the Communist (Counter) Intelligence Program, the COIN-

TELPRO, were not only plausible suspects in the Kennedy and King assassinations, but in the transmission of AIDS to specific American and Third World populations. We based this seemingly bizarre assertion on the fact that McCarthy mania, which raged overtly during the 1940s and 1950s, continued covertly throughout the 1970s. Most suspiciously, it consumed gays, blacks, and anyone accused of communist inclinations—roughly the same populations devastated by the AIDS epidemic.

The following summarizes what we learned about the early targeting of minority America.

Early McCarthyism and Its Homosexual Focus

In the mid-1940s, as post WWII reconstruction began, Governor Thomas E. Dewey, the New York GOP presidential candidate, accused the Truman administration of harboring sex offenders. GOP Republican party officials, quick to take advantage of the "homosexual angle," mailed thousands of newsletters to party aides explaining that "sexual perverts" were "perhaps as dangerous as the actual Communists" who allegedly supported them. They encouraged a campaign to rid government of the "queers" who had "lodged themselves in the tissues of the bureaucracy."[2]

Soon thereafter, the U.S. Senate formed a special "pervert committee," to investigate the allegations that led to a report charging that homosexuals tend "to have a corrosive influence upon . . . fellow employees. These perverts will frequently attempt to entice normal individuals to engage in perverted practices. This is particularly true in the case of young and impressionable people who might come under the influence of a pervert. . . . One homosexual can pollute a government office," the report said.[2]

By 1952, ninety-one homosexuals had been fired from the State Department allegedly for links to communism and immorality. Such stories dominated the press and fanned fears that affected every government agency. Even the FBI and CIA was stricken with "perverts" and infiltrated by "communists" according to Hoover.[2]

Reflecting on *Deadly Innocence*

More than thirty years of "gay bashing" apparently foreshadowed Dr. David Acer's efforts to get even, I suddenly realized.

It was 1987 when Acer and Edward Parsons viewed Strecker's videotape and learned that in 1978 the allegedly tainted hepatitis B vaccine was administered to more than 1,000 homosexuals as a "Trojan horse" experiment.[4-6]

"But Hoover himself was a homosexual," Jackie argued. "Surely he wouldn't have wanted other gays to be so brutally affected. And he couldn't have had anything to do with the hepatitis B experiments. He had been dead for several years!"

"Right, Hoover died in 1972, but Gallo synthesized AIDS-like viruses in 1970. Hoover controlled the FBI and was a powerful influence in the CIA until shortly before his death. He may or may not have been dead at the time a plan to deal with the "homosexual problem" may have been decided. Either way, it would be naive to think that the political and commercial powers that Hoover represented would have changed their agendas simply because of his death. His extensive intelligence files on domestic and foreign enemies—gays, blacks, and communists—would have been passed on to his heirs.

"And so far as his homosexuality is concerned, Acer was a homosexual too. That didn't stop him from threatening the lives of dozens of other gay men by exposing them to his virus through unprotected sex. There are good and bad people of every background.[6]

"Also, the antics of Hoover and Cohn are well documented." Being farther ahead in my reading than Jackie, given her constant attention to our toddler Alena, I explained, "Cohn, Hoover, and Acer were all 'closet' homosexuals who disrespected other gays. Cohn, in particular, was famous for persecuting homosexuals.[2]

"Surrounded by CIA and FBI officials who, at the time, believed the civil rights movement as well as the gay rights movement was a communist conspiracy to be squelched at whatever cost, Hoover would not likely have defended his sexual preference or interfered with plans to target gays, blacks, or other politically left groups."

"I suppose you're right," Jackie admitted. "It seems that Hoover hated minorities about as much as Hitler. He was also an impassioned power monger who apparently stopped at nothing to destroy his enemies. . . ."

"Right. Given *his* history," I interrupted, "even if he had been alive, he wouldn't have risked being compromised to defend the American gay community."

More "Gay Bashing"

To further substantiate my point, I showed Jackie a segment of von Hoffman's book which noted that persecution against homosexuals discovered in public office was so fierce, many took their lives rather than bear the shame. Examples included the famous English mathematician, Alan Turing, who broke Germany's "Enigma" code during World War II and subsequently contributed greatly to the development of computers. He was arrested for homosexual acts, pleaded guilty, and was sentenced to receive hormone injections. The treatment caused him to become impotent and grow breasts. Shortly thereafter, he committed suicide.[2]

John Montgomery, manager of the State Department's Finnish Desk, suffered a similar fate. He ended his life by hanging himself by a rope tied to the balcony of a Georgetown house he shared with his lover.

Episodes like these reinforced widespread homophobia. As a result, the media exploited the Republican-directed purging of homosexuals in public service. In *Washington Confidential*,[7] a book published in 1951 by Crown, readers were told in Chapter 15, "Garden of the Pansies," that:

> More than 90 twisted twerps in trousers had been swished out of the State Department. . . . [T]here are at least 6,000 homosexuals on the government payroll, most of them known, and these comprise only a fraction of the total of their kind in the city. . . .

> Aware of the seriousness of the problem, the State Department has a highly hush-hush Homosexual Bureau, manned by trained investigators and former counterespionage agents, whose duties are to ferret out pansies in Foggy Bottom. . . . With more than 6,000 fairies in government offices, you may be concerned about the security of the country. Fairies are no more disloyal than the normal. But homosexuals are vulnerable; they can be blackmailed or influenced by sex more deeply than conventional citizens: they are far more intense about their love-life.[7]

It was opinions like these, wrote von Hoffman, that accounted for more than 1,000 annual arrests in D.C. alone during the early 1950s. "Thousands more were forced out of federal jobs in both the civilian and military service, and unknown numbers were refused employment for the same reason. . . ."[8]

Social historian John D'Emilio also wrote about the FBI's involvement in this homosexual inquisition:

The FBI sought out friendly vice squad officers who supplied arrest records on morals charges, regardless of whether convictions had ensued. Regional FBI offices gathered data on gay bars, compiled lists of other places frequented by homosexuals, and clipped press articles that provided information about the gay world. Friendships with known homosexuals or lesbians subjected anyone to an investigation. . . . Postal inspectors subscribed to pen pal clubs, initiated correspondence with men who they believed might be homosexual, and, if their suspicions were confirmed, placed tracers on victims' mail in order to locate other homosexuals.[8]

Though both Hoover and Cohn denied their homosexuality, vulnerability to blackmail was part of the reason they persecuted homosexuals. "In many minds, homosexuality and communism were entwined."[2]

Thus Nebraska's Republican Senator Kenneth Wherry was calling for measures to guarantee "the security of seaports and major cities against sabotage through conspiracy of subversives and moral perverts in government establishments." It was thought by the senator and others that Adolf Hitler had made a "world list" of homosexuals who could be reached and enlisted one way or another for espionage, sabotage, or terrorism. The list was supposed to have fallen into Stalin's hands when the Nazi capital was captured in 1945 and now the Communists were updating and using it. Small wonder that Wherry was moved to tell newspaperman Max Lerner that "You can't . . . separate homosexuals from subversives. . . . Mind you, I don't say every homosexual is a subversive, and I don't say every subversive is a homosexual. But a man of low morality is a menace in the government, whatever he is, and they are all tied up together."[2]

"Oddly enough, 'they' were, to a very limited extent, all tied up together," von Hoffman analyzed. He argued that what we know of civil rights for homosexuals came from the pens of American left-wing radicals, and "especially the anarchists." He recalled that Paul Goodman, an admitted anarchist and bisexual was among the first to argue publicly that "gay might be good."

Anarchism, von Hoffman argued, is tainted with libertarianism, which opposes any form of communist rule. Also on the left, briefly following the revolution, Marxist-Leninism delayed its execrations, tolerating homosexuality for a few years before Stalin outlawed such behavior. So it was that capitalistic and Marxist puritanism marched to the same beat.

Early History of Gay Rights: Links to Communism?

The first, enduring public organization for gays was founded by Henry Hay, an outspoken communist in Los Angeles in 1951—the Mattachine (from the French word *masque*) Society. Hay had tried to follow the communist line of remaining a heterosexual but felt uncomfortable trying to be something he was not. He brought the matter and desire to start the Mattachine to the attention of his higher-ups in the U. S. Communist Party, CPUSA. Here's what Hay wrote:

> About the fall of 1951 I decided that organizing the Mattachine was a call to me deeper than the innermost reaches of spirit, a vision quest more important than life. I went to the Communist Party and discussed this "total call" upon me, recommending to them my expulsion. They rejected "expulsion," and in honor of my eighteen years as a member and ten years as a teacher and cultural innovator dropped me as "a security risk" but [praised me for being] a lifelong friend of the people.[2]

Von Hoffman commented, "it seems that the only thing the Communist Party and the American Government agreed on was that homosexuals were security risks."[2]

> Ultimately, it was an article in the Los Angeles *Mirror*, which provided the Mattachine Society its communist label. The piece stated that the organization's attorney had been an antagonistic witness during House Committee hearings on un-American activities. The reporter theorized that one day, homosexuals, who were "scorned" by the American majority, "might band together for their own protection. Eventually they might swing tremendous political power. A well-trained subversive could move in and forge that power into a dangerous political weapon."[2]

Mattachine members became as alarmed as the newspaper reporter at the "possibility of subversive influences among them," von Hoffman wrote:

> Hay recalled that the men in the organization were straight, middle-class types, who insisted they were exactly like everybody else, except in bed. They had no interest in or sympathy for Marxism, so in short order some Mattachine chapters were proposing loyalty oaths for prospective members; one leader threatened that if the organization weren't sterilized of "communistic" notions, he would give the FBI names of the members.[2]

Cohn's Deadly Denial

"For a young, Jewish, homosexual, anti-Communist prosecutor," von Hoffman continued, "these must have been strange, dangerously confusing, and exciting days." Cohn is remembered as having frequented Washington's gay bars. It is unknown if he considered himself a homosexual. "It appears that for Roy the definition of a homosexual was a man with womanish mannerisms."[2]

During an interview with Ken Auletta in the 1970s, Cohn denied his homosexuality yet became embarrassed and thick-tongued in the process:

> Anybody who knows me . . . and knows anything about me or who knows the way my mind works or knows the way I function . . . would have an awfully hard time reconciling ah, ah, reconciling that with ah, ah, any kind of homosexuality. Every facet of my personality, of my, ah, aggressiveness, of my toughness, of everything along those lines, is just totally, I suppose, incompatible with anything like that. . . . [T]here have always been normal-appearing men who were homosexual [though] never or seldom practiced, while the other type—what you call Teutonic—was not so much in evidence and we knew very little about them and thought they were just trade, you know, the truck driver who enjoyed being had but pretended that he was really interested in women and money.[2]

In the final years of Cohn's life, people from all walks of life pointed angrily to his hypocrisy. "How can the man go on denying what he is?" many asked. Von Hoffman explained:

> [T]here was a recognizable type of manly male, a Roy type, who had sex with other men but did not consider himself a homosexual. . . . That pretension could be a pretending to the self with a young man like Roy who was out to show that Jews were not Communists, but who also had to face the overlap between Communist and homosexualist.[2]

Cohn ultimately died of AIDS.

Black Hate and American Intelligence

The effect of McCarthy mania on the fledgling civil rights movement and the plight of blacks struggling to overcome racial burdens in post-Reconstruction America was onerous.

In the early days following World War II, the National Association for the Advancement of Colored People, the NAACP, approached President Eisenhower with a petition for ending segregation and discrimination in

America's capitol, the District of Columbia. Historian Dorothy K. Newman recorded many of the events during this time:[9]

> Black federal workers were fired for participating after work in NAACP-spon-sored picketing of discriminating retail stores, and on the strength of unproved allegations that they attended Communist-inspired meetings. A black postal worker in Santa Monica, who was also head of the local NAACP, was fired from his job for organizing a drive, after hours, to increase black employment at a local department store. His crime, and that of black postal and govern-ment employees in other states, was simply membership in the NAACP. These were the early Cold War years, and an atmosphere of prying and recrimination pervaded government. . . . In that atmosphere, fighting discrimination became nearly synonymous with disloyalty, and black employees everywhere became especially vulnerable—particularly since there was no need to prove the charges before firing a worker. Time and time again, the NAACP was called on to defend black government workers accused of disloyalty after pressing for black rights.[9]

In keeping with the racist nature of the time, the "first offensive re-search" lab at Fort Detrick, which was just beginning to produce biological weapons, was christened the "Black Maria"—adopted from the old high german term *mare,* meaning the black incubation chamber for evil "ex-ceeding what is natural or regular."[10]

Fears of black communist collusion continued throughout the Kennedy years and beyond. Before being forced to propose comprehensive civil rights legislation because of pressure from northern liberal and southern black leaders, the Kennedys served Hoover's racist agenda.

In 1963, for instance, John Kennedy's Assistant Attorney General Burke Marshall told Martin Luther King that he had to divorce himself from two chief advisors—Stanley Levison, the New York attorney, and Hunter Pitts O'Dell, one of King's executive assistants. The bureau had concluded the two men were communists. "A paid agent of the Soviet Communist apparatus," Marshall called Levison. King resisted the charge and demanded proof. With that, Bobby Kennedy, then attorney general, took charge of the case. He considered the possibility that King—being linked to communists—might bring down the president as well.[11]

In an effort to persuade King to obey, the attorney general mentioned Bayard Rustin, the man A. Philip Randolph had chosen to organize the 1963 March on Washington, who had been a registered communist and had once been arrested for sodomy. Bobby also approached King supporters in an effort to undermine King's leadership. Leaning toward Marietta Tree, a friend and UN delegate, Bobby said, "So, you're down here for that old black fairy's anti-Kennedy demonstration."[11]

When it was clear that King wouldn't be moved by either Bobby or his assistant, the president took over. He asked King to take a walk with him in the Rose Garden, where he put a hand on King's shoulder, something he rarely did, and said: "I assume you know you're under very close surveillance." He mentioned Levison and O'Dell by name and said, "They're communists, you've got to get rid of them."[11]

After the Kennedys

Following the Kennedy and King assassinations, on April 27, 1965, President Johnson's advisor George Bundy requested that Hoover provide information linking blacks and communists to the antiwar movement. At a White House meeting the following day, Johnson told Hoover:

> that he was quite concerned over the anti-Vietnam situation that has developed in this country and he appreciated particularly the material that we sent him yesterday containing clippings from various columnists in the country who had attributed the agitation in this country to the communists as there was no doubt in his mind but that they were behind the disturbances that have already occurred. [The CIA had] stated that their intelligence showed that the Chinese and North Vietnamese believe that by intensifying the agitation in this country, particularly on the college campus level, it would so confuse and divide the Americans that our troops in South Vietnam would have to be withdrawn in order to preserve order here and it would enable North Vietnam to move in at once.[12]

In response to Johnson's concerns and request for expanded intelligence, Hoover ordered his staff to prepare a report for Johnson "containing what we know about the Students for a Democratic Society. . . . What I want to get to the President is the background with emphasis upon the communist influence therein so that he will know exactly what the picture is. . . . I believe we should have . . . proper informant coverage similar to what we have in the Ku Klux Klan and the Communist Party itself."[13]

Shortly thereafter, the black riots in Watts in the summer of 1965, followed by similar aggression in Chicago, Newark, Brooklyn, Cleveland, Omaha, Jacksonville, Baltimore, San Francisco, and finally the "cataclysmic Detroit riots" in July 1967, prompted an expanded attack on the civil rights and black power movements by Johnson, Hoover, and the American intelligence community.

In September 1967, Hoover received word from Attorney General Ramsey Clark to "use the maximum resources, investigative and intelligence, to collect and report all facts bearing upon the question as to whether there has been or is a scheme or conspiracy by any group of whatever size, effectiveness or affiliation, to plan, promote, or aggravate riot activity." In response, Hoover recruited a network of "ghetto-type racial informants"— over 4,000 contacts in a ghetto informant program, which supplied the FBI and White House with intelligence reports about the activities and sentiments of black America.[14,15]

Hoover's response to the race riots of the late 1960s, however, was not limited to intelligence gathering. Dr. King's harassment since 1963 primed the FBI to expand its Communist (Counter) Intelligence Program, the COINTELPRO, into a Cold War against black power. Leaders like Stokely Carmichael who warned "the white establishment" to "move on over or we'll move on over you," and appealed to blacks across the land to "take over" through violence, were attacked like King with death threats and disinformation campaigns designed to discredit them.[14,16]

In an effort to maximize effectiveness and prevent wasted effort, as the Nixon administration took office in the spring of 1968, Hoover set "long-range goals" for the Black Nationalist COINTELPRO, and instructed his agents to:

> 1. Prevent the coalition of militant black nationalist groups. In unity there is strength; a truism that is no less valid for all its triteness. An effective coalition of black nationalist groups might be the first step toward a feared "Mau Mau" in America, the beginning of a true black revolution.

> 2. Prevent the rise of a "messiah" who could unify and electrify the militant black nationalist movement. Malcolm X might have been such a "messiah," he is the martyr of this movement today. Martin Luther King, Stokely Carmichael, and Elijah Muhammed all aspire to this position. King could be a very real contender ... should he abandon his supposed "obedience" to "white liberal doctrines." Carmichael has the necessary charisma to be a real threat in this way.[14,16]

Hoover thus ordered his agents to "prevent militant black nationalist groups and leaders from gaining respectability" and to prevent black nationalist organizations from growing, especially among black youth.[14,16]

In response, the FBI created 360 disruptive operations under the COINTELPRO Black Nationalist Hate Group's umbrella, including the dissemination of media propaganda and some affirmative action programs to dissuade black youth from joining the militant movement. Richard Powers, the author of *Secrecy and Power: The Life of J. Edgar Hoover*, wrote that their counterintelligence campaign included:

> rumors to the media about Elijah Muhammad's sexual conduct, alerting the IRS to possible tax fraud by black organizations, and planting stories that portrayed the 1968 Poor People's March on Washington as dominated by violence-prone radicals. In November 1968, COINTELPRO—Black Hate, concentrated its attention on the Black Panther party, a black radical organization led by Bobby Seale, Fred Hampton, and Eldridge Cleaver that had adopted some of the trappings of the counterinsurgency Green Berets. The Bureau deliberately tried to incite confrontation between this group and its militant rivals within the black radical movement. It has been impossible to prove conclusively that the Bureau was responsible for specific acts of violence, but a Senate investigative committee concluded that "the chief investigative branch of the Federal Government, which was charged by law with investigating crimes and preventing criminal conduct, itself engaged in lawless tactics and responded to deep-seated social problems by fomenting violence and unrest."[14,15]

Black Nationalist Hate

Between 1968 and 1973, even after Hoover's death, the Nixon administration's dirty tricks against blacks gained momentum. Efforts to "expose" Martin Luther King, Jr., persisted more than a year after King's death. Hoover personally directed a conservative attack against King's memory and tried to block attempts to honor the fallen leader. At the same time, the COINTELPRO Hate Groups launched a major offensive against the Black Panther party, the BPP. Having issued the "Panther Directives" aimed at disrupting the BPP, Hoover intensified the Bureau's involvement in the most dangerous COINTELPRO initiative ever launched against any group.[16]

Some anti-Panther operations encouraged violence. In its effort to destroy the 3,000-member-strong organization, the Bureau encouraged local police departments to mount Panther offensives. One such operation led to the deaths of Illinois Panther chairman Fred Hampton and Peoria chairman Mark Clark. The December 4, 1969, raid by the Chicago police department was directed by Hampton's bodyguard, an FBI informant.[17,18]

In the course of attacking Hollywood Panther supporters, including celebrities such as Leonard Bernstein and Peter Duchin, the "Bureau caught an unstable young screen actress, Jean Seberg, in its net."[19,20]

Fig. 9.1. FBI Memorandum From J. Edgar Hoover Regarding the "Negro Question" During COINTELPRO

UNITED STATES GOVERNMENT

Memorandum ROUTE IN ENVELOPE

TO : Mr. A. H. Belmont   DATE: January 27, 1964

FROM : Mr. W. C. Sullivan   J U N E

SUBJECT: COMMUNIST PARTY, USA
NEGRO QUESTION
COMMUNIST INFLUENCE IN RACIAL MATTERS
INTERNAL SECURITY - COMMUNIST

Memorandum 1/23/64 from Mr. F. J. Baumgardner to myself advised of authority given to the Milwaukee Office for a microphone surveillance (misur) to cover the activities of Martin Luther King, Jr., and his associates while in Milwaukee, Wisconsin, where he is scheduled to appear for a talk tonight (1/27/64).

SAC Baker of the Milwaukee Office phoned me this morning to advise that King had arrived in Milwaukee and checked into the Shroeder Hotel as scheduled and that the misur was activated at 10:30 a.m. today. Symbol numbers assigned are   and

Baker also advised that the local police have taken a room close to the suite of rooms engaged by King so that protection might be afforded King. In view of this, it was the conjecture of Baker that the likelihood of King's going ahead with any plans is greatly minimized. I agree with this observation.

Milwaukee is to keep the Bureau promptly advised of all developments and upon receipt of additional information you will be further informed.

ACTION:

None. For information.

100-3-116
1 - 100-106670 (Martin Luther King, Jr.) (JUNE)

1 - Mr. Belmont
1 - Mr. Sullivan
1 - Mr. Baumgardner
1 - Mr. Bland
1 - Mr. Forsyth
1 - Mr. Ryan
1 - Mr. Donohue
1 - Mr. Phillips

WCS:kmj

[handwritten note:] I don't share the conjecture. King is a "top cat" with obscene, degenerate sexual urges.

REC-53

22 FEB 8 1964

Hoover expanded COINTELPRO—his covert anticommunist undertaking—to include attacks on black activists. Martin Luther King, Jr., in particular, was intensively hated and targeted during this period. Hoover's handwritten note here urges his agents to keep close tabs on King, whom he called a "'tom cat' with obsessive degenerate sexual urging." Source: Powers, RG. *Secrecy and Power: The Life of J. Edgar Hoover.* New York: The Free Press, 1987.

Seberg had gotten interested in black radicalism while in Paris pursuing her film career. She had a lover, a North African, who was friendly with the Black Panthers in Los Angeles, and through him Seberg got to know Panther leader Bobby Seale. She became a supporter and financial contributor to the Panthers, and thus a subject of interest to Hoover and the Bureau.

. . . a culture of racism had so permeated the Bureau and its field offices that the agents seethed with hatred toward the Panthers and the white women who associated with them. "In the view of the Bureau" [according to one FBI agent stationed in Los Angeles], " . . . Jean was giving aid and comfort to the enemy, the BPP . . . [and] giving of her white body to a black man was an unbearable thought for many of the white agents."[19,20]

Ultimately, the Bureau targeted the pregnant Seberg with a disinformation campaign through its contacts with the *Los Angeles Times* and *Newsweek*. The slanderous articles ultimately resulted in the premature birth of her child and the baby's death. Three years later, Seberg committed suicide, and her ex-husband, shortly thereafter, also killed himself.[21]

The COINTELPRO attack on Seberg, wrote Powers, was "no different from hundreds of other documented attacks on obscure radicals and their friends, stories that were never told because the victims were not glamorous, not famous, and, in many of the worst cases, not white."[21]

A campaign as vicious and lawless as the one against Seberg proves there was nothing Hoover would not do to destroy black radicalism.[21]

Two other celebrities with black and communist ties marked for foreign and domestic denigration by the COINTELPRO was the French feminist, philosopher, and author Simone de Beauvoir and her lifelong companion, existentialist philosopher Jean-Paul Sartre. The couple served in the vanguard of French intellectual life for nearly four decades, much of the time as members of the French Communist Party.

Between 1961 and 1966, Sartre devoted much of his time to political activity while Beauvoir accompanied him to the Soviet Union on seven different occasions—events considered "a boon for Soviet propaganda." They also visited Cuba and became personal friends of Castro and his closest friend Che Guevara who escorted the couple on their guided tour of the island. On their return trip, Cuban officials planned for the couple to fly via New York.[22,23]

[U]nknown to them the Cuban press attaché had arranged a conference in which Sartre was expected to render a further snub to the United States by praising the glories of Castro's Cuba. He did not disappoint them. . . . Beauvoir [repaid] her Cuban sponsors for their hospitality . . . through an interview in *France-Observateur*, praising Castro as the incarnation of a tremendous emotional power and calling his leadership "not only a success but an example."[24]

Beauvoir, maintained another serious relationship with Nelson Algren, an American communist who was "being investigated by the FBI for his left-wing political activities."[21] The two repeatedly vacationed in North Africa, which is believed to have ignited Beauvoir's love for the African continent. Finally, in 1960, she became an outspoken proponent of Algerian independence from France.[25]

During the next decade, with the increasing threat of Third World revolution on their minds, American intelligence agencies saw Africa struggle to define and assert its native identity. Ultimately, the continent emerged largely socialist, procommunist, and staunchly anticapitalist.

The African American Connection

During the period when the domestic war against black radicals was raging, the African continent became a principal target of COINTELPRO and other covert CIA anticommunist operations.

As early as 1966, the CIA was ordered to "search for alien influence in the antiwar movement." The Johnson and Hoover directive resulted in the launching of "Operation Chaos," which ran from 1966 to 1974. During this initiative, the FBI and CIA agreed to share the fruits of each other's intelligence-gathering labors. Midway through Operation Chaos, the U.S. Army formally established a domestic intelligence section with similar objectives. Orders undoubtedly came from National Security Advisor Dr. Henry Kissinger, who during the Nixon era, personally oversaw major CIA and FBI intelligence operations and directed the military chiefs of staff.[26]

During this operation, "the CIA established a new file or case entitled "Activities of United States Black Militants."

Field offices were instructed to forward to headquarters, by memorandum, information which came to their attention "concerning the activities of United States Black Militants either in the United States or abroad."[27]

The Rockefeller Commission Report on CIA Wrongdoing reported:

CIA's interest [was] primarily to ascertain the details of foreign involvement/ support/guidance/training/funding or exploitation of the above groups or movements, particularly through coverage of the foreign travel, contacts and activities of the Americans involved.

Although the emphasis was clearly on information establishing a foreign link with these groups, the division's field officers were also requested to report—for background purposes—on the purely domestic activities of these groups and their members. The Operation CHAOS representative explained that this purely domestic information was necessary to compile a data base essential to full understanding of possible connections between these groups and hostile elements abroad.[27]

The purpose of foreign espionage efforts in Africa was considered both urgent and multifaceted. Within the highest circles of American government, officials feared that American civil rights groups and militant organizations such as the Black Panthers had received direct aid from communist supporters in Russia, Asia, and Africa. Concern over the exploding Third World population, and the inherent threat this posed to white supremacist ideology and capitalistic expansion abroad, directly influenced the CIA's targeting of the "New Left."[27]

Given this knowledge, the possibility that AIDS-like viruses, once developed by Gallo and coworkers during the early 1970s, may have been used for population control loomed ever larger. This awareness directed our attention to the next area we investigated—population control in the Third World.

Chapter 10
African Foreign Policy
and Population Control

TO the displeasure of American political and corporate interests, by 1970, Africa had succeeded in defining its "culture."[1] Despite a recognized diversity of native beliefs and practices, an anti-American consensus emerged for most African nations that clearly alarmed the entire allied intelligence community.

Jackie and I first became aware of this state of affairs from a 1971 *WHO Chronicle* article. In May of that year, the WHO held its Twenty-Fourth World Health Organization Assembly in Geneva, Switzerland. With Nixon staffers poised to administer the famous Watergate break-ins, COINTELPRO forces expanding widely into foreign capitals,[2] and the CIA beginning paramilitary operations in Zaire and Angola under direct orders from Dr. Henry Kissinger,[3] a spokesman for Africa's political consensus, Professor T. Adeoye Lambo, brought international attention to Africa's need to keep American powers and corporate greed from infecting the "African mind."[1]

"African Culture" and American Displeasure

Lambo's opening remarks before the entire WHO assembly were indeed noteworthy. The Vice-Chancellor of the University of Ibadan, Nigeria, where he was formerly Head of the Department of Psychiatry and Dean of the Faculty of Medicine, Lambo praised socialized medicine, disease prevention, and natural–spiritual healing, as opposed to other forms of health care inspired by western medical industrialists. Openly attacking the American way of life and economically driven medicine, he declared that in contrast to African ways of life:

> men in many advanced countries at the present time are so engrossed in their various occupations, in manufacturing superfluous goods, in buying and selling, in searching for affluence, in accumulating wealth, in altering their environment, in building for the future, and in rushing hither and thither, that they have no time left to wonder what it is all about.[1]

Believing that capitalism led only to mass "disillusionment," Lambo expressed the African position of "doubt whether material prosperity is necessarily synonymous with successful living."[1]

> There is no doubt that this preoccupation with affluence tends to destroy traditional cultures, or at least to transform them.
>
> . . . Yet in all cases the modified cultures weaken dependencies of individuals on family, clan, shrine, and community, and it is this break in the affective bond which is at the root of the contemporary conflict agitating the mind of the African.[1]

Lambo cautioned against the negative "impact of the western style of life, including technology, on the family 'tradition' or 'atmosphere,' its interests and amusements, its resources for occupying and developing rather than repressing the growing mind, its social ideals and customs."[1]

> It is important to remember that the fundamental basis of African cultures attributes all values, categories of thought, and significant content of thought to the group. Because of the nature of this cultural environment, intellectual and affective [emotional] factors are closely interwoven (a form of autoplastic adaptation), but the affective sector predominates and it overshadows the African's life: he does not interpret reality in relation to the temporal environment but in terms of the relations of men to other men, and of men to the supernatural. . . .

Despite acknowledging western medicine's "remarkable development" in providing drugs to combat "infectious diseases and disorders of metabolism," Lambo cited its weaknesses in Africa:

> The patient himself was provisionally ignored; he was merely the incidental battlefield of a bacteriological conflict, or the irrelevant container of fascinating biochemical processes. The prestige of discoveries made along these lines encouraged the injudicious to formulate practically all ailments, even the psychoneuroses, in terms of internal medicine, with no reference to the integrative levels of the instincts, the emotions, the personality, and the ecology.[1]

Largely rejecting western medicine and WHO pharmaceutical campaigns, Lambo urged the adoption of "a well-designed programme of preventive medicine in many fields, involving the social sciences and mental health . . . in order to obviate the necessity of building expensive institutions for curative purposes."[1]

"This must have alerted Afro-American policy analysts and infuriated lobbyists for the American medical–industrial complex," Jackie concluded.

A moment of thought later I replied, "Had the AIDS virus been deployed in Africa through WHO-directed vaccination programs, it would have killed three birds with one stone: The Defense Department could see how well their $10 million biological weapon—HIV—functioned; COINTELPRO forces could put a damper on the alleged black population explosion and the growing communist–socialist–anticapitalist Third World threat; and the pharmaceutical barons and lords of the medical industrial complex could prove to "the African mind" how important germs are while securing the black continent's dependence on western medicine."

Lambo continued his tirade against westernization:

> The state of mind engendered in those most exposed to the stress of rapid social change, as characterized by formal . . . major intrusions of the western style of life, would seem to be compounded [by] various feelings: complete lack of interest in, or lack of capacity to control, events on which well-being depends; overt human responses to change, including anxiety and fear; an extreme sense of insecurity, lack of purpose and direction; severe manifestations of depersonalization and derealization, including confusion of identity; conflicts generated by incompatible values characterized by the sense of social isolation, [and] self-estrangement. . . .[1]

> Africa's development must be based upon a deep commitment to a profound value system, even to the exclusion of affluence. Only in this way can Africa make an important contribution to human civilization. It must retain its identity, its particularity, and its singularity. It is not inconceivable that our relative poverty in Africa may force us to have the courage to find ways and new methods of raising the standard of living of the African, of liberating him from the shackles of disease for creative work, without losing those fundamental human values that are so important for the dignity of man and for the progressive and positive development of his society. I believe that Africa's apparent disadvantages could be converted to a wealth of advantages, thereby becoming the source of its strength.[1]

In retrospect, we realized, it was ironic that Lambo closed by praising the WHO—"there is no organization better qualified and better equipped to attend to these human problems with expert understanding, to guide the transition and adaptations which must attend the introduction of modern technological, economic, and political ideas than the World Health Organization"—the organization that, mounting evidence suggested, played a minor role in developing genocidal germs and possibly a major role in delivering them to the Third World.

The Roots of Third World Foreign Policy

Two years before Lambo's critical remarks before the WHO general assembly, and only days after the DOD requisitioned the $10 million from

Congress to fund the development of AIDS-like viruses,[4] on July 29, 1969, the House Republican research committee task force on earth resources and population, chaired by the Honorable George Bush of Texas, cited the urgent need for population control activities to fend off a growing Third World crisis.[5] Earlier in the week, their committee had heard from General William H. Draper, Jr., national chairman of the Population Crisis Committee, and Dr. William Moran, president of the Population Reference Bureau. Mr. Bush brought the House of Representatives up to speed on their discussions:

> General Draper stated, "Our strivings for the individual good will become a scourge to the community unless we use our God-given brain power to bring back a balance between the birth rate and the death rate.
>
> The governments of Latin American countries realize the significance of their own population growth rates, but cannot politically support family planning programs due to the opposition of the Roman Catholic Church. . . .
>
> General Draper pointed to three areas which are related to population control, which have not been adequately covered: (1) the 1970 and 1971 censuses should be supported on a worldwide basis, (2) contraceptive research should be accelerated both here and abroad, [and] (3) the World Health Organization should step up its proposed international programs. . . .
>
> Referring to a possible trend to liberalize abortion laws, General Draper pointed out that the Executive Committee of Planned Parenthood World Population has adopted a policy resolution claiming that abortion is not a legal matter, but rather one for the husband, wife and doctor to decide without the help of the state.
>
> Col. Frank Borman, the famous [NASA Apollo program] astronaut, added that he personally couldn't see any hope for a meaningful life on earth, "living in a cubical apartment with a bowling alley in the basement."[5]

Borman's anxiety was apparently felt at the highest political levels. Following his speech, population control was thought so urgent that President Nixon "proposed a major transformation in the foreign assistance program of the United States."[6]

Graphic illustrations depicting exploding Third World populations were developed, under USAID contract, and distributed to the press. Samples of these are shown in figs. 10.1 and 10.2.

The president, in his Message to the Congress on Population Matters of July 1969, and then again in April 1971, appealed for more urgent action. Secretary of State William P. Rogers quoted the president who said:

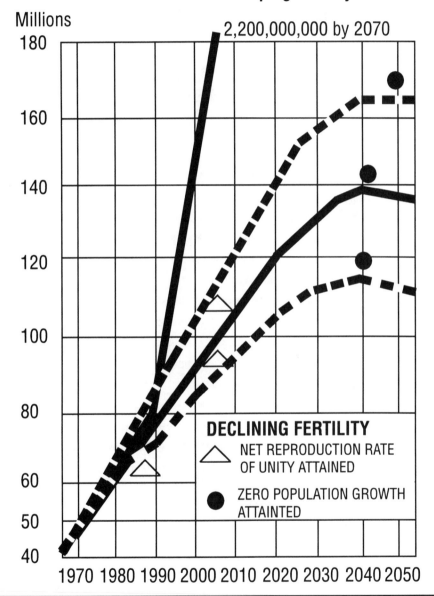

Fig. 10.1. Persuasion Graphic Illustrating An Urgent Need For Population Control in Third World Countries

Momentum of Population
In an Illustrative Developing Country

Millions

2,200,000,000 by 2070

DECLINING FERTILITY

△ NET REPRODUCTION RATE OF UNITY ATTAINED

● ZERO POPULATION GROWTH ATTAINTED

This diagram was presented by Secretary of State William P. Rogers to promote emergency funding of population control programs by the U S Congress. The graphic, typical of the persuasion tools used, depicts theoretical population explosion in an undefined country. Source: Rogers W. P. Report of the Secretary of State, U.S. Foreign Policy 1971, Washington, D.C.: U.S. Govt. Printing Office, Dept. of State Publication 8634, 1972, p. 325.

Fig. 10.2. One of a Series of Persuasion Graphics Intimating the USA Would Be Overrun By Third World Populations

Birth Rates in Selected Developing Countries: 1965 and 1975

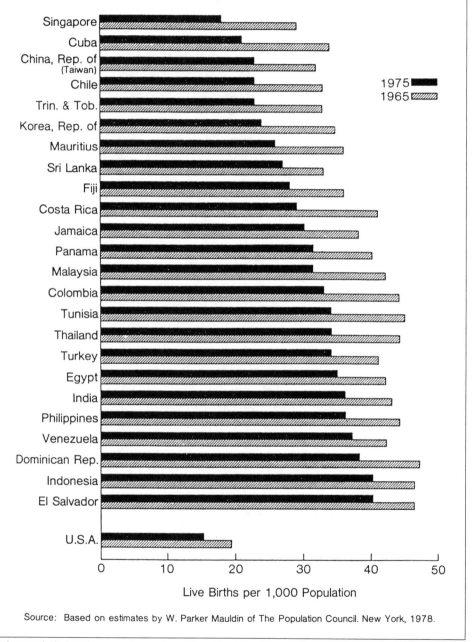

1975 ■
1965 ▨

Live Births per 1,000 Population

Source: Based on estimates by W. Parker Mauldin of The Population Council. New York, 1978.

Another graph designed to promote an alleged threat to national security interests from "exploding" Third World populations. This chart was one of dozens prepared by a Washington, D.C.-based consulting firm under contract with USAID. Source: *Department of State Bulletin.* World population: The silent explosion—Part 2 (of a three part series which ran Oct.–Dec.), November, 1978, p 8.

"... few subjects will so deeply affect the lives of this and future generations as the challenge of population growth. It is important also that we recognize the need to meet this challenge with an extreme sense of urgency. The momentum already built into the world's population growth means that delay in acting now will greatly increase the burden of the problems which must be borne later.

"But if our people, with your educational help, and if all the peoples of the world will join in doing what is needed without delay, then mankind may indeed successfully surmount this serious challenge.

"Otherwise, I truly fear the consequences for all of humanity."[6]

All these warnings came during Nixon's first term in office when Third World military advantage, economic development, health policy, and population control were lumped together under one foreign policy umbrella over which Henry Kissinger ruled.[7]

Not long after Bush gained added congressional support for Third World population control programs, Nixon stressed that economic progress in Africa was vital to western world interests. As the Vietnam War was winding down, the "energy crisis" was revving up, and Americans waited in long lines for gas. Soon thereafter, Nixon reported to Congress:

Our interest in supporting Africa's development efforts rests on many bases. . . . We also believe a developing African economy will mean expanding potential markets for American goods. Moreover, Africa is becoming a major source of energy for the United States and Western Europe. . . .[7]

To stress America's humanitarian deeds, Nixon added:

The United States can be proud of its record of direct development assistance to Africa. We have assisted Africa both through bilateral aid and by contributing over 30 percent of the funds provided to Africa by international agencies. . . . In 1972, our bilateral and multilateral aid was $600 million—up from $550 in 1971 and $450 million in 1970. . . . Two thousand four hundred Peace Corps volunteers are currently serving in Africa. . . .[7]

American direct *private investment* in Africa, Nixon recalled, had about doubled between 1968 and 1972, "reaching a total of $4 billion." American firms, Congress was told, have been a "conduit for the transfer of skills, resources, and technology" to the region. "The productive impact of these enterprises" was seen by the administration as "the most direct as well as the most reliable outside stimulus to the raising of living standards in developing Africa. . . ."[7]

Nixon also hailed America's response to Africa's health and education needs. For decades, he said:

Americans have worked—through private and voluntary agencies and public programs—to help Africans combat illiteracy, starvation, disease, and the effects of natural disasters. We can take particular pride in our contribution to a major seven-year campaign to control smallpox throughout Central and West Africa. Working with the World Health Organization and twenty African Governments, we helped virtually to eliminate the disease from the area. We are continuing efforts to reduce the prevalence of measles in the area [again, through vaccination programs]. . . . [7]

"Where civil strife has occurred, the United States" Nixon added, "has responded with generosity and impartiality" to the basic needs of the people living in Africa's war-torn areas. He cited as examples, once again, central African countries, including those hardest hit by the AIDS epidemic—Ethiopia, Nigeria, Zaire, and Sudan.[7]

Nixon also cited Burundi and Uganda, wherein American diplomatic efforts were still in progress. Both countries were also in the AIDS belt of central Africa, and both were adjacent Zaire.[7]

The president concluded his speech this way:

The United States continues to enforce—more strictly than many other countries—an embargo on sales of arms to all sides in South Africa and in the Portuguese territories. While we favor change, we do not regard violence as an acceptable formula for human progress.[7]

We soon learned that this last remark—including both arms sales to the region, and nonviolent conflict resolution—was, respectively, a complete misrepresentation of the facts and a downright lie.

Sahel African Disaster Relief

Six months after President Nixon articulated his administration's African foreign policy objectives before Congress, Maurice J. Williams, the Deputy Administrator of USAID and the president's Special Coordinator for Emergency Relief to Sub-Sahara Africa, submitted a report to the president summarizing his agency's "Disaster Relief and Recovery Assistance for Sahel Africa." The response was allegedly needed in the wake of "immense devastation and dislocations" that had occurred due to a regional drought. He noted that widespread starvation had been averted because of "relief food and medical supplies from the U.S."[8]

We have sent a special AID [Aid for International Development] Task Force to the area to help design concrete programs of action to cope with drought-related problems. . . .

Nutritional problems, particularly for women and children, are a growing concern. U.S. epidemiologists from the Center for Disease Control have helped identify pockets of distress. In response we are supplying medicines, vitamins, blankets, shelter and specially fortified foods for these camps. . . .[8]

The World Bank made available a special, "flexible credit" program. Other major donors included the Germans, French, Canadians, and European Economic Community.[8]

Williams reinforced U.S. willingness to help Africa's drought-stricken nations with "both technical and material resources in meeting the region's needs." Specifically, Williams said he had engaged:

—NASA to explore the use of such advanced technology as the Earth Resources Technology Satellite [ERTS] and Sky Lab to analyze from photos the cropping and water resource potential;

—Massachusetts Institute of Technology [MIT] to analyze major development options for this region;

—the National Academy of Sciences [NAS] to provide scientific advisory services covering a spectrum of disciplines during the recovery period.[8]

"All this for drought relief?" Jackie questioned.

Apparently not. The following month, the *Department of State Bulletin* published statements by David D. Newsom, Assistant Secretary for African Affairs. "We have a clear and compelling interest in the natural resources and markets of Africa on terms consistent with Africa's independence," Newsom said. "We need energy fuels and . . . we need development and expanding markets for our products." And in an effort to secure such African treasures, Newsom recommended "new foreign aid legislation" that emphasized "areas of particular importance to the African countries: agriculture, population and health, and education and human resources."[9]

Kissinger's Comments

Henry Kissinger, however, best articulated America's motivation for granting African assistance in the broader context of world affairs. Speaking before the House Committee on Foreign Affairs on June 4, 1974, Secretary Kissinger said America's foreign policy assistance program served a larger "global situation in which America must pursue its national interests." He envisioned world "peace sustained by the growing realization on the part of all nations that they have a stake in stability and that stability is insured by acting from a sense of justice and moderation." In such a world, he said, "all nations would share the benefits of stability, and all would have an incentive to maintain it through cooperation."

Americans have a vital stake in the realization of this prospect. In a world made interdependent—by nuclear weapons, instant communications, and a global economy—Americans can preserve their security, their values, and their prosperity only by nurturing the shoots of stability and cooperation. Our policies are shaped to that purpose. . . .[10]

Next, the foreign affairs director cited the "unprecedented opportunity for American diplomacy . . . to make progress on the central issues which have threatened world peace. . . ." He stated that "hopes for a peaceful, cooperative, and just international order can only be realized with the strong participation of this nation. . . ." He also said "security and economic assistance programs" were "essential instruments as we seek to shape a cooperative international order that reflects our interests."[10]

Kissinger then discussed his "foreign assistance and security proposals for fiscal year 1975," which he proposed would place us in a better position:

—To enlist the developing nations' cooperation in sustaining an open global economy;

—To promote a long-term balance between demand for goods and their supply; and

—To be responsive to the concerns of countries and areas of importance to us. . . .[10]

Regarding his "security assistance programs apart from those in Indochina and the Middle East," Kissinger stated "long-term food, population, and education programs," and the International Development Association (IDA), which concentrates on the needs of the poorest" nations was especially needed in Latin America and Africa.[10]

We must provide adequate credit levels to our friends and allies as we reduce direct government assistance. The foreign military sales program promotes the self-sufficiency we seek and our partners are pursuing.[10]

Military Buildup in Zaire

The following year, Kissinger again appealed to a House committee for foreign security assistance funding. This time he cited "two significant programs" that were addressing the needs of African "partners." Since "stability in the Horn of Africa" had "wider geopolitical meaning, . . . to help maintain that stability" he proposed "$12.6 million in grant aid and $10 million in credits for Ethiopia, a strategically located nation."

"Zaire," he explained, needed "$19 million in credits to help modernize its forces and meet its legitimate defense needs in view of increased threats to its security, particularly that posed by the instability in Angola. Our aid," he concluded, "would help meet a defensive force need recommended by a U.S. military study team after careful observation and consultation with the Zaire military."[11]

Congress typically granted Kissinger everything he alleged Zaire needed in terms of military hardware and "humanitarian aid," including one NASA ERTS-Zaire reconnaissance station. The project, which required a written treaty, was signed by Zairian and American officials on January 6, 1975 (see fig. 10.3).[12]

The Silent Explosion

A few years later, shortly after George Bush's retirement as CIA director,[13] the State Department issued a three-part series of publications entitled "World Population: The Silent Explosion."[14] The reports, accompanied by a series of graphs, predicted disastrous effects of the burgeoning Third World populations on the world's resources.

"Nearly 2 billion people in developing countries are continually undernourished, with resultant low vitality, vulnerability to disease, and low life expectancy," the State Department said. "A 1977 U.N. Food and Agriculture Organization (FAO) survey found that in 23 developing countries, per capita daily caloric supplies, in fact, declined between 1961-63 and 1972-74. . . . The FAO estimates that food deficits for developing countries (excluding Communist Asia) can be expected to increase fivefold between 1970 and 1990."[14]

The Carter administration's report continued:

> It is sometimes said that there is no food problem, only a population problem. This is an oversimplification—there would be food problems in many developing countries even if their populations were suddenly much reduced. But, unquestionably, the severe undernourishment of two-fifths of mankind is attributable, in major part, to the handicap of too many mouths to feed. And the number grows daily.[14]

"That's clearly a mixed message," Jackie observed. "On the one hand, the officials were citing the need to provide more aid to feed and immunize

4964   *U.S. Treaties and Other International Agreements* [29 UST

A.I.D. Project No. 660–0059

Project Loan Agreement

Dated JANUARY 27, 1977

Between

THE REPUBLIC OF ZAIRE (*"Borrower"*)

And

THE UNITED STATES OF AMERICA, ACTING THROUGH THE AGENCY FOR INTERNATIONAL DEVELOPMENT (*"A.I.D."*)

ARTICLE 1: The Agreement

The purpose of this Agreement is to set out the understandings of the parties named above ("Parties") with respect to the undertaking by the Borrower of the Project described herein, and with respect to the financing of goods and services needed for the Project by the Parties. Annexes I and II [1] are integral to this agreement.

ARTICLE 2: The Project

SECTION 2.1. Definition of Project. The Project which is further described in Annex 1 shall identify major factors of environment and traditional crop production techniques, including transportation and marketing methods in the project area, which adversely affect Zaire's ability to achieve self-sufficiency in maize production, and attempt to develop new techniques, or to modify existing production techniques, so as to increase substantially maize yields. Under the Project the system will consist of six components as follows:

(a) A Sub-system for Research and Extension Operations under which goods, services and training will be financed to establish a research and training center where basic farming systems in use in the Project Area will be replicated, agronomic research will be conducted, innovations will be tested for dissemination to farmers, and agricultural assistants will be trained in collaborative extension methods emphasizing maximum farmer involvement.

[1] Not printed herein. Annex II is deposited in the archives of the Department of State where it is available for reference.

MEMORANDUM OF UNDERSTANDING

BETWEEN

ERTS-ZAIRE

AND THE

UNITED STATES NATIONAL AERONAUTICS AND SPACE ADMINISTRATION (NASA)

1. The purposes of this agreement are to set forth the responsibilities of the parties and the procedures for providing for: (a) direct access, by a ground station to be built and operated in Zaire by ERTS-Zaire, to NASA ERTS-1 and ERTS-B satellite data and to the data from any future ERTS experimental satellites which NASA may launch, and (b) availability to NASA of data acquired by the Zairian station pursuant to (a) above, subject to the provisions which follow.

2. For its part, ERTS-Zaire will use its best efforts to:

    (a) Develop and operate a facility near Kinshasa, Zaire for acquisition and processing of ERTS data as well as other non-space data of interest to ERTS-Zaire entirely at its own cost, including the cost of the necessary communication links with the NASA ERTS OCC/NDPF (Operations Control Center/NASA Data Processing Facility) at the Goddard Space Flight Center.

    (b) Provide during Phase B, as described below, processed data to ERTS Principal Investigators duly selected by NASA whose test sites are in range of the Zairian data acquisition station for the period of coverage promised to them and under the same conditions as NASA provides data to Principal Investigators. Should another country in the region establish ERTS facilities, ERTS-Zaire's obligation to provide data to Principal Investigators in that country will terminate as soon as the new facilities are capable of providing this service. ERTS-Zaire will continue to serve Principal Investigators in countries within range of the Kinshasa Station which do not have ERTS facilities, unless and until alternative arrangements are concluded.

(c) Provide, to the best of its ability, any support requested by NASA in a spacecraft emergency condition, such as the provision of data indicated in paragraph 2(e) below, should the on-board tape recorders fail.

(d) Provide quarterly reports in English to NASA on the progress and results of the ERTS-Zaire experimental program with respect especially to the ability to apply data and analyses obtained to real-time decision making, and the principal applications made.

(e) Make available to NASA, on a cost-free basis and in the NASA-preferred format (negative imagery format with identifying annotation) such copies of the ERTS data it acquires and processes as NASA may request in reasonable quantities (except in emergency conditions as noted in paragraph 2(c) above). These data provided to NASA by ERTS-Zaire will be made available to the public from US sources on precisely the same terms as data acquired directly by NASA. These provisions apply as well to selected duplicate computer compatible tapes. Public requests (for data) from the area covered by Kinshasa Station will be referred as appropriate to ERTS-Zaire, or to other regional facilities which may be established in the area. Coordination among such facilities would be highly desirable.

(f) Include as output data from the Kinshasa Station computer compatible tapes (CCT's) and 70mm roll film.

3. For its part, NASA will use its best efforts to:

(a) Program ERTS-1 and any subsequent experimental ERTS-type satellite to acquire data in areas accessible for direct read-out by the Zairian Station. The frequency of such programming will be subject to mutual agreement by the Project Managers (see below). It will be limited to test purposes in Phase A, and expanded as agreed in Phase B.

(b) Provide to ERTS-Zaire as necessary antenna pointing elements for acquisition of the ERTS spacecraft transmitted signal and updated definitive orbital information for use in processing the data.

(c) Process, on a time-available basis and as may be agreed by the Project Managers, a limited number of data tapes acquired by the Zairian Station in Phase A for initial evaluation and calibration of the station's performance.

(d)   Provide, during Phase A, ERTS data to any
NASA-selected Zairian Principal Investigators to the
extent of the time-coverage promised for them.

(e)   Make available, for comparison purposes, a
limited number of selected NASA data tapes covering
portions of the area accessible to the Kinshasa Station.

(f)   Keep ERTS-Zaire informed of other prospective
ERTS facilities in the area so that regional coordination
can be effected.

4.   The course of the project will be divided into two
phases.   Phase A is for the test and checkout of the
Kinshasa Station.   Phase B is for the following period
of routine data acquisition and processing at the
Kinshasa Station.   Phase A will begin when the Project
Managers agree on the readiness of the technical and
operational interfaces required to carry out the project
and on a schedule for accomplishing Phases A and B.   Phase A
will be concluded and Phase B begun by mutual agreement
of the Project Managers.

5.   To implement the agreement, ERTS-Zaire and NASA will
each designate Project Managers to be responsible for
coordinating the agreed functions and responsibilities
of each side with the other.   The Project Managers will
be co-chairmen of a Joint Working Group which will be
the principal instrument for assuring the execution
of the project and for keeping both sides continuously
informed of the project status.   The Joint Working Group
may establish such committees as required to carry out
the project.

6.   The following additional understandings are confirmed:

(a)   ERTS-Zaire will resolve any radio frequency
difficulties in the region to the satisfaction of the
parties concerned so this cooperation can proceed without
difficulty.

(b)   The responsibility for spacecraft control, health
and status will remain with NASA throughout the program.

(c)   There will be no exchange of funds between
ERTS-Zaire and NASA for ERTS-1 operations.   This agreement
assures ERTS-Zaire access to the ERTS-B satellite without
charge for a six month period from the date the ERTS-Zaire
ground station begins to acquire ERTS data.   It is understood,
however, that NASA may thereafter establish some cost-sharing
arrangement, such as users' fees, for participating Ground
Stations.

(d)   It is understood at this stage that NASA cannot make a firm commitment for future ERTS-type satellites.

(e)   Decisions taken by the International Telecommunications Union require that radio frequencies for future operational ERTS satellites will differ from those currently used for experimental satellites.

(f)   It is understood that ERTS-Zaire and the other Zairian agencies participating in the program will pursue an ERTS open-data policy comparable to that of NASA and other US agencies participating in the program, particularly with respect to the public availability of data.   ERTS-Zaire will thus ensure unrestricted public availability of the earth resources satellite data at a fair and reasonable charge based on actual cost.

(g)   Training and exchange of technical personnel will take place as mutually agreed.

(h)   ERTS-Zaire and NASA will freely share and exchange technical information as mutually agreed, and consistent with the export regulations of the two countries.

(i)   It is understood that this project is experimental in character and subject to change in accordance with changes in technical requirements and opportunities.

(j)   ERTS-Zaire and NASA may each release general information to the public regarding the conduct of their own portion of the project as desired and, insofar as participation of the other agency is concerned, after suitable coordination.

(k)   ERTS-Zaire and NASA will assure that the project is appropriately recorded in still and motion picture photography, and that the photography is made available to the other agency upon request for public information purposes.

(1)   It is understood that the ability of ERTS-Zaire and NASA to carry out the responsibilities of this agreement is subject to the availability of appropriated funds.

7. This Memorandum of Understanding shall enter into force upon signature by ERTS-Zaire and NASA and shall continue in force for four years, subject to extension as may be agreed by ERTS-Zaire and NASA.

For ERTS-Zaire

_____

BISENGIMANA RWEMA,
Directeur du
Bureau du Président

Date : 31 janvier 1975.

For the National Aeronautics
and Space Administration

_____

James C. Fletcher
Administrator

1/6/75
_____
Date

TIAS 8129

Source: Department of State. Memorandum of Understanding Between ERTS-Zaire and the United States National Aeronautics and Space Administration (NASA). Diplomatic List. Washington, D. C.: U. S. Governement Printing Office, (1977) 1975 pp. (4964) 1700-1704.

the starving and diseased masses. On the other hand, if the starving masses died, there would be less of a problem."

I agreed.

Superficially, chief administrators of USAID reconciled the conflict this way. "Neither death nor birth control action can or should proceed far independently, the one without the other."[15]

This message was initially advanced and clarified during a policy statement made during the Nixon administration by USAID mass immunization program analyst Dr. R. T. Ravenholt:

> The confluence of needed policy change, adequate fiscal resources, large numbers of trained and experienced personnel, more effective means of controlling fertility, and more effective program strategies (distilled from far-flung program experience) provides a strong basis for optimism that highly effective fertility control programs and activities will soon be operating in all countries to counter any too-rapid population growth that might otherwise result from highly effective mass immunization programs.

> As one now fully engaged in work concerned with fertility-control programs in developing countries, I do not view the promise of more effective control of microparasitic disease by immunization with alarm; I look upon such disease and death control programs as partners in our common endeavor to move traditional societies from their inefficient pattern of high birth rates balanced by high death rates to a modern and more efficient developmental pattern of low birth and death rates.

> Neither death nor birth control action can or should proceed far independently, the one without the other. Together they can provide a sound basis for the achievement of man's ultimate goal—a prosperous and peaceful world in which everyone will have the best possible opportunity of attaining his own unique potential.[16]

Later, the Carter administration's State Department published a related report expressing more clearly their fundamental national security concern:

> In centuries past, millions of poor have accepted their lot with resignation and political apathy. This situation is changing, as expanding communications instill greater awareness that there can be a better life. Some can be expected to seek radical prescriptions in violence, including terrorism. There is real danger that violence will grow and spread unless more effective means can be found for improving conditions of life for the masses.

> Overpopulation has been an underlying factor in certain international conflicts and major internal disorders. This danger continues and may intensify as populations burgeon and the scramble for scarce raw materials intensifies.

> Such pressures seem destined to produce an increasingly turbulent and dangerous international environment for the pursuit of peace, stability, and improved conditions of life for all people.[14]

"WHAT IS BEING DONE?" [Emphasis not added.] The report explained:

> To a large extent, farsighted, public-spirited private individuals and organizations have taken the lead in sounding the alarm and initiating national and international population programs. The United Nations and its concerned specialized and associated agencies, including the World Bank, have become more and more involved. In mid-1974, a U.N.-sponsored World Population Conference was held in Bucharest. The conference adopted a World Population Plan of Action (WPPA) which reflected a consensus of 136 participating governments and which stands today as a charter and beacon for effective, morally, and culturally acceptable population policies and programs. (The Holy See did not participate in the consensus.)
>
> The WPPA . . . advocates a two-pronged approach in which development is pursued in mutually reinforcing conjunction with population programs.
>
> Such population programs have come to center in two broad areas—motivation of couples to desire small families and the provision of modern family planning services.[14]

The report explained organized efforts to advance activities in these two areas. Then the role of the United Nations was articulated:

> The U.N. Fund for Population Activities (UNFPA) is the largest multilateral source of external funding for population action programs in developing countries. In its 9 years' existence, UNFPA has provided over $250 million in support of more than 1,200 population projects in more than 100 countries. In 1977 the Fund's annual budget, obtained from voluntary contributions, exceeded $100 million. The major donors have included Canada, Denmark, the Federal Republic of Germany, Japan, the Netherlands, Norway, Sweden, the United Kingdom, and the United States. [Essentially the NATO alliance, I quickly realized.] The United States in recent years has provided about 30% of total UNFPA funding.
>
> Most of the projects that UNFPA supports are implemented through organizations and specialized agencies of the U.N. system, acting in their respective fields of competence. Among these are the U.N. Office of Technical Cooperation, the U.N. Development Program (UNDP), World Health Organization (WHO), [the] U.N. Children's Fund (UNICEF) . . . [and others].
>
> The World Bank and its soft-loan affiliate, the International Development Association (IDA), entered the population assistance field in 1968. This reflected the Bank's conviction that rapid population growth is a major barrier to the economic and social progress of many developing countries. Supported projects have included a widening range of activities relevant to an effective population program. Assistance is provided on conventional Bank terms or, in the case of especially weak economies, on highly subsidized soft-loan terms. [Meaning repayment was not required.][14]

Bilateral assistance, the report continued, came from the NATO countries and Japan. The U.S. program comprised about "two-thirds of the total over the 1965-78 period," and the entire operation was "administered by the Agency for International Development (USAID)."[14]

And who were the "voluntary" contributors funding the lion's share of the operation? The State Department said:

> The United States has provided substantial financial support, through USAID, to a number of NGO's [non-governmental organizations] in recognition of the need for many-sided efforts for effective overall population assistance to developing countries. The Ford and Rockefeller Foundations have been major supporters of world population programs since 1965.[14]

Califano on Health and Population Control

In May 1978, shortly before the AIDS epidemic began, Mr. Joseph A. Califano, Jr., Secretary of Health, Education and Welfare, headed a U.S. delegation to the 31st assembly of the WHO in Geneva.

Califano's role as government lawyer and "public health policy educator" began shortly following his receipt of a law degree from Harvard in 1955. Over the next decade, he served as special assistant to the general counsel of the DOD, special assistant to the secretary of the Army, general counsel for the Army, and then between 1964 and 1965, he became special assistant to the secretary, and ultimately, deputy secretary of the Defense Department.[17]

"It is my honor to speak today," he said, "as the first Cabinet officer ever to head the U.S. delegation to the World Health Assembly. I come as President Carter's personal emissary to underscore the commitment of the Government and people of the United States to the World Health Organization (WHO)."[18]

The expert in health and military justice then reviewed the WHO's achievements and challenges. The achievements, he said, "striking as they are, are dwarfed by the unmet challenges that confront us."

Chief among the unmet challenges Califano noted, besides food and water shortages and infectious diseases, was rapid population growth, which "retards social and economic progress in many nations and burdens many families and communities."[17]

To help resolve these woes, he pledged activities that "will be conducted in close cooperation with international agencies, and in partnership with other nations." The emphasis, he said, "will be on prevention of ill health, including malnutrition and infectious diseases. Our own national resources will be more fully mobilized—our universities, industries, and private organizations—and we will coordinate more closely the various international health activities within our government."[17]

Regarding America's role in international health, "President Carter announced publicly his intention to strengthen the role of the United States in international health," Califano said. "We want to commit new resources to the battle against infectious diseases. The United States is already deeply involved in combating the major infectious diseases." He cited the tropical diseases, including cholera and diarrheal diseases, and malaria. "To this end, we are conducting significant work to develop a malaria vaccine . . ."

Califano continued his address explaining it was his intention to improve research in countries where tropical diseases were a problem. The NIH and the WHO he said would collaborate in developing a "global epidemic surveillance service," and that this was "indispensable" for public health. "We stand ready to help the World Health Organization develop a program for training physicians and field officers from developing countries," he said. Then he mentioned that "Tropical Disease Research Centers" would be established in two countries in particular—Ndola, Zambia and Kuala Lumpur, Malaysia.[17]

Zambia, we realized after surveying a map, lies between Zaire and Angola, just below the militarily active Shaba region of Southern Zaire. We noted the timing and placement of the NIH/WHO "global epidemic surveillance outpost" here just before the AIDS epidemic.

Yaws, Califano said was another controllable infectious disease, though it resurged in several African and Asian countries. In one African country, reported cases had risen "from less than 3,000 in 1969 to more than 70,000 in 1976." It appeared to be increasing in 12 other African nations.[18] This admission seemed odd as I considered the period coincided with increased USAID and WHO public health research, education, and vaccination programs. One might have expected less of this most treatable disease, especially with such a sharp focus on African health at that time. "Why the 1,000 plus percent increase?" I asked Jackie rhetorically.

Then he said:

The expanded program on immunization is an endeavor we believe highly important. . . .

In the developing world, despite the fact that effective vaccines exist, less than 10% of the children receive immunizations against preventable diseases. . . . Our concern for these preventable diseases abroad has led us to develop bilateral immunization programs in cooperation with the World Health Organization—programs designed to help countries strengthen their own preventive health capacities.

We stand ready to go beyond our present participation in WHO's immunization program by increasing the numbers of our epidemiologists and other international health workers available to join in the efforts of developing nations. Moreover, I can announce that, in addition to the services we are already providing, we will make available a further $200,000 in direct support to the WHO expanded program on immunization through a contribution to the Voluntary Fund for Health Promotion [VFHP]. Our Agency for International AID [USAID], in cooperation with my own Department, is exploring with WHO the possibility of undertaking a multiyear immunization program for the African region.[18]

Califano then called for joint efforts to achieve one overriding objective—"to immunize the children of the world by 1990." There could be no greater gift to the next generation," he cheered, than to celebrate this event as it came to pass.[18]

The public celebration Califano anticipated, however, never occurred. There were those, though, who in 1990 found cause to celebrate. AIDS had devastated many of the most populated areas of central Africa.[19]

Repackaging Population Control

During the Fall of 1994, Jackie, Alena, and I visited friends and family in San Francisco. There, in a newsstand adjacent Fisherman's Market, I came across an issue of *Covert Action Information Bulletin* that contained a fascinating article by British journalist Helen Simons entitled "Repackaging Population Control." The article, which we read on the plane ride back to Boston, explained that despite official claims to the contrary, African overpopulation was not a prime motivation behind family planning and maternal and child health programs.[19-21] Nor was population control even a desire among African women.

As Nicholas Eberstadt, foreign policy analyst for the American Enterprise Institute for Public Policy Research, noted, "in most of sub-Saharan Africa it is infertility—not unwanted pregnancies—that women rank as their top priority." The fate of barren women throughout the region, he continued, "is a pitiable one. . . . While fertility enhancement in the industrialized north is a multi-billion dollar industry, little attention is accorded to the population problems that most concern Africans themselves."[21]

For almost four decades, we learned, Third World countries had held American population control policies accountable for diverting attention from the central problem—too much poverty, not over-population.[22] Many leaders charged that such policies were "nothing short of blackmail and coercion directed against the people of the Third World."[19] Linda Gordon, author of *Woman's Body, Woman's Rights: A Social History of Birth Control in America,* argued:

> Coercive population control is stimulated and then made acceptable by racism. . . . Nonsensical ideas about the cheapness of life among Asians and highly documented analyses of the different structure of the black family such as matriarchal theory have served to justify coercion to reduce non-white birth rates.[23]

This view predominated during the first United Nations conference on population control held in Bucharest in 1974. The meeting ended in shambles after delegates from Africa, Latin America, and Russia denounced the entire concept of Third World population control as imperialist and racist.[23]

To make her point, Simons quoted Pentagon consultant and National Defense University associate dean Gregory D. Foster who wrote:

> [P]olicy makers and strategic planners in this country, have little choice in the coming decades but to pay serious attention to population trends, their causes and effects. Already the United States has embarked on an era of constrained resources. It thus becomes more important than ever to do those things that will provide more bang for every buck spent on national security. . . . [Policy makers] must employ all the instruments of statecraft at their disposal (development assistance and population planning every bit as much as new weapons systems).[24]

Alternative Views of Population Policy

Despite the State Department's hailing of the Bucharest conference as consensus building, it was in reality an "embarrassing failure." In its wake, U.S. policy makers scrambled to reformulate population control strategies as discussed in a secret National Security Council report published four months later.[20,25]

The document suggested new language be used. It warned against actions that gave the appearance that "the policy was directed against the Less Developed Countries." Instead, it recommended the use of leverage through more neutral organizations like the U.N. and NGOs to assist developing countries "in integrating population factors in national plans, particularly as they relate to health services, nutrition, agriculture, education, social services, organized labor, women's activities and community development." In essence, population control was repackaged to overcome the opposition.[20,25,26]

The report revealed the true motives underlying the representational changes in U.S. foreign population control policy:

> The U.S. can help minimize charges of an imperialist motivation behind its support of population activities by repeatedly asserting that such support derives from a concern for: a) the right of the individual to determine freely and responsibly their number and spacing of children. . . . and b) the fundamental and economic development of poor countries.[26]

Thus, the tarnished image of U.S. population control policies in the Third World largely ceased. It was replaced by the perception that America sought only to promote basic rights for women. In doing so, it became possible to present population control as a legitimate concern for developing countries. International feminist groups, NGOs, and foreign leaders all endorsed the principals and practices of "family planning."[20]

Over the next two decades, U.S. population policy makers repeatedly refined their messages so that family planning activities and their impact would be more broadly accepted. A USAID commissioners' report urged that population activities "should be integrated with maternal and health care delivery." The move was motivated by concerns that USAID programs "only increase suspicion in the host country" if they were too narrowly focused on family planning.[20,27,28]

"Since the mid-1970s," Simons wrote, "much of the aid from Western governments, the World Bank, and the European Union has been channelled through" NGOs that "are prepared to toe the line on population control."[20] Thus, American-backed donor agencies, including AID and the World Bank, have used their economic power to influence NGO policy.[29,30]

> The World Bank, which was present [at the September 5-13, 1994 Cairo, Egypt 'International Conference on Population and Development' meeting] . . . in full force, . . . emerged as a major funder of population control. During 1969-70, it only spent $27 million on population programs. In 1987, the then president promised to increase the amount to $500 million by 1990. In 1993, it had already shot up to $1.3 billion. [Additional funds are] . . . now promised to jack it up further to an annual $2.5 billion by 1995.[20]

A position paper transmitted over the Internet entitled, "Was Cairo a step forward for Third World women?" by Drs. Vandana and Mira-Hiva, warned:

> The World Bank has cleverly redefined the "population and development" sector as "population and women," thus making invisible the destructive impact of its policies on the lives of Third World women and ironically appearing as a champion of women's rights.[20]

Simons also noted, when appeals for stricter "maternal and child health policy" failed, environmental concerns were then successfully used to "dress up old racist rantings."[20] Their argument was eloquently expressed in an article in *Atlantic Monthly* by author, Robert Kaplan:

> Mention "the environment" or "diminishing natural resources" in foreign-policy circles and you meet a brick wall of skepticism or boredom. To conservatives especially the very term seems flaky . . . [but] it is time to understand "the environment" for what it is: the national security issue of the early twenty-first century. The political and strategic impact of surging populations spreading disease, deforestation and soil erosion, water depletion and possibly rising sea levels in critical overcrowded regions like the Nile Delta and Bangladesh—developments that will prompt mass migration and in turn incite group conflicts—will be the core foreign policy challenge from which most others will ultimately emanate.[31]

Thoreau's warning darted through my mind—"Nothing is so much to be feared as fear."[32]

Simons concluded:

> Wrapped up in the language of women's empowerment and environmental concerns, the establishment's old arguments about there being too many non-white babies in the world have finally won the day.[20]

RAPID Disinformation and Deterioration

Betsy Hartmann, Director of the Population and Development Program at Hampshire College and author of *Reproductive Rights and Wrongs: The Global Politics of Population Control and Contraceptive Choice* (New York: Harper and Row, 1987), noted the World Bank's key device for administering population policy was "leverage over other forms of development finance." She noted that governments often burdened by massive foreign debt are persuaded to "devalue their currency, privatize their industries, open their doors to foreign investment, freeze wages, raise food prices, slash social services *and* implement Bank-sanctioned population programs."[28,33]

Hartmann reported that the Futures Group, a Washington, D.C.-based consulting firm was funded by USAID to develop RAPID (Resources for the Awareness of Population Impacts on Development), the source of the alleged disinformation seen in figs. 10.1 and 10.2.[19]

RAPID analyses urged Third World economies to follow a Western-style development model and thus become dependent on external markets and Western technology. For example, in Zaire's eastern neighbor, Tanzania, a RAPID study concluded the country must abandon traditional labor-intensive farming for more "scientific and commercial agriculture." The report warned that the ensuing population growth and "entry of large numbers of new workers into the agricultural sector" hinder the country's development since "traditional patterns of small holder production with land-intensive and resource-intensive cultivation" are probably not "the most feasible means of employing so many additional people."[34]

Unfortunately, RAPID consultants failed to look in their own backyard—the heartland of America—to predict this policy's most tragic outcome. Jackie and I discussed the fact that once upon a time, American families who worked their farms, were bonded by the labor and service to society. Generally speaking, family farmers maintained a great sense of purpose. Most appreciated God for providing nature, and therefore the family, its sustainance. The social and work environments supported family values as families depended on one another to survive. When automated farming methods forced many small farm owners to sell their land, the vast majority of family owned farms were lost. This also forced many families apart. Children left home to earn a living elsewhere. This added to the country's political burdens, not the least of which is the perceived breach in family values.[35] As Lambo predicted 1970, what might happen if western capitalists were allowed to dictate African economic policies and "development," happened in America—mass disillusionment accompanied by the destruction of traditional cultures, the preoccupation with money, and a weakened dependence on "family, clan, shrine, and community."[1]

Women's Rights or Malthusian Eco-Fascism?

Before concluding, Hartmann provided an example of USAID's "cavalier" approach to population control in disregard of health and safety.[29] The use of Norplant was cited:

> Developed by the *Population Council in New York*, Norplant is a progestin implant system inserted under the skin of a woman's arm, which prevents pregnancy for at least five years. Common side effects of Norplant include menstrual irregularity, headaches, nervousness, nausea, acne and weight gain. Both insertion and removal require local anesthesia and medical skill. Ethical use of the drug depends on adequate medical screening and follow-up, and most importantly on access to removal on demand.

> An internal Population Control report provides chilling evidence of how Norplant has been misused in the Indonesian population program. Nearly half million women have had Norplant inserted, often without counseling on side effects, alternative contraceptive options, pregnancy screening, or proper sterilization of equipment. Many have not even been told that the implant must be removed after five years to avoid increased risk of life-threatening ectopic pregnancy.

> Moreover, removal on demand is not guaranteed, not only because of lack of trained personnel, but more importantly to serve the . . . government's demographic objectives. According to the Population Council report, "Recent government policy encourages use of Norplant for the duration of the full five years of effectiveness, which is communicated to the client as a form of commitment. . . ." Or as one Indonesian population official put it, "People are told it has to last five years, they give their word . . . and rural people don't go back on their word. If they request removal, they are reminded that they gave their word."[28,36] [Emphasis added]

Hartmann then noted, "coercive use of Norplant is not restricted to the Third World." Similar programs in California, Kansas and Texas have been proposed or sanctioned for use in special populations.[28,37]

Finally, in addressing what she considers "Malthusian Eco-Fascism," Hartmann considered the moral decay of population strategists, among whom Dr. Maurice King established prominence in Britain. King, in *The Lancet*, endorsed what Hartmann adversely labeled "a 1990s variant of triage: try family planning, but if it doesn't work, let the poor die because they are an ecological menace."[28]

According to King, in countries where there is unsustainable pressure on the environment from overpopulation, "such desustaining measures as oral rehydration [a simple lifesaving method of treating diarrheal disease] should not be introduced on a public health scale," he concluded, "since they increase the man-years of human misery, ultimately from starvation. . . . Such a strategy needs a name," he wrote. "Why not call it HSE 2100—Health in a sustainable ecosystem for the year 2100?"[37]

Why not call it "MEF—Malthusain Eco-Fascism," Hartmann rebutted after contacting Dr. King in Leeds to confirm that his statements in *Lancet*—believed by some to have been a parody—were "dead serious."[28]

Hartmann concluded:

In much of Africa where AIDS threatens tragic human and demographic consequences, the present emphasis on population control and de-funding of health systems amount to indirect triage—no less morally repugnant than Dr. King's twisted vision.[19]

Some extremist U.S. ecologists go so far as to see AIDS as a blessing. According to a letter from "Miss Ann Thropy" printed under an open-letter policy in *Earth First!* journal, "If radical environmentalists were to invent a disease to bring human population back to ecological sanity, it would probably be something like AIDS. . . . We can see AIDS not as a problem, but a necessary solution. . . ."

Fig. 10.4. Selected USAID Summary Reports Regarding Immunization and Population Control Programs in Africa Between 1963 and 1980 Including Funding Data for Fiscal Years 1973 and 1974

Table 4   Funds obligated for A.I.D. activities and amount and percentage for health, population and nutrition projects by country or other allocation, Africa Region, FY 1973 and FY 1974.

FY 1973

Allocation	Total	Health Population & Nutrition	Percentage for Health, Population & Nutrition
	(thousands of dollars)		
Total	162,143	20,572	13.0
Regional	15,600	5,161	33.0
Botswana	57	–	–
Cameroon	80	–	–
Central Africa Republic	188	–	–
CWARP*	17,200	1,472	9.0
Chad	109	15	13.7
Dahomey	126	–	–
East Africa Regional	962	–	–
Ethiopia	8,800	4,821	55.0
Gabon	30	–	–
Gambia	45	15	33.3
Ghana	21,433	1,034	5.0
Ivory Coast	35	–	–
Kenya	12,200	155	2.0
Lesotho	111	11	9.9
Liberia	16,100	1,372	9.1
Malawi	155	49	31.6
Mali	27	–	–
Mauritania	84	24	28.5
Mauritius	26	–	–
Morocco	11,700	510	5.0
Niger	84	19	22.6
Nigeria	10,600	830	8.0
Rwanda	74	11	14.8
Senegal	65	5	7.6
Seychelles	5	–	–
Sierra Leone	75	–	–
So. Africa Reg. OSARAC	20,623	510	3.0
Sudan	11,000	–	–
Swaziland	107	49	45.7
Tanzania	7,200	3,064	43.0
Togo	119	–	–
Tunisia	2,465	1,019	41.3
Uganda	1,120	125	11.1
Upper Volta	115	–	–
Zaire	3,592	301	8.3
Zambia	35	–	–

*Central West Africa Regional

```
COUNTRY       :  Central West Africa Regional
Project Name:  Measles Control - Smallpox Eradication
Project No.  :  625-11-510-116
Contract No  :  AFR (HA) 18-67
Began        :  Fiscal Year 1963
Estimated Termination Date:  Fiscal Year 1974
```

Description:

This project was designed to assist 20 West and Central African countries in the eradication of smallpox and the control of measles.

Smallpox is one of the most lethal diseases known to man and in Africa kills approximately 25% of those stricken. The smallpox portion of the project represents a U.S. contribution to the global program sponsored by the World Health Organization (WHO) to eradicate the disease throughout the world. The measles portion of this dual campaign was intended to reduce a major cause of death and disability among young Africans.

Technical direction of the project was carried out for A.I.D. by the Center for Disease Control of the PHS under a PASA. Commodities were provided by A.I.D. through grant agreements with the Organization for Cooperation and Coordination in the Fight Against Major Endemic Diseases (OCCGE) and by the Organization for the Control of Endemic Diseases in Central Africa (OCEAC). Planning and operations in West Africa were coordinated by the OCCGE and by the OCEAC, by the governments of participating countries and with WHO, as required.

Phase I included one mass smallpox vaccination of the entire population of the 20 countries and a simultaneous measles vaccination of all susceptible children between the ages of six months and six years, later reduced to four years in most countries. Phase II was limited to a maintenance program consisting of smallpox vaccinations for persons not vaccinated in Phase I, and surveillance.

Phasing out of U.S. assistance began in FY 1971. During this period U.S. advisors were engaged in activities aimed at bringing about an orderly transition of the program into health services of the participating countries. The project was concluded in FY 1974.

Funding:

```
FY 1973 - No grant funds were obligated by A.I.D.
FY 1974 - No grant funds were obligated by A.I.D.
Total through 6/30/74:  $24,248,000
```

```
COUNTRY      :  Central West Africa Regional
Project Name:  Onchocerciasis Control Program
Project No. :  625-11-510-908
Began        :  Fiscal Year 1974
Estimated Termination Date:  Fiscal Year 1980
```

Description:

This program is aimed at alleviating human suffering and at rehabilitating the onchocerciasis infected areas. Onchocerciasis (river blindness) affects over one million persons in the zone covered by the proposed control program (a river basin area shared by Dahomey, Ghana, Ivory Coast, Mali, Niger, Togo and Upper Volta). Fear of the disease has led to abandonment of extensive areas of fertile river valleys in the Volta River Basin. These valleys are badly needed for production of staple food supplies.

In July 1968 a conference convened by WHO with the West Africa OCCGE and AID concluded that control of the disease was technically feasible. Following that conference the seven governments of the affected Volta River Basin area confirmed their desire to participate in an onchocerciasis program.

A Preparatory Assistance Group prepared a plan of work to achieve control of the disease in the affected zone and to work out expected costs and benefits of the scheme. At the end of June 1973, the World Bank and WHO, the fiscal and executing agencies for the proposed program, convened a preliminary meeting in Paris of the participating African countries, interested donor Governments, and concerned international agencies for purposes of organizing the programming and implementation of an international effort with regard to onchocerciasis. Total costs for the twenty-year control program are estimated at $120 million. The total cost for the first six years is estimated at $54 million. The Onchocerciasis 1974 Fund Agreement was promulgated, in which initial funding of $7.5 million has been committed by Canada, France, the Federal Republic of Germany, the Netherlands, the United Kingdom, the United States, the WHO, UNDP, and the World Bank. The total U.S. contribution to the six-year phase of the program is estimated at $8.2 million, or not to exceed 20 percent of total program costs. The participating governments will provide the program with full support including priority consideration for socioeconomic development in the sectors freed from onchocerciasis.

Funding:

FY 1974 - $2,000,000 grant funds were obligated by A.I.D.
Total through 6/30/74 - $2,000,000

ZAIRE

FY 1973 Foreign Assistance funds totaling $3.592 million were obligated for A.I.D. activities. Of this amount, $301,000 was obligated for one health project, Maternal and Child Health, 660-11-531-049.

In FY 1974, $1.087 million was obligated for A.I.D. activities which included $336,000 for the above project.

HEALTH, POPULATION AND NUTRITION
AFRICA REGION
FY 1973 - FY 1974

Area	Project Number	Title	Contractor Loan No.	FY 1973 Funds	FY 1974 Funds
Regional	698-11-490-363	Labor Project		1,605,000	1,775,000
Regional	932-11-570-360	Univ. Teaching of Population Dynamics	U. of N. Carolina AFR 797	600,000	500,000
Regional	932-11-570-374	Marketing Research	Population Services Inc. AFR 827	245,000	---
Regional	932-11-580-166	Regional Population Support	AAMC, csd-1171	435,000	---
Regional	698-11-580-189	Regional Population Planning	Pathfinder Fund AFR-575	---	---
Regional	698-11-580-346	Regional Population Planning	Population Council AFR-629	---	---
Regional	932-11-580-358	Maternal and Child Health Extension	Univ. of Calif. (Santa Cruz), ORT AFR-799	685,000	---
Regional	932-11-580-359	Family Planning Courses in Health Training Institutes		1,180,000	---
Regional	932-11-580-373	MCH & FP Training and Research Development	Meharry Med. Col. AFR-373	796,000	---
Regional	698-11-590-381	Science Health Care	African American Scholars Council AFR-1076	---	82,000
Regional	932-11-570-337	Regional Demographic Survey Workshop	Bureau of Census	15,000	---

15

Area	Project Number	Title	Contractor Loan No.	FY 1973 Funds	FY 1974 Funds
Regional	698-11-999-135	Howard University Conference	Howard U. AFR-G-1077	---	35,000
CWAR*	625-11-510-116	Measles Control/Smallpox Eradication		---	---
CWAR*	625-11-540-510	Regional Public Health Training	U. of Pittsburgh AFR-756	461,000	549,000
CWAR*	625-11-550-531	University Center for Health Sciences		80,000	---
CWAR*	625-11-590-904	Strengthening Health Delivery Systems		1,011,000	436,000
CWAR*	625-11-510-908	Onchocerchiasis Control		---	2,000,000
CWAR*	625-11-550-809	Albert Schweitzer Hospital		---	1,000,000
Chad	677-11-580-500	Special Population Activity		15,000	---
Ethiopia	663-11-510-006	Malaria Eradication	(L) 663-H-013C	4,800,000(L)	---
Ethiopia	663-11-530-170	Training in MCH Care		21,000	---
Gambia	635-11-580-200	Special Population Activity		15,000	45,000
Ghana	641-11-580-055	Danfa Rural Health Development/ Family Planning	U.C.L.A. AFR-697	800,000	740,000
Ghana	641-11-580-064	Population Program Support		234,000	224,000
Ghana	641-11-590-068	Rural Health Management Services		---	340,000
Kenya	615-11-580-141	Population Dynamics		155,000	335,000

*Central West Africa Region

16

Area	Project Number	Title	Contractor Loan No.	FY 1973 Funds	FY 1974 Funds
Lesotho	632-11-580-500	Special Population Activity		11,000	19,000
Liberia	669-11-540-054	National Medical Center	DHEW/IHS PASA AFR 36-85	1,276,000	1,274,000
Liberia	669-11-540-110	Maternal and Child Health Training		96,000	---
Malawi	612-11-580-500	Special Population Activity		49,000	48,000
Mauritania	682-11-580-500	Special Population Activity		24,000	---
Morocco	608-22-521-096	Water Supply	608-H-040 (L)	---	---
Morocco	608-11-570-109	Demographic Research Center	U. of N. Carolina csd-2495	200,000	140,000
Morocco	608-11-580-112	Family Planning Support		310,000	270,000
Niger	698-11-580-500	Special Population Activity		19,000	5,000
Nigeria	620-22-521-720	Ibadan Water Supply	(L) 620-H-004	---	---
Nigeria	620-11-580-789	Family Health Training	Johns Hopkins U.	830,000	225,000
Rwanda	696-11-580-500	Special Population Activity		11,000	51,000
Senegal	685-11-580-500	Special Population Activity		5,000	5,000
Southern Africa Regional	690-11-540-932	Maternal & Child Health, Family Planning Training	Meharry Med. Col. AID/CM/pha C-73-8	510,000	74,000

Area	Project Number	Title	Contractor Loan No.	FY 1973 Funds	FY 1974 Funds
Somali	649-52-520-037	Mogadiscio Water System	(L) 649-H-005	---	---
Swaziland	645-11-580-500	Special Population Activity		49,000	15,000
Tanzania	621-11-580-121	Manpower Training Project (MCH Aides)		3,064,000	1,165,000
Togo	693-11-580-500	Special Population Activity		---	17,000
Tunisia	664-11-580-224	Family Planning		870,000	562,000
Tunisia	664-11-560-255	Food and Nutrition: Lysine Fortification Study		149,000	347,000
Uganda	617-11-570-057	Program Assistance Grant, Maternal and Child Health Training		125,000	---
Zaire	660-11-531-049	Maternal and Child Health		301,000	336,000
Zambia	611-11-580-500	Special Population Activity		---	29,000

18

The above selected items show a wide array of contractors, including The Population Council of the City of New York, and related projects, including several called "Special Population Activity." The word "special," in intelligence circles, typically indicates "secret" or "covert." Source: *Report on the Health, Population and Nutrition Activities of the Agency for International Development.* Department of State for Fiscal Years 1973 and 1974. U.S. Government Printing Office, Washington, D.C. 1975

Chapter 11
Henry Kissinger's
"New World Order"

NOT long after our return to Boston, I needed to fly out to the west coast again to give a presentation in Bellingham, Washington. The following day, while killing time at the Village Bookstore, a discounted hardcover caught my eye—*Kissinger* by Walter Isaacson.

At the time, Jackie was spiritually engaged in *The Celestine Prophecy.* Following our San Francisco trip, she had relinquished her investigative chores for a good reason. We were pregnant. On entering her first trimester, a naturally protective maternal instinct arose. What we had so far discovered in our search of the origin of AIDS was so disturbing that the stress, we feared, might have an adverse effect on our developing child. Our concern was magnified by the fact that Jackie had miscarried twice during the past year. The intensity of our *Deadly Innocence* investigation that exposed the Florida dental AIDS cover-up, sifting through stacks of sickening testimony, obtaining and analyzing FBI reports on dozens of serial killers, and the constant reminders from caring friends and loving family that we were placing our lives at risk, would have scared off any soul searching for the comforts of a nurturing womb. It was obvious she'd be better off focusing her attention on more soothing subjects. So as I purchased *Kissinger,* I knew I would be perusing it alone.

From this point on, though Jackie maintained an interest in the investigation, and frequently asked about my ongoing discoveries, what had been largely our cooperative labor was now my sole passion.

Trauma and Escape From Nazi Germany

I found Isaacson's book fascinating. The meticulously referenced text quickly taught me that Heinz Alfred Kissinger had been a key player in U.S. foreign policy from the late 1950s to the time of this writing. Naturally the author began by reviewing Kissinger's early history.

Henry Kissinger was the first-born son of German Jewish parents—Louis and Paula. The couple led their family to freedom in August 1938, less than three months before the Kristallnacht riots destroyed most of the Jewish institutions in Nazi Germany.[1]

"My life in Fürch seems to have passed without leaving any lasting impressions," Kissinger told a German reporter more recently. "That part of my childhood is not a key to anything." Minimizing the trauma he faced as a fifteen-year-old refugee, the statesman added, "I was not consciously unhappy. I was not acutely aware of what was going on. For children, these things are not that serious."[2]

Give me a break. I thought on reading this. He's either got to be kidding or steeped in massive denial.

I too was a first-born son of a German Jewish father and Austrian mother who were also fortunate to have survived the holocaust. I could relate to Kissinger's plight better than most. Given this background, plus my postdoctoral degree in behavioral science, I understood well the role persecution can play on the development of personalities and personality disorders.

My mother, at age sixteen, was among the last group of Jews to leave Nazi Austria. Her immortal picture can be seen in The National Holocaust Museum, where she, among dozens, was photographed on her knees, scrubbing the streets of Vienna at Nazi gunpoint. She along with her brother, who was thirteen at the time, and the other refugees in our family never forgot those nightmarish days. Understandably, they lived a largely paranoid life. My mother and I argued for decades about what I judged (perhaps in retrospect incorrectly) to be her unjustified paranoia that Nazis could once again assume power and control over world events.

Though Kissinger may have been spared the worst, I found it incomprehensible that he could have left Nazi Germany, at that age and time, unfazed.

Denial and Paranoia

I was not alone in this view. Kissinger's childhood friends also felt his denial was a form of "self-delusion." Isaacson wrote:

> Some of them see his escape from memory as a key to his legendary insecurities. The child who had to pretend to be someone else so that he could get into soccer games, they say, became an adult who was prone to deceit and self-deception in the pursuit of acceptance by political and social patrons. . . .[1]

Whereas Kissinger's childhood friends recalled numerous traumas, young Heinz allegedly felt nothing. "We couldn't go to the swimming pool, the dances, or the tea room," Werner Gundelfinger said. "We couldn't go anywhere without seeing the sign: *Juden Verboten*. These are things that remain in your subconscious." Frank Harris argued, "We all grew up with a certain amount of inferiority." Otto Pretsfelder added, "You can't grow up like we did and be untouched. Every day there were slurs on the street, anti-Semitic remarks, calling you filthy names."[3]

"The Hitler Youth, which included almost all the children in Fürch, sang in ranks in the streets and paraded in uniform, and Henry and his brother would watch them, unable to understand why they didn't have the right to do what others did," recalled Lina Rau Schubach.[4] "Anti-Semitism was a feature of Bavaria and did not start with Hitler," Menachem Lion added. "We didn't have much, if any, contact with non-Jewish children. We were afraid when we saw any non-Jewish kids coming down the street. We would experience things that people couldn't imagine today, but we took it for granted. It was like the air we breathed."[5]

Despite Kissinger's denials, the Nazi atrocities "were able to damage his soul," said Fritz Kraemer, a German gentile who resisted Hitler and later became Kissinger's student in the U.S. Army. "For the formative years of his youth, he faced the horror of his world coming apart, of the father he loved being turned into a helpless mouse."[6]

Kissinger's most obvious personality traits, Kraemer argued, could be traced to his Nazi experience. "It made him seek order, and it led him to hunger for acceptance, even if it meant trying to please those he considered his intellectual inferiors."[6]

His drive for social acceptance, and his paranoid tendencies were both reasonable reactions to a childhood "violated by one of the most gruesome chapters in human history." As a result, during his career, he was often known to compromise his beliefs to impress those he feared.[7]

For Kissinger, the Nazi experience severed the connection between God's will and historic evolution—a basic principle of the Jewish faith and one of its most important contributions to Western philosophy. For faithful Jews, historic meaning is linked to divine justice. After witnessing Hitler's horror, Kissinger abandoned his religion and embarked on an intellectual journey to find an alternative way to interpret history.[8]

Kissinger's traumatic childhood also instilled in him "a deep distrust of other people." He felt compelled to establish secret wiretaps on the phones of even his closest aides.[9]

Another symptom of Kissinger's holocaust rearing was his tendency to disguise, as an adult, any sign of personal weakness. This consistent compulsion of his had been commonly observed; particularly in his approach to foreign policy negotiations. Kissinger's father, "whom he loved deeply, was graced by gentleness and a heart of unquestioning kindness. But such virtues served only to make him seem weak in the face of Nazi humiliations." Thus, as Kissinger matured, he "repeatedly attached himself to forceful, often overbearing patrons with powerful personalities," including Nelson Rockefeller and Richard Nixon.[9]

Still another childhood legacy was his "philosophical pessimism." He maintained a dark and verboten world view "suffused with a sense of tragedy." He embraced the view that civilization's tendency is toward decay, and "statesmen must continually fight against the natural tendency toward international instability."[9]

> The Nazi experience could have instilled in Kissinger either of two approaches to foreign policy: an idealistic, moralistic approach dedicated to protecting human rights; or a realist, realpolitik approach that sought to preserve order through balances of power and a willingness to use force as a tool of diplomacy. Kissinger would follow the latter route. Given a choice of order or justice, he often said, paraphrasing Goethe, he would choose order. He had seen too clearly the consequences of disorder.[9]

As a result, Nixon's secretary of state became a philosophical, intellectual, and political conservative. He developed an intuitive aversion to change through revolution and became "uncomfortable with the passions of democracy and populism." In essence, Kissinger never embraced "the messy glory of the American political system" particularly since it constrained his "realpolitik" approach to administering foreign policy.[9]

Throughout his career, Kissinger confronted a recurring tension that in his view existed between realism and morality. Survival, he argued, at times required that moral standards be disregarded. This he noted was "inconceivable" to people who had lived "sheltered" lives. He contrasted the callous realist, who survived, with "the men of high morals," who, during rough times, had no chance. In his later years, Kissinger equated moral sensitivity to personal weakness.[10]

Chief Intelligence Officer and Nazi Hunter

When the 84th Infantry Division received its order to embark for Europe in September 1944, private Kissinger was with the 335 Infantry Regiment. Six years after his escape from Hitler, he and his G Company invaded Germany though he never fired a shot.

Thanks to Fritz Gustav Anton Kraemer, a proud aristocratic German expatriate who took a shining to the overflattering private, Kissinger was soon assigned to a safer position in General Bolling's Army Intelligence unit. Kraemer got him assigned to translate for the general, and "instigated his selection as a chief administrator overseeing the occupation of captured towns." In essence, Kraemer paved Kissinger's way "into the Counter-Intelligence Corps." From there, he was selected to teach "military intelligence" in Germany.[11]

During his German stint in Army Intelligence, Kissinger refrained from expressing any animosity toward the Germans. "In fact," his biographer noted, "he reserved his anger for those Counter-Intelligence agents—particularly Jews—who gave vent to anti-German feelings. "I remember one occasion when some of these refugee interpreters were being a little abusive to a civilian couple," one army colleague, Ralph Farris, recalled. "Henry began yelling at the questioners thusly: 'You lived under the Nazis! You know how abusive they were! How can you turn around and abuse these people the same way?'"[12]

> Kissinger went even further: he kept quiet, insofar as it was possible, about the fact that he was Jewish. He no longer practiced his religion and never brought it up. And though his army colleagues of course knew him as Kissinger, he called himself Mr. Henry among the Germans in his jurisdiction because it sounded more American than Jewish. "I used the name Mr. Henry," he later explained, "because I didn't want the Germans to think the Jews were coming back to take revenge."[12]

As the chief Army Counter-Intelligence administrator with jurisdiction over more than twenty towns, Kissinger honed his diplomatic skills. Frequent dinner guests included the mayor of Bensheim, "the pre-Hitler police chief, who helped Kissinger identify and arrest the local Nazi leaders," and others who might serve American intelligence interests.[13] "Henry was an excellent diplomat," said Bechhofer. "He was able to get along with German officials and make them do his bidding. In short order, the towns were working and the region had been de-Nazified."[12]

Fig. 11.1. Declassified Document Explaining The CIA's Project Paperclip and PROJECT 63—Programs to Locate, Recruit, and Exfiltrate Nazi Scientists To Serve American Intelligence Interests

Project Paperclip

Subject: Civilian Personnel Spaces to Accommodate the PAPERCLIP and PROJECT 63 Programs.

SECURITY INFORMATION

1. The Department of Defense has two classified projects, deemed of utmost importance, that result in the employment and exploitation of foreign scientists by the Department:

a. The first, PAPERCLIP, provides a means of obtaining services of foreign specialists for specific assignments within the technical services of the Departments of Army, Navy, and Air Force. The primary function of this program is the utilization of the individual, the denial aspect being a highly desirable, although secondary feature. Such specialists sign a year's contract for a specific assignment prior to leaving their place of residence.

b. PROJECT 63 is primarily a denial program with utilization as a desirable feature. The aim of this program is to secure employment in the United States of certain preeminent German and Austrian specialists, thus denying their services to potential enemies. Such specialists sign a six-month Department of Defense contract which guarantees them an income until permanent employment is arranged with Department of Defense agencies or industry within the United States.

Project Overcast, later renamed Project Paperclip, was the top-secret program set up in 1945 by the War Department to locate, recruit, and exfiltrate to the United States hundreds of Nazi scientists, specialists in rocketry, biological warfare, aviation medicine, wind tunnels, and the like. This declassified document is dated June 2, 1953 and signed by Air Force Chief of Staff (and former Director of Central Intelligence) Hoyt S. Vandenberg. It indicates that at least 820 Nazis were brought to the U.S. under Paperclip, seen as "a means of obtaining the services of foreign specialists" for the U.S. military. (Reliable accounts indicate they numbered in excess of 900.) Another parallel program was "Project 63," to bring "certain preeminent German and Austrian specialists" to the U.S., with the primary intent of denying their services to potential enemies. Vandenberg acknowledged however that their "utilization [was] a desirable feature."

Many of these hundreds of Nazis, including SS and SA officers, were provably guilty of war crimes and prosecutable before the Nuremberg Tribunal. To get them out of Germany and into the United States the Joint Intelligence Objectives Agency, responsible to the Joint Chiefs of Staff for the administration of Paperclip, shamelessly set about altering, hiding, and destroying the evidence of their recruits' atrocities. Security reports researched and written by U.S. military intelligence were located and changed. When some State Department officials discovered the changes, further changes were made and lies were told.

An extremely valuable account of the exfiltration program by freelance journalist Linda Hunt, who spent 18 months using the Freedom of Information Act to obtain the relevant files, appears in the April 1985 *Bulletin of the Atomic Scientists.*

Source: Preston W. The real treason. *Covert Action Information Bulletin* 1986;25:23-26. Reprinted with permission.

Shortly thereafter, Kraemer played patron to Kissinger again and promoted him to teach Allied military officers "how to uncover Nazis and restore German civil authority at the European Command Intelligence School in Oberammergau."[12]

The Nazis uncovered by Kissinger and his students were evaluated for their potential to serve as American military and industrial assets. In particular, Allied intelligence was looking for Nazi scientists who maintained special expertise in rocketry, biological warfare, and other areas of military medicine. More than 900 Nazi scientists were eventually recruited under this Department of Defense secret "PROJECT 63."[13] Figure 11.1, published by Covert Action Publications, Inc., a Washington, D.C.-based, nonprofit CIA watchdog organization, describes this project in more detail.

The Harvard Experience

In the fall of 1947, Kissinger returned from Germany to join Harvard's class of 1950 as a twenty-four-year-old mentally gifted sophomore. Harvard, at the time, was bristling with excitement. McGeorge Bundy, then a government professor recalled, "International affairs was expanding as a discipline . . . [and] Harvard believed it had a new role because the country had a new role." During his 1947 commencement speech in Harvard Yard, Secretary of State George Marshall inaugurated his postwar European revival plan. That semester, a forum featuring Joseph Alsop and I. F. Stone, debated the issue "Must We Stop Russia?" The Carnegie Foundation heralded its funding of the university's "area studies" program in which the first task was to establish a Russian Research Center to support America's emergence from isolationism.[14]

At Harvard, though discrimination evaded extinction in some departments, it was least noticed in the Government Department wherein Kissinger majored.

"We never, ever discussed our Jewishness," recalled Arthur Gilman, Kissinger's roommate. But during late-night discussions, Kissinger strongly opposed Israel's creation. "He said it would alienate the Arabs and jeopardize U.S. interests. I thought it was a strange view for someone who had been a refugee from Nazi Germany. Herbert Engelhardt, another dormitory resident said, "I got the impression that Kissinger suffered less anti-Semitism in his youth than I did as a kid in New Jersey."[15]

Kissinger's university acquaintances described him as an intensely driven, excessively mature, incessant reader who bit his fingernails and established his own rules. Despite his expressed interest in sports, the young immigrant skipped all athletic events, avoided drinking and partying with his housemates, failed to join clubs or societies, contributed nothing to school publications, and made no effort to participate in student activities. "Henry could be charming if he decided he wanted to be," said Gilman, "but he was really a loner."[15]

Englehardt, while claiming a grudging affection, confessed, "he was deadly serious all the time. He never liked to chase after women. His famous wit and nuance were not in evidence when he was an undergraduate. He had no judgment, no feel for what was happening around him, no empathy for people he was with. He was clumsy, socially awkward, I guess a little shy. Basically, he was a very limited person."[16]

With his interests peaked in government and philosophy, the straight-A student became fascinated with William Yandell Elliott, his first-semester course professor in "The Development of Constitutional Government." Owing to outstanding academic achievements, Kissinger was entitled to have Elliott serve as his senior faculty tutor. And in recommending Henry for Phi Beta Kappa, Elliott's endorsement read:

> I would say that I have not had any students in the past five years, even among the summa cum laude group, who have had the depth and philosophical insight shown by Mr. Kissinger. On the other hand, his mind lacks grace and is Teutonic in its systematic thoroughness. He has a certain emotional bent, perhaps from a refugee origin, that occasionally comes out. But I would regard him as on the whole a very balanced and just mind.[17]

Though Kissinger became attached to Elliott, he diplomatically paid homage to Professor Carl Friedrich who with Elliott represented the "twin pillars of the Government Department." In fact, the aspiring diplomat became famous for his ability to transcend the political rivalry Elliott and Friedrich demonstrated.[18]

Kissinger's "Meaning of History"

"In Harvard's 350-year history," wrote Isaacson, "it has learned to take in stride the peculiar combination of intellectual brilliance and quirkiness that occasionally blossoms among its undergraduates. Even so, Henry Kissinger's senior thesis is still described in awed tones."[19]

The 383-page "Meaning of History" introduced themes about freedom, morality, revolution, creativity, and bureaucracy that recurred throughout Kissinger's life. It provided a taste of the intellectual haughtiness for which he became famous; it provided an impression of how the future statesman waged the pursuit of peace as "a constant balancing act that lacked larger meaning."[19,20]

In his chapter covering the early twentieth-century political philosopher Spengler, titled "History as Intuition," Kissinger paraphrased the nationalistic German scholar: ". . . amidst a repetition of cataclysmic wars the civilization petrifies and dies." [21]

Thus Kissinger advanced Spengler's portrayal of history as an incessant and existentially doomed power struggle: "a vast succession of catastrophic upheavals of which power is not only the manifestation but the exclusive aim."[21]

"It would be wrong," Isaacson cautioned, "to identify Spengler's gloomy views with those of Kissinger," who sought to "find a more palatable meaning" in history. But it would be inaccurate to ignore "the perverse fascination that the brooding German refugee had for Spengler. Kissinger's historic pessimism, inbred as a boy, set him apart from the traditional American mavens of manifest destiny."[22]

Then Kissinger provided a stark portrayal of historic determinism: "Life is suffering, birth involves death. Transitoriness is the fate of existence."[21]

The cure for this moribund state of affairs, according to his thesis, lies in the development of personal awareness and "inward conviction" of each individual's freedom—a philosophy advanced most notably by the famous French existentialist Jean Paul Sartre who, following the lead of Karl Marx, became a principal promoter of communism. Odd that neither Kissinger nor Isaacson acknowledged that, I thought.

Kissinger also appreciated Kant but only partially embraced the philosopher's European liberalism, republicanism, and idealism. Kant's "Perpetual Peace" advocated a League of Republics that cooperated according to international law, much like that which is practiced by the United Nations.

Alternatively, Kissinger was also drawn to European conservatism, which focused on national sovereignty and balanced powers. "Youthful fascination with Kant's political writings could have moved Kissinger toward a Wilsonian view of America's interests and mission," explained Peter Dickson in his study of Kissinger. "Instead, the émigré turned to Metternich and Bismarck—the prime practitioners of power politics."[23]

The Harvard International Seminar

Besides being an intellectual mentor to the fledgling diplomat, Professor Elliott became one of Kissinger's most influential mid-career patrons. To his credit, the flashy Southern educator overcame the academic jealousy that caused most other Harvard colleagues to snub Henry. Elliott knew his bright student could readily surpass his intellectual prowess, so he dedicated himself to helping him when he needed it.

With Elliott's aid Kissinger found work, made extra money, and established an academic and political base at Harvard. As the university's summer school director, Elliott helped Kissinger start a project that served him well—the Harvard International Seminar.[24]

The program, which invited some of the world's most promising young leaders to Harvard, ran successfully from 1951 to 1968. During that time, Kissinger personally selected hundreds of young elected officials, civil servants, and journalists to participate. As America assumed greater influence in the Western alliance, aspiring leaders from around the globe hungered for an invitation to visit Cambridge for the summer. Henry obliged dozens of them.[24]

As the program evolved, Kissinger solicited Harvard's power elite to participate. "At twenty-eight," wrote Isaacson, "he was developing a power base within the academic bureaucracy." There was even money to dispense. The seminar was "well funded . . . [and Kissinger] could offer a fat fee to the professors [he] invited to lecture."[25]

> Kissinger was not shy about calling famous professors, both at Harvard and around the country, pouring on doses of flattery, and asking if they would be kind enough to lecture his students. Those who spoke at Kissinger's behest ranged from Eleanor Roosevelt to Southern poet John Crowe Ranson, from sociologist David Riesman to the labor leader Walter Reuther. . . .
>
> Money [for the International Seminar] came from the university, the Ford Foundation, the Rockefeller Foundation, and elsewhere. Kissinger spent much of his time hustling funds. Beginning in 1953, a group named Friends of the Middle East began giving grants that eventually totaled just under $250,000. Later it was revealed that the group was a CIA front. Kissinger was panicky at first, fearing that this might ruin his reputation. He stormed into his office the day the story broke and flew into a rage. But the controversy soon blew over.[25]

Might his military background and service to Army intelligence have boosted his concerns? I questioned in the silence of my Bellingham hotel room.

Additional Links to Domestic Intelligence

By the time Kissinger set sail for Cambridge, he had established vital connections to the military intelligence community. In fact, his intelligence contacts included not only Fritz Kraemer and General Bolling, but Helmut Sonnenfeldt, who later became Kissinger's counselor at the State Department, and Henry Rosovsky, "who attended Kissinger's class on German paramilitary organizations," when the two were stationed in Oberammergau. Rosovsky later became a "noted economist and dean at Harvard."[11,12]

In summary, Kissinger was at the center of a good old boy intelligence network even before the Ford and Rockefeller Foundations funded his International Seminar, I realized.

So in July 1953, when a batch of forty envelopes addressed to foreign seminar participants arrived at Kissinger's office, he curiously opened one. To his dismay, it contained literature critical of American military policy and "ban-the-bomb propaganda." Enraged, he phoned Boston's FBI field office, and an agent was sent to investigate. The final part of the investigator's confidential report read: "KISSINGER identified himself as an individual who is strongly sympathetic to the FBI . . . Steps will be taken . . . to make KISSINGER a Confidential Source of this Division." As a result, Kissinger was occasionally contacted at Harvard for information valuable to domestic intelligence.[26]

In return for his kindness, many of the International Seminar participants extended their host invitations to visit them in their native lands. This, coupled with Kissinger's intelligence interest provided numerous opportunities for overseas travel. In 1951, for instance, the Operations Research Office of the Army sent Kissinger as a graduate student to Korea to assess the impact of the U.S. military presence on civilian life. The following summer, Kissinger returned to Germany and met with "leading German industrialists in Dusseldorf and was feted at a dinner in his honor—held in the dining room of the Krupp munitions plant. 'Who would have thought?' he joked to his parents."[27]

Kissinger's Realpolitik: Visions of a New World Order

Kissinger's "realpolitik"—his practical philosophy of political history—as described in his Harvard thesis and demonstrated by his diplomatic behavior, showed that throughout his career he sought to "preserve [and even define a] world order." His approach to peace implied "artfully tending to balances of power."[28] World peace was, therefore, not the defining policy objective for Kissinger.

Kissinger believed that a "balance of power" was the best that could be obtained. This he believed could be achieved through the acceptance and control of limited conflicts—"small wars." With this in mind, the diplomat's mission was to assure that the United States and not the Russians would lead and win many of these.[28]

> Kissinger's conservative realpolitik . . . was based on the principle, taught by realists from Karl von Clausewitz to Hans Morgenthau, that diplomacy cannot be divorced from the realities of force and power. But diplomacy should be divorced, Kissinger argued, from a moralistic and meddlesome concern with the internal policies of other nations. Stability is the prime goal of diplomacy. It is served when nations accept the legitimacy of the existing world order and when they act based on their national interests; it is threatened when nations embark on ideological or moral crusades. "His was a quest for a realpolitik devoid of moral homilies," said his Harvard colleague Stanley Hoffman.[28]

From the beginning of his thesis, the political historian established a premise that would define his career's work. "Whenever peace—conceived as the avoidance of war—has been the primary objective of a power or a group of powers," Kissinger wrote, "the international system has been at the mercy of the most ruthless member of the international community." A more appropriate goal, he advanced, was for "stability based on an equilibrium of forces."[21]

In one instance, Stoessinger asked Kissinger his preference between a revolutionary state committed to justice versus a ruling state that sought unjust ends? Kissinger replied by paraphrasing Goethe: "If I had to choose between justice and order, on the one hand, and injustice and order, on the other, I would always choose the latter."[29]

Kissinger believed that summit conferences with the other superpowers only served a propaganda objective. In his first article in the lay press, "The Limitations of Diplomacy" published in *The New Republic* in 1955, he contended that summit meetings with the communists could only raise false hopes; yet, they should be conducted to win neutral nation confidence and assuage allies concerns.[30]

Later, he advanced the belief that China's and Russia's "revolutionary" tendencies could be mitigated by offering them a legitimate stake in the international system. Thus, the game plan for the New World Order was established.[28]

The Foreign Affairs Minister

In April 1955, Kissinger's first major national security policy paper appeared in *Foreign Affairs*, a prestigious quarterly published by the Council on Foreign Relations in New York. The report, developed at the request of Harvard history professor Arthur Schlesinger, advanced Kissinger's critique of the "massive retaliation" doctrine that proposed an all-out nuclear response to Soviet attack.[31]

In the report, Kissinger argued that the massive retaliation doctrine acquired during the Eisenhower years was dangerously outdated. The Soviets now had their own bomb. Threatened all-out nuclear retaliation for Soviet expansion into the "gray areas" of the world was, therefore, no longer credible. "As Soviet nuclear strength increases," he wrote, "the number of areas that will seem worth the destruction of New York, Detroit, or Chicago will steadily diminish. An all-or-nothing military policy therefore makes for a paralysis of diplomacy." Kissinger called for policy change in which the capacity to wage localized "little wars" was emphasized.[31]

> The Foreign Affairs piece had two notable consequences. It laid the groundwork for Kissinger's theory that the U.S. should be prepared to fight "limited nuclear wars"—a doctrine that became the intellectual precursor to the Kennedy administration's "flexible response" strategy and NATO's decision to deploy intermediate-range nuclear weapons in Europe.[31]

"In addition," Isaacson noted, "the article helped get Kissinger a job at the Council on Foreign Relations, a post that would catapult him from the obscurity of an untenured instructor to the celebrity of a best-selling nuclear strategist."[31]

The Council on Foreign Relations

The Council on Foreign Relations (CFR) was founded in 1921 "by members of Manhattan's internationally minded business and legal elite. . . ."

Contrary to what I had assumed, the CFR is a "private organization that serves as a discussion club for close to three thousand well-connected aficionados of foreign affairs. Beneath chandeliers and stately portraits in its Park Avenue mansion, members attend lectures, dinners, and roundtable seminars featuring top officials and visiting world leaders."[31]

Isaacson further revealed:

> The most exalted enterprises at the Council are the study groups, which consist of about a dozen distinguished members and wise men who meet regularly for a year or so to explore a particular subject. Each has a study director, often a rising star in the academic world. The group that Kissinger was asked to direct had been formed in November 1954 to probe the topic of "nuclear weapons and foreign policy."[31]

Kissinger's group met almost monthly and was chaired by the former head of the Atomic Energy Commission, Gordon Dean. Included in the evening discussions was such foreign policy mavins as Paul Nitze, a previous director of the State Department's policy planning committee; the department's director Robert Bowie, who later became Kissinger's academic antagonist at Harvard; Lieutenant General James Gavin, "whose belief in the potential of nuclear technology to cure American military deficiencies proved infectious. . ."; and David Rockefeller, who was enthralled by Gavin's recommendations for military industrialization, and soon thereafter acquired two chairmanships: one of the Council and the other of the Chase Bank.[31]

Graduated Deterrence Doctrine

Among Kissinger's first invited guests was Harvard's dean McGeorge Bundy who arrived in December 1955 to lead a fascinating discussion on NATO strategy. "It was one of the first times that abstract theorizing about limited nuclear war was related to the defense doctrine that later became known as flexible response," wrote Isaacson.[31]

When Nitze—Kissinger's cohort on the topic of "limited nuclear war"—argued that threatened massive nuclear retaliation might be considered a "bluff," Bundy replied, "Can we not develop a concept for the graduated application of power? It is essential that we find some flexible policy." Six years later, as national security advisor during the Kennedy administration, Bundy helped activate this "flexible response" doctrine.[31]

"Kissinger, with some discomfort" had by then accepted the view that "for the foreseeable future, the U.S. would have to rely on nuclear weapons in fighting even a limited war."[31]

> It would be "extremely dangerous," Kissinger argued, to become paralyzed by the belief that any use of nuclear weapons would automatically escalate to an all-out war. Like Nitze, he endorsed the concept of graduated deterrence, which meant being willing to fight limited wars with tactical nuclear weapons.[31]

"One of the crucial problems facing the U.S.," Kissinger said at the time, "was to develop a doctrine for the graduated employment of force."[32]

On reading this, I wondered—Could the incredible proliferation of chemical and biological weapons during the late 1960s and early 1970s have been the result of Kissinger's articulated need for nuclear alternatives; a broader weapons arsenal that might allow for more "graduated deterrence" and "flexible response" capabilities?

I reflected on the fact that the order for AIDS-like viruses came during Nixon's years in office when Henry Kissinger ran the National Security Council (NSC).

Early Rockefeller Influence

Among Kissinger's most influential patrons as he worked his way up the ladder of success to become Nixon's "Deputy to the President for National Security," was Nelson Aldrich Rockefeller, the son of Standard Oil heir John D. Rockefeller, Jr.[33]

The Rockefeller family's involvement in the medical–industrial complex, health science research, and American politics, deserves some background.

Before World War II, major administration of medical research, or financing by federal agencies, had been generally opposed by America's scientific community. In fact, it was only during times of war that organizations like the NAS or the NRC received major funding. Both the NAS, established during the Civil War, and the NRC, set up during the First World War, were largely ignored in times of peace.[34]

Between 1900 and 1940, private foundations and universities financed most medical research. According to Paul Starr, author of *The Social Transformation of American Medicine: The rise of a sovereign profession and the making of a vast industry*, "the most richly endowed research center, the Rockefeller Institute for Medical Research was established in New York in 1902 and by 1928 had received from John D. Rockefeller $65 million in endowment funds." In contrast, as late as 1938, as little as $2.8 million in federal funding was budgeted for the entire PHS. Therefore, it is easy to see that Rockefeller family investment in health science research predated, and far surpassed, even the federal government's.[34]

More than the New Deal, the Second World War created the greatest boom in federal government and private industry support for medical research. In 1938, the NIH took up residence in "a privately donated estate" in Bethesda, Maryland, which is still its home today.[35]

Prior to the war, American science and medicine was heavily influenced by German models. This precedent, however, changed during the 1930s when the Nazis purged Jewish scientists from German universities and biological laboratories. These changes, according to Starr, significantly altered the course of American health science and medicine. Many of Germany's most brilliant Jewish researchers emigrated to the United States just as the movement burgeoned to privatize war related biological and medical research.[34]

At this time, the Rockefeller led medical–industrial complex was fully poised to influence, and take advantage of, Congress's "first series of measures to promote cancer research and cancer control." In 1937, the new federal legislation authorized the establishment of the National Cancer Institute under the NIH, and, for the first time, "the Public Health Service to make grants to outside researchers."[34]

According to Starr:

> The war gave medical research priority. In July 1941 President Roosevelt created an Office of Scientific Research and Development (OSRD) with two parallel committees on national defense and medical research. The Committee on Medical Research (CMR) undertook a comprehensive research program to deal with the medical problems of the war. The work, costing $15 million, involved 450 contracts with universities and another 150 with research institutes, hospitals, and other organizations. Altogether, some 5,500 scientists and technicians were employed in the enterprise.[36]

Moreover, according to E. Richard Brown's *Rockefeller Medicine Men*, the Rockefellers exercised significant control over the outcomes of these efforts through the foundations they established.[37]

Rockefeller Befriends Kissinger

Following the war, Nelson Rockefeller remained active in the CFR, and, in 1955, while serving as President Eisenhower's assistant for international affairs, invited Kissinger to discuss national security issues at the Quantico (Virginia) Marine Base. Following their meeting, according to Isaacson, the diplomat became Rockefeller's "closest intellectual associate," and soon after, Kissinger authored several military proposals for Eisenhower to consider. Unimpressed, Eisenhower turned them down.[33]

As a result, Rockefeller sent Eisenhower his resignation and then launched a Special Studies Project that explored the "critical choices" America faced militarily in the coming years. Kissinger agreed to direct this new project and published a 468-page book on his findings. The treatise proposed that tactical nuclear weapons be developed and "a bomb shelter [be built] in every house" in preparation for limited thermonuclear war. "The willingness to engage in nuclear war when necessary is part of the price of our freedom," Kissinger argued.

I suddenly realized that the anxiety I felt in grade school while drilling for possible nuclear attacks was part of Kissinger's price for freedom.

Eisenhower had warned America that the gravest threat to world security, democracy, and even spirituality, was the growing military–industrial complex, I recalled. And the Rockefellers and Kissinger played leading roles in its expansion.

For more than ten years, Nelson Rockefeller's nuclear policy guru remained a well-paid Chase Bank consultant and Harvard faculty member. During that time, Kissinger continued writing numerous books and articles on subjects related to the practical application of his realpolitik in the nuclear age. He also continued to provide favors and advice to White House dignitaries and Rockefeller executives until late 1968. After Rockefeller lost the Republican presidential nomination to Nixon, Kissinger then joined Nixon's staff.[33,38]

The National Security Council Job

Following the 1968 Republican convention, Richard Allen, Nixon's foreign policy adviser, contacted Kissinger to serve on his advisory board. The invitation was not only in deference to Kissinger's formidable intelligence on the subject, but as remuneration for helping keep Nixon abreast of the latest developments in the Paris peace negotiations, which ended the bombing in Vietnam.

"During the last days of the campaign," Nixon noted, "when Kissinger was providing us with information about the bombing halt, I became more aware of his knowledge and his influence." Kissinger had served as Nixon's spook in the Johnson camp. He kept the Republican presidential candidate abreast for campaign speeches and meetings with the press. In appreciation, Nixon rewarded him with the top position in national security.[39]

Nixon's aim in appointing Kissinger to be in charge of the National Security Council was to "run foreign policy from the White House." Undoubtedly, the chief executive intended to emasculate the State Department.[39]

As vice president under Eisenhower, Nixon felt abused by members of the State Department who "treated him with contempt." In retaliation, he intended to "usurp the power of the State Department bureaucracy," by establishing a "strong National Security Council staff in the White House that would take over from State the responsibility for developing policy options." Kissinger agreed with Nixon's mission, and the two men struck a bond.[39]

Besides Kissinger, three other candidates for the national security post were interviewed by the president. They included Robert Strausz-Hupe and William Kinter of the University of Pennsylvania, and Roy Ash, president of Litton Industries.

"Holy smoke!" I burst. "Will you look at that. Litton Industries's president Roy Ash was Kissinger's alternate for the national security job." I immediately realized Litton Industries was the parent company to Litton Bionetics—the firm Gallo and his co-workers often cited as their funding source. "Now when was that?" I searched *Kissinger* for the date—January 1969. "Just six months before Congress was asked to fund the DOD contract for AIDS-like viruses."[40]

The following week back from the west coast, and on tour in New York, I stopped in the public library to look up Roy Ash in *Who's Who*. The business executive and co-founder of Litton Industries, Inc., in Beverly Hills, California, had directed the military megacontractor from 1953 to 1972. In 1969, instead of the NSC directorship, Nixon appointed him chairman of the President's Advisory Council on Executive Organizations, on which he served until 1971. Then he was elevated to the rank of "Assistant to the President of the United States." He served the Nixon and Ford administrations in this capacity as well as directed the Office of Management and Budget for the White House until 1975.[41]

The Silent Coup Begins

In order to direct foreign policy from the White House, Nixon needed to "sap the traditional powers of the State and Defense departments and centralize control in the West Wing, specifically in the hands of Nixon and Kissinger," Isaacson wrote.[42]

The principal purpose of this strategy was not only to appease Nixon's megalomaniacal insecurity, but to punish the agency that had irresponsibly guided America through its worst international embarrassment—Vietnam.

To establish new policy in the old State Department, painstaking negotiations among countless bureaucrats were required for even the simplest decisions. Institutional input from dozens of agencies, including the CIA, FBI, Pentagon, and State Department resulted in "glacial changes, fuzzy conclusions swathed in murky language, and a resistance to reopening issues once a bureaucratic consensus had been reached."[43]

Nixon wanted to revisit a horde of issues and, like Kissinger, tended to circumvent instead of confront immovable bureaucracies. The National Security Council became their vehicle for securing this liberty.

> The NSC had been created in 1947 during the Truman administration in response to Franklin Roosevelt's habit of leaving certain agencies in the dark when he made decisions. Its membership—known as the NSC "principals"— included the president, vice president, secretary of state, secretary of defense, and other top officials [such as the director of central intelligence] designated by the president.[42]

During the Kennedy and Johnson years, the significance of the NSC waned, but the importance of a separate but related entity—the NSC staff— grew to assume the most powerful role in American government. "Headed by a special assistant who eventually became known as the national security 'adviser,' the staff became a personal minibureaucracy that could analyze policy, devise tactics, and carry out operations for the president—often without the other principals of the NSC being informed. . . ." That was precisely what Kissinger and Nixon wanted.[42]

Following their reorganization of the agency, Kissinger gained: veto power over State Department or other agency proposals; virtual control over NSC meeting agendas; the ability to hold secret meetings with State,

Defense, and other department directors so that he alone could privately negotiate with them without revealing his purposes to others.[42]

"From the start," Undersecretary of State U. Alexis Johnson recalled, "it was obvious that Kissinger was extremely insecure and had an obsession, which persisted throughout his White House years, that the State Department and Foreign Service were determined to undermine him." The result concluded Isaacson, "was a national security apparatus well crafted for a diplomacy based on bold new approaches, secrecy, surprise, and tactical maneuvering. On the other hand, it was not as well suited for building a bureaucratic and public consensus for major policies, nor for creating institutional checks on a defiant president who was prone to acting on impulse."[42]

All of Kissinger's Men

When Kissinger began to look for an NSC military assistant, Colonel Alexander Haig was recommended by Robert McNamara (defense secretary under Kennedy) and Joseph Califano—Secretary of Health and Human Services under Jimmy Carter. Califano, according to Isaacson, had known Haig "from his days as a staff officer in the Pentagon."[44] In fact, Califano had been Haig's boss at the Pentagon in the early 1960s. On further research in New York Public Library, I learned that both had received law degrees. Califano received his from Harvard in 1955—the year Kissinger submitted his *Meaning of History* for his Ph.D. What's more, all three had served in the army during the war.

From 1964 to 1965, Haig served as Deputy Special Assistant to the Secretary of the Army, and as Deputy Secretary of Defense of the Army while Califano was at the Pentagon as Special Assistant to the Secretary and Deputy Secretary of the DOD.[41]

Kissinger's old mentor Fritz Kraemer also urged him to tap Haig, whom he later called "my other great discovery."[44]

Unlike the myriad other NSC staff Kissinger had sent to the Executive Office Building, Haig and personal assistant Eagleburger set up shop in the basement of the White House just outside Kissinger's West Wing office. Soon Haig began administering the most sensitive projects in his quest to become the NSC director's deputy. "Haig's duties were manifold. . . ." explained Isaacson:

> He served as the emissary to FBI Director J. Edgar Hoover and others who might suspect Kissinger of being soft. He taught Kissinger about the perks of power, . . . [and] soon came to handle . . . overseeing a secret FBI program to

wiretap the home telephones of other members of the NSC staff. [Morton] Halperin and [Helmut] Sonnenfeldt [two Kissinger NSC appointees, both of whom had designs on the vacant deputy director position] . . . would be the first two victims of that program.[44]

Kissinger became convinced that Haig would never threaten his relationship with Nixon or become disloyal.

Matching Nixon's White House austerity, an air of secrecy surrounded the NSC in those days. The president and Kissinger both were paranoid that underlings were out to get them. So they labored to make themselves invincible. They severed channels of communication and routinely destroyed paper trails to limit their accessibility and vulnerability. Their staff, in essence, operated with information provided only—as in the CIA—on a need-to-know basis.[46]

Compared to President Johnson, who maintained "a bank of phones" and sought information from a variety of sources within and beyond his administration, Nixon was a loner who trusted few others. "If I needed to get hold of somebody," Johnson bragged to an aide on leaving his replacement's Oval Office, "all I had to do was mash a button. And I mean anybody—even some little fellow tucked away in one of the agencies." Nixon, he reported with wonder, "had just one dinky phone" with three buttons. . . . "That's all! Just three buttons! And they all go to Germans."[42]

Likewise, Kissinger's paranoia drove him to make unparalleled demands on the staff. He ended the practice of allowing chief administrators to share their expertise with Nixon in his absence. Isaacson reported he would not even allow high-level staff "to accompany him to meetings with the president except in rare cases." Winston Lord, a former Kissinger aide believed this behavior "reflected his tremendous mixture of ego and insecurity." Ultimately, White House morale suffered as the anticipation and thrill of presidential encounters eroded.

For instance, when Morton Halperin provided CIA director Richard Helms a routine summary of the NSC's first meeting agenda, Kissinger protested. He did not object to what was said, only that an underling had presumed to address a cabinet official. Kissinger ordered Haig to rule "No staffer is to talk to principals."[46]

The White House Wire Taps

Kissinger's angst that members of his staff would undermine his leadership and violate the secrecy he needed to carry out his realpolitik transformed into full-blown paranoia when the *New York Times* broke the story about

American B-52 bombers hitting North Vietnam. Kissinger then ordered Haig to Hoover's office to direct the FBI to wiretap "six of Kissinger's aides, eight other officials and four prominent journalists."[47,48]

> In all there would be seventeen FBI wiretaps ordered by the White House under the justification of national security—thirteen of them on government employees, four on newsmen. The program would last for twenty-one months, until February 1971. . . . As the summaries came to Kissinger's office, Haig would read them, show his boss the interesting parts, and then store them in a safe. . . .
>
> Other aides began to suspect something. Soon after the wiretaps had begun, Roger Morris went to the hospital to visit Lawrence Eagleburger, Kissinger's personal assistant who had collapsed from nervous exhaustion. Tears came to Eagleburger's eyes as he told his old friend from the foreign service about the tapping. "Don't say anything you don't want Haldeman or Henry to read over breakfast," Eagleburger warned. Anthony Lake, another idealistic staffer, stumbled across a wiretap summary involving one of their colleagues, and he told Morris about it. "Roger and I decided not to confront Kissinger," he recalled. "We were fighting on enough fronts. But every now and then, when we were talking on the phone, we'd wish J. Edgar Hoover a merry Christmas."[47]

To protect his flanks, Hoover had Attorney General John Mitchell sign the wiretap authorizations.

Likewise, Kissinger targeted Hoover and Haig for his alibi. He used a written defense to incriminate Hoover. He wrote in his memoirs: "J. Edgar Hoover invariably listed some official outside the FBI hierarchy as requesting each wiretap, even in cases where I had heard Hoover himself specifically recommend them to Nixon."[48] Though he had instructed Haig to deliver the wiretap order to Hoover, Kissinger later told friends that Haig originated the plan. Isaacson wrote that much of what was requested in Kissinger's name, "he insisted was done on Haig's own initiative." And there was "some truth to the charge; Haig used the program to further his own interests and spy on his rivals."[47]

He also rationalized the surveillance as something previous administrations had done. "I don't think there was any more or less wiretapping" during the Nixon administration than in previous years, the FBI's intelligence division chief James Adams said. However, "what was unusual about this [was] that it involved wiretaps on the NSC staff, on individuals that were part of the White House family." Administration officials had previously ordered wiretaps to spy on potentially criminal union leaders and organized mobsters. A wiretapping program set against one's own staff was, according to another top FBI official, Thomas Smith, "unprecedented."[47,49]

Deputy FBI director William Sullivan was charged with overseeing Kissinger's wiretap operation. Hoover later discharged Sullivan for insubordination since he was suspected of plotting against the FBI director for the benefit of the CIA and Nixon White House officials—particularly Haig and Kissinger.

The surveillance program reflected "quite a natural temptation, especially for two people with a touch of paranoia," Isaacson concluded. "To eavesdrop on what others are saying—colleagues, subordinates, rivals, and enemies—gives a heady sense of power that has tempted people even more ethically fastidious than Kissinger and Nixon."[47]

> The program—which ultimately led to the plumbers, which led to Watergate—illustrated what can happen when a White House is intent on pursuing policies, such as the bombing of Cambodia, that it feels it cannot dare let the public discover.[47]

"It is the part of my public service about which I am most ambivalent," Kissinger said, referring to this phase of his career. This was as close as he ever came to saying he was sorry.

The Great Power Grab

For Nixon, National Security Council meetings quickly became bothersome. Rather than having to deal with issues and objections raised by State Department director William Rogers and Defense Secretary Melvin Laird, both of whom threatened Kissinger's power and ego, Nixon directed Haldeman to announce a decision he and Kissinger had been considering for five months: the new role of the NSC adviser would be to oversee the departments of Defense and State. Thereafter, rather than exploring foreign policy matters during full NSC meetings, Nixon and Kissinger decided them alone.[50]

"Cut NSC to one every two week[s]—or once a month," read Haldeman's notes of the great power grab. "More brought privately to President for his discussion with Kissinger." Later in the meeting, Nixon informed Haldeman that from now on, Kissinger should direct NSC agenda discussions directly to him before informing agency chiefs during council meetings. In this way, the two came to decisions without Rogers and Laird being informed. "No appeal," Nixon ordered, as he frequently did, for emphasis.[51]

"This suited Kissinger just fine," wrote Isaacson who chronicled:

> From the start, he had been seeking to make foreign policy in private with Nixon whenever possible. For the very first NSC meeting, which dealt with Vietnam options, he had Halperin do a two-page cover memo summarizing the plans put forth from State and other agencies. There were little boxes for Nixon to initial. Kissinger looked at it and told Halperin, "Fine, but now tell him what to do." Halperin was a little taken aback, having heard all of Kissinger's pronouncements about how the NSC staff would merely pass along options. The summary documents, with Kissinger's recommended course of action, were to become another of the secrets that Kissinger had to keep from the State Department and the rest of the government.[50,52]

The power shift was quickly announced by the press. After only three weeks at the White House, *Time*'s cover story featured Kissinger. Already the article said, "Kissinger is . . . widely suspected in Washington of being a would-be usurper of the powers traditionally delegated to the State and Defense departments [and] . . . Humility is not his hallmark." Likewise, The *New York Times* reported that Kissinger "is taking over the responsibility for coordinating foreign policy in the Nixon Administration, a mandate formerly assigned to the Secretary of State."[50,53]

At this point I questioned: What were Kissinger's responsibilities? Might they have included directing Defense Department research activities. Did he order the request for appropriations for the development of AIDS-like viruses? Could he have discussed with Roy Ash the award granted to Gallo through Litton Bionetics for the development of immune-system-destroying viruses following Nixon's signing of the Geneva accord? Had Roy Ash informed Kissinger about such possibilities from his company's R & D reports?

Isaacson quickly answered the first of my questions with a resounding yes. As chairman of the NSC's Senior Review Group, he was in the most powerful position to determine what issues reached the president as well as the agency directors. As shown in figure 11.2, Kissinger quickly "set up a covey of other committees, all of which he chaired, to give him better control over specific topics. They included:

- *The Defense Program Review Committee, which considered the funding requests for weapons and other military needs.*

- *The 40 Committee, a new name for an older panel, which was in charge of authorizing covert actions by the CIA and other agencies.* [emphasis added.]

- The Vietnam Special Studies Group, set up in September 1969, which coordinated military and diplomatic policy regarding the war.

• The Verification Panel, formed in July 1969, which ostensibly analyzed whether compliance with different arms control proposals could be verified by U.S. intelligence, but which was soon in charge of managing all arms negotiations.

• The Washington Special Action Group, set up after North Korea's downing of the EC-121 plane, which handled breaking events and crises."[50]

From 1968 to 1971, the Kissinger-directed NSC annual budget jumped from $700,000 to $2.2 million as its staff almost doubled to 105 administrative aides.[50,54]

In essence, during Nixon's years in office, Kissinger dictated foreign (as well as domestic) policies, procedures, and programs to everyone, including those in command of the military and intelligence communities. In one case, CIA director Richard Helms bore the brunt of Kissinger's power. Kissinger had never felt comfortable with aristocrats like Helms. So he ordered the CIA patrician to supply raw intelligence data rather than summary reports for the NSC director to personally interpret. "It skewed our way of writing estimates, especially about the Soviets," Helms complained. "The estimates had to provide a vast amount of data so Kissinger could make up his own mind."[50]

In another instance, Kissinger pressured military directors, including Laird, to fall in line. *In early 1969, he phoned Admiral Zumwalt,[55] chief of naval operations, over an issue regarding Africa.* Laird was outraged. He insisted that all NSC military dealings should run through him. Kissinger argued that as the president's representative, he held the power to command military operations.

> A few weeks later, when Zumwalt and Kissinger met at a social event, the navy chief noted that he shared Laird's objections to dealing outside of the chain of command. But Kissinger was adamant. It was a matter of both power and principle, he felt, and he insisted that he had the right to deal with all members of the Joint Chiefs of Staff directly. "From then on," says Zumwalt, "every time we got together for business, he referred to it as a 'nonmeeting.'" Without Kissinger's knowledge, Zumwalt kept Laird fully informed.[50]

"Kissinger's desire to control foreign policy," Isaacson wrote, "was not wholly unwarranted." By keeping close tabs on the bureaucracy, "he was able to dispel some of the stale thinking that permeated the State and Defense departments."[50]

My distrust of Kissinger for having played a key role in the development and possible deployment of AIDS-like viruses was not unwarranted according to Isaacson's record:

In the summer of 1969, he ordered a study on chemical and biological weapons. He was dubious about whether they had much use in a war-fighting strategy, and assumed correctly that little thought had been given to the issue. By asking for a range of feasible options, Kissinger guaranteed that the possibility of eliminating the program would be listed, if only as an extreme option to set off the policy the military preferred.[50]

What returned to Kissinger's desk was a "mass of opaque prose" that even he couldn't understand. "I can't even read this paper," he bellowed.

"But he knew that an opportunity had been uncovered," Isaacson concluded. "He had his staff sharpen the wording so that the options became clearer. In making his decision to renounce first use of chemical weapons and to dismantle production of biological ones, Nixon stressed the novelty of the review process and how well it had worked."[50] He also effectively misled the media and world powers that the United States had turned away from the evils of biological warfare. Nothing could have been further from the truth.[56]

That night, from my New York hotel room, with *Kissinger* on my lap, and military intelligence on my mind, I telephoned Jackie. "Jack, get this." I said. "Kissinger undoubtedly ordered the DOD appropriations request for the AIDS-like viruses."

"How do you know that?" she asked.

"It's apparent from what I just read. I'll tell you about it when I get home."

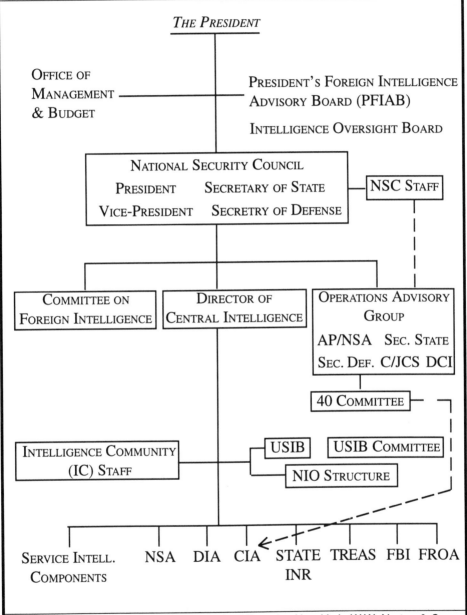

Fig. 11.2. Control and Direction of U.S. Foreign Intelligence Within the National Security System

Adapted from John Stockwell's *In Search of Enemies.* New York: W.W. Norton & Company, Inc., 1978, p. 261. Mr. Stockwell was the Chief of the CIA's Angola Task Force during the late 1960s and early 1970s.

Chapter 12
Silent Coup in
American Intelligence

MY attention focused on *Kissinger* for the duration of the New York trip. It was inconceivable how little I knew and how much I learned about the man whose power not only challeged presidents, but the greatest American demagogue—J. Edgar Hoover.

Isaacson revealed that Kissinger and Hoover were virtually at war with each another, and though Kissinger may not have known it, he too, was a target of the FBI director's wiretaps.[1] Might anything less be expected from the man who, through blackmail, made his way to the "seat of government" and stayed there for more than four decades? Would Hoover bow to the forces of change Kissinger so easily applied against his State and Defense Department counterparts? Not likely.

Hoover and Nixon both distrusted Kissinger as much as he did them. But to Kissinger's advantage, Nixon distrusted Hoover more.[2]

Besides, Kissinger—the NSC director—held power over the Justice Department, and his supporters were a lot wealthier than Hoover's gang of union leaders and mafia chiefs.

The Kissinger–Hoover–Nixon triangle of power, cunning, and deception became one of the most disturbing secrets in political history. To relieve the strain this unholy trinity bore, something had to give. Ultimately, when the smoke cleared, Kissinger led, Hoover was dead, and Nixon may as well have been.

The biggest winners of this Pennsylvania Avenue war were Kissinger's patrons and disciples who seized all the opportunities they could from backing a winner—one whose expressed purpose was global economic and political domination in quest of a New World Order.

Nixon's Perspective

When Kissinger became rabid over the press leaks that announced the North Vietnam bombing operation, Nixon and Haldeman believed Kissinger was one of the leakers. "Get Kissinger away from the press," Haldeman quoted Nixon as saying. "He talks too much."[1]

Throughout their relationship, Nixon bated Kissinger about his heritage. Isaacson wrote that "Nixon seemed to take a fiendish glee in launching into diatribes against Jews and watching as Kissinger shifted feet nervously, afraid to contradict him."[3]

"Nixon shared many of the prejudices of the uprooted, California lower-middle class from which he had come," Kissinger later said regarding the president's anti-Semitism."[3]

During one telephone conversation overheard and recalled by Winston Lord, Nixon bated Kissinger about Jews and blacks. After they hung up, Lord asked, "Why didn't you say something?" Kissinger responded, "I have enough trouble fighting with him on the things that really matter; his attitudes towards Jews and blacks are not my worry."

Hoover's Untenable Position

During the Nixon years, the FBI labored on a project code named "Inlet" to supply Nixon and Kissinger with smut on counterintelligence targets.[4]

When the dirt was finally received, Kissinger and Haig ridiculed Hoover's work. "The FBI investigative work I saw was of poor quality," John Ehrlichman said later, "rumor, gossip, and conjecture . . . often hearsay, two or three times removed. When FBI work was particularly bad, I sent it back to Hoover, but the rework was seldom an improvement."[4]

In the spring of 1970, with Nixon strained by an unprecedented domestic terrorism epidemic wherein highly organized revolutionaries dedicated themselves to "the violent destruction of our democratic system," the president proposed a complete reorganization of U.S. intelligence services.[5]

Years earlier, Hoover had called for more rigorous counterintelligence activities against blacks and the Nation of Islam. In the late 1960s he had terminated many of the illegal programs and espionage policies that Nixon and Kissinger now felt needed to be expanded. There was much talk among White House and CIA officials that the aged Hoover had grown too weak and timid to effectively lead an invigorated anticommunist campaign at home and abroad. CIA Director Richard Helms's request for the deployment of additional FBI support and surveillance of targeted groups was rebuffed by an angry Hoover who saw this as a breach of command and a threat to his autonomy.[5]

In February 1970, with Kissinger now at the helm of the NSC, this rift between the FBI and CIA grew. When the CIA refused to turn over information about a Denver FBI agent who turned CIA informant, without Hoover's knowledge or permission, Hoover ended regular liaison with the CIA.

Then, when the feud was criticized by administration chiefs, Hoover ended "liaison with all other external agencies except the White House."[5,6]

On June 5, 1970, a concerned President Nixon ordered the directors of America's intelligence community to the White House—Hoover, Richard Helms of the CIA, General Donald V. Bennett of the Defense Department, and Admiral Noel Gayler of the National Security Agency—and gave them a dressing down. He told them they were disorganized, inefficient, and unproductive. He wanted them to reorganize themselves into a single, streamlined unit that could keep him informed. . . . Hoover was to be chairman; the staff was to be directed by the White House's Tom Charles Huston, who had been in charge of the administration's campaign to mobilize the Internal Revenue Service against its enemies. Huston had also had the responsibility of collecting information about foreign involvement in campus disturbances, and in the course of this work had formed an alliance with the FBI's assistant director in charge of Domestic Intelligence, William C. Sullivan.[6]

According to author Richard Powers, in the months that followed, Huston attempted to usurp Hoover's power and position as domestic intelligence agency chief, and White House officials attempted to gain Hoover's resignation. Both efforts failed as the director applied the same tactics he had successfully used for almost a half century—blackmail.

About this time, Haldeman, who had evaluated information on U.S. politicians supplied by Hoover, became uneasy. He believed the FBI director was "lobbying" for Nixon's affection, and "trying to pique the President's curiosity," rather than providing quality intelligence. He also became concerned about Hoover's potential for eavesdropping on the Oval Office. Rose Mary Woods, Nixon's secretary, who was later made famous by her "accidental" erasure of a Watergate tape, was in Haldeman's eyes too friendly with Hoover. He insisted the president "minimize the connection" he had with Ms. Woods. This, according to political investigator and author Anthony Summers, became a turning point in Nixon's relationship with Hoover:

"FBI Director Hoover, *Newsweek* reported in May 1969, "no longer enjoys direct access to the White House. . . ." Realizing Nixon's advisers [including Kissinger] were responsible for the change, Edgar struck back in characteristic fashion. That month, using Rose Mary Woods to ensure the message got through, he passed on an astonishing allegation—that Haldeman, Ehrlichman and a third aide, Dwight Chapin, were homosexual lovers.[4]

Haldeman said, Hoover's report allegedly "came from a bartender who was a source for the FBI on stuff like this. We were supposed to have attended homosexual parties at the Watergate complex. There were dates, places, everything. Well, every factual allegation he made was totally false and easily disproven." John Mitchell advised the accused staff to give depositions to the FBI, to help in their defense should the need arise. They did what he suggested.[4]

"Mitchell's conclusion," continued Haldeman, "was that this was an attempt by Hoover to lay a threat across our path, to keep us in line, remind us of his potential."[4]

"This was just the start of the game," Summers chronicled. "In midsummer, after more bizarre statements by Edgar about Robert Kennedy and Dr. King, former Attorney General Ramsey Clark—and an editorial in *The Washington Post*—called for his resignation. The President, it was reported, was looking for a way to dump him."

"Nixon, of course, denied the rumors," Erlichman recalled.[4]

Sullivan's Switch

While contemplating ways to diplomatically remove Hoover from office, the president and Kissinger were also needed to fend off the growing threat of domestic violence over Vietnam. As a result, they challenged Hoover to step up his antiblack dissident campaign. Then, something strange happened in June, 1971. Sullivan also began quarreling with Hoover and other FBI executives over a decision to increase the "legal attachés"—FBI agents—attached to American embassies abroad. After initially supporting the proposal, Sullivan suddenly reversed himself with a scathing attack on the "lack of objectivity, originality and independent thinking" among Hoover's executives." Powers wrote:

> He charged that because of "racial conflict, student and academic revolution, and possible increase in unemployment, this country is heading into ever more troubled waters and the Bureau had better be fully prepared. . . . This cannot be done if we spread ourselves too thin." Puzzled by Sullivan's attack on a policy he had supported a few days before, Hoover had one of his aides analyze Sullivan's memo. The conclusion was . . . that he is more on the side of CIA, State Department and Military Intelligence Agencies, than the FBI."[4]

Hoover's assessment was accurate. Sullivan had turned coat. According to Summers, he became "frustrated by Edgar's stonewalling over domestic intelligence, and by the ending of COINTELPRO," a program NSC advisor Kissinger desired to expand. He was also allegedly angry about "Edgar's latest empire building abroad."[4]

Having lost patience with Hoover, Sullivan established covert contacts with Nixon officials, particularly Assistant Attorney General Mardian.[8]

Sullivan supplied Mardian with stacks of Hoover's internal correspondence. Mardian passed several of the most select to Attorney General Mitchell, then filed the remainder away in a folder he simply marked "Jones." The administration knew that Hoover would undoubtedly find out about the theft.[8]

Then, at the height of the furor over the Pentagon Papers (the forty-seven-volume DOD report, leaked to the *New York Times* by Rand Corporation's Vietnam expert Daniel Ellsberg, that traced America's involement in Vietnam—a study in which Kissinger participated), Sullivan told Mardian that Hoover was "not of sound mind," and that Hoover possessed "documents that were 'out of channel,' wiretap information." Hoover, he said, was likely to use these documents to blackmail Nixon, and as long as he held those records, Nixon could not "relieve him."[8]

The wiretap files to which he was obviously referring were those ordered by Kissinger, directed by Haig, administered by Hoover and the FBI, authorized by Mitchell, and signed off by the president. The Bureau's copies—taps on at least four newsmen and thirteen government employees—were then locked away in Sullivan's office.[8]

Though Summers failed to mention Kissinger's apparent involvement, he noted that Mardian passed word of the blackmail threat to the president. Then orders were sent to Haig most likely by Kissinger to request the FBI (Sullivan) to destroy all such "special coverage."[8]

In response, Sullivan turned over two satchels containing the tap summaries to Mardian. He locked them up in his vault, then waited for further instructions.

At the FBI, Sullivan and Hoover finally butted heads. On August 28, after discussing his concerns with numerous FBI colleagues, Sullivan addressed a letter to Hoover defining their differences. "I would like to convince you," he wrote, "that those of us who disagree with you are trying to help you and not hurt you. . . . This letter will probably anger you. In view of your absolute power you can fire me . . . or in some other way work out your displeasure with me. So be it. . . ."[8]

Hoover began "the ensuing meeting with Sullivan," Summers revealed, "with a harangue. He said he had given the matter 'a good deal of prayer.' Then he began to sputter and stammer. When Sullivan advised him to retire [as Nixon through Mardian undoubtedly advised Sullivan to do] he said he would not. On the contrary, it was Sullivan" who was forced to leave. . . .[8]

Pretending that he was unaware that Sullivan had passed the incriminating wiretap transcripts over to Mardian, Hoover ordered his aides to search for them in Sullivan's office. The aides pulled every drawer and file but found nothing. When Sullivan returned, Hoover ordered him to reveal their whereabouts. He refused. "If you want to know more," he abruptly said, "you'll have to talk to the Attorney General."[8]

> Months later, following Hoover's death and the total significance of the wiretap program emerged, Mark Felt, Sullivan's replacement wondered: "It is very strange that Hoover did not explain the entire situation to me." Despite ordering Felt to search fruitlessly for the missing wiretap records, Hoover "knew the whole story."[8]

Ending an Intelligence Career

On October 3, 1971, Assistant Attorney General Mardian asked Ehrlichman for advice. Having custody of the dangerous wiretap transcripts made Mardian nervous.

"Mardian was very afraid," Ehrlichman recalled, "not only of the integrity of the files but also of his own personal safety. He felt he was being surveilled by Hoover, that it was only a matter of time before Hoover caused agents of the FBI to break into his office vault and recover the records. . . ."

Days later, in the Oval Office, Ehrlichman and Attorney General Mitchell requested the president's advice. Not until 1991, with the release of the Nixon tapes, was their conversation disclosed:

> MITCHELL: Hoover is tearing the place up over there trying to get at them. The question is, should we get them out of Mardian's office before Hoover blows the safe . . . and bring them over here?
>
> EHRLICHMAN: My impression from talking with Mardian is that Hoover feels very insecure without having his own copy of those things. Because, of course, that gives him leverage with Mitchell and you.
>
> NIXON: Yeah.

EHRLICHMAN: Because they're illegal. Now he doesn't have any copies and he has agents all over this town interrogating people, trying to find out where they are. He's got Mardian's building under surveillance.

NIXON: Now, why the hell didn't he have a copy, too?

EHRLICHMAN: If he does, he'll beat you over the head with it.

NIXON: Oh . . . you've gotta get them out of there.

MITCHELL: Hoover won't come and talk to me about it. He's just got his Gestapo all over the place.

NIXON: Yeah . . . just say [to Mardian] that we want to see them. Put them in a special safe.[9]

The troop complied with their general's demand.

For nearly a year, Nixon and his aides discussed how they might neutralize the Hoover risk or remove him from office. Initially, discharging him had seemed too risky given his popularity. But later polls showed that the public's enthusiasm for the aging FBI chief had waned. This was reinforced by a constant barrage of criticism Hoover received from the press.[9] Much of this was likely contrived by the CIA under the Kissinger and Haig NSC staff chain of command.

In response, the director had charged the media with being "journalistic prostitutes" and ordered FBI personnel to avoid all contact with *The Washington Post*, *The New York Times*, the *Los Angeles Times*, *CBS* and *NBC*—organizations that Hoover knew maintained strong ties to the CIA.[10]

"I'm willing to fight him," said the president lamely during a meeting on October 8, 1971 in the Oval Office. "We've got to avoid the situation where he could leave with a blast. . . . If he does go, he's got to go of his own volition. . . ." The president had struck out in his previous efforts to dismiss Hoover. Now he was undoubtedly shy about trying again.

Two weeks later, the president received a special report on Hoover from Ehrlichman. Further delay, it cautioned, might be disastrous. Blackmail was suggested:

> Morale of FBI agents in the field has deteriorated badly. . . . All clandestine activities have been terminated. Liaison with the intelligence community has been disrupted and key men forced out. . . . Hoover has reportedly threatened the President. . . . Years of intense adulation have inured Hoover to self-doubt. He remains realistic, however, and on June 30 his most trusted confidant, Clyde Tolson, stated to a reliable source, "Hoover knows that, no matter who wins in '72, he's through."

Sullivan has been "keeping book" on Hoover for some time. He is a skilled writer. His book could be devastating should he choose to expose such matters as the supervisor who handled Hoover's stock portfolio and tax matter; the painting of Hoover's house by the FBI Exhibits Section; the ghostwriting of Hoover's books by FBI employees; the rewriting of FBI history and the "donation" by "admiring" facility owners of accommodations and services which are often in fact underwritten by employee contribution. . . .[9]

The report recommended Hoover's retirement before the end of the year. Nixon wholeheartedly agreed. "Hoover," he said, "has to realize that he can't stay forever. . . . I think I could get him to resign, if I put it to him directly that without it he's going to be hurt politically. . . . But I want this closely held—it's just got to be."[9]

Despite lengthy preparation, scripting, and rehearsals, the president attempted and failed again. The reason was explained by Summers:

Contrary to what Nixon had imagined at first, the threat [of the White House wiretap transcripts] had not evaporated when Sullivan handed over the FBI copies . . . to Assistant Attorney General Mardian. When Mardian checked the list, he discovered some of the transcripts were missing. They had been retained, all along, by Edgar.[9]

Though Nixon openly claimed to his death that "Hoover never gave any indication to me of blackmail," the truth was known to his intimates. Months after his meeting with Hoover, Nixon confided with Ehrlichman: "The meeting was a total strikeout. He told me I'd have to force him out." "It was my conclusion," Ehrlichman said, that the president believed, "that Hoover's resignation before the election would raise more problems than it would solve." Likewise, Kissinger recalled, "Nixon thought Hoover was quite capable of using the knowledge he acquired as part of his investigations to blackmail the president."[9]

So rather than heralding his dismissal, the press reported that Nixon wanted "Hoover to remain in office."[9]

In one of the final interviews of his life, Hoover declared himself fit and determined to carry on: "Many of our great artists and composers," he said, "did their best work in their eighties. They were judged on performance, not age. . . . Look at Bernard Baruch; he was brilliant in his nineties—and Herbert Hoover and Douglas MacArthur in their eighties. That is my policy. . . . "[9]

Consequently, with COINTELPRO on ice, the FBI stupefied, the CIA cut off from domestic intelligence, the administration blackmailed, and Kissinger's authority blocked along with his patron's economic interests,

Nixon was at his wits end. Besides everything else, he was certain his White House still harbored a mole—someone who might again leak secrets to the press. What's more, the president was still outraged that Hoover had blocked the investigation of a perceived traitor and suspected communist—Daniel Ellsberg. Hoover had apparently befriended Ellsberg's father-in-law, so he felt obliged to come to the family's aid.[9]

"If the FBI was not going to pursue the [Ellsberg] case," Nixon wrote in his memoirs, "then we would have to do it ourselves."[9]

Beyond Watergate

In June 1971, seated in his Oval Office, Nixon told his aide Charles Colson, "I don't give a damn how it is done, do whatever has to be done to stop these leaks and prevent further unauthorized disclosures. . . . I want to know who is behind this . . . whatever the cost."

The directive led to the formation of the Plumbers and then to Watergate:

> The cast of characters is now well known. The chain of command went from Nixon to Ehrlichman to Krogh and Young, with Colson and the President's Counsel, John Dean, putting in their nickel's worth. In the field, assigned to do the White House's dirty work, were Howard Hunt and Gordon Liddy. Hunt was a fifty-two-year-old career CIA officer who had, technically, retired from the Agency and gone free-lance. [Previous to Watergate, he had been investigated by the Warren Commission for his CIA connections and possible role in the assassination of JFK—he was allegedly seen on the grassy knoll behind a puff of smoke at the time the shots were fired and had no alibi.[11]] Liddy had served as an Assistant District Attorney in New York, then as a special assistant in the Nixon Treasury Department, since leaving the FBI in 1962.[9]

Interesting that Kissinger wasn't in the Plumber's chain of command, I thought. Particularly since he was in charge of the 40 Committee, the group that took charge of authorizing covert actions by the CIA.[12] He would have likely known about the entire affair since it was essentially a CIA-run operation according to the Rockefeller Commission. But his name failed to appear in the report and CIA reprimand.[11]

I considered that Nixon may have suspected Kissinger's involvement in the Ellsberg case, and purposely kept him in the dark about the Plumbers. But that wasn't likely either, I realized. Kissinger's intelligence network exceeded Hoover's and infiltrated the CIA's by then. If anything went on, Kissinger most likely knew about it.

A Kissinger/Rockefeller Coup?

Then it occurred to me how Kissinger came out on top. He outlasted everyone. In fact, he's still considered the most powerful foreign policy adviser in the world.

Had a Kissinger/Rockefeller coup actually occurred?

I reflected on the fact that Nixon held Nelson Rockefeller in disregard, and snubbed him—Nixon's 1968 presidential contender—by giving Kissinger the job Rocky expected.[13] When Kissinger was selected instead of the banking mogul, Rockefeller's staff "were shocked." Kissinger himself suggested that Nixon reconsider Rockefeller rather than him to lead the Defense Department. Before that, Kissinger told Gloria Steinem that the only way he would go to Washington is if Rockefeller became his boss. In retrospect, that's what happened. Rockefeller remained Kissinger's patron before, during, and after the Nixon era.[14]

I reflected on the fact that it was largely Rockefeller's influence and contacts that helped catapult Kissinger to the top of the business consulting industry. A partial list of his international clients was remarkable to say the least: American Express, Anheuser-Busch, Atlantic Richfield, Coca-Cola, GTE, Chase Manhattan and Midland Banks, Bell Telephone, H.J. Heinz, Revlon, Union Carbide, and Volvo to name just a few. And then there was Merck and Co.[15]

Isn't that interesting! I thought, reflecting on my knowledge of George Merck's leadership of America's biological weapons industry[16] as well as the experimental hepatitis B vaccines Merck and Co. prepared for the American gay community.[17]

I considered the fact that Nixon and Hoover stood in the way of both Kissinger and Rockefeller—financially and politically. Hoover was overtly hostile toward Kissinger, he hated jews, wouldn't take orders, and catered to organized crime. And neither Kissinger nor Rockefeller thought much of Nixon. At best they perceived him as inept. At worst, they considered him a paranoid maniac and a mutual threat.

Moreover, both Nixon and Hoover had potentially dangerous intelligence data on Kissinger as well as Rockefeller. Hoover held "a big file of dirt" on Rockefeller. And the two held wiretap transcripts that could have incriminated Kissinger as well as his closest aides.[18]

Rockefeller, I also recalled, served as President Eisenhower's international affairs assistant. He resigned when Eisenhower refused to endure his Vietnam war plans—billions in military–industrial revenue. That's when

Eisenhower issued his warning about the evil "military–industrial complex." Now Kissinger was playing the same role for Nixon with the "East Coast establishment, the Rockefellers, the media and banking elite pulling the strings.[19]

Moreover, after Nixon was ousted and Ford became president, Kissinger petitioned Ford to select Rockefeller to be the new vice president. Having hundreds of political colleagues, Isaacson reported, "Kissinger felt the most trust and affection of anyone in public life" for Rockefeller.[19]

Then following their White House communion, the "Kissingers and the Rockefellers spent New Year's together at the outset of 1975 at Dorado Beach in Puerto Rico." Isaacson reported that Henry felt very good about himself at the time: "Relaxing in the sun, and married to a socially impeccable former Rockefeller aide, Kissinger seemed more at peace with himself than he had been for a long time."[19]

Naturally, he seemed more at peace, I observed, their principle political rivals were destroyed. They now maintained sole control of the White House.

Had they played a determining role in discrediting Nixon. Could they have been behind the Plumbers getting caught? And what about Hoover's untimely and mysterious death?

Haig as Deep Throat?

I flashed back to watching a CBS special I had seen a few years ago. The program cited Haig and Kissinger among the likeliest suspects to have played the role of "Deep Throat." Since Kissinger and Haig allegedly had alibis, Mike Wallace concluded Deep Throat was Patrick Gray, a former assistant attorney general "who was appointed acting director of the FBI six weeks before the break-in at the Watergate." Neither Woodward nor the 76-year-old (in 1992) Gray confirmed the report, however, and two sources outright denied it— Charles Bates (the former assistant director of the FBI at the time of the break-in) and Howard Hunt (one of the CIA operative Plumbers).

It wouldn't be the first or last time CBS and Mike Wallace spread lies to cover up government incriminating truths, I realized.[20]

It was Rockefeller, I considered, who enlisted Kissinger to join his international military–security business during their meeting at Quantico in 1955. Kissinger's Quantico report laid out Rockefeller's, that is, America's foreign policy objectives and foreshadowed over four decades of violent American history. Most important, it contained military proposals that required, of course, far more spending.[20]

And it was Kissinger who drafted Haig to be his chief aide at the NSC. *And Joseph Califano recommended Haig.* The recollection suddenly took on greater meaning. Califano, the former secretary of the Department of Health, Education and Welfare (DHEW) during the Carter administration. The man who gave the U.S. surgeon general his orders when I was completing my M.P.H. at Harvard! Isn't that interesting.

My mind raced to consider the possible role Califano played during this perilous period of American history. Califano became Secretary of DHEW in 1977, I recalled.[21] That was just when the large Merck and USPHS gay hepatitis B study was getting underway. As the secretary of DHEW, Califano was empowered to direct both foreign and domestic vaccination programs for the USPHS, USAID, as well as the WHO.

After letting the Califano connection sink in a bit, I continued to consider Deep Throat. Deep Throat fed Woodward and the *Washington Post* the inside poop on Kissinger/Rockefeller political enemies. That was traditional CIA counterintelligence operations over which Kissinger was in charge at the time. That was why Hoover ordered the FBI to break ties with *The Washington Post* which he knew was being influenced by Kissinger, most likely through his Washington Special Action Group. (See fig. 11.2 for an organizational chart of the U.S. national security system under Kissinger; also see reference 10.) With the score of CIA- and FBI-sponsored break-ins that went unreported during that time, maybe it's not so astonishing they caught the Plumbers at the Watergate. Deep Throat was most likely Haig.

I searched the library shelves once again in an effort to investigate my hunch. In Len Colodny's fascinating book *Silent Coup: the removal of Richard Nixon*, I learned that my suspicions were well founded. Not only was Haig exposed for his virtually certain role as Deep Throat, but Bob Woodward, who himself published a treatise on the CIA, was revealed to be a communications specialist for American intelligence. In fact, Colodny provided substantial documented evidence that Woodward routinely briefed Haig at the Pentagon prior to their Nixon White House assignments.[22]

Then, in Summers's book, I read that many believed Watergate was "only the tip of the iceberg." During the Nixon era, the CIA conducted hundreds of break-ins into people's homes and businesses; all of "whom the administration considered to be its 'enemies.' Their spectrum of targets ranged from radicals and subversives to high ranking diplomats and politicians. One such victim, Summers assures us, was J. Edgar Hoover.[18]

Why had the Plumbers gotten caught at the Watergate and nowhere else? Could it have been a play, perhaps with Haig as quarterback, to initiate Nixon's downfall, thus, facilitating a Kissinger/Rockefeller coup?

Prelude to the Sting

Isaacson's book revealed that Nixon's relationship with Kissinger had steadily deteriorated:

> During his five and a half years in office, Nixon's admiration for Kissinger would gradually become more infected by jealousy and suspicions of disloyalty. With no personal affection to serve as a foundation for their relationship, what had been a love-hate alliance eventually tilted toward the latter. As the president's dependency on Kissinger grew, his resentment and bitterness increased.[23]

Ultimately, when the Plumber's failed to find evidence of the inside leak they expected to find in the office of Ellsberg's psychiatrist, Nixon was in deep trouble. Not only did the media begin chasing "all the president's men," but Hoover knew the truth about the whole affair. Nixon had informed the director personally of his intention to enter Ellsberg's office. (Hoover would have learned this anyway. By that time, his intelligence network had thoroughly infiltrated the White House.)[9]

Push finally came to shove when Hoover learned of Liddy's written report calling for the director's forced removal. Since it was clear he would not go gracefully, nor would Nixon be able to shame him from office, Hoover's assassination became a clear option.[9]

The director recognized his predicament. On New Year's day 1972, while awaiting his flight back to Washington, Hoover spent forty-five morose minutes discussing his problems with Kenneth Whittaker, his special agent in charge of the city. Parked in his limousine outside Miami's international airport, Whittaker got an earful about how upset Hoover was about his trouble with Nixon. It was the last time he saw Hoover alive.[9]

Back home, Hoover took a curious step. He asked Andrew Tully, a trusted journalist, to lunch in private. "I have some things to say," he told

Tully, "but I don't want you to publish it until after I'm dead." Tully agreed. Then the reporter asked, "Is the President pressuring you to retire?"

"Not anymore he's not," Hoover replied. "I put the kibosh on those jaspers who want to get rid of me. . . . The President asked me what thoughts I had about retirement and I said none, then I told him why. I told him he needed me around."[9]

Having secured intelligence and illegal wiretaps on virtually all White House notables, Hoover likely suspected a Kissinger/Rockefeller coup was underway. Perhaps this is what he meant when he said Nixon "needed me around."

Later, Hoover threatened to expose the administration's ongoing domestic snooping ring. This fit the story relayed by James McCord, another former FBI and CIA agent. He said, Hoover "resolved that he would have to go to Congress with the facts" regarding the "wiretapping of the news media, the National Security Council staff and of Ellsberg." Undoubtedly, Nixon, Kissinger, Haig, and other NSC staffers feared this as well.

The last straw was a Nixon-damning exposé that Hoover fed *Life*. It spilled the beans on how "the White House had intervened to help" Arnholt Smith, "one of Nixon's best friends, and a bookmaker called John Alessio, another Nixon backer, to shake off corruption and tax charges." Hoover, the article said, had "used his personal influence to help defeat the White House moves," to assure "that Alessio faced trial." This, McCord believed, was what "really set Nixon at Edgar's throat."[9]

The Assassination of J. Edgar Hoover?

Summers filed an intriguing investigation report along with a startling conclusion—J. Edgar Hoover was very likely assassinated:

> A year after Watergate, Mark Frazier, a young reporter working in Washington, was to pick up an intriguing lead. Three sources, he learned, had given affidavits to the Senate Watergate Committee referring to two break-in operations at Edgar's home in Rock Creek Park. They were, allegedly, "directed by Gordon Liddy."
>
> In the welter of news arising from Watergate [or possibly because of official media censorship], Frazier was unable to get the story published in a Washington paper. Instead, it ran in a university publication, *The Harvard Crimson*.

Hoover's home, the article said, had been targeted twice for break-ins. The first operation, in "late winter of 1972," was intended to "retrieve documents that were thought to be used as potential blackmail against the White

House." This attempt failed, but was followed by another which succeeded. "This time," Frazier reported, "whether through misunderstanding or design, a poison of the thiophosphate genre was placed on Hoover's personal toilet articles."[22]

Thiophosphate, a chemical commonly found in insecticides, is extremely toxic to human beings if ingested, inhaled, or absorbed through the skin. Exposure can cause fatal heart attacks, and can only be detected by an autopsy performed within hours of the lethal poisoning.

> Gordon Liddy today denies knowledge of any break-in at Edgar's house. Hunt, contacted in Mexico, said curtly it was "a matter of total disinterest to me." Nixon's former Chief of Staff, Haldeman, however, accepts that something of the kind may have happened. "I have to concede the possibility," he said. "I think Nixon was capable at the time of saying to Colson, 'I want this done. I don't want any arguments about it. I don't want you to talk to Haldeman because he'll just say, Don't do it. Just go ahead and get it done. . . .'"

> Watergate burglar Felipe DeDiego, who today claims ignorance of the Hoover break-ins, . . . [at first said] he knew about the operation and hoped soon to be able "to talk about everything." Then, questioned again, he withdrew his comments. At home in Florida, however, he told Dade County State's Attorney Richard Gerstein that he had information on "other burglaries of a political nature."

> Another of the Watergate burglars, Frank Sturgis, said in 1988 that DeDiego told him about the Hoover break-ins immediately after Edgar's death. "Felipe told me about it," he said. "I suspected the CIA was behind it. I told him, 'I guess our friends probably wanted to go over there and see what kind of documents Hoover had stashed away.' Felipe laughed and said, 'That's dangerous. It's dangerous. . . .' And we didn't talk about it anymore."

> Sturgis admitted that the burglars were active in Washington earlier than emerged from the official Watergate investigation. Asked if he himself was involved in the Hoover break-ins, he hedged. "I'm not saying yes to my involvement. Let me say 'no' to that. It opens up a can of worms."[22]

Chief Plumber Krogh coincidentally served time where former Congressman Neil Gallagher was jailed as a result of Hoover's malicious attack—in Allenwood Pennsylvania's minimum security prison. In 1991, Gallagher signed a sworn affidavit which testified:

"I was the prison librarian, and Krogh would come in. . . . One night, when I was about to close the place and there were only the two of us there, we talked about Hoover.

"I said I thought the circumstances of Hoover's death were a bit strange. Because of my war with Hoover, I'd followed everything about him closely. I said to Krogh, 'Hoover knew everything that was going on in

Washington. He must surely have known about the Plumbers and everything. Do you think Hoover was blackmailing the President?' And then I said, and it surprises me now, 'Did you guys knock Hoover off? You had the troops to do it, and the reason. . . .'

"It took several seconds for it to sink in. Then Krogh literally jumped out of his chair. And in a highly charged voice he sort of screamed, 'We didn't knock off Hoover. He knocked himself off.' And I said, 'My God, that explains a lot about the bastard's death coming the way it did.' And with that Krogh . . . rushed out of the library. We never had another conversation the rest of the time we were in Allenwood."[24]

After Hoover's body was discovered by his housekeepers, and his lover Clyde Tolson was alerted, Robert Choisser, Edgar's physician arrived on the scene. "Mr. Hoover had been dead for some hours," he recalled. "I was rather surprised by his sudden death, because he was in good health. I do not recall prescribing him medication for blood pressure or heart disease. There was nothing to lead anyone to expect him to die at that time, except for his age."

Later that morning, two medical examiners, Dr. Richard Welton and Coroner James Luke, surveilled the situation. "It was totally normal," Welton recalled. "There was nothing to suggest trauma. Hoover was in an age group where it could be expected. . . . It is common for such a person to be found dead after apparently trying to get to the bathroom during the night."

On his way out, considering the need for an autopsy, Welton said to Luke "What if someone should pop up six months from now and say someone had been feeding Hoover arsenic? We'll think we should have done an autopsy."

Summers concluded that, "Neither pathologist had any reason to suppose anyone had been feeding Edgar arsenic, or any other poison."

No one knew that the Watergate burglars even existed, let alone that two of them had consulted a CIA expert about ways of killing columnist Jack Anderson, including the option of planting poison in his medicine cabinet. They knew nothing of alleged break-ins at Edgar's home, nothing of the suggestion that a poison might have been "placed on Hoover's personal toilet articles"— a poison capable of inducing cardiac arrest. . . . They knew nothing of the call Nixon had reportedly made to Edgar late the previous night, telling him it was time to step down.[24]

Three days after Hoover's demise, having decided against the autopsy, Luke signed the certificate of death:

John Edgar Hoover, male, white.
Occupation: Director, FBI.
Immediate cause: Hypertensive cardiovascular disease.

Life After Hoover

All of this meant that from mid-1970 to mid-1973, the CIA operated without any interference from the Justice Department. During this time, and following Hoover's death, the CIA grew in strength as the nucleus of foreign and domestic espionage operations. Despite the embarrassment of getting caught playing a central role in the infamous Watergate break-ins,[25] the CIA was hardly chastised by Congress.[11] It continued to expand agency operations at home and abroad under Kissinger and soon to be Chief of Staff Haig.[26] The two Nixon administration survivors ran the CIA, State, and Defense departments. They reinstated COINTELPRO-like operations,[27] expanded its covert operations in Africa,[28] and increased biological as well as chemical weapons research.[29,30]

In 1973, the CIA labored to maintain its positive public image. International condemnation over ongoing American biological warfare "experiments" was imminent. The Rockefeller Commission Investigation on CIA Wrongdoing was also about to begin as was a Congressional investigation in the aftermath of Watergate. It was then that CIA director Richard Helms, succeeded shortly thereafter by William Colby, ordered Mr. Sidney Gottlieb, Chief of the CIA's Technical Services Division, and former head of its MKULTRA—drug and mind control operation—to destroy all records pertaining to the "formulation, the development and the retention of" illegal biologicals that were used to wage war and experiment widely on Third World populations. Helms's orders apparently came from his superior—Dr. Henry Kissinger.[29-31]

By May 1973, in the wake of the Watergate scandal, as international attention focused on Nixon's fall from grace, a shadow government took control of America. The interim administration—which formed before President Ford was confirmed—was largely powered by Rockefeller, and commandeered by Kissinger and Haig.[32]

During the following presidential campaign, Brzezinski, Jimmy Carter's campaign manager and old-time Kissinger nemesis from Harvard, launched an embittered attack against the incumbent's foreign policy. Publishing in *Foreign Affairs* he described Kissinger's tactics as:

Covert, manipulative, and deceptive in style, it seemed committed to a largely static view of the world, based on a traditional balance of power, seeking accommodation among the major powers on the basis of spheres of influence.[33]

Cold and accurate as it was, the irrepressible fact is Kissinger and his realpolitik survived.

While campaigning for the presidency, Carter hailed Kissinger as the real "foreign policy . . . president of this country." "Under the Nixon–Ford administration," he said in a speech, "there has evolved a kind of secretive . . . closely guarded and amoral . . . , 'Lone Ranger' foreign policy, a one-man policy of international adventure." To these attacks, Carter added his standard refrain. "Our foreign policy should be as open and honest as the American people themselves."[33,34]

One year later, under the more "open and honest" policies established by Carter, Ray Ravenhott, the director of population control programs for USAID, revealed his agency's intention to help sterilize one quarter of the world's women. He argued that this need stemmed from the administration's desire to protect U.S. corporate interests from the threat of Third World revolutions spawned by chronic unemployment.[29]

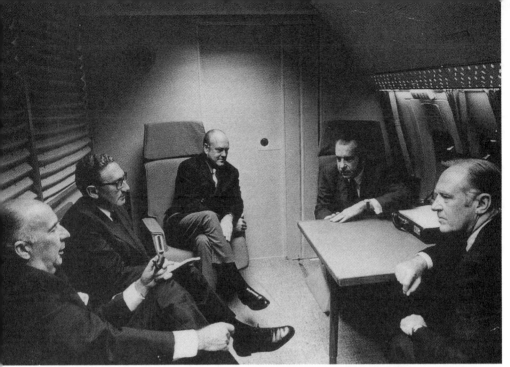

TWO PHOTOS: NATIONAL ARCHIES, NIXON PROJECT

John Mitchell, Henry Kissinger, Melvin Laird, Richard Nixon, and William Rogers aboard Air Force One, 1969. After feeding Nixon intelligence for his 1968 campaign, Kissinger was appointed national security adviser. Not long after, he ordered Defense Secretary Laird to reassess America's biological weapons capabilities, and then discovered the option of viruses for covert operations.

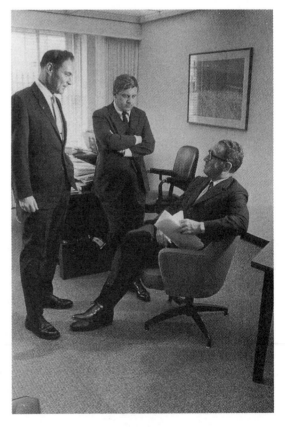

Chief deputy Alexander Haig, Lawrence Eagleburger and Kissinger, 1969. Colonel Haig, the evidence indicates, was most plausibly "Deep Throat." He coordinated secret projects including the White House wiretaps, Cambodian bombings, and very likely the assassination of J. Edgar Hoover along with the downfall of Richard Nixon.

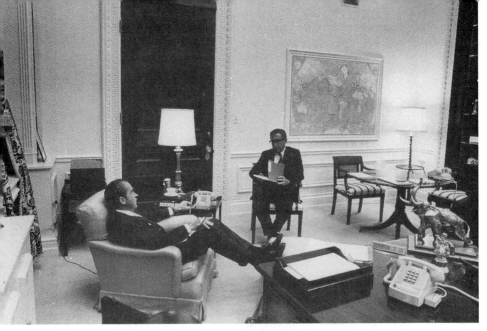

Executive Office meetings, 1969. Nixon and Kissinger rambled for hours, engaged in underhanded fantasies, plotted conspiratorial intrigues, and made numerous contradicting decisions. Nixon was openly antisemitic, racist, and homophobic. Both men believed Black nationalism was a communist plot, and population control was a national security necessity.

Kissinger with Rogers, Ehrlichman, Colson, and Haldeman, 1971. Ehrlichman and Haldeman administered an informal "Henry Handling Committee" to help relieve Kissinger's paranoid fits. Colson organized the Plumber's Unit. This led to Watergate. Oddly then, Kissinger and Haig escaped recrimination.

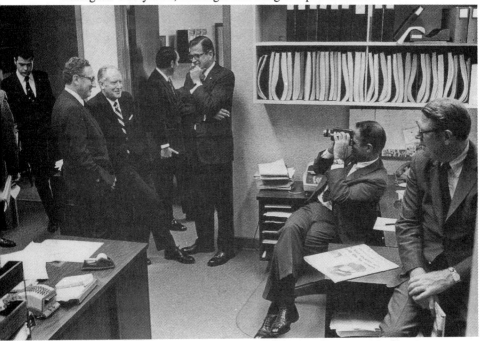

TWO PHOTOS: NATIONAL ARCHIES, NIXON PROJECT

Chapter 13
USAID and New York Blood

AS soon as I was able to free myself from the work that had piled up while in New York, I made a return trip to Countway's on-line center to continue my search for clues as to how HIV broke out, as it did, among specific populations.

Knowing that USAID, especially during the 1970s, had focused vast resources on controlling Third World populations, I typed "USAID" into the subject field and pressed "Enter." The computer then gave me several categories from which to choose, including "Population Control," "Vaccines," and "World Health Organization." First I selected "Population Control," and then the period before 1975. In less than a minute, the search located 733 "USAID-Population Control references."

Then I attempted the same search after 1975. To my absolute amazement, the entire field of "Population Control" had vanished! The subject heading had been terminated.

Could the whole field have been censored? I questioned. Califano and the Carter administration, apparently, replaced the term "Population Control" with the more comforting phrase "Maternal and Child Health."

Then I did the same period searches for USAID vaccine and WHO reports. During the later, I was directed to a *Department of State Bulletin* article wherein Califano addressed the WHO general assembly. "Rapid population growth," the Secretary of DHEW warned, "retards social and economic progress in many nations and burdens many families and communities."[1]

At the time Califano spoke, I was on the verge of joining the faculty at Harvard's School of Dental Medicine. I wondered at the time, why they were changing the name of the "Population Studies" department at the School of Public Health to "Maternal and Child Health." After reading Califano's speech, and reflecting on the disappearance of "Population Control" from MEDLAR, the influence of America's intelligence community on public health policy took on far greater meaning. I learned that by doing away with the phrase "Population Control," Califano and his subordinates was able to conduct similar programs under the less stigmatized "Maternal and Child Health" venue.

Looking for Merck and USAID in Africa

Next, I considered whether there was a direct link between Califano and Merck. It was certainly a good possibility. After all, Merck was the world's largest supplier of AIDS-related drugs and hepatitis vaccines,[2] with documented connections to military intelligence and biological weapons research and development,[3] and Califano had his military, intelligence, and public health background. The fit seemed natural. Moreover, Califano was part of the politically ignoble elite. The Rockefeller led military–medical–industrial complex held Kissinger's confidence as he held Califano's.[4] Kissinger was also a paid consultant of Merck, Sharp and Dohme (MSD).[5] That Califano heralded population control and oversaw many such projects in the Third World just prior to the AIDS outbreak, I felt, deserved further investigation. Had Califano authorized USAID funds for Merck-related hepatitis B vaccine studies in central Africa during his stint as secretary of DHEW?

I followed my intuition and entered a new search path—"USAID"—"Viral Vaccines." In about a minute, the computer retrieved 2,498 viral vaccine study reports from 1975 to 1985. I shuttered over the task of reviewing each entry. So instead, I chose to limit my search to hepatitis vaccine studies. That way, I could investigate my suspicions about Merck–African hepatitis B vaccine research.

Seconds later, MEDLAR produced dozens of abstracts describing various viral hepatitis vaccine experiments. One drew my immediate attention: "Whither immunization against viral infections?" by the chief of Merck's Division of Virus and Cell Biology Research, Dr. Maurice Hilleman.[6]

The paper was published in the *Annals of Internal Medicine*, the journal that during my *Deadly Innocence* investigation, had published absolutely ridiculous speculations offered by the CDC regarding the Acer case.[7] I read the abstract quickly and then retrieved the document.

Hilleman's article argued for the economic and social benefits of preventing infectious diseases through the use of vaccines. By the end of the report I realized, USAID—that is, the American taxpayer—and the WHO was undoubtedly supporting Hilleman's research on behalf of Merck.[6]

A Slight Conflict of Interest

Next, a report titled, "Hepatitis B [HB] vaccine: evidence confirming lack of AIDS transmission" drew my attention. The source was the CDC's *Mor-

bidity & Mortality Weekly Report. I ran to the stacks again and within minutes retrieved the article by "Anonymous" MSD and CDC authors.[8]

This December 14, 1984, publication was the CDC's official response to "concerns" that had "been expressed that the etiologic agent of AIDS might" have been transmitted by MSD hepatitis vaccines. The report noted that questions arose because the vaccines had been developed from pooled blood plasma, some of which had come from homosexual males who volunteered for the study. "HB vaccine acceptance in the United States," the authors wrote, "has been seriously hindered by the fear of possible AIDS transmission from the vaccine."[8]

To consider the possibility of HIV tainted HB vaccines, Merck researchers provided the company's vaccine to two groups of researchers—one at the Hepatitis Branch, Division of Viral Diseases at the CDC—a group specializing in Don Francis's (and as I would shortly learn—Dr. Robert Purcell's) area of expertise; the other to a group of researchers at the State University of New York led by Dr. B. J. Poiesz. Poiesz, the article noted in a reference, had worked closely with Robert Gallo in the late 1970s. Together, the two virologists had isolated type-C cancer viruses from patients with lymphomas—a blood cancer common among AIDS patients.

Despite the groups' best efforts, the report stated, they were unable to find any trace of the AIDS virus in any of the Merck supplied samples.

Next, to put an end to the damaging claims, the CDC reported:

> Epidemiologic approaches to detect an association between HB vaccine and AIDS have included an analysis of data on AIDS cases reported to CDC concerning their receipt of HB vaccine and monitoring rates of AIDS in groups of homosexually active men who did or did not receive HB vaccine in the vaccine trials conducted by CDC in Denver, Colorado, and San Francisco, California. To date, 68 AIDS cases have been reported among approximately 700,000 U.S. HB vaccine recipients; 65 have occurred among persons with known AIDS risk factors, while risk factors for the remaining three are under investigation. In addition, *the rate of AIDS for HB vaccine recipients in CDC vaccine trials among homosexually active men in Denver and San Francisco does not differ from that for men screened for possible participation in the trials but who received no HB vaccine* because they were found immune to HB.[8] [Emphasis added.]

After carefully considering their work, I recognized the authorities had, once again, misrepresented the facts and concealed evidence in a fashion reminiscent of their Kimberly Bergalis case investigation.[9]

Behind the Smoke and Mirrors

The fact is the homosexual men who received the first batches of experimental HB vaccine did not live in Denver or San Francisco. They lived in New York. Szmuness's *New England Journal of Medicine* report stated:

> We report here the initial results of a placebo-controlled, randomized, double-blind clinical trial to evaluate the efficacy of a hepatitis B vaccine in 1083 homosexual men from New York City.[10]

Undoubtedly, New York City was the hotbed of new AIDS cases in the late 1970s and early 1980s. There was no other place in America like it. In fact, the same trend observed in gay men from *New York* was also observed in intravenous drug users living there. I recalled a startling graph depicting this geographic pattern (see fig. 13.1) in the *American Journal of Public Health*.[11]

Why the report by Poiesz's team and anonymous CDC authors included Denver and not New York City study participants was highly irregular and suspicious since: (1) the volunteers were from the "Gay Men's Health Project of New York City and other gay organizations in New York"; (2) Poiesz and his co-workers were also in New York and neighboring states; (3) nineteen months into the AIDS epidemic, 501 of the 1,025 AIDS case fatalities were from New York (California had the second highest mortality rate with 221 AIDS victims);[12] and (4) Denver was not considered an especially high AIDS case area.

Moreover, the "experts" presented a flawed contention when they said, "the rate of AIDS for HB vaccine recipients in CDC vaccine trials among sexually active gay men in Denver and San Francisco does not differ from" those who did not receive the vaccine or placebo. I noted the distortion, as did Robert Lederer, a seasoned journalist and AIDS investigator. Lederer pointed out that the CDC's insistence that the vaccine was safe was explained using "circular logic, that all but four of the 64 recipients who developed AIDS had 'other risk factors,' i.e., they were gay. Yet medical follow-up studies of vaccine recipients specifically excluded persons with AIDS, preventing a resolution of this controversy."[13]

Technically, Lederer's objection about the Merck/CDC authors use of "circular logic" is accurate. The authorities simply used the risk factor—homosexuality—as a scape goat. The fact is the authorities should have and could have controlled for this as they worked to prove or disprove their "null hypothesis"—that HIV was not transmitted via the Merck/CDC vaccines, but in some other way.

Fig. 13.1. Geographic Patterns In the Spread of HIV and AIDS in the United States Showing New York City's Uniqueness

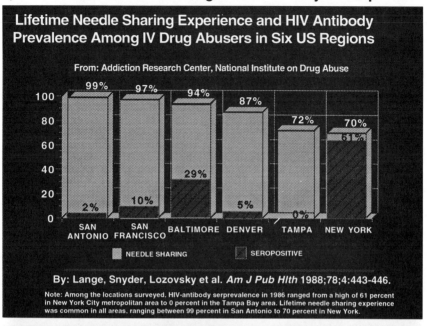

Lifetime Needle Sharing Experience and HIV Antibody Prevalence Among IV Drug Abusers in Six US Regions

From: Addiction Research Center, National Institute on Drug Abuse

NEEDLE SHARING   SEROPOSITIVE

By: Lange, Snyder, Lozovsky et al. *Am J Pub Hlth* 1988;78;4:443-446.

Note: Among the locations surveyed, HIV-antibody serprevalence in 1986 ranged from a high of 61 percent in New York City metropolitan area to 0 percent in the Tampa Bay area. Lifetime needle sharing experience was common in all areas, ranging between 99 percent in San Antonio to 70 percent in New York.

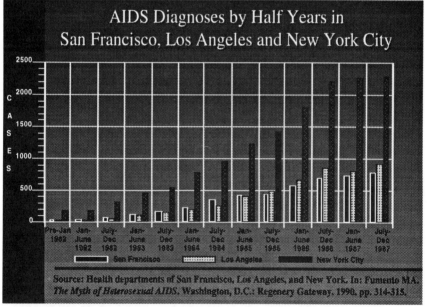

AIDS Diagnoses by Half Years in San Francisco, Los Angeles and New York City

Source: Health departments of San Francisco, Los Angeles, and New York. In: Fumento MA. *The Myth of Heterosexual AIDS*, Washington, D.C.: Regenery Gateway, 1990, pp. 314-315.

Graphs depict the number of HIV-positive persons among IV drug users in New York City as well as those diagnosed with AIDS was far greater than in other major cities. These trends could be explained by the theory that homosexual males and drug users in Manhattan had received tainted-experimental hepatitis B vaccines during the early to mid 1970s. Sources are cited in the graphs.

Equally distorted and suspicious was the report by Dr. Robert Hirsch, medical director of the Greater New York Blood Program published that same year. Hirsch insisted that "no [HB vaccine] recipient has been reported to have contracted any disease, including AIDS."[14] A study published two years later, in 1986, in the *Journal of the American Medical Association* provided conflicting evidence, some of which follows:[13]

Nathaniel Lehrman, a medical physician and Life Fellow of the American Psychiatric Association, noted with suspicion that the percentage of gay men from the San Francisco hepatitis B study group who became infected with the AIDS virus rose dramatically and too quickly—from "4 percent in 1978 to 68 percent in 1984 among the 6,875 members." The rate of HIV infection among homosexual men reported in 1989 varied across the U.S. from 10 percent in some communities to 70 percent in few others. Most telling, five years earlier, and only six years into the AIDS epidemic, the upper range was reached in New York and San Francisco. Lehrman correctly concluded that this oddity lent additional support to the tainted HB vaccine premise.[15]

More persuasive knowledge came from Pasteur Production—the Pasteur Institute's pharmaceutical company. Principals of the firm—which generated a good portion of the revenue that financed the privately run institute—were frantic over rumors that the Merck-manufactured hepatitis vaccine was tainted.[16] In 1982, Don Francis assured Luc Montagnier that "no link between AIDS and the vaccine inoculations" had been found. Yet, a year later, Francis sent Montagnier thirteen blood samples to test for the presence of the AIDS virus. The samples came from gay men in the San Francisco study who were dying of AIDS, and who had received the experimental hepatitis B vaccine.[17]

Additionally, in 1985, Harold Jaffe, deputy director for AIDS science at the CDC and co-worker Andrew Moss "presented data from the San Francisco hepatitis B study that found the virus was present in blood of 4.5 percent of the study's subjects in 1978, 20 percent in 1980, and 67 percent by late 1984."[18] In contrast, Randy Shilts wrote:

> In Pittsburgh, a city with a relatively low incidence of AIDS, 25 percent of gay men in one study were infected with the virus, and an additional 2 percent of local gay men were being infected every month. A Boston study found that 21 percent of a sampling of gay men were HTLV-III positive. To a large extent, all these studies were biased by the fact that subjects were selected from more sexually active men who went to VD clinics. [Meaning that a much lower prevalence of the virus was likely infecting the general homosexual popula-

tion throughout the United States.] *In San Francisco, for example, only about 40 percent of a randomly selected sample of gay men were infected, compared with the 67 percent infected in the hepatitis cohort.* [18] [Emphasis added.]

Dr. Jaffe's revelation should have called greater attention to the Merck HB vaccines as a suspect in the growing AIDS mystery. Jaffe, however, was not the only CDC researcher to present alarming facts.

Don Francis examined the "blood he had collected from the 6,800 [gay] men" who participated in the Merck/CDC study. He "selected 110 blood samples drawn in 1978 and about 50 taken in 1980. Only 1 percent in the 1978 study had LAV antibodies, while 25 percent of the group studied two years later were infected. Since then, the infection rate had more than doubled. The retrospective testing bolstered the hypothesis that a new viral agent had appeared among San Francisco gay men in 1976 or 1977 and spread rapidly. . . ."[19]

In following that logic, it seemed most plausible that the New York infections had not begun with the famous "Patient Zero"—Gaetan Dugas—around 1980 as was promoted by the CDC.[20]

More likely, I speculated, gay men from New York were being infected before 1976—sometime between 1973 and 1975 was my guess. My next thought was I wonder whether Szmuness's group conducted any hepatitis B vaccine trials in New York City in the early 1970s? I decided to look into that possibility posthaste.

Saul Krugman and Company

I quickly returned to the computer terminal I had left a few hours earlier. I typed in the new search path, "USAID"—"Vaccines"—"Hepatitis," and entered the database prior to 1975. The search retrieved numerous sources; the most frequently recurring name on this list was S. Krugman—a name I remembered seeing in Szmuness's report.

I'll have to reread that again when I get home, I thought. Then I spent the rest of the day finding and photocopying other references cited during the search.

Later that evening, after telling Jackie about the CDC's and Merck's "Anonymous" vindication of their hepatitis B vaccine experiments, I pulled out Szmuness's *New England Journal of Medicine* report and found the New York University Medical Center (NYUMC) affiliate's name all over it. "Krugman" appeared four times on the first page alone; five times in the reference section, and again in each of two acknowledgment sections.

Krugman, in fact, was acknowledged as being the chairman of the advisory committee overseeing the entire homosexual hepatitis B vaccine program.[10]

Additionally, I recalled the name "New York University Medical Center" was on the list of biological weapons contractors the Army had turned over to the House appropriations subcommittee (see fig. 6.7).[21]

Then it dawned on me that Szmuness and his colleagues from the New York Blood Center had conducted the gay HB vaccine study in cooperation with researchers from the Division of Epidemiology at Columbia University's School of Public Health—where Joseph Califano was employed.[22]

I reread Szmuness's report carefully to consider Krugman's contributions to the field of hepatitis B virology. "*Bingo!* There it is." I shouted from the library alterting Jackie to my find. She came over and sat beside me on the arm of the recliner. "Krugman and his colleagues had been investigating various concoctions of live and disabled hepatitis B viruses on monkeys and men in New York City since the early 1970s," I said.[10]

"In fact," I continued, "Krugman and his colleagues—R. H. Purcell and J. L. Gerin—had injected homosexual males with various research reagents during their 1976 and 1977 vaccine trials. The report states that 'Krugman et al., in a classic series of studies [between 1969 and 1978], found that a 1:10 dilution of hepatitis B infective serum (strain MS-2) . . . prevented or modified hepatitis B in about 70 percent of vaccinated subjects who were later challenged with infectious material.'"[23]

"God help the poor souls in the other 30 percent of the group," Jackie replied, then got up and walked off towards the nursery.

I continued reading the report which also stated:

A more sophisticated vaccine, in principle similar to Krugman's, has subsequently been developed by Hilleman and his colleagues at the Merck Institute of Therapeutic Research. This vaccine consists of highly purified, formalin-inactivated HB_sAg [HB surface particles capable of prompting an immune response] derived from the plasma of chronic carriers of the antigen. The vaccine has been extensively evaluated for safety, immunogenicity, and efficacy in chimpanzees, and its safety and immunogenicity were confirmed in human volunteers. A similar vaccine has been developed by Purcell and Gerin [colleagues of Krugman and Hilleman with ties to Merck, Sharp & Dohme]. By mid-1978, data obtained from these Phase I and II studies were sufficient to permit efficacy testing in a large-scale field trial with human subjects.[10]

In essence, the "Phase I and II studies" had been conducted in New York City from 1976 to 1977. Just the right time for prompting a small homosexual outbreak of AIDS cases in Manhattan in 1978.

Figure 13.2 shows how gay male volunteers were solicited for these hepatitis B vaccine experiments through newspaper advertisements.

It was also clear that Krugman—affiliated with NYUMC—did the initial studies, and then passed his innovations on to Hilleman and others at Merck.

I walked into the nursery to find Jackie putting together Alena's old crib in preparation for our new arrival. "No doubt Merck paid Krugman a fee for his labor and discoveries," I said. "What bothers me is, here again, the American taxpayer was left footing the bill and holding an empty bag. Government grants, that is, our taxes, undoubtedly funded the discovery of the hepatitis B vaccine; then the rights to it were sold off."

The realization that Merck had been making billions a year from AIDS-related drugs, and fortunes more from hepatitis B vaccines, made me momentarily ill. Particularly since April 15—tax day—was close at hand.

Fig. 13.2. Advertisement Placed in New York Newspapers to Recruit Homosexual Men Into Experimental Hepatitis B Vaccination Program

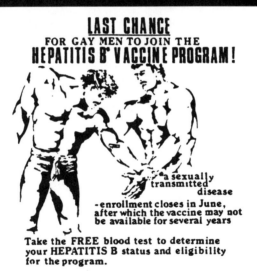

This 1979 ad recruited volunteers for hepatitis-B vaccine experiments conducted by W. Szmuness and other investigators associated with the New York City Blood Center, Merck, Sharp & Dohme, and the CDC. Credit: *Gaysweek.* Source: Lederer R. Origin and spread of AIDS: Is the West responsible. *Covert Action Information Bulletin* (Winter) 1988;29:60.

Purcell and Gerin: Merck's NIAID Connection

Szmuness's report revealed that the pilot surveys, Phase I and II, were conducted by "M. R. Hilleman . . . and his colleagues at the Merck Institute of Therapeutic Research," and by R. H. Purcell and J. L. Gerin. Therefore, the following day, I decided to investigate their interconnections.

Robert H. Purcell, I learned by digging up one of his grant proposals (see fig. 13.3), was Head of the Hepatitis Viruses Section in the Laboratory of Infectious Diseases of the National Institute of Allergy and Infectious Diseases (NIAID) in Bethesda, Maryland.[24]

Dr. Gerin, who frequently published with Purcell on the subject of hepatitis, was affiliated with the NIAID and "MAN Laboratory."[24]

From a NIAID Task Force report entitled *Virology: Control of Viral Infections* published by the USPHS's DHEW at the time Califano was the agency's chief, I learned that Gerin was credited for having prepared "two pilot lots of the hepatitis B vaccine, one subtype adw and the other subtype ayw. . . . Following extensive safety testing in chimpanzees," Purcell wrote, "both vaccines are currently undergoing safety testing in humans." The human test subjects were the homosexual males who had volunteered for the Merck/CDC HB vaccine trials.[24]

Purcell, leery of vaccine production costs, explained the complexity of their experiments on monkeys and gay men in advance of Szmuness's New York City HB vaccine trials. He wrote in his 1977–1978 grant proposal:

> Although a hepatitis B vaccine . . . purified from the plasma of chronic carriers of the antigen is feasible and probably cost-effective for its contemplated uses in the United States, such a vaccine probably will not be cost-effective for the people most in need of a vaccine in the developing world. Therefore, additional studies on alternative methods of purification and inactivation, comparisons of monovalent vs bivalent or polyvalent [that is, different combinations of] vaccines, studies of different vaccine dosages, different vaccination schedules, different routes of administration, studies of possible adjuvants [substances that might be added to enhance the main ingredient's strength] and their interaction with vaccine preparations and further characterization of the immunizing antigens themselves will be carried out [during the human trials for which this grant proposal was written].
>
> In addition, one important observation associated with the vaccine trials in chimpanzees was that type B hepatitis could be prevented in chimps by vaccination after exposure. . . . Additional studies in chimpanzees to confirm and extend these observations [to humans] are planned.[24]

Fig. 13.3. NIAID Grant Summary Report: Hepatitis Virus Experiments Conducted on Monkeys and Homosexual Males in N.Y.C.

SMITHSONIAN SCIENCE INFORMATION EXCHANGE PROJECT NUMBER (Do **NOT** use this space)	U.S. DEPARTMENT OF HEALTH, EDUCATION, AND WELFARE PUBLIC HEALTH SERVICE **NOTICE OF** INTRAMURAL RESEARCH PROJECT	PROJECT NUMBER
		Z01 AI 00026-11 LID

PERIOD COVERED
October 1, 1977 through September 30, 1978

TITLE OF PROJECT (80 characters or less)

Laboratory and Epidemiologic Studies of Viral Hepatitis Agents

NAMES, LABORATORY AND INSTITUTE AFFILIATIONS, AND TITLES OF PRINCIPAL INVESTIGATORS AND ALL OTHER PROFESSIONAL PERSONNEL ENGAGED ON THE PROJECT

PI:	R.H. Purcell	Head, Hepatitis Viruses Section	LID, NIAID
	Y. Moritsugu	Visiting Scientist	LID, NIAID
	V. McAuliffe	Research Associate	LID, NIAID
	Y. Shimizu	Visiting Fellow	LID, NIAID
	G. Hess	Guest Worker	LID, NIAID
	J. Slusarczyk	Visiting Fellow	LID, NIAID
	L. Mathiesen	Guest Worker	LID, NIAID

Other:

P. Holland, H. Alter (CC, Blood Bank, NIH)   L. Barker, D. Lorenz,
K. Soike (Delta Primate Center)   E. Tabor, R. Gerety (FDA)
J.L. Gerin (MAN Laboratory)
W. London (NINCDS)
J. Maynard (CDC)

COOPERATING UNITS (if any)

None

LAB/BRANCH
Laboratory of Infectious Diseases

SECTION
Hepatitis Viruses Section

INSTITUTE AND LOCATION
NIAID, NIH, Bethesda, Maryland

TOTAL MANYEARS: 99/12	PROFESSIONAL: 51/12	OTHER: 36/12

CHECK APPROPRIATE BOX(ES)

☒ (a) HUMAN SUBJECTS   ☐ (b) HUMAN TISSUES   ☐ (c) NEITHER

☐ (a1) MINORS ☐ (a2) INTERVIEWS

SUMMARY OF WORK (200 words or less - underline keywords)
This project consists of continuing studies of the chemistry, structure, epidemiology, immunology and pathology of the human hepatitis viruses. The goal of such studies is the control of human viral hepatitis by application of the most appropriate methods, including active and passive immunization, chemotherapy and interdiction of spread of the viruses. Progress: The biophysical and biochemical characterization of hepatitis A viral antigen has begun, and studies of the immunopathology of hepatitis type A in non-human primates, using defined pools of virus, are in progress. An inactivated subunit vaccine for hepatitis type B has been developed and is undergoing extensive tests of safety and efficacy in chimpanzees and man. A third hepatitis B antigen, e antigen, is being characterized and its relationship to infectivity is being explored. Evidence that populations of hepatitis B viruses may contain defective interfering particles has been obtained, and this finding is being utilized in renewed attempts to isolate the virus. A newly recognized clinical syndrome, type non-A, non-B hepatitis has been further defined and attempts to identify an etiologic agent intensified through transmission studies in chimpanzees.

Source: USDHEW. *Virology: Volume 4—Control of Viral Infections. NIAID Task Force Report.* Bethesda, MD: Public Health Service, National Institutes of Health (NIH) 79-1834, 1979, p. 20-65.

In other words, in Gerin's lab, chimps were being experimentally infected *and then* vaccinated (as the CDC and Merck currently recommend for healthcare workers following risky body fluid exposures[25]). Undoubtedly, human trials of this nature were planned and apparently conducted "in the developing world" and in New York City. Were gay males from New York given the honor of volunteering during the mid-1970s? I would soon find out.

On the next page of his grant application, Purcell discussed his plan to isolate, modify, and transmit liver cancer viruses in efforts to create a vaccine, he wrote:

> [P]reparations of high density and intermediate density HB virions [viruses] are being purified . . . under conditions of high containment in Dr. Gerin's laboratory. [The same Dr. Gerin who prepared the vaccines for experimentation on New York's homosexual population]. These preparations are being aliquoted and titered [fractioned and standardized] for infectivity in chimpanzees; they will be used for attempts to isolate HBV in a number of tissue culture cell lines.

> Cell lines that can be certified as being of ["fetal human or chimpanzee"] liver origin will be inoculated with partially purified HBV that is being titered in chimpanzees. These inoculated cultures will be monitored. . . .

> [R]ecently a hepatoma [liver cancer] cell line was isolated . . . in South Africa. . . . It is recognized that this cell line cannot serve as a source for hepatitis B vaccine because of its malignant origin, but it may yield important information on HBV-cell interaction. Attempts to recover the virus . . . are in progress.[24]

What frightened me was that these recovered viruses were being injected into chimpanzees that might have contacted other monkeys or chimps in Gerin's lab enroute to gay hepatitis B vaccine production and testing. Again, I would soon learn, these fears too were not unfounded. Related concerns were raised by research colleagues of Purcell and Gerin.

"Inner Circle" Interest in Central Africa

What struck me most about Purcell's report, however, was reference to an African connection to Merck-funded researchers in New York and Bethesda. If my suspicions were accurate, the literature held many more.

Merck, the U.S. Army, USAID, Litton Bionetics, and the NCI were all in the same business, I realized—cancer research. All were interested in vaccines and studies in which cancer-causing viruses were isolated and transported from Africa to the United States and visa versa. I suspected all were financially interconnected as well. My next job was to locate evidence to prove or disprove my suspicions.

I was now beginning to assess the relatively small "inner circle" of researchers running the planet's hepatitis and liver cancer research programs. It included the three Roberts from Bethesda—Gallo, Manaker, and Purcell—who were charged with overseeing the NCI and NIAID cancer cell biology programs. Saul Krugman and Maurice Hilleman were their counterparts at NYU Medical Center and the Merck Institute.

My suspicions that they worked together were fueled by several sources of information. First, Dr. Poiesz's arbitrary *MMWR* report "confirming lack of AIDS transmission" through Merck vaccines.[8] From this document, it was clear the SUNY researcher, Poiesz, had worked closely with Gallo in the late 1970s on T-cell leukemia/lymphoma.[26] Both sought to isolate cancer-causing viruses under military contracts, and both were apparently supported by Merck.

Indeed, the Poiesz–Gallo connection was so intimate, Poiesz led Gallo's research team in characterizing and reporting HTLV-I and HTLV-II—Gallo's two allegedly discovered leukemia viruses. Combined, the two military contractors reported the AIDS virus relatives were associated with T-cell malignancies. This work was done in the late 1970s, allegedly prior to the identification of the AIDS virus HTLV-III.[26] And when the time came to disclose the "complete nucleotide sequence of the AIDS virus," Gallo and his team cited Poiesz among the investigators who established, "human T-cell leukaemia (lymphotropic) viruses HTLV-I, -II and -III," the "family of exogenous retroviruses . . . associated with T-cell disorders, including adult T-cell leukaemia lymphoma and the acquired immune deficiency syndrome (AIDS)."[27] In essence, Poiesz was among the most intimate of Gallo supporters, and this bias alone could explain but not excuse his Merck-vaccine-vindicating *MMWR* report—as an expression of conflicting interest.

Two reports I had already read by Gallo and his colleagues thanked "Merck and Co., Incorp." for supplying them with experimental reagents, including a drug known as cordycepin.[28,29] Recalling the channel for one such contribution was the "Drug Development Branch" of the NCI, I realized this was a conduit of experimental reagents and drugs, including vaccines to and from MSD to Gallo and company.[29]

And now, here were other reports documenting the inner circle—New York, Bethesda, African researchers'—connections to experimental vaccines. The many Krugman papers I had photocopied earlier in the day provided clues as to how and why these researchers gathered cell lines from African natives—cell lines "successfully" infected with cancer viruses.[30]

The first Krugman report I read was his 1974 presentation before the "International Symposium on Viral Hepatitis." The conference, held in Milan, Italy, was "very generously" supported by Merck, Sharp and Dohme.[31] The report reiterated much of what had been published in Szmuness's report with one exception: Krugman acknowledged that his main source of funding, besides the Health Research Council of the City of New York, was the *United States Army Research and Development Command.*[31]

Krugman, I then realized, aside from his lucrative connections to Merck, was likely among the benefactors of the $142,000 the United States Army gave the NYUMC for biological weapons in 1969.[32, 33]

Most interesting, in this symposium report, was a discussion between Drs. Hilleman, Krugman, their colleague Dr. A. M. Prince, who was in charge of their monkey facility at the Laboratory of Virology at The New York Blood Center, (310 East 67th Street, New York, NY 10021), and three other participants—Dr. G. N. Vyas from the University of California, San Francisco, Dr. Desmyter from Belgium (where the NATO symposium on "entry of foreign nucleic acids into cells" was held in 1970), and Dr. J. E. Maynard from the CDC's Phoenix Laboratories Division (where Don Francis, several years later, became involved in the hepatitis B vaccine trials that these men were discussing). Their conversation revealed the New York group had tested their first batches of experimental HB vaccine even earlier than their other reports indicated. Here they discussed the fact that their initial HB vaccine trials were conducted on chimpanzees in the late 1960s, and "serosusceptible unimmunized persons" between 1970 and 1974.[31]

Moreover, they were preparing for extensive human trials in the mid-1970s. During the beginning of their discussion, Hilleman said:

> We have prepared 4 lots of vaccine that would amount to perhaps 200,000 human doses and we hope this can soon be put on initial limited clinical test for establishing safety and measuring antibody response.[31]

Soon thereafter, Hilleman evaded a question from Maynard about "who ought to be given the vaccine" by saying "This is a question better answered, perhaps, by Dr. Krugman," who also evaded the question by responding:

> Our preliminary studies with a heat-inactivated hepatitis B vaccine (JAMA, 217: 21–45, 1971) revealed evidence of protection. . . . If the hepatitis B vaccine proves to be safe and immunogenic in susceptible adults during the initial trials . . . , subsequent studies could be carried out . . . at a later time.[31]

The "who ought to be given the vaccine" question was finally answered by Szmuness a decade later. In his 1980 HB vaccine trial report, Szmuness wrote:

> Several populations in the United States with a high risk of HBV infection were considered for such a trial: patients institutionalized for mental retardation, patients undergoing hemodialysis, members of the medical staff of dialysis centers, American Indians, and homosexual men.[31] Of these groups, a population of HBV-susceptible homosexual healthy young men appeared to be the most suitable. Their risk of HBV infection is unusually high, they are readily accessible through numerous gay organizations, and their cooperation in previous studies has been excellent.[10]

Undoubtedly, with "200,000 human doses," which Krugman and company hoped in December 1974, to soon test, it is *highly* unlikely they vaccinated only 1,083 as reported by Szmuness.[10,34] After all, 7,000 local gay men took part in the hepatitis study conducted in San Francisco alone. Homosexuals who, according to Dr. Paul O' Malley, the health investigator who had headed up the Merck/CDC hepatitis B study, suffered "an inordinate number of GRID victims. . . . Of the first twenty-four GRID cases in San Francisco, in fact, eleven were in the hepatitis B cohort."[35]

Monkeying Around with Cancer for Profit

During the early 1970s, these researchers were experimenting with various heat treatments for preparing hepatitis B vaccines from infected chimpanzees and humans. Some inactivation methods were effective, they reported, and others were not.[31] In any case, the rush was on for immediate human trials.

Following Krugman's evasive statement, regarding who should be tested, Dr. Desmyter responded to concerns that a viral outbreak might occur from these experiments. He and other inner circle researchers knew that Krugman, since the mid-1960s, had been using children at the Willowbrook State School for the mentally retarded as human guinea pigs for Army and Atomic Energy Commission funded hepatitis B studies.[36] In an effort to determine the lowest concentration of HBV needed to immunize against hepatitis, Krugman inoculated dozens of New York children with, what was believed to be possible liver-cancer-causing viruses. At the time, their rationale was that the children were likely to become exposed to hepatitis B viruses anyway, in that setting, so little more consideration was given to the bioethics of such experimentation.[36]

"In relation to Dr. Prince's problem of quarantine for chimpanzees," Desmyter argued, "it is certainly not unavoidable that chimpanzees become infected before or after captivity. We have been monitoring two colonies for about 4 years. In one, more than 60% of the animals have [become infected with the hepatitis virus during holding]. . . ." He then told the group of another monkey colony that fared much better; to which the New York Blood Center's Dr. Prince replied, "Most of the animals that we have examined at the Laboratory of Experimental Medicine and Surgery in Primates in New York, that have been held for use in other programmes for a year or more, I would say more than 70% have [been environmentally infected with hepatitis B]. . . ."[31]

Prince's admission that 70 percent of their quarantined caged monkeys had sustained hepatitis infections in some unknown way was exactly what I had feared. Being "held for use in other programmes for a year or more," the monkeys were undoubtedly infected with more than just hepatitis B virus. The New York group I learned had, in fact, been experimenting with various types of viruses and mutant strains, just as Gallo and his Litton Bionetics associates had been doing. (The only difference is Gallo focused more on "type-C" cancer virus suspects, including RNA retroviruses that produced leukemia, lymphomas, and sarcomas, whereas Krugman's and Purcell's groups concentrated somewhat more on the herpes-type (DNA) viruses and "type B" RNA viruses associated with various forms of hepatitis and certain cancers of the liver, breast, nasopharynx, and lymph nodes. These included the yellow fever virus, cytomegalovirus, herpes simplex virus, and Epstein Barr virus (EBV) thought to be associated with Burkitt's lymphoma (BL)—most commonly seen in central Africa.[37]) Their work overlapped so much that they often shared their expertise and resources including *viruses*.

As documented during my USAID literature search, during the late 1960s and early 1970s, Krugman, Hilleman, and Purcell held a virtual monopoly over viral hepatitis research.[41] Yet their vaccine studies were not limited to hepatitis. Their quest for lucrative grants and contracts included studying dozens of virus strains in search of highly profitable vaccines. This created a grave laboratory and outbreak threat. Their chimps became natural breeding grounds for deadly contagions including hepatitis, herpes simplex, cytomegalovirus, EBV, measles,[38] mumps,[39] rubella,[39] tetanus,[40] diptheria,[40] smallpox,[38] and polio viruses.[40] Any number of mutant viruses might have been formed as the apes lived captive in Gerin's and Prince's labs. This, then, was one plausible way in which slow acting AIDS-like viruses, developed in Gallo/Bionetics labs, may have been accidentally transmitted to experimental hepatitis B vaccines developed in Gerin's lab—the vaccines tested in New York on humans, including homosexual males, kidney dialysis patients, the mentally retarded, and other high risk persons, during the Phase I and II studies discussed by Purcell.[24]

In 1974, during a virology symposium sponsored by the Gustav Stern Foundation, Purcell and Krugman discussed their problems and progress in developing, what would later become, Hilleman's and Merck's hepatitis B vaccine.[41] Purcell stated his failure to culture hepatitis B virus—the MS-2 strain that Krugman had pulled from "HAM," a mentally retarded child—in human cell cultures.[42] Likewise, rhesus monkey cell cultures failed to grow the monkey adapted hepatitis B virus. To overcome this problem, live chimpanzees were selected to grow all the different types of hepatitis B virus the researchers needed for their human experiments.[41]

"To avoid duplication of experiments and wastage of seronegative [scarce and expensive] chimpanzees, we are collaborating with Dr. Barker of the Bureau of Biologics, Food and Drug Administration, and Dr. Maynard of the Center for Disease Control, in an interagency study of hepatitis B infection in chimpanzees," Purcell wrote. "A high priority of these studies is the establishment of pools of hepatitis B virus. . . . Human serum or plasma containing HB_sAg of subtype *adw*, *ayw*, *adr*, or *ayr* has been inoculated into [the] chimpanzees. . . . The inoculum chosen to represent subtype *ayw* was serum supplied by Dr. Saul Krugman from the MS-2 pool of hepatitis B virus."[41]

"Cross-challenge experiments, and evaluation of various aspects of passive and active immunization against hepatitis B infection," Purcell explained, then proceeded in chimpanzees, rhesus monkeys, *and* humans. I later learned that Krugman's affiliated NYUMC was the world's leading institution for testing simian-to-man organ transplants, blood transfusions, and *vaccine research*.[43]

The final piece of the iatrogenic theory of AIDS puzzle fell into place when Purcell admitted the FDA–CDC–NIAID–NYUMC–AEC–Army and later Merck collaborative experimental hepatitis B vaccines, destined for humans, included viruses grown in chimpanzees containing any number of monkey virus contaminants that could have given rise to HIV-2 or 1.

Further implicating their hepatitis B vaccine, as Shultz explained, "a lentivirus isolated from chimpanzees (SIV_{cpz})" is "the closest primate relative of HIV-1."[44] SIV_{cpz} likely evolved, then, because the chimps had been: 1) used to develop experimental hepatitis B and other vaccines largely because they were primates bearing the greatest similarity to humans; and 2) among the first creatures to be exposed to the man-made retroviruses by way of direct inoculation or experimental monkey cohabitation.

It also occurred to me that even if Merck's human experimental hepatitis B vaccine hadn't included chimpanzee serum, only serum taken from New York's retarded children or gay men, live viral contaminants injected around 1970 could have combined with the simian viruses—SV40, SIV_{agm}, or SFV—the "volunteers" likely carried following vaccination with Merck's polio vaccines administered during the previous decade.

In 1976, the Willowbrook State School, under intense criticism for publicized cases of child abuse and neglect, was closed. The children, many possibly carrying the world's first AIDS viruses, dispersed back into the communities from which they came. "Only the State Institute for Basic Studies in Neuroscience stayed open on the campus," explained Leonard Ciaccio, a local biology teacher and historian. "The neuroscience lab conducted microbiological and biochemical studies . . . they were studying how cells were affected by various toxins."[45]

Though now the accidental theory of AIDS seemed highly plausible, since major funding for all this work came from Merck, the U.S. Army, CDC, NCI, NIAID, USAID, and AEC, given the Army and Merck connections to Kissinger *et al.*, BW research, and COINTELPRO targeting of gays and blacks, the intentional transmission theory remained to be disproven.

Though now I had identified the "self-serving bureaucracy" strong evidence indicated had brought AIDS into the world (see fig. 13.4),[46] I realized the hardest evidence still remained to be analyzed—the Krugman–Purcell–Hilleman Phase I and II hepatitis B vaccine lots allegedly in safe keeping at the FDA. Also, look-back studies of AIDS cases among Willowbrook alumni, and others who received these vaccines, were clearly warranted.

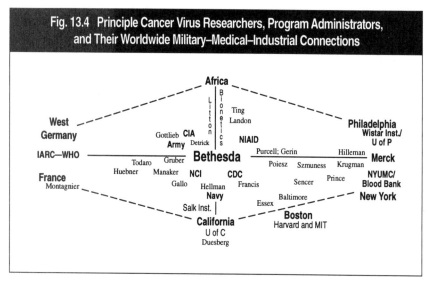

Fig. 13.4 Principle Cancer Virus Researchers, Program Administrators, and Their Worldwide Military–Medical–Industrial Connections

Chapter 14
Central West African Vaccine Trials

THE time had come to investigate the vaccine/immunization studies conducted in Central West Africa during the 1970s. Acknowledging that tainted HB vaccine was the prime suspect in transmitting the AIDS virus to homosexuals in New York, I now suspected the same was true for central west African natives.

By now I also knew the major players in America's vaccine and cancer research effort were closely knit and well funded by the military–medical–industrial complex. My next task was to investigate the specific African vaccine studies and immunization campaigns waged by the human suspects since this information might provide details on how AIDS viruses might have been accidentally or intentionally transmitted there as well.

The USAID MEDLAR search I had conducted days earlier provided numerous abstracts and references, among which were reports published by the International Association for Research in Cancer (IARC). Two IARC abstracts I immediately accessed detailed USAID-supported studies describing "HB vaccine" trials in Central Africa. One report acknowledged large-scale pilot studies carried out on children in order to test the safety and efficacy of Merck's hepatitis B vaccine. The report from Senegal stated:

> In 1978 it was suggested that hepatitis B (HB) vaccine should be used to prevent the early hepatitis B surface antigen (HB$_s$Ag) carrier state in children. Immunization was effected by 3 injections of HB vaccine at one-month intervals followed by a booster injection after one year. Children in a control group were immunized with DT-polio vaccine according to the same schedule. . . . In addition, an investigation was carried out on the immune response to HB$_s$Ag and tetanus toxoid . . . when administered simultaneously to [hundreds more] children in HB vaccine and DT-polio vaccine. In Africa, immunization teams have a limited amount of time to devote to each rural community. . . . These results demonstrate that 2 doses of 5 micrograms of HB vaccine are sufficient to obtain a high immunogenic effect in infants.[1]

The second abstract described another USAID HB vaccine study that was launched in Burundi, Zaire's eastern neighbor. A hospital setting was used this time to test new vaccines on infants. The abstract stated:

Vaccination against hepatitis B is carried out at birth in the Bujumbura Hospital in Burundi. The vaccination protocol comprises only two injections, the first being given during the first 48 hours after birth and the second two months later. A booster is given at the age of one year. The results of this vaccination programme are compared with those obtained in a control population. At the time of the booster, 82% of vaccinated subjects had anti-HBs antibodies, compared with 3% of control subjects. Six months after the second injection, all vaccinated subjects had anti-HBs antibodies.[2]

So it was clear, hepatitis B vaccine studies, similar to those conducted in New York on gay volunteers, proceeded in Africa on children and infants during the same period. Moreover, some of these studies used various combinations of live and inactivated viruses to immunize the test subjects. This could have created additional mutant germs and unusual "tropical diseases."

The Cream of International Vaccine Research

Next, I followed Krugman's paper trail to the WHO office in Washington, D.C. Here on December 14–18, 1970, the WHO held an "International Conference on the Application of Vaccines Against Viral, Rickettsial, and Bacterial Diseases of Man." Once again, the meeting was generously funded by Merck, Sharp and Dohme.[3]

The Pan American Health Organization, quartered in the WHO's Washington office building, co-hosted the event that made the world's cream of vaccine research rise to the occasion. Among the 330 researchers in attendance was Dr. Robert Manaker—Gallo's senior at the NIH.[3] Manaker, I learned from the proceedings report, had studied lymphoid-leukemia viruses at the NCI—Gallo's claim to fame—while Gallo was still studying to be a doctor at Jefferson Medical College.[4] That was 1960— more than ten years before Gallo allegedly discovered HTLV-I.

Also in attendance was Dr. S. Paul Ehrlich, Jr. representing the USDHEW. Ehrlich later became the acting surgeon general when Califano became secretary of the department in 1976. At the time, Congress was investigating the DOD for its open-air biological weapons experiments on unsuspecting human subjects in San Francisco, New York, and elsewhere. Ehrlich's department then defended the Army by issuing a statement that read: "We do not know of any evidence that would indicate an association between the deaths reported in the press . . . and the organisms reported to have been used in the atmospheric tests."[5]

Other famous researchers present were Hilary Koprowski and Stanley Plotkin from the Wistar Institute, Dr. Albert Sabin from the Weitzmann Institute of Science in Israel, Hilleman from Merck, Purcell from NIAID, and Krugman from NYUMC. Hilleman and Krugman were acknowledged for working on the ten-member Program Committee, and Hilleman was given special credit for being a "Consultant" to the organization.[6]

The most well-represented organizations at the conference included Merck, who had sent a total of ten delegates, the Wistar Institute in Philadelphia, the United States Department of the Army in Washington and the Biological Defense Research Center in Fort Detrick, and the Navy Department in Washington. The Behringwerke AG in Marburg/Lahn, the Paul Ehrlich Institute in Frankfort/Main, and the Institute of Immunology (Sera and Vaccines) in Zagreb, Yugoslavia, were also well represented. These three research centers were where, in 1967, the Marburg virus outbreak occurred.

Other organizations represented included the USAID, the CDC, and the NIH.[6]

Twenty-Country Central West African Experiments

The conference highlights included several presentations and discussions about numerous vaccine trials conducted *specifically* in Central West Africa. The researchers discussed testing vaccines against the myriad ailments for which Merck and the others maintained huge financial interests. Vaccines, the presenters noted, had been developed for yellow fever, measles, mumps, poliomyelitis, smallpox, diphtheria, pertussis, tetanus, and rubella. Central West African natives were largely the subjects of the researchers' experiments.

Dr. William Foege from the CDC described the breadth of initial USAID and CDC vaccine trials in the region.[7] Although "Measles vaccination in Africa" was his topic, his discussion included smallpox. Foege reported that:

> In 1961, recognizing the public health significance of measles, the Government of Upper Volta conducted an immunization trial. Because of its success, in 1963 the Government conducted a nationwide immunization program, with assistance from the U.S. Agency for International Development ([US]AID). Projects were soon started in other countries, and by 1966 eleven West African countries were engaged in such programs. Early in 1967 measles immunization programs were started as part of a coordinated twenty-country regional

program for smallpox eradication and measles control, with technical assistance from [US]AID and the U.S. Center for Disease Control.[7] The original objective in regard to measles was stated to be control rather than eradication. The methods to be employed consisted of village-by-village programs carried out by mobile teams using jet injectors. Children from 6 months to 6 years of age were to be immunized during the first cycle; the upper age limit for subsequent cycles would be 6 months plus the interval since the previous cycle.[7]

Foege's statement and article was particularly interesting for three reasons:

First, he cited many of the twenty countries that had participated in the Central West African vaccine trials (see figs. 14.1 and 14.2). This I felt was suspicious evidence. As Shilts wrote in *The Band*:

> The spread of AIDS in Africa most likely outpaced the spread in any other region in the world . . . one in six [European] AIDS patients was African. These cases could be traced to eighteen sub-Saharan African nations. Two-thirds of the African-linked AIDS cases in Europe, however, came from one country, Zaire, and 11 percent came from the nearby Congo. . . . In Zaire, the virus was so widespread that scientists had a hard time constructing studies on risk factors. It was difficult to find a control group that was not infected. . . . [9]

And despite this epidemiologic evidence that the disease had followed a specific path previously worn by multicomponent vaccine trials, "Belgian scientists reported only one major risk factor in the victim nations: heterosexual promiscuity."[9]

My thoughts diverted to the few scientists who voiced concern about this arbitrary conclusion. The CDC/Merck rebuttal to hepatitis B vaccine suspicions was insufficient at best and at worst scientific fraud. Why, after all, were the New York City AIDS cases spared from HB vaccine analysis? Why had the scientific community not acknowledged their flawed study design? The only educated guess I could render was that anyone in the international scientific community even remotely dependent on grants from the NIH, USPHS, CDC, NCI, NIAID, USAID, and WHO or pharmaceutical industry contracts wouldn't dare object. To buck the system in this way would be like committing academic and economic suicide for anyone dependent on the establishment for their livelihood, and that was almost everyone with the wherewithal to evaluate the hard facts.

Second, Foege's paper documented the extent to which the African smallpox eradication campaign was used to test other experimental vaccines that would eventually be licensed by Merck.[10] This was important because: (1) According to comments by Hilleman, Merck ended up owning the licensing rights to various vaccines even though federally funded

Fig. 14.1. Combined Measles/Smallpox Immunization Campaign By Agencies Suspected of Spreading AIDS to Central West Africa

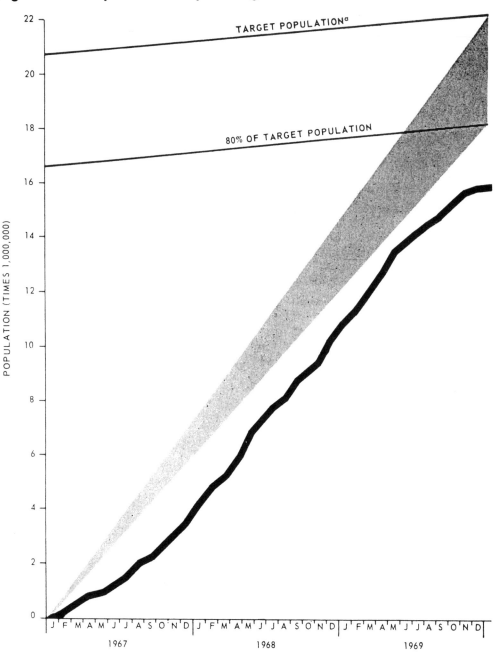

Graph depicts cumulative measles/smallpox immunization in the estimated target population of 20-22 million West and Central Africa natives from 20 countries. Source: William H. Foege, Center for Disease Control. Reprinted from "Measles Vaccination in Africa"— presented during the Pan American (World) Health Organization International Conference on the Application of Vaccines Against Viral, Rickettsial, and Bacterial Diseases of Man, December 14–18, 1970, p. 208.

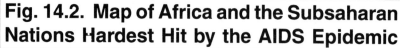

Fig. 14.2. Map of Africa and the Subsaharan Nations Hardest Hit by the AIDS Epidemic

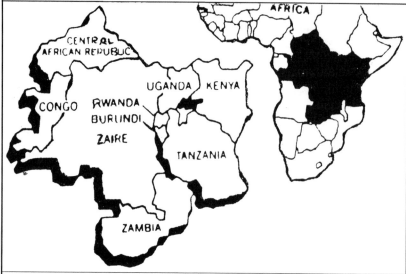

Map of Africa shows the nations in central Africa hardest hit by the AIDS epidemic where those in which experimental vaccines were administered. This work was supported by USAID, the CDC, the WHO, Merck and Co., Inc., and the NCI. Source: Lederer R. Origin and spread of AIDS: Is the West responsible? *Covert Action Information Bulletin* 1987;28:43

investigators did the lion's share of the primary research;[10] and (2) As was documented when Gallo acknowledged the NCI's "Drug Development Branch" for relaying Merck's experimental reagent Cordycepin, there was obviously a channel from Merck to the NCI, and therefore, from Africa to the United States, through which experimental drugs and immune-system-impacting biologicals, like vaccines, flowed;[11] and (3) These African multiviral vaccine tests were clearly dangerous. As numerous scientists had shown, the AIDS virus appears to contain several recognizable components from other viruses.[12,13] This, according to Strecker, strongly suggested that AIDS "was constructed." Therefore, vaccine experiments in which particles from different types of viruses were combined in humans, animals, or cell cultures, provided a plausible explanation for new "emerging viruses" from this region of the world.[13]

Strecker's theory of man-made HIV development from bovine and visna viruses, however, failed to consider one important fact—the principal NCI viral researchers implicated by the scientific evidence, were not experimenting with sheep or cow lentiviruses in Manhattan in the early 1970s. They were experimenting with various primate cancer viruses and vaccines. Moreover, Russian researchers were not implicated whatsoever by the paper trail. The spotlight of suspicion focused primarily on Merck,[7,10] Gallo's group at the NCI and Litton Bionetics, and their New York colleagues.

The Heart of the Military–Medical–Industrial Complex

Within minutes of Foege's presentation, Saul Krugman stood up and reported that, in Africa and elsewhere, their measles vaccine studies had been "supported by the Health Research Council of the City of New York" and his organization—the New York University Medical Center. Who was behind the Health Research Council of the City of New York, I wondered? Why were they interested in vaccinating black Africans overseas?

Hilleman had already openly admitted he and his group at Merck followed Krugman's lead in developing the hepatitis B vaccine.[14] This was evidence to support the theory that the African AIDS "party" began in New York and was hosted by key players in America's military–medical–industrial complex. Besides the Army, Krugman credited Merck and Dow Chemical Company, both Army bioweapons contractors, for the vaccines used in his trials (see fig. 6.7).[15,16]

On reviewing the Army's list of principal biological weapons contractors once again, I realized Dow Chemical had just topped Hazelton Laboratories by a few thousand dollars and was closing ground on Bionetics Research Laboratories, which held sixth place. In fourth place was the University of Chicago, where Gallo interned and began to publish his blood cancer research.[17] Stanford University, where Gallo had sent his cell cultures to have them examined for bacterial and fungal contamination, was in thirteenth place.[18] And last on the list was New England Nuclear Corp., which delivered experimental reagents to Gallo on his request in 1965.[17]

I then realized that Gallo documented receiving support from at least a third of the Army's top-eighteen biological research contractors, including Bionetics, Hazelton, the U. of Chicago,[17] Stanford University,[18] Dow Chemical,[19] and New England Nuclear Corp.[17]–not including his documented connection to Krugman's staff at the NYUMC or Hilleman's colleagues at Merck.[15]

Objections and Predictions for Unnatural Disaster

I sat glued reviewing discourses between several conference participants, including Merck's Hilleman, Dr. Frederick Rasmussen, Jr. of the University of California School of Medicine—another certified bioweapons contractor with links to Gallo and immunosuppressive germ warfare, Dr. Alexander Langmuir of Harvard University Medical School, and the NCI's Manaker, who along with Hilleman held a driving desire to develop a vaccine for cancer.

Hilleman initially stated that new viral vaccine combinations were being prepared for mass immunization campaigns based on studies of soldiers and prisoners, and that "we have measles–mumps–rubella vaccines in various combinations that are up for licensing right now."[10] To which Dr. Langmuir replied:

> I am very much in favor of a good vaccine. . . . I hope they can be licensed, but before a product can be promoted for general use in 200 million people, there needs to be reasonably consistent and solid evidence that it not only produces antibodies . . . [but] protects. I insist that this has not been delivered. It is not a question of whether the product protects troops in a military camp or inmates of a certain institution. It should protect the high-risk group: the aged and the chronically ill.
>
> Studies have been made, and some have shown rather good results, but they are anything but consistent. It seems to me that we cannot yet say we have a product that should be promoted for general use. Furthermore, let us not go adding a lot of things to vaccines that themselves are still questionable and hope to give them a little extra aura of authenticity.[10]

Here, Langmuir objected to the inconsistent efficacy of some vaccines that, when combined with other vaccines, might reduce even more the overall benefit or even produce harm. One example of the less than ideal results achieved from a mass immunization campaign is shown in fig. 14.3.

More incredibly, Rasmussen added his concern that a slow virus immune-system-destroying disease, essentially identical to AIDS, would be a likely outcome of multiple mass vaccination programs due to the way viruses reproduce by altering their host's immune system:

> In view of the complexity and diversity of immunizing antigens and the possible host responses, an occasional adverse interaction should not surprise us. Such proved, widely-used vaccines as pertussis and BCG are known to increase and modify immunological reactivity profoundly. A number of viral immunogens, notably measles, consist of or are prepared from viruses. . . . There must also be biological interactions, genetic among sufficiently closely related viruses and through sharing of virus coded mechanisms for the synthesis of subunits [viral components and new viruses].

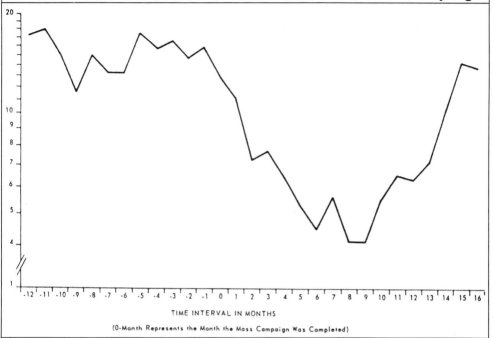

Fig. 14.3. Measles Incidence Rate Per 100,000 in Central and West Africa Before and After Mass Immunization Campaign

TIME INTERVAL IN MONTHS

(0-Month Represents the Month the Mass Campaign Was Completed)

Graph shows measles incidence rate per 100,000 population 12 months prior to the mass campaign and 16 months after the mass campaign in West and Central Africa. Data shows a return to precampaign disease levels by month 15 in Cameroon, Chad, Gabon, the Gambia, Ghana, Guinea, Nigeria, Senegal, Sierra Leone, and Togo . Source: William H. Foege, Center for Disease Control. Reprinted from "Measles Vaccination in Africa"—presented during the Pan American (World) Health Organization International Conference on the Application of Vaccines Against Viral, Rickettsial, and Bacterial Diseases of Man, December 14–18, 1970, p. 210.

The dangers confronting us in the development and use of new vaccines, together with those known to exist with the present vaccines, may have been overemphasized, but they are very real. . . .

Like Strecker, Rasmussen went on to cite the sheep visna virus as an example of the risk of creating slow progressive immune system and nervous-system-destroying epidemics. He explained:

Among the dangers, . . . the possible potentiation or activation of certain slowly progressive viral infections is particularly difficult to combat, because untoward reactions may be so few or so distantly related to the initiating immunizing procedure as to be overlooked unless rigorous and sustained surveillance is undertaken—and, even if recognized, may not become clearly evident until large numbers of people have been placed at irreversible risk.

If we are to anticipate unknown dangers it is imperative that all facets of the immune response and other host responses to any new product be exhaustively studied. . . .

Furthermore, Rasmussen even warned that vaccines may actually potentiate the cell killing properties of some RNA viruses, and that bizarre, unpredictable, nervous system disorders and lymph cancers, like those associated with AIDS, might be expected from this research.[20]

Manaker then replied largely in agreement with Rasmussen's concerns, but quickly steered the focus of their discussion away from the controversy and toward the "control of cancer with vaccine." Explaining his work at the NIH and that of his colleagues at the NCI, the cancer virus expert presented some of the challenges they faced with "selective" defining of "populations or groups at higher risk" through blood collection and analysis programs.[20]

Preventing Liability and Evading Accountability

Next, conference participants discussed their legal and financial concerns in the event their vaccines caused illness, disability, and death.[21] Dr. Dull from the CDC directed discussion on "the question of indemnification of persons unforeseeably or unavoidably injured by immunization or other processes in preventive medicine." He noted his "concern over court awards of large money settlements and the fear that the makers may not only discontinue the production of vaccines but also turn their attention from research and development, on which we rely a good deal for advancement in this field." Moreover, he offered a way out through "legislative mechanisms." He argued:

> As many of us recognize, the current attitudes have resulted from the fact that we are now much better able to interpret the risks and benefits of immunization than formerly and that we also have a population increasingly desirous of sharing in health decisions and unwilling to assume the risks of injury from the unknown and unavoidable aspects of preventive medicine.

> The law, speaking for the consumer or in this case the patient, looks commonly to the deepest pocket, which is often the producer's or the insurance company's, for compensation for injuries possibly related to immunization. If we acknowledge that the benefits of immunization accrue not only to the recipients of vaccines but also to the community, as well as to the producers, it is quite reasonable for us to seek administrative or legislative mechanisms that will spread the costs of unavoidable injuries to all who benefit and will attempt to educate patients so as to enable them to balance in their own minds some of the risks and benefits.

> Such mechanisms could prevent the discrediting of the practices of immunization and preventive medicine, the costly litigation of personal injury claims, and the suppression of the imaginative development of new vaccines, drugs, or other preventive medical procedures. At the same time they could increase the public's confidence in acknowledging risks and benefits, reporting adverse reactions, and thus extending our knowledge of the field of preventive medicine.

Many other countries are far ahead of us in these areas. Some in Western Europe and in the Far East already have legislation to this effect or are developing it. Perhaps some of the participants from those countries would like to comment. . . .[21]

Dr. von Magnus from the Statens Seruminstitut in Denmark responded:

Some years ago in Denmark a number of cases of a polio-like disease occurred that were related in time to the oral polio vaccination campaign and were considered compatible with a diagnosis of vaccine-induced polio. Since the vaccine had been given to a large segment of the population (about 2.7 million doses) within a very short time, these cases were very conspicuous. Claims were made for compensation for the damage considered to have been caused by the vaccine.

The Minister of the Interior, who is the man responsible for our health services, immediately promised indemnification for the damage if it was caused by the vaccine. An expert committee set up for the purpose decided that some six to eight of the cases were actually compatible with such a conclusion, and financial compensation was awarded according to the incapacity suffered.

Since then the whole problem of vaccine-induced incapacity has been raised, particularly with respect to smallpox and pertussis vaccination. A committee has been set up to consider this problem and is at present working on it. Up to now, over a period of about 10 years, we have received about 20 claims for indemnification, mostly from parents of children who had received pertussis vaccination and also two or three cases of encephalitis following smallpox vaccination.

The general plan is to prepare legislation under which the government must take care of these people and pay them financial compensation for their disability in accordance with their reduced earning capacity if it is considered due to the vaccination. This will be handled in much the same way as workmen's compensation. The current idea is that these payments will be made only to people who have become incapacitated from vaccinations that are recommended or required. . . . I believe that the recommendation will be to create a law whereby those who suffer lasting incapacity from vaccination will receive financial support from the state in the form of an annual pension somewhat higher than is available to persons suffering handicaps caused by other factors.[21]

Thus, vaccine manufacturers were freed from accountability and liability. Instead, taxpayers shouldered the burden once again. Whatever happened to the Hippocratic oath—"above all do no harm"—I wondered?

Immunization Procedures and Propaganda

Another revealing soliloquy came from Dr. James Gear, director of The South African Institute for Medical Research's vaccine studies in Johannesburg. Describing the broad extent of South African vaccination and "propaganda" programs, a paternal spirit may also be recognized in his comments:

> South Africa produces or has the facilities to produce nearly all the vaccines required for its own use and helps to meet the needs of the neighboring territories and islands. Vaccines for protection against poliomyelitis, smallpox, diphtheria, whooping cough, and tetanus are available and free to all. Vaccines against measles, yellow fever, and cholera are available to all in special need of them. Some local authorities, such as the City Council of Johannesburg, have decided to offer rubella vaccine to all schoolgirls above the age of 10 years. Several vaccines, such as those against herpesvirus [specifically the rage in cancer research at that time], varicella, and cytomegalovirus, trachoma, and bilharzia are under investigation.
>
> Extensive serological surveys have been carried out and are being continued to determine the immunity of different age groups of the population to the enteroviruses and respiratory viruses, including measles and rubella and the arbovirus infections [among Merck's prime research areas]. The findings are of value in determining their needs for vaccine. . . .
>
> The jet gun has been extensively used in this campaign and is a most valuable timesaving weapon; but it has to be handled by someone expert in its use.
>
> It was our experience that it was essential to launch a propaganda campaign to convince parents of the value of and need for vaccinating their children and also of the dangers of neglecting to have them vaccinated. The most effective means was found to be the radio; it seems that every family in Southern Africa has at least one transistor radio. . . .[22]

Jet Guns, Mosquitoes, and Marginal Advantages

Jet injectors, according to Dr. Paul Wehrle of the University of Southern California School of Medicine, were developed for "more efficient population coverage" and were largely credited for "the apparent success of the smallpox program."[23]

The jet guns, Wehrle explained, "make for efficient administration of vaccines requiring parenteral inoculations of large volume—for example, diphtheria, tetanus, and typhoid—and for immunization programs conducted in more concentrated populations such as the larger villages and cities."[23]

The device, manufactured in different sizes to accommodate various age groups, "is comparatively expensive, and breakage and maintenance problems are certain to occur unless the operators are carefully selected and trained."[23]

The chief of arbovirus diseases—including yellow fever—for the World Health Organization further explained the way jet gun programs were administered by USAID teams during their "Smallpox-Measles Program."[24]

The basic problem Dr. Bres explained was that viral research, initiated in Uganda "in 1936 by the Rockefeller Foundation and continued by the East African Virus Research Institute of the East African Community," was unable to keep up with the flight path of *Aedes aegypti*—a mosquito that Bres stated was "the classic vector of urban yellow fever. . . ." He noted, however, since it "breeds far away from human dwellings . . . [i]n East Africa, *A. aegypti* only rarely bites man." Monkeys he explained were believed to be the likeliest "vector species" despite his acknowledgment that mosquitoes, more often than monkeys, bit humans.[24]

Bres also reviewed the "epidemics in the past decade" and noted that yellow fever had broken out several times between 1958 and 1966 in eight Central West African countries. "230 cases with 216 deaths" were recorded during this period, where "2,000 to 20,000 cases were suspected."[24]

As a result, the WHO yellow fever expert reported:

Nearly 2 million vaccinations were carried out in a period of two months on the 3 million inhabitants of Senegal. A total of 125,000 doses of 17-D [the yellow fever] vaccine were available at that time to vaccinate nearly a million children under 10 years of age. The use of FNV vaccine instead of 17-D in many children in this age group was followed by 240 complications with 25 fatal cases of encephalitis. 'Ped-O-Jet' injectors were on trial for the first time in an African epidemic and were judged to be very efficient.[24]

Another example Bres gave was the Ghana, Upper Volta and Nigerian outbreak of 1969. Here he reported five cases in Ghana with two deaths and possibly 250 other jaundiced patients of which 73 died. The cause of death as yellow fever, however, could not be confirmed. Moreover, "on the opposite side of the common border, 87 confirmed cases with 44 deaths" occurred in Upper Volta, but the authorities estimated as many as 3,000 unconfirmed cases with 100 deaths occurred. "As in Senegal," Bres admitted, "the country had previously been vaccinated, and 90 percent of the victims were young children. This "urban-type epidemic he believed was easily controlled by vaccinating 600,000 people with 17-D "carried out by well trained teams of USAID."[24]

Altogether, during these 1969 epidemics, Bres explained, 4 million doses of 17-D vaccine were administered, "including 1 million supplied by WHO. Most were administered with 'Ped-O-Jet' injectors by USAID teams." In conclusion, he reported:

> It is quite easy to protect an individual using 17-D vaccine, but difficulties arise if we aim at the protection of a whole country.
>
> Eradication of *A. aegypti* is impossible in Africa, because the mosquito breeds in the brush as well as in towns. . . . Eradication of other possible vectors is equally impossible: mass vaccination therefore appears the most effective method for countrywide protection. . . . [Such programs] are a question of speed. Several teams are necessary. One team can perform 500 to 1,000 vaccinations an hour. As the vaccine requirements may be considerable in a short time, WHO has constituted a reserve of 2 million doses of 17-D. . . .[24]

Several conference delegates thought it interesting that so much vaccine was being administered in an effort to save so few lives. Arguably, even a single life is precious, but the fear was that fatal vaccine reactions were being under-reported by the same ten-fold factor that cases were.[24]

Finally, the knowledge that the New York City based Rockefeller Foundation's earliest investments in viral research occurred in Uganda, bordering eastern Zaire, I noted as potentially relevant. Could Rockefeller funding have been behind the Health Research Council of the City of New York? I wondered.

Gaining Public Acceptance

Radio advertising was not the only method needed and used to persuade families to accept western vaccination recommendations. Dr. Carl Taylor, from Johns Hopkins School of Hygiene and Public Health, advanced a complete campaign designed to overcome the "cultural blocks . . . influencing acceptance of immunization programs in developing countries."[25]

Some of Taylor's recommendations reviewed standard WHO policies regarding "propaganda and vaccination teams." The WHO's Epidemiological Research Laboratory headed by Dr. T. M. Pollock had, in 1966, advised that "the *propaganda team*" should be "headed by the chief health educator, who will distribute the work. . . . The work of the team is arranged in such a way as to ensure the full cooperation of the public with the vaccination team. The vaccination team consists of four members: its *leader-orga-nizer* (a physician) . . . the *registrar* (a clerk) . . . the *physician-vaccinator* . . . [and] the *assistant*."[26]

And in response to concerns that mass vaccination campaigns may be more risky and costly than they're worth, Dr. Abram Benenson from the University of Kentucky chastised the congregation:

> We developed and published statistics of the high rate of [vaccination] complications, but the vast bulk of these complications are entities that have no prognostic significance whatsoever. Part of the discussion . . . has borne on the fact that successful immunological control of a disease is based on acceptance by the public and by the medical profession, but from our debates on what is best or what is wrong we are conditioning the public to reject measures that sometimes, in some situations, are very important.

In warning against open communication regarding the risks of vaccination, Benenson said:

> We can indeed argue today whether the hazards equal or outweigh the value of vaccination in the United Kingdom or the United States, but as we argue these things we impress those in less developed countries that there is a great danger here, and I am concerned whether we are not doing the total program a disservice.[27]

Racism and Immunization for National Security

Moreover, Dr. J. D. Millar from the CDC explained the gravest danger posed by a lack of public acceptance of mass immunization programs was the threat posed to whites by "Spanish-Americans and Negroes." This he said was "the greatest motive for supporting mass vaccination campaigns at home and abroad."[28]

Millar had worked closely with Dr. Foege at the CDC. Together, they administered extensive smallpox and measles vaccination campaigns in West and Central Africa shortly after Hilleman's group at Merck standardized the "mass application of combined live measles-smallpox vaccines" on the same continent.[29]

Millar drew the group's attention to excerpts from two 1970 issues of *Morbidity and Mortality Weekly Report*. The first heralded "a marked resurgence" of measles cases in 1969. "Of the 261 cases, 255 were Negroes," which he said showed "the development of new populations of susceptibles in the younger age groups who have not been immunized."

The second excerpt reported "ninety-six cases of tonsillar or pharyngeal diphtheria" in San Antonio through September 6, 1970. He read:

> The outbreak is centered in the lower socioeconomic areas of the city and in a few census tracts. The highest attack rates have been in the 5-9 and 10-14 year age groups. Of the 80 patients whose immunization status was known, 43 (54 percent) had no previous immunization against diphtheria, 23 (29 percent) had lapsed for inadequate immunization, and 14 (18 percent) were reported fully immunized.

The table Millar presented depicted that attack rates among Spanish-Americans and Negroes ten times higher than those reported in the rest of the population.

Immunizable diseases such as diphtheria and poliomyelitis, Millar said had also increased substantially in 1970 as had measles among "unvaccinated preschool children residing in poverty areas of major cities." It is apparent he said that "the immunizable diseases are more and more restricted to the disadvantaged peoples in our nation and that the incidence of immunizable disease among these groups is increasing."

Millar then argued that the central issue and greatest risk to public health was one of race, class, and "the crucial group." He said:

> It is apparent that race, residence, and riches are factors affecting immunization status. Being nonwhite, residing in the central city, and being poor all [work against immunization practices]. . . . Activities to maintain high levels of immunization in the population have failed most dramatically among the urban poor, who are predominantly nonwhite. [This] . . . medically disadvantaged group, variously described as the 'hard core' or 'hard-to-reach' is at least two decades old. . . . Reaching them is the fundamental problem that must be solved to control communicable diseases in developed countries.

Millar's motives, it seems, were not singularly humanitarian. Some were coldly utilitarian—designed to protect the interests of the whites in both the United States and Africa. Immunization programs, according to Millar, served above all to protect the "middle-class suburbanite" who, in light of his earlier remarks, was not at high risk for these diseases.

"The problem," maintained Dr. Millar, was the threat posed by the transmission of diseases from nonwhite minority populations to Anglo-American children and families. The resurgence of disease in 1969 and 1970—as Nixon, Kissinger, and Rockefeller began restructuring government to facilitate an international allignment of power—Millar said, was caused by "an accumulation of susceptibles" for which additional immunization services were needed.

Before closing, he referred to the U.S. Vaccination Assistance Act of 1962, the year, I later learned, the NCI and Litton Bionetics began intense cancer virus vaccine studies (see fig. 22.5). The legislation had encouraged partially successful "community-wide immunization activities across the nation." Reaching the nonwhite "susceptibles," he concluded, was vital in preventing a resurgence of diseases, including polio, diphtheria, whooping cough, tetanus, and measles.

This he concluded:

> . . . is the fundamental problem that must be solved to control communicable diseases in developed countries. In the United States, the central cities will continue to seethe with immunizable diseases and thereby create a significant risk to other parts of the society until these people are regularly included in immunization practice.[28]

Part III
Covert Operations

Chapter 15
The CIA/Detrick Operation

IN 1975, following a storm of public outrage over the CIA's involvement in Watergate, the agency was investigated and indicted by several groups. These included the Rockefeller Commission for numerous incidents of wrongdoing,[1] a House review of the CIA's role in the Watergate break-ins,[2] and a Senate inquiry into the illegal storage of biological weapons.[3]

Word had leaked from the Army's special (that is, secret) operations division at Fort Detrick that the CIA was still storing supplies of deadly bacteria, viruses, and other toxins—biological weapons for offensive uses—five years after the drafting and signing of the Geneva accord by Kissinger and Nixon, respectively.[3] As a result, a Select Committee to Study Governmental Operations with Respect to Intelligence Activities formed and met at the U.S. Senate on Tuesday, September 16, 1975, to investigate the matter. Senator Frank Church presided over the meeting. Also present were Senators Tower, Mondale, Huddleston, Morgan, Hart (of Colorado), Baker, Goldwater, Mathias, and Schweiker.[3] I obtained and read my copy of the testimony at the Boston Public Library.

The chairman opened the meeting by providing an overview of the issues at hand:

CHAIRMAN CHURCH: The Senate Select Committee on Intelligence Activities opens its public hearings today with an inquiry into a case in which direct orders of the President of the United States were evidently disobeyed by employees of the CIA. It is the purpose of this hearing . . . to illuminate the need to make certain in the future that Federal law enforcement and intelligence agencies perform their duties in ways which do not infringe upon the rights of American citizens.

The committee has not held public hearings prior to this time, because of its concentration on charges that the CIA has been involved in assassination plots directed against certain foreign leaders. . . .

Because of the serious damage that protracted public hearings on such a subject could do to the United States in its relations with foreign governments, the committee chose to conduct these hearings behind closed doors. . . .

It is the right of the American people to know what their Government has done—the bad as well as the good—and we have every confidence that the country will benefit by a comprehensive disclosure of this grim chapter in our recent history.

Today as a member of the Foreign Relations Committee, I am fully aware of the great value of good intelligence in times of peace. . . . [The CIA and the FBI] were established to spy on foreign governments and to fend off foreign spies. We must know to what degree they have turned their techniques inward to spy on the American people instead. If such, unlawful and improper conduct is not exposed and stopped, it could, undermine the very foundations of freedom in our own land. . .

The particular case under examination today involves the illegal possession of deadly biological poisons which were retained within the CIA for 5 years after their destruction was ordered by the President, and for 5 years after the United States had entered into a solemn international commitment not to maintain stocks of these poisons except for very limited research purposes.

The main questions before the committee are why the poisons were developed in such quantities in the first place; why the Presidential order was disobeyed; and why such a serious act of insubordination could remain undetected for so many years. . . .[4]

TESTIMONY OF WILLIAM E. COLBY, DIRECTOR OF CENTRAL INTELLI-GENCE, ACCOMPANIED BY SAYRE STEVENS, ASSISTANT DEPUTY DI-RECTOR, SCIENCE AND TECHNOLOGY, CIA; AND MITCHELL ROGOVIN, SPECIAL COUNSEL, CIA. [Emphasis not added]

COLBY: Mr. Chairman. . . . The subject today concerns CIA's involvement in the development of bacteriological warfare materials with the Army's Biological Laboratory at Fort Detrick. . . . The project at Fort Detrick involved the development of bacteriological warfare agents—some lethal—and associated delivery systems suitable for clandestine use. . . .

CIA association with Fort Detrick involved the Special Operations Division (SOD) of that facility. This division was responsible for developing special applications for biological warfare agents and toxins. Its principal customer was the U.S. Army. Its concern was with the development of both suitable agents and delivery mechanisms for use in paramilitary situations. Both standard biological warfare agents and biologically derived toxins were investigated by the division.

The CIA relationship with SOD was formally established in May 1952 . . . in the laboratory facilities of the Special Operations Division of the Army's Biological Laboratory at Fort Detrick. . . .

From its outset, the project was characterized by extreme compartmentation, or a high degree of secrecy within the CIA itself. Only two or three Agency officers at any time were cleared for access to Fort Detrick activities. Though some CIA-originated documents have been found in the project files, it is clear that only a very limited documentation of activities took place.[5]

I immediately realized there would be little if any paper trail to follow here. And with only two or three high-level military scientists at any one time with access to the CIA's Detrick facility, the operation was very tight.

The intentional transmission theory of AIDS, however, remained to be disproven. A few military scientists, I realized, were all that was needed to transport a vile of viruses from Fort Detrick, or for that matter Gallo's lab, to Hilleman's hepatitis B vaccine lab in West Point, Pennsylvania, or directly to Krugman's group in New York. The African supplies could have easily been tainted the same way, while making their way through the NCI's Drug Development Branch, or somewhere enroute to USAID teams in the field.

Colby: . . . By the late sixties, a variety of biological warfare agents and toxins were maintained by the SOD for possible Agency use. . . . Though specific accounting for each agent on the list is not on hand, Department of Defense records indicate that the materials were, in fact, destroyed in 1970 by SOD personnel, except for the 11 grams of a substance in small medical bottles labeled shellfish toxin, plus the 11 milligrams of cobra venom, which were found on May 20 of this year.[5]

Why would they have only saved the shellfish toxin, and no other biological weapon? I questioned.

Then I reflected on Hearing Exhibit No. 1—an addendum cited on page III of the publication entitled, "February 16, 1970 DDP memorandum from Thomas Karamessines to Director of Central Intelligence [Richard Helms]." Here Karamessines requested from Helms explicit orders to destroy or maintain in storage a long list of biological weapons that were stockpiled. Karamessines cited the option of transferring the stockpile to "the Huntingdon Research Center, Becton-Dickenson Company, Baltimore, Maryland" where "arrangements have been made for this contingency and assurances have been given by the potential contractor to store and maintain the agency's stockpile at a cost of no greater than $75,000 per annum."

Obviously, Karamessines and his higher-ups had developed contingency plans to store the whole array of biologicals well after Nixon and Kissinger publicly heralded their destruction. The list included biological toxins, several kinds of deadly bacteria, lethal viruses, including Venezuelan equine encephalomyelitis virus, and the smallpox virus variola (see fig. 15.1).[6]

In addition to exhibit 1, there were two memos from President Nixon, reiterating U.S. biological weapons policy following his signing of the Geneva accord. One stated:

The United States will confine its military programs for toxins, whether produced by bacteriological or any other biological method or by chemical synthesis to research for defensive purposes only, such as to improve techniques of immunization and medical therapy.[7]

Fig. 15.1 Hearing Exhibits—Exhibit 1

189

HEARINGS EXHIBITS [1]

EXHIBIT 1

Attachment D

MEMORANDUM FOR: Director of Central Intelligence

SUBJECT : Contingency Plan for Stockpile of
Biological Warfare Agents

1. On 25 November 1969, President Nixon ordered the
Department of Defense to recommend plans for the disposal
of existing stocks of bacteriological weapons. (On 14
February 1970, he included all toxin weapons.)

2. On 15 January 1970, the Special Operations Division
of Fort Detrick, Maryland prepared a requested agent inventory, less toxins, and submitted it to the Scientific
Director, Fort Detrick. This inventory was a required input
to assist the Commanding Officer, Ft. Detrick to prepare
a comprehensive plan for demilitarization on site of all
biological agents/munitions which are stockpiled in support
of operational plans.

3. Under an established agreement with the Department
of the Army, the CIA has a limited quantity of biological
agents and toxins stored and maintained by the SO Division
at Ft. Detrick. This stockpile did not appear on the inventory list. The agents and toxins are:

  Agents:

    1. Bacillus anthracis (anthrax) – 100 grams

    2. Pasteurella tularensis (tularemia) – 20 grams

    3. Venezuelan Equine Encephalomyelitis virus
       (encephalitis) – 20 grams

    4. Coccidioides imitis (valley fever) – 20 grams

    5. Brucella suis (brucellosis) – 2 to 3 grams

    6. Brucella melitensis (brucellosis) – 2 to 3
       grams

    7. Mycobacterium tuberculosis (tuberculosis) –
       3 grams

[1] Under criteria determined by the Committee, in consultation with the White House, the Department
of Defense and the Central Intelligence Agency, certain materials have been deleted from these documents, some of which were previously classified, to maintain the integrity of the internal operating procedures of the agencies involved and to protect certain information of a national security nature.

8. Salmonella typhimurium (food poisoning) – 10 grams

9. Salmonella typhimurium (chlorine resistant) (food poisoning) – 3 grams

10. Variola Virus (smallpox) – 50 grams

Toxins:

1. Staphylococcal Enterotoxin (food poisoning) – 10 grams

2. Clostridium botulinum Type A (lethal food poisoning) – 5 grams

3. Paralytic Shellfish Poison – 5.193 grams

4. Dangerus Candidia Venom (Krait) (lethal snake venom) – 2 grams

5. Microcystis aeruginosa toxin (intestinal flu) – 25 mg

6. Toxiferine (paralytic effect) – 100 mg

This stockpile capability plus some research effort in delivery systems is funded at $75,000 per annum.

4. In the event the decision is made by the Department of Defense to dispose of existing stocks of bacteriological weapons, it is possible that the CIA's stockpile, even though in R&D quantities and unlisted, will be destroyed.

5. If the Director wishes to continue this special capability, it is recommended that if the above DOD decision is made, the existing agency stockpile at SO Division, Ft. Detrick be transferred to the Huntingdon Research Center, Becton-Dickinson Company, Baltimore, Maryland. Arrangements have been made for this contingency and assurances have been given by the potential contractor to store and maintain the agency's stockpile at a cost no greater than $75,000 per annum.

Thomas H. Karamessines
Deputy Director for Plans

FROM

FEB. 23 1975

CIA

Source: Hearings before the Select Committee to Study Governmental Operations With Respect to Intelligence Activities of the United States Senate, Ninety-Fourth Congress, First Session, Vol. 1: Unauthorized Storage of Toxic Agents, Intelligence Activities Senate Resolution 21, Washington, D.C.: U.S. Government Printing Office, September 16, 17, and 18, 1975, pp. 189–190.

Exhibit 6 was a 1967 memorandum from Chief, Technical Service Division, Biological Branch to Chief, Technical Services Division: PROJECT: MKNAOMI, which covered the gamut of activities undertaken by the CIA in cooperation with the Army SOD at Fort Detrick to develop and covertly deploy their wide assortment of biological weapons. The vast majority of text in this document was illegible. This seemed odd since most of the exhibits before and after were much easier to read. Perhaps not coincidentally, for the lay reader, under the description of this document on page III, it read:

> Under criteria determined by the committee in consultation with the White House, the Department of Defense and the Central Intelligence Agency, certain materials have been deleted from these documents, some of which were previously classified, to maintain the integrity of the internal operating procedures of the agencies involved and to protect certain information of a national security nature.[6]

Additional exhibits included two NSC memos from Henry Kissinger to all agency chiefs reiterating the president's policy (see figs. 15.2 and 15.3).[8]

Exhibit 11 listed some 184 medical researchers who "received toxins from Fort Detrick." It was not implied these were biological weapons contractors. Moreover, the CIA failed to mention the doctors who were involved in the most important and secret project ongoing at the time of the inquiry, the Special Virus Cancer Program (SVCP)[9], or those involved in experimental vaccine research.[10]

Among the doctors listed were four who served at Rockefeller's Institute or University, one from New York University Medical Center, one from Columbia University, and several from the U.S. Public Health Service, including several of its institutes. Most of the individuals cited were university-based researchers, but a couple were independent or corporate. One was Dr. James L. Haynes from the Applied Science Division of Litton Systems, Inc. in Minneapolis.[10]

Haynes's citation was the first documented evidence of a direct connection between Fort Detrick and Litton Systems, Inc.—Dr. Gallo's patron—a connection that I suspected for months (see figs. 6.6 and 15.4).

Later I discovered that during the 1960s, fourteen biological-weapons-testing contracts were carried out by Litton Bionetics for the Defense Department (see fig. 17.1),[11] and during the same period, the NCI was paying

Fig. 15.2. Hearing Exhibits—Exhibit 7

207

EXHIBIT 7

NATIONAL SECURITY COUNCIL
WASHINGTON D C 20506

November 25, 1969

National Security Decision Memorandum 35

TO: The Vice President
          The Secretary of State
          The Secretary of Defense
          The Director, Central Intelligence Agency
          The Director, Arms Control and Disarmament Agency
          The Director, Office of Emergency Preparedness
          The Director, Office of Science and Technology

SUBJECT: United States Policy on Chemical Warfare Program
          and Bacteriological/Biological Research Program

Following consideration by the National Security Council, the President
has decided that:

1.   The term Chemical and Biological Warfare (CBW) will no longer
be used. The reference henceforth should be to the two categories
separately -- The Chemical Warfare Program and The Biological
Research Program.

2.   With respect to Chemical Warfare:

      a.   The objective of the U.S. program will be to deter the use
            of chemical weapons by other nations and to provide a
            retaliatory capability if deterrence fails.

      b.   The renunciation of the first use of lethal chemical weapons
            is reaffirmed.

      c.   This renunciation is hereby applied to incapacitating
            chemical weapons as well.

      d.   This renunciation does not apply to the use of riot control
            agents or herbicides. A special NSDM on authorization for
            their use will be issued.

g. The Secretary of Defense, in cooperation with the Director of the Office of Science and Technology, shall continue to develop and improve controls and safety measures in all Chemical Warfare programs.

h. The Under Secretaries Committee shall conduct an annual review of United States Chemical Warfare programs and public information policy, and will make recommendations to the President.

3. With respect to Bacteriological/Biological programs:

a. The United States will renounce the use of lethal methods of bacteriological/biological warfare.

b. The United States will similarly renounce the use of all other methods of bacteriological/biological warfare (for example, incapacitating agents).

c. The United States bacteriological/biological programs will be confined to research and development for defensive purposes (immunization, safety measures, et cetera). This does not preclude research into those offensive aspects of bacteriological/biological agents necessary to determine what defensive measures are required.

d. The Secretary of Defense will submit recommendations about the disposal of existing stocks of bacteriological/biological weapons.

e. The United States shall associate itself with the principles and objectives of the Draft Convention Prohibiting the Use of Biological Methods of Warfare presented by the United Kingdom at the Eighteen-Nation Disarmament Conference in Geneva, on 26 August 1969. Recommendation as to association with specific provisions of the Draft Convention should be prepared by the Secretary of State and the Director of the Arms Control and Disarmament Agency, in coordination with other interested agencies, for the President's consideration.

f. The Secretary of Defense, in conjunction with the Director of the Office of Science and Technology, shall continue to develop controls and safety measures in all bacteriological/biological programs.

g. The Under Secretaries Committee shall conduct an annual review of United States Bacteriological/Biological Research Programs and public information policy, and will make recommendations to the President.

Henry A. Kissinger

cc: Chairman, Joint Chiefs of Staff

Fig. 15.3. Hearing Exhibits—Exhibit 8

EXHIBIT 8

NATIONAL SECURITY COUNCIL
WASHINGTON C 20506

February 20, 1970

Nationial Security Decision Memorandum 44

TO: The Vice President
           The Secretary of State
           The Secretary of Defense
           The Director, Central Intelligence Agency
           The Director, Arms Control and Disarmament Agency
           The Director, Office of Emergency Preparedness
           The Director, Office of Science and Technology

SUBJECT: United States Policy on Toxins

Following a review of United States military programs for toxins,
the President has decided that:

1.   The United States will renounce the production for operational
purposes, stockpiling and use of toxins of all types produced
either by biological or biochemical processes or by chemical
synthesis.

2.   The United States military program for toxins will be confined
to research and development for defensive purposes only.

3.   The Secretary of Defense will submit recommendations concerning the disposal of existing stocks of toxin weapons and/or
agents. These recommendations should accompany the recommendations pursuant to National Security Decision Memorandum 35
regarding the disposal of bacteriological/biological weapons.

4.   The Under Secretaries Committee's annual review of United
States chemical warfare program and public information
policy, as directed by National Security Decision Memorandum 35,
will include a review of United States military toxins programs.

Henry A. Kissinger

cc: Chairman, Joint Chiefs of Staff

NSC

Litton Bionetics to conduct a variety of biological and chemical carcinogen studies.[12]

Here, however, Congress only learned that Dr. Haynes was contracted to help evaluate the effects of human exposure to botulism toxin.[10]

Finally, exhibit 12 was heavily edited. The official study title had been deleted, and it now read: "Excerpt from 'Summary Report, Working Fund Investigations' from the Special Operations Division." The remaining memo provided an overview of a human study involving the use of a virus that was not listed on exhibit 1—presumably because the CIA did not stockpile it—the colibacteriophage. This is a bacterial virus that attacks human intestinal tract bacteria to produce a variety of stomach, bowel, and digestive disorders.

The CIA, along with the SOD, was interested in studying the effects of contaminating the water supply of a government office building to see how far and fast the viruses would spread and how many people would be infected. The population involved in the study were unsuspecting workers and visitors who took a drink at the Food and Drug Administration Building in Washington, D.C. one day in mid-1969.[13]

Colby continued his prepared statement:

COLBY: [Over the years] a project approval memo of 1967 identified four functional categories of project activity: maintenance of a stockpile of temporary incapacitation and lethal agents in readiness for operational use; assessment and maintenance of biological and chemical dissemination systems for operational use; adaptation and testing of a nondiscernible microbioinoculator—a dart device for clandestine and imperceptible inoculation with biological warfare or chemical warfare agents—for use with various materials and to assure that the microbioinoculator could not be easily detected by later examination of the target; and providing technical support and consultation on request for offensive and defensive biological warfare and chemical warfare.[5]

Discussions with Mr. Helms, Director of Central Intelligence, and Mr. Karamessines, the Deputy Director for Plans in 1970, have established that both were aware of the requirement that such material be disposed of. They recall that clear instructions were given that the CIA stockpile should be destroyed by the Army, and that, in accordance with Presidential directives, the Agency should get out of the biological warfare business.

With the discovery of the shellfish toxin this year, a complete inventory of the vault in which it was found was taken. The inventory consisted of a stock of various materials and delivery systems accumulated over the years, including other lethal materials, incapacitants, narcotics, hallucinogenic drugs, irritants and riot control agents, herbicides, animal control materials, and many common chemicals.

Fig. 15.4 Selected References From Exhibit 11—"Persons Who Received Toxins From Fort Detrick"

Dr. William H. Beers[†]
Rockefeller University
New York, NY 10021

Mr. Thomas Burton[§]
Department of Hth., Ed. & Welfare,
Food & Drug Administration
1521 W. Pico Boulevard
Los Angeles, CA 90015

Dr. Ezra Casman[†]
Food & Drug Administration
U.S. Public Health Service
Washington, DC

Dr. M. Dickie[†]
Dept. of National Health & Welfare
Food & Drug Directorate
Tunney's Pasture
Ottawa, Ontario, Canada

Dr. V. R. Dowell[†]
National Communicable Disease Center
(CDC), Atlanta, GA

Dr. Gary Dykstra[§]
Department of Hth., Ed. & Welfare,
Food & Drug Administration
1560 East Jefferson Avenue
Detroit, MI 48207

Dr. Arthur Eberstein[†]
New York University Medical Center
Institute of Physical Medicine
400 East 34the Street
New York, NY

Dr. H. E. Hall[†]
Robert A. Taft Sanitary
Engineering Center
U.S. Public Health Service
Cincinnati, OH

Dr. William K. Harrell[†]
Chief, Microbiological Reagents Unit
Communicable Disease Center (CDC)
Atlanta, GA 30333

Dr. James L. Haynes[†]
Litton Systems, Inc.
Applied Science Division
Minneapolis, MN 55413

Dr. Bortil Hille[§]
The Rockefeller Institute
New York, NY

Dr. Toshikaru Kawabata[§]
Department of Food Control
National Institute of Health
284 Kamiosaki-Chojamaru
Shinagawa-Ku, Tokyo, Japan

Dr. John T. Meacham[§]
Food & Drug Administration
U.S. Public Health Service
850 Third Avenue
Brooklyn, NY 11232

Dr. Richard L. Masland[†]
Department of Neurology
College of Physicians and Surgeons
Columbia University
New York, NY

Dr. Edward Reich[§]
Rockefeller University
66th Street & York Road
New York, NY

Dr. Martin Rirack[§]
Rockefeller University
New York, NY 10021

Dr. B. T. Tozar[§]
Microbiological Research Establishment
Porton Down, Salisbury
Wiltshire, England

Dr. John F. Winn[†]
Chief, Biological Reagents Section Communicable Disease Center (CDC)
Atlanta, GA 30333

Types of biological weapons received:
[†] Botulinum Toxin   [§] Shellfish Poison   [‡] Staph Ent A & B

Source: Hearings before the Select Committee to Study Governmental Operations With Respect to Intelligence Activities of the United States Senate, Ninety-Fourth Congress, First Session, Vol. 1: Unauthorized Storage of Toxic Agents, Intelligence Activities Senate Resolution 21, Washington, D.C.: U.S. Government Printing Office, September 16, 17, and 18, 1975, pp. 216–239.

The small size of the vault (about 8 by 10 feet) and the few shelves limit the extent of this stockpile. The materials are, for the most part, the residue of a number of different CIA programs . . . many different materials were obtained and stored for provision to contractors who did the actual scientific research involved. . . . *These involved CIA's effort to keep a close watch on emerging technology—in this case pharmaceutical technology—to insure* that we did not encounter an unanticipated threat from hostile intelligence services with which we could not contend.[14] [emphasis added]

With that, Colby ended his remarks and passed out copies of his prepared statement.

"Pharmaceutical technology?" I questioned, recognizing the "emerging technology" at the time was cancer-causing immunosuppressive viruses. Colby might have mentioned the $10 million DOD appropriation in 1970 for five additional years of mutant virus research. He could have, at least, shared his opinion regarding Exhibit 12 as it discussed the delivery of a virus into a study population as early as 1967, or regarding the outcome of contingency storage plans for the deadly viruses on Karamessines's inventory list. Instead, he left it up to the committee to gather the hidden intelligence.

The chairman thanked Colby and then opened the hearing to questions from committee members. Mr. Schwartz went first. He suggested that the CIA held lethal biologicals other than shellfish toxin and questioned why the CIA would directly violate an order from the president:

SCHWARTZ: You agree, do you not, that the retention of shellfish toxin, and probably certain other materials, violated that order.

COLBY: I think it was in a quantity which certainly is excessive for research purposes.

SCHWARTZ: And, in fact, no research was done on it after it was delivered to the CIA facilities. Is that right.

COLBY: Right.

SCHWARTZ: And, in fact, it was not for defensive purposes only, was it!

COLBY: No. I do not think you can say it . . . .[15]

CHAIRMAN CHURCH: Mr. Smothers, do you have any supplemental questions?

SMOTHERS: Yes. Maybe we could clarify the point that the chief counsel just raised. Mr. Colby, could you be more clear on the responsibility of the people who are involved with these toxins. . . . In the course of their duties, would these persons have had the opportunity to employ these substances in any manner against individuals or targets, if you will, that they might have selected?

COLBY: I do not quite understand the question.

SMOTHERS: The scientists we are talking about—would they have had the opportunity in the normal course of their duties with the Agency to determine how these materials might in fact be employed?

COLBY: Oh, they would certainly conduct experiments at Fort Detrick in various forms, but not on people.

"What about exhibit 12?" I wondered outloud, startling my BPL neighbors.

SMOTHERS: Would they be responsible for any employment of these materials beyond experimentation in a laboratory?

COLBY: Generally, no, although they would probably participate to some degree in the detailed planning of an operation. This will vary from operation to operation. Some operations cannot be established without a very close relationship between the technical people and the operational people. . . .

SMOTHERS: To the best of your knowledge, either during the time of your tenure or that of previous Directors, was there any effort made by any of these persons who had knowledge of the toxins either to urge employment of them or to seek in some manner to use them against persons, or to use them in a non-experimental manner?

COLBY: There were various suggestions made over time, yes. As a matter of fact, I had a job at one time when the idea was proposed to me, and I turned it down.

SMOTHERS: Yes; but was it proposed by these persons who had knowledge of the toxins?

COLBY: It was proposed by an expert. It was not a toxin in that case, but it was a very similar chemical. He was offering a capability, trying to see whether we were interested in using it.

SMOTHERS: How may people work in this laboratory, Mr. Colby?

COLBY: This particular laboratory was really a storeroom in recent years, and it is a very small room. The people who had access to it were only the chief and deputy chief and the secretary of that particular section, except that some additional people would sometimes visit it. But it is in the neighborhood of nine, something like that, in that particular branch.

SMOTHERS: Now, in addition to the lethal substances indicated on the inventory of exhibit 2, were there not, in fact, other substances and materials kept in this storage area?

COLBY: Yes, there are a number of other materials, and I tried to refer to that in my statement. . . .

SMOTHERS: Finally, to the best of your knowledge, Mr. Colby, as indicated by both your investigative efforts and any other information you may have, was any unauthorized use made of these materials at any time since their storage in the facility in question?

COLBY: Not to our knowledge.

SMOTHERS: Thank you. I have nothing further, Mr. Chairman.[16]

After a lengthy discussion about shellfish toxin, its delivery through a pistol that "fires a small dart," the chairman asked Colby if the CIA had any use for shellfish toxin supplies in amounts capable of killing hundreds of thousands of people:

COLBY: I certainly can't today, Mr. Chairman, in view of our current policies and directives.

CHAIRMAN CHURCH: Well, even at the time, certainly, the CIA was never commissioned or empowered to conduct bacteriological warfare against whole communities; and quantities of poison capable of destroying up to the hundreds of thousands of lives—it seems to me to be entirely inappropriate for any possible use to which the CIA might have put such poison.

COLBY: I think the fact that we were jointly doing this with the Army, Mr. Chairman, probably led into this kind of quantitative approach to it. . . .

CHAIRMAN CHURCH: Well, who paid for . . . the maintenance of a stockpile, about $75,000 a year?

COLBY: Yes; [the CIA] in collaboration with Fort Detrick, that was the sum that was involved.[17]

CHAIRMAN CHURCH: . . . Thank you. Senator Mondale.

MONDALE: Mr. Colby, in your opening statement you observed that the Agency which you head must operate in a secret environment. I think most of us would accept that fundamental concession and serious concessions in a society which is based upon the theory that the American people must know what is going on. But what troubles me is that this record seems to disclose an additional concession, namely, the lack of accountability, so that we not only have a secret agency, but we have an agency about which there is some question as to its accountability to the authority of the President or to the authority of the National Security Council. The record seems to disclose that there is no Presidential or National Security Council order in the first place directing the CIA to establish this program at all.

But in 1969 Kissinger ordered Laird to file a report on America's biological weapons capabilities. Thus, he had to know about their inventory, research, and ongoing projects. Next, MacArthur, Laird's Deputy Director of the Department of Defense asked Congress for $10 million to develop and test AIDS-like viruses.[18] As the director of the NSC staff, Kissinger surely knew what the CIA was up to.

MONDALE: Second, there appears to be no report by the CIA to higher authority of the existence of these toxins or biological weapons.

Third, there seems to be no evidence that those in charge of the CIA inquired of subordinates as to the existence of toxins or biological weapons, or that following the Presidential order decreeing destruction of such toxins, that any formal order went forth within the CIA to require their destruction.

In short, the record is a mess and we may never know just exactly what happened. Does it bother you that this kind of record could be available to us and should exist in something as serious as this?

COLBY: It certainly does, Senator Mondale. And I think we have taken some steps to try to overcome the problem. . . . the theory of the intelligence operations in the fifties—and that gradually has changed—but at that time, clearly those matters were not made in a great deal of record. There was some severe compartmentation of sensitive matter, things of this nature. This, then, reduced the amount of record keeping, the amount of involvement of other people in sensitive activities, and you reduced it down to a very small group who knew anything about it.

I think this then explains the difficulty today of reconstructing some of these matters.

MONDALE: But it also apparently created situations where the Agency, or someone in the Agency, pursued a course which violated a fundamental order of the President of the United States and the spirit of a solemn international convention against biological and toxic warfare.

COLBY: There is no question about it that a middle-grade officer made a decision that was wrong.

Middle grade officer? I questioned.

MONDALE: The trouble is we have seen this same phenomenon with respect to other matters that are not before us today, where, if something happened, people at the top did not know about it, or claim they knew about it and said it shouldn't happen. Then someone lower did it, claiming higher authority, not knowing who, no documentation. So, as we seek to reach the issue of accountability in a secret agency, we are left repeatedly with a record which is utterly beyond understanding. And I wonder if that does not go to questions of management and control and Presidential authority in a profound way, as this record discloses.

COLBY: I think it goes to a question of the cultural pattern of intelligence activities and the traditions, the old traditions of how they were conducted. And those are being changed in America and I for one am glad they are.[19]

CHAIRMAN CHURCH: Thank you, Senator Mondale. Senator Baker.

BAKER: Mr. Colby, it is clear to me from the evidence at hand that somebody authorized the formulation, the development and the retention of these toxic materials. Can you tell me who did it?

COLBY: The development, the research and development, I think, was begun in the sixties, the early sixties. I cannot tell you specifically who authorized it.

BAKER: Is there a record that would tell us who did it?

COLBY: The records are very incomplete, as you know sir.

BAKER: Why are they incomplete?

COLBY: Some of them apparently have been destroyed.

BAKER: Do you know who destroyed them?

COLBY: I do. I have a report that one set was destroyed by the Chief of the Division in question before his retirement.

BAKER: Is that Mr. Sidney Gottlieb?[17]

COLBY: Yes.

BAKER: What was his title at the time?

COLBY: He was Chief of the Technical Services Division.

BAKER: Have you interviewed Mr. Gottlieb?

COLBY: I have not.

BAKER: Has anyone at the Agency interviewed Mr. Gottlieb as to why these records were destroyed?

COLBY: There is a memorandum in the Agency between the Director and Mr. Gottlieb at that time.

BAKER: What does that mean? Does that mean yes they have or they haven't?

COLBY: That they were destroyed explaining—

BAKER: What I am asking you is, do you know; has anyone at the Agency interviewed Gottlieb as to why the material was destroyed?

COLBY: We have had one contact with Mr. Gottlieb in recent days. We have pretty much—

BAKER: Is it true that Gottlieb was at the Agency at Langley just a few days ago, going through his records and other material out there?

COLBY: He was.

BAKER: And did somebody at the time say, "What was it you destroyed, Sidney?" or "How come you did it?"

COLBY: Senator, we have taken the position with this committee, as we have with the other committees and with the Rockefeller Commission, that we would not go outside the current employees of the Agency to try to run down these stories. . . .

BAKER: Do you know what documents were destroyed?

COLBY: We are unsure as to the total. We do not have an inventory on it.

BAKER: Do you think they might have said who authorized the formulation or the retention of this stuff? Do you have any reason to think it might or might not contain that information?

COLBY: In this case, I doubt it would have very much, because this case, from the evidence we have at hand—

BAKER: Does it say anything or have any reason to indicate that it might say how, if at all, this material was used in an aggressive way against someone to kill someone?

COLBY: Well, there may well be some of that in the material.

BAKER: When was the documentation destroyed?

COLBY: In 1973.

BAKER: It did not happen to be destroyed at the same time as these [Watergate] tapes that the CIA destroyed.

COLBY: In 1972.

BAKER: In 1972? When in 1972?

COLBY: November, I believe it was.

BAKER: In November of 1972. Do you have any idea what volume or records were destroyed?

COLBY: I do not know.

BAKER: . . . May I ask you only this further question, then, in general, Mr. Colby. You have heard of the doctrine of plausible deniability?

COLBY: Yes, and I have rejected it now, Senator. I say we cannot depend upon that any more. . . . [Previously] if the United States could deny something and not be clearly demonstrated as having said something falsely, then the United States could do so.

BAKER: In the case of assassinations, in the case of any other—of domestic surveillance, in the case of the formulation of poisons, under that previous rationale, would the doctrine of plausible deniability have led the Agency to destroy records to conceal evidence or to compartmentalize to the point that it would be—that a committee such as this later would have been unable to establish what really happened?

COLBY: I think the plausible denial concept was used in the sense of international diplomatic relationships, that our country—

BAKER: And you saying by—that it would not have applied to the formulation of toxic materials?

COLBY: I would not say it did not have anything to do with it at all, but I think that the basic rationale for the doctrine of plausible denial was so our Nation could deny something and not be tagged with it.

BAKER: . . . Is that the sort of thing that would prevent us from finding records of responsibility and causal connection to this matter of the formulation and retention or the failure to destroy toxic materials?

COLBY: The effect of it would. . . .

BAKER: Thank you, Mr. Chairman.[20]

CHAIRMAN CHURCH: Thank you, Senator Baker. Senator Huddleston.

HUDDLESTON: . . . Mr. Colby, . . . I would like to refer you to a memorandum [exhibit 1] that was purported to have been prepared by Thomas H. Karamessines. . . . I understand that this memorandum was not signed by Mr. Karamessines, that the person to whom it was directed indicated that he did not, in fact, see it.

However, it sets out very specifically the situation at that time, in 1970, following the President's order to eliminate our activity in bacteriological and toxin warfare, . . . the CIA did have at Fort Detrick certain supplies. It then says that this stockpile did not appear on the inventory list. . . .

COLBY: . . . [A] certain officer wanted to save this material because it was very valuable.

HUDDLESTON: Mr. Colby, it has already been established that the cost of this research work and development was in the neighborhood of $3 million. . . . Now, most of the material there, the toxic material, was applied by some sort of injection. . . . Was there also material there that would be administered in some other way?"

COLBY: Oh, yes; there were various ways you could administer various of these materials, no question about it, both orally and under some kind of a guise and so forth.

HUDDLESTON: And what devices were prepared for that kind of administration?

COLBY: It was really rather the development—to see what the effect of putting the particular material into another substance, what chemical reactions and stabilities were.

Like putting viruses into vaccines, and seeing if they were stable enough to spread plagues? I wondered.

HUDDLESTON: Now, the inventory for the first set of materials that were held at Fort Detrick included an agent that, I presume, was designed to induce tuberculosis. Is that correct?

COLBY: Yes, there is that capability.

HUDDLESTON: What application would be made of that particular agent?

COLBY: It is obviously to induce tuberculosis in a subject that you want to induce it in.

HUDDLESTON: For what purpose?

COLBY: We know of no application ever being done with it, but the idea of giving someone this particular disease is obviously the thought process behind this.

Considering the resurgent tuberculosis epidemic associated with AIDS-related immunosuppression, I wondered whether CIA scientists had entertained this result also.

HUDDLESTON: You mentioned earlier in your testimony that the primary purpose for collecting this material was to induce a temporary situation to prevent harm?

COLBY: That certainly does not apply to the lethal agents.

HUDDLESTON: I would not think it did.

COLBY: No.

HUDDLESTON: What about brucellosis, which we are trying to eradicate in Kentucky. It affects cattle. That was also on the inventory. What was the purpose of that?

COLBY: I think we were talking about an experiment. We were talking about what its capabilities were, what the reactions were, and so forth. I do not think anyone had gone down the trail to a particular use, a particular purpose there. They were dealing as scientists with the different materials available to them.

HUDDLESTON: Was this at the direction of the CIA to develop this or for scientists just looking around trying to find out?

COLBY: These were CIA officers who were responsible for keeping up with the state of the art in various kinds of technical and pharmaceutical areas to see what applications might be appropriate for intelligence-related purposes.

Clearly then, some of the scientists with access to Fort Detrick actually worked for the CIA. A part of me did not want to believe that health professionals who had taken the Hippocratic Oath would work for an agency that covertly killed people. Yet, here was the possibility that some scientist like Gallo, with CIA or SOD clearance, could have easily walked in, accessed the merchandise, and done whatever his or her little heart desired with it.

HUDDLESTON: Thank you. I believe my time has expired, Mr. Chairman.[21]

CHAIRMAN CHURCH: Thank you, Senator Huddleston. Senator Goldwater.

GOLDWATER: Thank you, Mr. Chairman. I only have one question, Mr. Colby . . . have other countries developed bacteriological warfare ability?

COLBY: Certainly Senator; that is one aspect of bacteriological warfare that the President's directive in 1969 and 1970 tells CIA to continue, and that is to follow the activities of other nations. . . .

GOLDWATER: But you are now prevented from—

COLBY: No; we can follow the foreign ones, that's no problem.

GOLDWATER: You can follow them, but can you do anything to offset them?

COLBY: I think that the defensive against those possible things is a matter for the Department of Defense.

GOLDWATER: Do you feel you are safe in that field?

COLBY: I think in cooperation with the Department of Defense, and advising the Department of Defense of foreign developments in this area, we are giving them the basis for developing such defense efforts as we need them.

GOLDWATER: Thank you, that is all I have, Mr. Chairman.[22]

CHAIRMAN CHURCH: Thank you, Senator Goldwater. . . . Senator Mathias.

MATHIAS: Mr. Colby, . . . We wanted to be sure we had the best intelligence system that was available. But I think we also had in mind John Adams's warning that a frequent recurrence to the principles of the Constitution is absolutely necessary to preserve the advantages of liberty and to maintain a free government. I think the discovery of [these] toxin[s] raises some interesting questions. . . . For example, I accept your statement that this [shellfish] toxin was never used except in the one instance that you described. . . . If you had used the toxin, what provision in the Constitution would have afforded authority to do so?

COLBY: I think CIA's operations are certainly overseas operations. They fall under the National Security Act of 1947 and they fall, consequently, under the provisions of the Constitution that call for a national defense and the foreign relations of the United States.

MATHIAS: The use of a toxin of this sort is, of course, the use of force.

COLBY: It is a weapon; yes.

MATHIAS: . . . And so it seems to me that the discovery of this toxin raises very fundamental questions about the relationship of covert activities of any intelligence agencies, be it the CIA, the FBI, or others, with the constitutional process on which this Government is conducted. . . . Let me say this imposes responsibilities on the Congress that I do not think have always been discharged very well. I can recall members of Congress who recoiled from the responsibility of knowing what was happening, members of Congress who said, "Don't tell me, I do not want to know." I think that is an indictment of the Congress, just as severe an indictment as those labeled against any of the intelligence agencies.

COLBY: I would not call it an indictment of the Congress, Senator. I think it rather reflected the general atmosphere, political atmosphere, toward intelligence that was the traditional approach and I think we Americans are changing that. This act is an example of that change, as is this committee.[23]

CHAIRMAN CHURCH: I must say, Senator Mathias, I agree fully. We have been victimized by excessive secrecy, not only with respect to intelligence activities, but also excessive secrecy has created this kind of mischief within the executive branch. . . .

Church obviously meant the Nixon/Ford White House and the NSC under Kissinger.

CHAIRMAN CHURCH: Our next Senator is Senator Hart. . . .

HART: Thank you Mr. Chairman. Mr. Colby, can you be absolutely sure that there are not in other vaults any poisons in this town or in this country or in our possession in some part of the world?

COLBY: I cannot be absolutely sure, no Senator. We obviously are conducting such investigations and releasing such orders as possible, but I cannot be absolutely sure that some officer somewhere has not requested something.

HART: Could you concisely as possible state for the committee your understanding of the practice of compartmentation?

COLBY: Well, the compartmentation process is merely the strict application of the "need-to-know" principle. If an employee in the intelligence business needs to know something in order to do his job, then he has a right to the information. But if he does not need to know that particular information, he does not have a right to the information. And if the information is one which is required for large numbers of employees, then large numbers of employees will be allowed to know it.

If the particular activity is a very sensitive matter and only a very few employees need to know it, then it will be known to only a very few employees. We make a particular effort to keep the identities of our sources and some of our more complicated technical systems restricted very sharply to the people who actually need to work on them. And many of the rest of the people in the Agency know nothing about them.

Thus the intentional transmission of HIV into vaccines could have happened, and only a single technical person and one or two program directors might have known about it.

HART: . . . Mr. Colby, one brief line of inquiry in connection with the case under study. Are you familiar with a reported series of so-called vulnerability studies that were conducted probably sometime in the sixties in connection with this program of toxic weapons and so forth?

COLBY: I think this was a Defense Department activity of determining what possible vulnerabilities our country might have to these kinds of weapons.

HART: To your knowledge, were CIA personnel involved in this?

COLBY: CIA was aware of some of them because they were conducted with Fort Detrick and sometimes there are lessons to be learned from it that were picked up.

HART: But to your knowledge, your employees did not participate?

COLBY: They reported on the activities to us, but it was my impression that they did not actually participate in the experiment itself.

HART: And you are familiar with the fact that one of these experiments was conducted in the Food and Drug Administration here in Washington?

COLBY: I am aware of a report to that effect, yes sir.

HART: And you are also—

COLBY: There were other installations around the country that we looked at to determine what possible vulnerabilities large installations would have.

HART: Major urban subway systems and so forth.

COLBY: Yes.

HART: Did any of these studies in any way jeopardize human life and safety?

COLBY: According to my records . . . they were not conducted with hazardous substances. They were simulated rather than real.[23]

Apparently, Colby maintained additional records that Mr. Gottlieb had not destroyed.

HART: So, to your knowledge, no actual jeopardy occurred to any individual during any of these tests?

COLBY: I do not know of any that were in these studies. I do not know any. Obviously we did have the problem of the testing of LSD on unwitting subjects. That would fall within the category of your question.

HART: I am talking more about the mass—

COLBY: No, the mass ones, it is my impression that they did not risk the lives and health of the people involved.

HART: Thank you, and as far as you know, that one study on the subway system was conducted in New York City?

COLBY: I have seen a report to that effect. That is all I know about that particular program.

HART: There was further indication that some of these toxic elements might have had something to do with the destruction of crops in parts of the world. Do you know if that was ever implemented?

COLBY: I believe it was not. I know it was considered but it was decided not to do it.

HART: That is all I have, Mr. Chairman.[24]

As the hearing progressed, Senator Schweiker determined that the CIA's stockpile came from "somebody at the Army [who] decided they were going to slip their supply up to CIA."[25]

The chairman further noted that Karamessines's memo suggested that "the President's order be circumvented by taking the material out of the CIA laboratories and storing it with a private firm."[26] Considering this was illegal, he asked what right the CIA had for doing this, and if the National Security Council had ordered the CIA "to develop these quantities of poison?"

Colby said "no" and then felt the need to clarify:

COLBY: But the National Security Council certainly expects the CIA to be prepared to conduct paramilitary operations traditionally associated with the covert action areas, and in the process of preparing for those kinds of operations, the CIA has developed different weapons, has maintained different stocks of weapons, and I think that this incident came from the thought process that is represented by the development of that capability for the possibility of such covert operations."[27]

"*Wow,*" I again verbalized. Colby admitted having received orders from Kissinger to be prepared to conduct paramilitary operations using biological weapons in covert action areas of the world. That's why they kept the stockpile, and possibly moved it to a private firm. I now wondered if Zaire was such a covert action area?

Senator Tower continued Colby's interrogation:

TOWER: . . . Now, isn't the Agency expected to maintain the competence to perform any operation mandated by the President or the National Security Council?

COLBY: Any operation within the law.

TOWER: Any operation within the law. So in this connection, would specific NSC approval or knowledge be required from the standpoint of experimentation on weapons?

COLBY: On the experimentation, I would say no. . . . As to the use of such a weapon, either this or another weapons system, then I think it falls clearly within the provision of the memorandum which covers covert operations, which says that I am required to receive the approval for anything major or politically sensitive—and I think certainly this would fall into the category of politically sensitive.

TOWER: Thank you, Mr. Colby. No further questions.[28]

Chapter 16
PROJECT: MKNAOMI

AS the Congressional Select Committee's hearing continued, it became more and more obvious to the senators that the CIA was not accountable for any of its actions. It was operating above and obviously against the law. "What bothers me," Mondale said, "based on this evidence—the evidence we have had in other hearings—is this whole . . . [issue] of accountability, this difficulty of finding out what happened, and this gnawing fear that I have that things are occurring in deliberate contravention and disregard of official orders."[1]

The chairman, responded in kind. "In that connection," Church asked, "[are] any of those who failed to obey the President's order . . . still with the Agency?"

"Apparently so," Colby admitted.

"What disciplinary action has been taken?"

"I have not yet taken any. I have that under advisement right now, and I am coming to a decision."

The questioning went back to Senator Mathias:

MATHIAS: . . . [The] CIA had a continuing relationship at Fort Detrick which, in fact, [financially] supported the SOD division at Detrick. Is that not true?

COLBY: Yes.

MATHIAS: And that this was the facility in which experiments were carried out, in which research was done?

COLBY: Yes. It was not solely supported by CIA. It was also supported by the Army.

MATHIAS: But CIA was one of the principal customers.

COLBY: Principal participants, yes. It wasn't the principal, but it was a substantial customer.

MATHIAS: It was a principal customer. All right. . . . [But] Fort Detrick was not normally a production facility, though, was it?

COLBY: No. I think this particular material [shellfish toxin]—it is indicated it did come from elsewhere. It was actually produced somewhere else. . . . [and] I have a request now from a quite proper research interest not to destroy it, but to make it available to medical research.[2]

Soon thereafter Senator Hart chimed in with an important question.

HART: To your knowledge, was there any indication or any thought in the minds of those conducting these [population vulnerability] studies that we would make them operational or offensive at some time?

COLBY: I think the vulnerability studies conducted by the Department of Defense were basically defensive in their thought process. I think the intelligence people were observing them and watching them. I am not sure that they had a totally defensive approach toward the possibility of clandestine implementation of some such idea some day under some circumstances which might warrant it.

HART: I think in the memorandum of October 18, 1967 [exhibit 6], identified as MKNAOMI,[3] [it] clearly states that anticipated future use of some of these capabilities were certainly intended to be offensive.

COLBY: We are talking about a weapons system that the United States was developing," Colby replied, "and potential applications for it, and through regular military force or through secret methods and during times of war, and some such thing."

HART: So it was not purely defensive."

COLBY: No. I do not think it was purely defensive. I think particularly the intelligence people who were observing it were thinking of possible positive applications when appropriate."

Colby's honest and incriminating admission startled me. Surely the comment would have also startled Colby's higher ups—Kissinger and Ford.

I recalled reading a passage in Isaacson's book that said not long after Colby's testimony, the president and national security advisor met and decided to dump the CIA director. Kissinger was quoted as saying, "Every time that Bill Colby gets near Capitol Hill, the damn fool feels an irresistible urge to confess to some horrible crime."[4]

TESTIMONY OF NATHAN GORDON, FORMER CHIEF, CHEMISTRY BRANCH, TECHNICAL SERVICES DIVISION, CENTRAL INTELLIGENCE AGENCY.

GORDON: Gentlemen, I am appearing before this select committee freely and willingly. I am here, not as a mystery witness or a secret witness. I acknowledge that I have been served technically with a subpoena, but the record will show that I indicated to staff that I did not necessarily need a subpoena; I would be happy to appear before the closed session and the public testimony of my own free will. I would like to dispel the myth that has been circulating around with respect to a mysterious or secret witness.

CHAIRMAN CHURCH: May I say, Dr. Gordon, that a subpoena was issued by the committee with the understanding that it was necessary. The rule that has been invoked is based upon the issuance of the subpoena. Do you understand the subpoena, or are you here on some other basis? I want you to know your rights under the rule, and I think I should read the rule to you.

GORDON: Please do.

After reading Gordon his rights, including the right to prevent the broadcast media from filming, recording, or photographing him, Church looked to Gordon and said:

CHAIRMAN CHURCH: Do you accept the subpoena?

GORDON: Yes.

CHAIRMAN CHURCH: All right.

GORDON: May I continue?

CHAIRMAN CHURCH: Now you may continue.

GORDON: Let me start from the beginning, please, if I may.

I am appearing before this select committee freely and willingly to describe my involvement in a classified project known as MKNAOMI.

I wish to state that I was a CIA employee, specifically, a chemist, charged with the function of supporting and servicing operational requirements of the DDP—Deputy Director for Plans. Currently, I believe the designated title, since . . . September 30, 1972 . . . is the DDO—Deputy Director for Operations.

It was, and is, my belief that the Agency's policy in this field of behavioral materials was to maintain a potential capability—I emphasize, gentlemen, the phrase "potential capability"—in the event the need should arise to use these materials, biological and/or chemical, operationally. . . .

I would also like to emphasize, that to the best of my knowledge there was never a CIA directive, or any directive to my knowledge, that impinged on the CIA to destroy biological agents or toxins. . . .

I joined the TSD/CIA—TSD being Technical Services Division—in October, 1967, as the Deputy Chief of the Biology Branch of TSD. A few months later . . . I assumed the function of the [Branch] Chief . . . I held that position until April of 1970. . . .

SCHWARZ: At that time was the chain of command running from yourself to a Deputy Director of the TSD, then to Dr. Gottlieb, then to Mr. Thomas Karamessines, who was the Deputy Director for Plans, then from him to the Director of the Agency, Mr. Richard Helms?

GORDON: That is correct sir.

Misrepresenting MKNAOMI

Following a lengthy and unrevealing discussion, Mr. Gordon informed the group that he had personally informed the "Commanding Officer of the U.S. Army Biological Laboratories and the chain of command, [which included] the Chief of the Special Operations Division, the project officer for MKNAOMI . . . that it was our desire to cease operating the classified project MKNAOMI."

Some days later, Gordon was allegedly contacted by the Army's project officer, Mr. Charles Senseney, and asked whether the CIA would care to keep the toxins for "potential agency use." He thanked the officer and informed him he would consult with his superiors.

Gordon continued:

GORDON: After the consultation with my project officer and technical consultant, we agreed that the offer was valid for a number of factors. We knew that many years of hard, costly research had gone into the development of shellfish toxin and that those particular quantities, 5 grams or more, were realistic quantities for purposes of experiment, research and development, because if one had to really, in effect, study immunization methods for diseases vis-a-vis—who knows, cancer, anything of that particular ilk, it would take a considerable amount of this particular antigenic material to develop immunization. So that we know that was a reasonable quantity for that kind of purpose.

It certainly was not a reasonable quantity for [us] . . . However, I might add that that particular quantity . . . had been on a list of material held for . . . many years. . . . And in retrospect, I can see clearly now that our project officer just continued, including myself, to continue the listing, shellfish toxin being one of . . . a dozen or more different materials, never questioning the quantities that were being held.[5]

"Wait a minute!" I cried, "Hold everything!"

"Hush!" said a nearby reader.

"Sorry," I replied.

Gordon had Freudian-slipped and no one noticed. Where would he get the idea of studying "immunization methods for diseases vis-a-vis—who knows, cancer, anything of that particular ilk," from a 5-gram vile of shellfish toxin? I reflected on my knowledge of shellfish toxin learned two decades earlier as a Freshman at Tufts School of Dental Medicine. Shellfish toxin is a neurotoxin, not a carcinogen; that is, it is not a cancer-causing substance. The first thing that popped into Gordon's head was cancer and immunity. "Anything of that particular ilk," Mr. Gordon? How about the new cancer viruses that Gallo was describing before NATO audiences at that time?[6] How about mutant virus immunosuppression?

I quickly headed for the scientific reference section to look up the effects of shellfish poisoning just to be sure. The clinical features of exposure included numbness and tingling of the mouth, face, and arms and legs, visual disturbances, nausea, vomiting, diarrhea; in more severe cases, muscle weakness, paralysis, and respiratory arrest.[7] In essence, shellfish toxin made a great incapacitating agent for the CIA, but it held no benefit for studying immunity, cancer, or "anything of that particular ilk."

The cross-examination continued. At one point the chairman, obviously upset with Gordon's heightened sense of denial, got tough.

CHAIRMAN CHURCH: Let us be clear what we are talking about. President Nixon had decided that the United States should destroy biological toxins. Right! And you answered, 'right.' Then Mr. Schwarz said, 'the matter you discuss that some new President or administration official might come along and say, we would like to have such stuff in order to kill people. Is that right!' And you answered, 'that is right.'[8]

When I read this section, my question to Gordon would have been, "Did you have any inside knowledge that the Nixon White House might be quickly changing hands, and that the Kissinger/Ford administration might put some of these materials to immediate use in covert operations in Africa?

Still in a rage, the Chairman then blamed Gordon, as well as his higher-ups, for the whole messy MKNAOMI affair.

CHAIRMAN CHURCH: Where does the blame lie? You say it does not lie with you. If you say it does not lie with Mr. Helms, where does the blame lie?

GORDON: You asked the question, who in the CIA made the decision. Now you know that it was the Chemistry Branch Chief, the project director, and his technical consultant.

CHAIRMAN CHURCH: The blame lies with you!

GORDON: The blame lies with the group I have just specified.

CHAIRMAN CHURCH: Very well. . .

Later, toward the end of Gordon's testimony, questions were asked by Senator Schweiker about where the toxins originated. Angered by Gordon's hesitance to say or explain the role the United States Public Health Service played in MKNAOMI, Schweiker protested:

SCHWEIKER: Dr. Gordon, the part I have trouble comprehending, in view of your testimony is that labels on these cans are stuck on the top of the cans. You could not possibly pick a can up and put it in a file, without reading the label. One label says very clearly . . . paralytic shellfish toxin, working fund investigation Northeast Shellfish Sanitation Center. Then it says, USPHS—you do not have to be James Bond to figure out that means U.S. Public Health Service, Narragansett, R.I. And my question is why the U.S. Public Health Service is producing a deadly poison for this country, and who is paying for it, and you could see that by just reading the label on the can, so why all the mystery about where these 6 grams came from!

GORDON: Senator Schweiker, . . . insofar as the Public Health Service . . . being a source of the shellfish toxin material, this reflects a program that had been going on for some years. This is part of the cost in resources and value intrinsic in the quantity of shell toxin that was expended by those two particular Government agencies for many years. . . .

SCHWEIKER: Your testimony is that we have, in fact, been receiving deadly poison manufactured by the U.S. Public Health Service and delivered, indirectly at least, to Fort Detrick. It came to your hands, but first of all to Fort Detrick. And I am wondering whether our House subcommittee that appropriates money for health research is really aware that that is exactly where our health funds have been going.

GORDON: I understand your question, Senator. I do not have a response to it.

CHAIRMAN CHURCH: I understand your view that there is a suggestion here that the committee will have to fully inquire into whether other departments of the Government in addition to the CIA undertook to circumvent the Presidential order . . . and we will look into that because we really want to get to the root of the whole question presented here.[9]

I too wanted to get to the root of the USPHS link to biological weapons experiments. The combined role that agents from USPHS, the NCI, and Merck Inc. played in preparing and administering what was, very plausibly, HIV-tainted hepatitis B vaccines seemed worthy of further investigation.[10,11]

Naturally, I reflected on Szmuness's report[10] that the pioneering work on Merck's advanced formula hepatitis B vaccine was accomplished by "Krugman and his co-workers in 1970 to 1973."[12] Investigative journalist Robert Lederer keenly observed, as I did, that Krugman headed these initial studies, and that Krugman, like Gallo through Litton Bionetics, received funding for the project from the U.S. Army while serving in New York at the Willowbrook State School for mentally retarded children.[11] Despite a later publication by Szmuness and Purcell (from the CDC) describing hepatitis A and blood screening studies conducted on a group of mentally retarded children,[13] Szmuness's *New England Journal of Medicine* report said Krugman's experimental hepatitis B population was "healthy adults," and that Krugman's hepatitis B study began in 1974. Szmuness's report also noted that the Hilleman/Merck Institute hepatitis B studies began within twenty-four months of Krugman's efforts—more evidence, though circumstantial, that the early New York hepatitis B vaccine experiments could have been part of the CIA and Army's cooperative Project: MKNAOMI.[14]

Schweiker continued his assault on Gordon:

SCHWEIKER: Here is a toxin that could kill thousands of people. If you walk into the CIA building you have to be logged in. I do not know why we do not log a toxin that could kill many thousands of people.

I then realized that Fort Detrick logs might be checked to see if Gallo or any other suspects walked in or out with AIDS-like viruses during the early 1970s.

GORDON: I would like to make a comment with respect to what has been in the press a number of times. The only way admittedly, and unequivocally, that is a large amount of material for any purposes of applying it in a lethal form to people—the only way that you could kill those large numbers of people as related to the quantity of stockpile, is, in my humble opinion, to put some of them in one long line and inoculate each and every one.

Exactly the procedure recommended by the WHO and administered by USAID vaccination teams working within the twenty Central West African countries to immunize more than 20 million people from the mid-1960s through the late 1970s.[15,16]

Correctly Assigning Fault: Kissinger Ordered MKNAOMI

Finally, Senator Morgan surmised what I had about the origin of MKNAOMI. Giving Henry Kissinger a break and Gordon the benefit of the doubt, the senator from North Carolina said:

MORGAN: I think the President understood that there would be some problems in the disposal of biological and bacteriological weapons, and I think he must have understood that there would be some need to retain some for research, and I think this is why he asked the Secretary of Defense, who is on the National Security Council, to promulgate some guidelines for doing this very thing.

And according to this memorandum to the President, it appears to me that as of as late as January 25, 1973, these guidelines had not been promulgated. I think what I am saying, Dr. Gordon, is that somebody is trying to tree you, and I think we are treeing the wrong one. I think the fault lies at a higher level.

GORDON: Senator Morgan, I would appreciate some clarification as to how you see the Agency's role in that particular directive, sir.

MORGAN: I think the Agency role would have been to follow whatever guidelines the President and National Security Council may have set up after receiving recommendations from the DOD. I think you exercised your judgement, perhaps wrongly, but exercised it, based on the fact of what you understood it to mean—from what I read, this, as late as 3 years after the original order there had been no program devised or prepared or promulgated for the disposal of these bacteriological or biological drugs, and it was the responsibility of the President to enunciate this program.

In essence, Morgan pointed out that the secretary of defense, Melvin Laird, on or about January 25, 1973, had sent a memo to President Nixon asking for clarification as to what should be done regarding stockpiled biologicals. As Isaacson clearly noted in *Kissinger*, by that time—at the height of his Watergate embarrassment—Nixon was too depressed and dysfunctional to make any decisions. Virtually every important directive was made by Kissinger who sat atop the NSC, the President's Foreign Intelligence Advisory Board, the Intelligence Oversight Board, the Operations Advisory Group, the Committee on Foreign Intelligence, the CIA, the 40 Committee, and the Washington Special Action Group.

Therefore, it was Kissinger who had first ordered an interagency review of the nation's chemical and biological weapons capabilities. It was Kissinger who came up with the foreign policy recommendation that Nixon sign the Geneva accord for propaganda purposes. It was Kissinger who, having a vast amount of intelligence on the matter, plus having ordered the official CBW investigation report's rewrite, had to have turned a deaf ear to Gordon's and Karamessines's requests for orders to destroy the nation's deadly biological weapons.

Later in the hearings, Richard Helms, the former director of the CIA, also gave testimony. His statements also indicated that Kissinger oversaw MKNAOMI.

CHAIRMAN CHURCH: Mr. Helms, I am puzzled somewhat. It has been established by your testimony that the CIA had in its possession biological toxins that were subject to the President's order that they should be destroyed.

You have testified that a special study group was set up by the NSC pursuant to that order, and that that study group was not notified of the possession of these materials. And you have said that you did not think it was appropriate to give them that kind of information.

Since this was a study group of the NSC, and since, under the statute you are to take your directions from NSC in covert operations, why wasn't it appropriate to tell this study group that particular capability?

HELMS: Yes, sir, it is true that the statute reads that the Director of Central Intelligence reports to the National Security Council, which, in effect, is reporting to the President. . . . They do not necessarily report to the National Security Council staff.

This was the staff, of course, established by Kissinger with Nixon's blessing. Thus, the two men maintained complete control over the passage of intelligence and administrative authority. The NSC staff was considered a separate body from the NSC with different meeting agendas, and Kissinger ran them both (see fig. 11.2).

HELMS: Many of these study groups that were put together on a whole variety of matters over the years would not have been made privy to secret intelligence information unless there was some specific request on the part of Dr. Kissinger, or someone, that they should be so briefed. So this was the custom, not an exception to the rule.[17]

Thus, Kissinger never ordered Helms to report to the study group the CIA's stockpile of biological weapons. Apparently, he intended to use them on a mission not even the NSC discussed.

Chapter 17
The CIA's Human Experiments

IT was now clear that Kissinger and a few MKNAOMI scientists controlled the fate of AIDS-like viruses engineered for the Army for use in CIA-directed operations. Could the CIA really have gotten away with this? Their reprehensible history foreshadowed the likelihood.

Four months after the Church Committee hearings closed, the House Appropriations Committee renewed the CIA's entire chemical and biological weapons (CBW) budget. Despite revelations that the CIA had misused its authority and resources for the development, storage, and outlawed use of biological weapons, their association with Fort Detrick, the NCI, and the killer germs continued.[1,2]

The following month, in February 1976, the Senate added additional funds to the CIA's CBW coffer after hearing African intelligence reports alleging Soviet and Cuban aggression in Angola. The news was perfect for CIA and Army special operations division patrons. They combined their efforts, and once again, successfully gained Senate approval for additional BW program funding.[3]

The CIA's Human Experiments

Within a year, however, more military CBW misdeeds gained notoriety. Newspapers throughout North America carried stories about the joint Army–Navy–CIA germ warfare experiments conducted from 1953 to 1970. During this time, tens of thousands of people in New York City and San Francisco were experimentally exposed to airborne germs—*Serratia marcescens* and *Bacillus globigii.* The bacteria, first considered benign, were later determined to be pathogenic since at least one person died, and many came down with pneumonia-like symptoms. The intelligence leak once again prompted hearings before the Senate Subcommittee on Health and Scientific Research.[4]

This time, senators heard testimony that the CIA had secretly tested unsuspecting human subjects with pathogenic bacteria. The congressional investigating committee—the Subcommittee on Health and Scientific Research—was then led by the Honorable Edward M. (Ted) Kennedy. The Massachusetts senator at the time also served as vice president of NATO's Military Committee.[4,5]

Kennedy opened the session by rhetorically asking, "How can public accountability be maintained when secrecy is a legitimate and necessary component of research on human subjects?" He then called upon Senator Schweiker to advance his concerns about the program and testing of unsuspecting subjects:

SCHWEIKER: Many serious questions have been raised, particularly in regard to the biological simulant tests which have been widely reported in the press. Medical experts have told us that the Army was using simulant agents—live organisms which we know can infect human beings—in places like the New York subway system. There have been tests in my home state of Pennsylvania—in Mechanicsburgh, in the Kittatinny and Tascarora Tunnels on the Pennsylvania Turnpike and along Pennsylvania State Highway 16. Some experts have told me that the Army continued to use a certain bacterium long after it was known to cause infection. Officials from the Center for Disease Control have stated that many better alternatives to the known pathogenic fungus *Aspergillus fumigates* exist. It has been suggested that the fact that the organisms used as simulants do naturally occur in the environment does not at all insure their safety—in fact, because they are normally regulated by the environment, their efforts may be harder to detect and control. . . .

One thing seems clear, it is very risky indeed to assume that any living organism, reduced to germ warfare size and released in a populated area, is actually, theoretically, ever safe. . . .

Perhaps most importantly, have the tests ended? If so, could they start up again?

All these questions are vital as we attempt to come to grips with the key issue in these hearings—the use of Americans as unwitting human subjects for open-air germ warfare testing conducted in the public domain by officials of our own Government.

Since the original news reports appeared, my office has received a number of letters from people who want to know if our Armed Forces, charged with protecting us, could have injured them or their loved ones through indiscriminate open-air testing with disease-producing agents. They do not like the idea that they may have been guinea pigs in germ warfare experiments. In most cases, there is no reason at all to believe that the tests are implicated in these illnesses, and of course no direct proof exists. But I think it is tragic that in a free country like ours these sorts of questions have to occur to people at all. The American people have a right to know what is going on around them, and I hope this hearing will help resolve their lingering doubts.

Assistant Secretary of the Army for Research and Development, Mr. Edward A. Miller spoke next. He was accompanied by Brigadier General William S. Augerson, the Assistant Surgeon General for Research and Development; and Lieutenant Colonel George A. Carruth, Staff Officer for the Chemical and Nuclear Biological Chemical Defense Division, Office of the Deputy Chief of Staff for Operations and Plans. What follows was published in the *Congressional Record*:

MILLER: Thank you very much, Mr. Chairman and Senator Schweiker.

We appreciate the opportunity to appear before you today to present testimony concerning the Army's biological and chemical warfare programs.

It began in 1941 when the National Academy of Sciences, due to national concern, appointed a committee to make a complete survey of biological warfare (BW). In February of 1942, the committee completed its efforts and reported that BW as a weapon was not only feasible but that appropriate steps should be taken to establish a BW program for this country.

In August 1942, President Roosevelt approved the formation of the War Research Service (WRS), with George W. Merck, of the prominent Merck pharmaceutical firm, as its Director. . . . It became obvious early in the program that the United States was behind other nations in its chemical and biological warfare capabilities.

KENNEDY: Can you . . . give us what your assessment is about whether biological warfare is a usable and effective weapon at the present time?

MILLER: We believe that biological warfare could in fact be an effective weapon. . . . Our present feeling is that it could be effective unless we are well protected against it.

KENNEDY: We are really talking about a wide variety of different organisms or mechanisms under biological warfare, are we not?

MILLER: Yes; we are.

KENNEDY: . . . Just briefly, . . . give us the parameter of the type of danger we are talking about so that the people can understand. . . .

AUGERSON: Before referring to the conscious work of men, nature has indeed examples of biological warfare, amply demonstrated in plagues and epidemics. The nature of the beast consists of what the targets might be: people, animals, or plants. . . .

KENNEDY: Let me just ask you about the recombinant DNA issue as it affects this particular question. We have been interested in this subject matter. The committee will have to deal with that in later hearings, but as I understand, there is substantial research being done by the Soviet Union in the DNA area, recombinant DNA. What is the potential for recombinant DNA in this area or biological warfare? Is there significance to it?

AUGERSON: Yes, sir. As with most important scientific accomplishments, it has the potential of great harm as well as great good. There are dangerous applications of genetic manipulation that one can imagine. I would hasten to add, sir, that the Department of Defense has conducted in the last year an inventory, if you will, of the work that we have in hand, and I am aware of no work in recombinant DNA.[6]

Given the fact that the DOD had specifically requested five years of appropriations for AIDS-like virus development, Augerson apparently perjured himself. This work was obviously based on recombinant RNA and

DNA research, and in the interim the field literally exploded, with the Army funding numerous studies in the field.[7] His following remark shows how this work was concealed and rationalized.

KENNEDY: You are not doing the work?

AUGERSON: We participate with the National Institutes of Health in the studies and development of guidelines and intend, if we ever do such work, to conform to the established policies and guidelines.

KENNEDY: Just before leaving that subject matter, does the potential in the area of DNA research concern you, how it could be used in—

AUGERSON: Yes, sir.

KENNEDY: In an adverse way?

AUGERSON: Yes, sir; potentially very powerful way of altering the way living organisms work.

Miller then summarized the history of biological warfare. He said the Army's research was based on the "vulnerability of the military, the ground forces of the Army, in particular," and required the Army to work with the USPHS, the NIH, and the DHEW to "aggressively" overcome "those problems with respect to the known [biological] agents."[8]

Later in the hearings, senators learned that research and development efforts on medical aspects of germ warfare "have been extensive throughout the history of the program and have involved close cooperative efforts between Army, USPHS, and other HEW agencies. Major accomplishments in this program include development of vaccines," allegedly for protective use only.[9]

"The records" Colonel Carruth added, "indicate that there were 19 tests . . . conducted in the public domain using biological simulants. I will make a distinction, Senator, between biological simulants and nonbiological materials, for instance particles and other materials which were released to check dispersion patterns, but were not living materials. There were 27 of those tests conducted in the public domain (see fig. 17.1 for selected experiments)."[8]

BW tests, the officials testified had been conducted on unsuspecting Americans between 1950 and 1969. According to Senator Schweiker, Army officials were well aware that "there was a serious problem" and the public's health was at risk during the tests. [10]

The New York subway test and San Francisco open air experiments received the lion's share of discussion. Here Army special operations officers filled the air with *Serratia marcenscens* and *Bacillus globigii*, two

Fig. 17.1. Selected United States Biological Weapons Tests on Human Subjects

BIOLOGICAL FIELD TESTING
ANTI-PERSONNEL
BIOLOGICAL SIMULANTS
INVOLVING PUBLIC DOMAIN

LOCATION OF TEST	DATE(s) OF TEST	SIMULANT/AGENT USED
Washington, DC	18 Aug 1949 26 Aug 1949 12-13 Dec 1949 11 Mar 1950	Serratia marcescens
USS Coral Sea anchored in Kampton Rds, & USS F.D. Bailey at sea off entrance to Kampton Roads, Kampton Roads, VA 1 trial at anchor, 16 trials at sea off the entrance	1-21 Apr 1950	Bacillus globigii (Bacillus subtilis or niger); Serratia marcescens
San Francisco, CA	Sep 1950	Serratia marcescens; Bacillus globigii
Port Huenene, CA	10 Sep - 24 Oct 1952	Bacillus globigii
Panama City, FL	Mar - May 1953	Serratia marcescens Bacillus globigii
Off-shore, between Port Huenene and Point Mugu, CA near Santa Barbara	17-27 Aug 1956	Bacillus globigii
Pennsylvania State Highway #16 westward for one mile from Benchmark #193	7 Jan 1955	Bacillus globigii
Kittakinny and Tuscarora Tunnels, Pennsylvania Turnpike	Aug 1955	Bacillus globigii
Offshore Hawaii	Jan-June 1963	Bacillus globigii
Vicinity Ft. Greeley Alaska	Dec 1963 - Jan 1964	Escharicia coli
Central Alaska	Jan - Feb 1965	Escharicia coli
National Airport & Greyhound Terminal Washington, DC	May 1965	Escharicia coli
New York, NY	7 - 10 June 1966	Bacillus globigii
Key West, FL	1969	Serratia marcescens

Document recreated from library microfiche, some of which was illegible. These fourteen test sites were extracted from a total of twenty-three listed in Appendix IV-E-1-1 of "Biological Testing Involving Human Subjects by the Department of Defense, 1977." Hearings before the Subcommittee on Health and Scientific Research to examine Army biological warfare research programs, March 8, 1977 and May 23, 1977. Cong. Sess. 95-1, pp. 125–126.

Fig. 17.2. Fort Detrick Biological Weapons Contracts and Contractors 1951–1970

FORT DETRICK RDTE TYPE CONTRACTS

CONTRACTOR	NUMBER OF CONTRACTS	CONTRACT DATE	TERMINATION DATE
Bionetics Research Laboratories	2	Mar 1966 Jun 1967	May 1967 Sep 1968
Univ. of California	12	Apr 1950 Sep 1950 Mar 1951 Aug 1951 Aug 1952 Oct 1954 Jul 1962 Mar 1963 Mar 1964 Jun 1965 Jun 1966 Dec 1967	Sep 1953 Aug 1951 Jul 1953 Aug 1952 Oct 1954 Oct 1955 Dec 1965 Dec 1963 Feb 1965 May 1966 Nov 1967 Nov 1968'
Univ. of Chicago	13	Jul 1955 May 1956 Oct 1950 Jun 1951 Dec 1951 Jun 1952 Jun 1952 Dec 1953 Apr 1960 Aug 1962 Oct 1963 Nov 1964 Mar 1966	Mar 1957 Sep 1963 Feb 1953 Jun 1953 Dec 1953 Jul 1954 Mar 1954 Dec 1956 Apr 1963 Aug 1965 Oct 1964 Oct 1965' Jul 1966'
Litton Systems, Inc.	14	Jun 1960 Nov 1962 Mar 1964 Sep 1964 May 1965 May 1965 Jun 1965 Mar 1966 Apr 1966 Jun 1962 Aug 1966 Nov 1966 Mar 1967 Nov 1967	Sep 1965 Feb 1964 Nov 1965 Jan 1966 Oct 1965 Jan 1966 Sep 1965 Apr 1966 Jul 1966 Jun 1964 Dec 1966 Jan 1968 Mar 1967 Nov 1967
Merck & Co., Inc.	2	May 1955 Apr 1960	Dec 1956 Jun 1961
New York University	2	Nov 1951 Jan 1954	Nov 1959 Jun 1956
Research Fndn. of State Univ. of New York	3	Oct 1952 Jun 1963 Jun 1969	Mar 1965 Jun 1967 Jul 1969
Stanford Research Inst.	1	Mar 1964	Jan 1966
University of Texas	8	Oct 1951 Oct 1952 Sep 1955 Jun 1957 Feb 1951 Aug 1958 May 1963 Jun 1968	Oct 1954 Jul 1959 Jul 1958 Aug 1958 Feb 1953 Aug 1960 Oct 1965 Jun 1970'
University of Virginia	2	Jun 1965 May 1967	Apr 1967 Feb 1969'

Document recreated from library microfiche. These Fort Detrick contracts were extracted from twenty-one pages of contractor listings in Appendix I-C-1-21 of "Biological Testing Involving Human Subjects by the Department of Defense, 1977." Hearings before the Subcommittee on Health and Scientific Research to examine Army biological warfare research programs, March 8, 1977 and May 23, 1977. Cong. Sess. 95-1, pp. 80–100. † Denotes contract under which Robert Gallo and his colleagues may have worked.

pathogens not particularly lethal, but known by most experts as being capable of causing respiratory infections.

Past History Foreshadowing Current Events

Dr. Stepen Weitzman of the Department of Microbiology, School of Basic Health Science, at the State University of New York at Stony Brook was called in to testify that these tests may have killed many people, particularly "infants, elderly persons, people with cancer, [and] people with lung disease . . . [whose] ability to fight off infection by *Serratia marcescens* is difficult to estimate."[11]

"In summary," Weitzman continued, "too many uncontrolled variables are present to consider vulnerability testing safe for large civilian populations with a biological simulant."

Since such dangers were professionally recognized, and since the "Army used a number of consultants for the tests," Weitzman concluded that the Army researchers were ill advised.

The official Army report according to Weitzman, "never really dealt with, in any convincing detail, . . . the necessity for using actual cities for the open-air tests."

WEITZMAN: It is unclear to me what additional information was gained by releasing bacteria in the New York City subways, for example, that could not be gathered by a similar experiment done in the tunnels of a deserted mine shaft; or why in studying aerosolization patterns unpopulated areas could not be used, instead of populated cities. So, why the tests were conducted in populated cities certainly remains unclear to me.

The only unique information that can be concluded from these tests is that the cities are in fact obviously vulnerable to biological warfare attack. This vulnerability is so obvious that it leads to a consideration of the major point I would like to make.

Since the offensive biological warfare research program was dismantled in 1960, there would seem to be little purpose in spending time analyzing actions taken 20 years ago. Still, some degree of biological warfare research continues in the Department of Defense with a budget in 1975-76 of close to $18 million. While this research emphasizes "defensive research" the distinction between "offensive" and "defensive" is often no more than a semantic one. This was realized in Army reports where they quote as early as 1916 that: "it should be emphasized that while the main objective in all these endeavors was to develop methods for defending ourselves against possible enemy use of biological warfare agents, it was necessary to investigate offensive possibilities in order to learn what measures could be used for defense. Accordingly, the problems of offense and defense were closely interlinked in all the investigations conducted."

That biological warfare continues in this and probably other countries is disturbing, and that was noted also, in 1946: "It is important to note that, unlike the development of the atomic bomb and other secret weapons during the war, the development of agents for biological warfare is possible in many countries, large and small, without vast expenditures of money or the construction of huge production facilities. It is clear that the development of biological warfare could very well proceed in many countries, perhaps under the guise of legitimate medical or bacteriological research.[11]

Exactly as it had proceeded here, I considered.

WEITZMAN: The question was in fact discussed in great detail by Dr. Meselson in a Carnegie endowment report several years ago, in which they really made the point that in the context of a tactical and strategic war, it is very much in the U.S. interest to preserve and strengthen the restraints that prevent chemical warfare and the proliferation of chemical weapons. It seems that the wealth of the United States allows it to expend enormous quantities on weapons to be used, and in particular we are talking about conventional munitions and tactical combat; very few other countries approach this capability.

The lesson that was really learned from the San Francisco tests was the fact that an individual person, or a small group of people could, in fact, expose the population to large numbers of bacteria; and that once the technology of biological warfare has been developed, it becomes then easy for small countries, or small groups to use this technology. . . .

To summarize, I have tried to establish the following points:

The first point is that testing in offensive and defensive biological warfare research, and, in particular large-scale, open-air testing, is unpredictable and thus potentially dangerous. Unique conditions develop that are distinct from the usual laboratory or hospital experience.

The second point is that the Army acted irresponsibly in carrying out the vulnerability open-air tests on large urban populations in the 1950s and 1960s. They ignored the ethical problem of informed consent and the potential health problem we already discussed.

The third point is that the continuation of biological warfare research is not in the military interest of the United States since once the techniques are developed, biological warfare can be used by small countries, terrorist groups, and individuals. The proliferation of biological warfare weaponry and techniques can only erode military advantages that the United States now has since biological agents are cheap to produce and can be delivered by a small force in a clandestine manner.[11]

I paused for a moment to reflect: If it wasn't in the best interest of the U.S. military, then, in whose interest was it? Then it occurred to me that these most controversial, unethical, immoral, illegal, and potentially deadly tests were conducted in the same two cities hardest struck by AIDS. And for no apparent scientific reason. The same information could have been gained without placing the public at risk, Weitzman said.

There had to have been some payoff for these crimes against humanity. Certainly there was lots of money involved. The Army's input had come from covert operations officers serving within the USPHS, NIH, and DHEW—agencies intimately linked to private firms, like Merck and Litton Bionetics.

I shook my head in disgust. The financial motive and military–industrial connections I would have previously thought absurd, I now perceived as plausible. The harsh probabilities were reinforced as I surveyed the hearings addendum and noted that Merck & Co., Inc. had received two BW contracts during the period in which biological weapons tests involving the "public domain" had been conducted (see fig. 17.2).[12]

In his final remarks, as a marginally effective precaution, Weitzman recommended stronger informed consent laws be enacted to protect people from such military escapades. Then, most ironically, he recommended the senators pass a law requiring that BW testing programs be supervised by "the Department of Health, Education, and Welfare." He added, "At a time when Federal guidelines are being established for regulating recombinant DNA research conducted in universities and industries," the principle of providing "outside checks and balances . . . would seem appropriate."[11]

The Rockefeller Commission Overlooked the Worst

According to the Rockefeller Commission's Report on CIA Wrongdoing, in the late 1940s, the CIA "began to study the properties of certain behavior-influencing drugs (such as LSD) and how such drugs might be put to use by [American] intelligence. This interest was prompted [once again] by reports that the Soviet Union was experimenting with such drugs and by speculation that the confessions introduced during trials in the Soviet Union . . . might have been elicited by the use of drugs or hypnosis. Great concern over Soviet and North Korean techniques in 'brainwashing' continued. . . ."[13]

As a result, a drug program was developed by the CIA in an effort to explore human behavior modification: "Unsuspecting subjects within the United States" and Canada, the commission noted, were used by CIA operatives as guinea pigs in often lethal experiments designed to test weapons ranging from drugs, radiation, electric-shock, chemicals, and biologicals. Such experiments apparently continued until 1967 when allegedly "all projects involving behavior-influencing drugs were terminated."[13]

The facts, however, were impossible to determine since "all records concerning the program were ordered destroyed in 1973. . . . A total of 152 separate files" were wiped out.[13] The order apparently came once again from Kissinger.

In concluding the inquiry, the commission—headed by Nelson Rockefeller—admonished the CIA, as the Senate had done, for testing "potentially dangerous drugs on unsuspecting United States citizens," and recommended that future agency experiments should "adhere strictly to Department of Health, Education and Welfare guidelines concerning the use of human subjects."[13]

On the same page, the commissioners addressed another issue involving the Science and Technology Directorate—the "Manufacture and Use of [false] Documents." I read on with interest. Apparently the CIA had routinely issued medical scientists false names and identification documents for covert operations. The report stated:

> The Agency maintains a capability for producing and providing to its agents and operatives a wide range of "alias credentials. Most such documents purport to be of foreign origin. Some, however, are documents ordinarily issued by other branches of the U.S. government or by private United States businesses and organizations.
>
> Among the United States "alias" documents furnished from time to time to Agency personnel and operatives are Social Security cards, bank cards, professional cards, club cards, alumni association cards and library cards. The Agency has recently stopped producing alias driver's licenses, credit cards and birth certificates, unless needed in a particularly sensitive operation and approved in advance by the Deputy Director of Operations.
>
> While the Agency does not produce false United States passports, it has in the past altered a few. . . .
>
> The purpose of alias documents is to facilitate cover during CIA operations. . . .
>
> The Commission found no evidence that any Agency employee has ever used false documentation of this kind to his personal advantage.[13]

This information struck me as particularly sobering as I reflected on Henry Kissinger's role in gathering Nazis from post–World War II Germany while American intelligence offered many, with scientific training, lucrative positions. They undoubtedly gave the Nazi researchers alias names and backgrounds so they couldn't be traced or tried for war crimes, I recalled.

The CIA and "The Mad Doctor" in Canada

Despite its proprietary appearance, The Rockefeller Commission was anything but thorough in investigating and reporting CIA improprieties. Had they been, they might have discussed Operation MKULTRA, the agency's most notorious and barbarous mind control experiments.[14]

The McDonald Commission—the Canadian counterpart to the Rockefeller Commission—had investigated allegations that the CIA had supported Cameron, one of the most prominent research psychiatrists in North America. Cameron had conducted what he called "depatterning" and "psychic driving" experiments. The guinea pigs this time were psychiatric patients of the Royal Victoria Hospital—a teaching hospital affiliated with McGill University in Montreal.[15]

From 1957 to 1962, the CIA funneled grants totaling $84,820 to Cameron via the Society for the Investigation of Human Ecology (SIHE), a CIA front, for funding their "psychic driving" research, code-named MKULTRA Subproject 38.[14]

Cameron, the director of the Allan Memorial Institute (AMI) from 1943 to 1964, prescribed heavy doses of drugs combined with electro-convulsive (shock) therapy (ECT) in an effort to "depattern" unwanted behaviors, and "drive" into the psyche, alternative thoughts, beliefs, and habits. Although discredited today, ECT had been widely used in the 1950s and 1960s. Cameron, however, pioneered a distinct ECT protocol. Cameron's depatterning was described by John Marks, the author of *The Search for the "Manchurian Candidate": The CIA and Mind Control.* Cameron's treatment:

> normally started with 15 to 30 days of "sleep therapy." As the name implies, the patient slept almost the whole day and night. According to a doctor at the hospital who used to administer what he calls the "sleep cocktail," a staff member woke up the patient three times a day for medication that consisted of 100 mg. Thorazine, 100 mg. Nembutal, 100 mg. Seconal, 150 mg. Veronal, and 10 mg. Phenergan. Another staff doctor would also awaken the patient

two or sometimes three times daily for electroshock treatments. This doctor and his assistant wheeled a portable machine into the "sleep room" and gave the subject a local anesthetic and muscle relaxant, so as not to cause damage with the convulsions that were to come. After attaching electrodes soaked in saline solution, the attendant held the patient down and the doctor turned on the current. In standard, professional electroshock, doctors gave the subject a single dose of 110 volts lasting a fraction of a second, once a day or every other day.

By contrast, Cameron used a form 20 to 40 times more intense, two or three times daily, with the power turned up to 150 volts. Named the "Page-Russell" method after its British originators, this technique featured an initial one-second shock, which caused a major convulsion, and then five to nine additional shocks in the middle of the primary and follow-on convulsions. Even Drs. Page and Russell limited their treatments to once a day, and they always stopped as soon as their patients showed "pronounced confusion" and became "faulty in habits." Cameron, however, welcomed this kind of impairment as a sign the treatment was taking effect and plowed ahead through his routine.

The frequent screams of patients that echoed through the hospital did not deter Cameron or most of his associates in their attempts to "depattern" their subjects completely. Other hospital patients reported being petrified by the "sleep rooms," where the treatment took place, and they would usually creep down the opposite side of the hall.[17]

Occasionally, Cameron used an alternative method, including "sensory isolation." He placed patients in a large box for up to thirty-five days, depriving them of all sensory input. He covered their eyes, plugged their ears, or exposed them to a constant sound. Padding was used to prevent their sense of touch, and all ambient smells were eliminated. He sometimes combined ECT, sensory isolation, and drug-induced sleep. These evoked the "depatterning" phase of therapy. "At the end of up to 30 days of treatment—up to 60 treatments at the rate of two per day—the patient's mind would be more or less in a childlike and unconcerned state."[17]

Cameron then attempted to reprogram his literally unwitting subjects with his "psychic driving" techniques. Recorded messages were played for the patients thousands of times through pillow speakers or headphones. First, ten days of "negative signals" were used. These stressed the patient's presumed inadequacies. "Positive" messages were played the next ten days that encouraged the desired behavior. "Psychic driving would take place for continuous periods of up to sixteen hours per day. Taken together, the positive and negative messages might be repeated up to half a million times."[18]

Cameron's research apparently paralleled several goals set by the CIA's technical services staff. These included obtaining "materials which will render the induction of hypnosis easier or otherwise enhance its usefulness. . . ., materials and physical methods which will produce amnesia for events preceding and during their use. . . , and substances which alter personality structure in such a way that the tendency of the recipient to become dependent upon another person is enhanced."[19]

In his proposal to the CIA front, Cameron also said he would test curare, the South American arrow poison which, when liberally applied, kills by paralyzing internal body functions. In nonlethal doses, curare causes a limited paralysis which blocks but does not stop these functions. According to his papers, some of which wound up in the archives of the American Psychiatric Association, Cameron injected his patients with curare in conjunction with sensory deprivation, presumably to immobilize them further. Cameron also tested LSD in combination with psychic driving and other techniques.[20]

Marks further detailed, at the time Cameron was in charge of psychiatry at AMI, Dr. Donald Hebb headed McGill's Department of Psychology. Hebb minced no words when asked about psychic driving. "That was an awful set of ideas Cameron was working with," he testified. "It called for no intellectual respect. If you actually look at what he was doing and what he wrote, it would make you laugh. If I had a graduate student who talked like that, I'd throw him out." Warming to his subject, Hebb concluded, "Look, Cameron was no good as a researcher. . . . He was eminent because of politics."[20]

Following his retirement in 1964, Dr. Robert A. Cleghorn, Cameron's successor as AMI director, reviewed and then halted the mad scientist's work. Cleghorn's private notes described Cameron's research as "therapy gone wild."[21] Cameron died in 1967. "Twenty years later his victims are still fighting for redress, while the Canadian government is still trenchantly battling to shield itself and the CIA from blame."[14]

More Mad Medical Experiments

Many other studies, carried out on unsuspecting Americans, were detailed by Robert Lederer in *Covert Action Information Bulletin*. According to Lederer's well-documented work:

• In 1952 and 1953, clouds of zinc cadmium sulfide were sprayed over Winnipeg, Manitoba; St. Louis, Missouri; Minneapolis, Minnesota; Fort Wayne, Indiana; the Monocacy River Valley in Maryland; and Leesburg, Virginia. Despite claims of harmlessness, a military report noted respiratory problems [among some of those exposed].

• In 1955, the Tampa Bay area of Florida experienced a sharp rise in whooping cough cases, including 12 deaths, following a CIA bio-war test whose details are still secret, involving bacteria withdrawn from an Army CBW center.

• From 1956 to 1958, in the poor Black communities of Savannah, Georgia, and Avon Park, Florida, the Army carried out tests with mosquitoes that may have been infected with yellow fever. The insects were released into residential areas from ground level and dropped from planes and helicopters. Many people were swarmed by mosquitoes and then developed unknown fevers; some died. After each test Army agents posing as public health officials photographed and tested victims and then disappeared from town.[22]

• In 1976, the Humane Society of Utah questioned the mysterious deaths of 50 wild horses who had drank from a spring near the U.S. Army's Dugway Proving Ground, a CBW research center.[23, 24]

Lederer also advanced the 1978 "mass suicide" of 900 Black North Americans in Jonestown, Guyana, as a "highly suspicious incident that could bear scrutiny as a possible CBW test." He wrote that a Philadelphia activist who "extensively investigated the incident"—John Judge—found that many of the lethal drugs used at the scene "were the same ones tested under MKULTRA."[23]

> The Guyanese Chief Medical Examiner testified in court that 80 percent of the bodies he examined showed signs of forcible injections. Jim Jones, the self-proclaimed leader of the "People's Temple" which moved to Guyana from San Francisco, and one of his aides, had CIA connections. The father of Jonestown leader Larry Layton was head of CBW Research at the Army's Dugway Proving Grounds in the 1950s. The elder Layton admitted contributing $25,000 to the People's Temple. According to Judge, "Public exposure [in the mid-1970s] of experiments in U.S. prisons and mental institutions was, in all likelihood, a major impetus for relocating this testing to the jungles of a virtually unknown country."[23, 25]

Besides these events, directly or allegedly related to MKULTRA, the Army's history is replete with deadly "civilian" medical experiments most often practiced on southern blacks, prisoners, the mentally handicapped, and Third World populations.[23, 26, 27]

Marshall Shapo, the author of *A Nation of Guinea Pigs: The Unknown Risks of Chemical Technology,* reported that numerous new drugs had been tested in Third World countries long before similar tests were allowed in the United States. For instance, the birth control pill was first tested on

Haitian and Puerto Rican women who were not informed about the possible side effects. The trials were conducted by the G. D. Searle pharmaceutical company in 1956.[26]

Lederer also reviewed examples of horrific experiments involving prisoners exposed to infectious diseases and carcinogenic chemicals.[28] Between 1965 and 1968 "70 prisoners, mostly black, at Holmesburg State Prison in Philadelphia, were the subjects of tests by Dow Chemical Company of the effects of dioxin, the highly toxic chemical contaminant in Agent Orange." Dow, I recalled, a documented biological weapons contractor, had also supplied Gallo with experimental reagents used in his 1970s viral research, and in 1995 funded the development of AIDS-like monkey viruses by Dr. Narayan at the University of Kansas Medical Center. Lederer noted the Philadelphia study was "the second such experiment commissioned by Dow, the previous one carried out on 51 'volunteers,'" believed to also involve prisoners.[29,44]

> A series of experiments that bears particular scrutiny in light of AIDS were the mind-altering drug tests and aversion therapy measures, including electroshock treatment, used on prisoners in the California prisons of Vacaville and Atascadero in the 1960s.[30] Some of these were particularly directed against gay inmates, attempting to "convert" them to heterosexuality. Blanche Wiesen Cooke, a New York history professor, has raised question of whether AIDS may have developed as one result of such experiment. Clearly, these experiments need more investigation.[23]

Tuskegee Genocide in the Name of Science

Another outlandish example of scientific treachery carried out in the name of public health was the Tuskegee Syphilis Study.

In 1932, the USPHS, allegedly interested in studying untreated tertiary (final stage) syphilis, selected an experimental group consisting of 400 poor, uneducated black males from rural Tuskegee, Alabama, to serve as study subjects. The men were never told about their life threatening disease, and worse, they were consistently denied treatment. Another 200 healthy black men served as control subjects. Both groups were carefully observed for decades. According to James H. Jones, author of *Bad Blood*—the authoritative book on the case—"as of 1969, at least 28 and perhaps as many as 100 men had died as a direct result of complications caused by syphilis. Others had developed syphilis-related heart conditions that may have contributed to their deaths."[31] Additional study victims included the untreated men's wives, many of whom also became infected, and some of their children who "may have been born with congenital defects."[23]

A cartoon depicting the immorality, published in the *Denver Rocky Mountain News*, appears in fig. 17.3.

The experiment continued until 1972, when an outraged federal worker blew the whistle to the press, and nationwide condemnation forced the government to cancel the project. This employee had protested privately as far back as 1966, only provoking increasingly high-level secret meetings which resolved to continue the project. In 1972, as they reluctantly ordered its end, federal health officials hypocritically joined the press denunciations while implicitly defending the study as legitimate in its time. The survivors still received no

Fig. 17.3. "400 Untreated Syphilis Cases" In USPHS Study

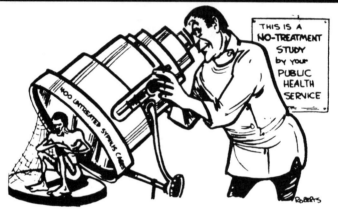

Under the USPHS's microscope were "400 untreated black syphilis cases" many of whom were observed until death. Source: Lederer R. Precedents for AIDS? Chemical-biological warfare, medical experiments and population control. *Covert Action Information Bulletin* 1987;28:35. Originally appeared in the *Denver Rocky Mountain News*.

treatment until eight months later, on the eve of congressional hearings. The federal office supervising the study was the predecessor of today's Center for Disease Control (CDC) unit in charge of the AIDS program. The CDC, a journalist wrote in 1972, "sees the poor, the black, the illiterate and the defenseless in American society as a vast experimental resource for the government."[23, 32]

Renewed Tuskegee Syphilis Study attention occurred during the confirmation hearings of Dr. Henry Foster, President Clinton's nominee for United States Surgeon General. Congress, following the national press, learned that Foster had served as an obstetrician at the Tuskegee clinic while the syphilis study was ongoing. He was also alleged to have attended a conference wherein the study was discussed. When questioned why he failed to intercede on behalf of the patients, Foster denied any knowledge of the experiment.[33]

Guardians of Ignorance

The Foster disclaimer was reminiscent of the congressional example set over a quarter century earlier at the height of Senate hearings on chemical and biological warfare.[34] On August 8, 1969, prior to his signing of the Geneva accord, President Nixon received numerous petitions. One plea came from Senator Yarborough, who warned Nixon about developing "a kind of 'super germ' or new strains of germs for which the body has not evolved antibodies and for which vaccines have not been developed." A genetic recombinant, he explained, was likely to produce "epidemic results" since it is "a self-replicating weapon—it proliferates itself, not only in the affected individuals but also in the entire population."[34]

Yarborough cited numerous examples of official negligence and ignorance in the face of impending disaster. In the text he sent Nixon was a story published in the July 25, 1969, edition of *Medical World News* entitled, "Biological Warfare: Off Limits to Doctors." The article relayed a conversation between a congressman and a prominent physician:

CONGRESSMAN'S QUESTION: What amount of VX nerve gas currently being tested in the open air over Dugway Proving Ground in Utah can kill a man?

PHYSICIAN'S ANSWER: I don't know.

CONGRESSMAN'S QUESTION: Were you aware that the Army's own maps show a permanent biocontaminated area about 17 miles outside Dugway?

PHYSICIAN'S ANSWER: Not until I read about it in yesterday's papers.

The doctor who was thus forced to admit ignorance . . . was the Surgeon General of the United States Public Health Service, William H. Stewart. . . . "I have primary responsibility within the federal government for the protection of public health," Dr. Stewart noted. To make the paradox more bitter, Dr. Stewart had served as chairman of the blue-ribbon committee set up to determine whether Dugway's testing programs, which killed some 6,000 sheep last year, have safety precautions adequate to protect humans, plants, and animals outside or inside the proving ground.

Much of the information about current U.S. biological warfare programs was apparently off limits to Dr. Stewart. . . . In the information that has been made available, there is no evidence of any substantial work on ways of protecting the civilian population against a biological attack, or against an air crash, train wreck, lab explosion, or earthquake involving U.S. research or storage facilities.[34]

More Links to New York Blood

One of Lederer's footnotes discussed what I realized was another incriminating link between CDC officials in charge of the Tuskegee Syphilis Experiment and public health officers in charge of the New York City Health Department and blood bank. I had already documented the research links between Bethesda hepatitis B investigators Purcell and Gerin, and Szmuness at the NYC Blood Center; and those between Krugman and Hilleman, who through Merck, Army, and Health Research Council of the City of New York contracts had direct access to New York's blood and homosexual vaccine supplies. Now Lederer footnoted that Dr. David Sencer, "the Director of the CDC who approved the continuation of the Tuskegee study in 1969"—the year Krugman began injecting experimental hepatitis B vaccines into human subjects from New York City[35]—"became New York City Health Commissioner, and a key player in AIDS policy, in the early 1980s."[23]

Undoubtedly anticipating the major focus of AIDS awareness would be on New York City, its blood bank, and health department, I realized, the CDC prudently placed an agency insider at the helm of the New York City Health Department. Sencer was the ideal candidate for the job—a veteran media bullet dodger and genocidal germ study administrator.

Later, I referenced *The Band* once again, seeking anything written about Sencer. I recalled that Shilts had liberally condemned the New York City Blood Center—America's largest blood bank—for resisting efforts to screen its stock. The "blood bankers" Shilts noted were "resolutely opposed" to testing the blood supplies even as late as 1984, "arguing almost solely on fiscal grounds."[36]

> Although largely run by non-profit organizations like the Red Cross, the blood industry represented big money, with annual receipts of a billion dollars. Their business of providing the blood for 3.5 million transfusions a year was threatened. Already the high cost of blood had created new markets for self-donation. Prices had to be competitive, blood bankers knew. The cost of testing for hepatitis antibodies, Kellner from the New York Blood Center suggested, would be $100 million annually for the entire nation. That was simply too much.[36]

As late as March 1984, Dr. Aaron Kellner, the president of the New York Blood Center had argued against testing their blood supplies for an AIDS factor. "Don't overstate the facts," Kellner said. "There are at most three cases of AIDS from blood donation and the evidence in two of these cases is very soft. And there are only a handful of cases among hemophiliacs."[36]

Besides, Kellner said, the proposed testing would cost his center $5 million to implement. False-positive test results would result in the unnecessary disposal of blood that wasn't infected with AIDS. "We must be careful not to overreact," he said. "The evidence is tenuous."[36]

At the same time, the National Gay Task Force had gathered its forces on the steps of the New York Blood Center. They denounced blood screening policies as Shilts wrote, despite their knowledge,

> . . . that virtually every gay man there had had hepatitis B and that most had engaged in the kind of sexual activities that put them at high risk for AIDS. Not one of them could in good conscience donate blood, [but] . . . here they were, exuding self-righteous indignation at the thought that someone would suggest they did not have the right to make such donations.[37]

Such were the facts when New York City Health Commissioner David Sencer announced the official decision to move confidentiality "to the top of their agenda." Blood screening dropped to the bottom. Shilts recalled how Sencer "spoke of the need to preserve confidentiality as the city's number-one priority. This pleased the Manhattan AIDS activists and took some of the sting out of the anger they felt about the lack of any city services or education programs. The city was very good on confidentiality, they assured each other." As a result, Shilts concluded, "Symbolism nearly always triumphed over substance in the world of AIDSpeak."[38]

Though Shilts clearly recalled the allegedly earnest manner in which the CDC had beseeched New York City Health Department and Blood Center officials to assist their federal efforts in identifying tainted blood lots as well as HIV-positive donors, it is extraordinary Shilts failed to realize Sencer's indelible connection to the federal authorities. Saying only that "a handful of cynics pointed out that confidentiality, like the gay bathhouses, was a perfect issue for David Sencer to champion, because it did not require spending a dime;" *The Band* failed to say that Sencer had quickly metamorphosed as the director of barbarous medical experiments to the protector of New York's most prosperous medical–industrial complex.

Equally suspicious was the fact that when the New York City Blood Center officials finally yielded to public outrage over their opposition to blood screening, the blood bankers selected the *hepatitis B core antigen* (anti-HBc) test to identify units suspected of HIV infection.[36] This radioimmunoassay had been licensed by Abbott Laboratories of Chicago. They had donated the radioactive experimental reagents to Szmuness for his now famous New York homosexual hepatitis B vaccine trial.[39] At the time, the less expensive ELISA test currently used to screen blood for HIV was being used successfully in Africa to detect antibodies to orthopoxviruses—those associated with smallpox. It had apparently been used successfully even years before that.[40]

Troublesome is the fact that Abbott Lab's principal hepatitis investigator was, like Hilleman at Merck, intimately connected to New York University Medical Center hepatitis B chief Krugman. Dr. L. R. Overby, of Abbott Laboratories, North Chicago, had not only attended the International Symposium on Viral Hepatitis in which the "Hepatitis B Virus Session II" was chaired by Professor Krugman, but Overby and Krugman combined their efforts between 1975 and 1978 to evaluate hepatitis B susceptibility and prevention methods among the gay men Szmuness later vaccinated in New York. Their co-authored paper was published in 1979 in the *New England Journal of Medicine.* [41,42]

The policy to employ the HBc antigen test to screen the nation's blood for AIDS—lucrative to the tune of tens of millions of dollars annually for Abbott and their affiliates—was set by Thomas Spira, one of the CDC's top viral immunologists. According to Shilts, Spira had spent a few weeks testing the blood of AIDS patients for markers that might identify the presence of a common infection. Though Shilts inaccurately claimed that "no test for AIDS itself yet existed," he recorded:

> The trait that distinguished the blood of AIDS sufferers was not difficult to find, considering that virtually everybody in AIDS risk groups—gay men, intravenous drug users, and hemophiliacs—had also suffered from hepatitis B at some point in their lives. Although the hepatitis virus usually disappeared after recovery, the blood still harbored antibodies to the core of the virus. Thus, Spira had found that 88 percent of the blood from gay AIDS patients contained hepatitis core antibodies, while all the blood from AIDS patients who were intravenous drug users had the antibodies, and 80 percent of people with lymphadenopathy carried the antibodies. The test might not screen out all AIDS carriers, Spira suggested, but it would eliminate enough to sharply reduce the threat of transmitting AIDS through transfusions.[36]

The 1984 finding that 88 percent of New York homosexuals carried the core HB antigen is somewhat confusing and questionable since it was appreciably higher than the 68 percent Szmuness recorded among Manhattan's gay men six years earlier in 1978.[39,43] Given that AIDS had been a wake-up call for safer sexual practices, particularly in New York's homosexual community, this large increase is remarkable. Instead, it allegedly increased by 20 percent. Had so many more gays been exposed to the hepatitis B virus during that time, and if so, how? If not, was the 88 percent falsely reported to make millions more on Abbott's core antigen test for a group of inside traders?

More Links to Rockefeller

A final nightmarish human investigation discussed by Lederer with potential relevance to my research was the Puerto Rican Cancer Experiment launched in 1931 by the Rockefeller Institute for Medical Investigations in San Juan. The program's director, Dr. Cornelius Rhoads, carried out the experiment in which thirteen Puerto Ricans died "after being purposely infected with cancer."[25] In a letter to a colleague, obtained by the Puerto Rican Nationalist Party, Rhoads wrote:

> the Porto Ricans [sic] . . . are beyond doubt the dirtiest, laziest, most degenerate and thievish race of men ever inhabiting this sphere. It makes you sick to inhabit the same island with them. . . . What the island needs is not public health work, but a tidal wave or something to totally exterminate the population. It might then be livable. I have done my best to further the process of extermination by killing off eight and transplanting cancer into several more. The latter has not resulted in any fatalities so far. . . . The matter of consideration for the patients' welfare plays no role here—in fact, all physicians take delight in the abuse and torture of the unfortunate subjects.[23, 44]

Lederer relayed the rest of a lengthy and horrifying story. I learned that Dr. Rhoads, rather than being held accountable for his crimes, was later awarded the Legion of Merit, and then appointed to the staff of the U.S. Atomic Energy Commission (AEC). This was during the 1950s when the commission was carrying out radiation experiments on unwitting hospital patients, mentally retarded children, prisoners, and soldiers.[23]

I later learned, the AEC was intimately involved in the NCI's cancer virus research program during the 1960s and early 1970s. Their "Joint AEC-NCI Molecular Anatomy Cancer Program," directed by Dr. Norman Anderson, extensively studied "human embryo tissues during early and mid gestation." Anderson, and a host of AEC and NCI researchers including Robert Gallo's superior Robert Manaker, injected human fetal specimens with various viral mutants in an effort to develop cancers and vaccines. Among their "major findings," announced in a 1971 DHEW publication, was that by bombarding fetuses with ionizing radiation, the researchers were able to cause tumorlike reactions in adults.[45,46]

Jackie, I considered, now in her second trimester, had no "need to know" what I had just learned about the CIA.

Chapter 18
Nazi Roots of
American Central Intelligence:
The Biological Warfare Industry

REALIZING now that anything was possible in the realm of CIA activity and biological experimentation, I continued to search back issues of *Covert Action Information Bulletin* for leads. I quickly located a fascinating article published in 1986 by Peter Dale Scott, Ph.D., a former Canadian diplomat, and Professor of English at the University of California. The political academician produced an eye-opening exposé on the Nazi medical officers who escaped prosecution through their service to American intelligence. His work, and several related articles, documented "the excessive zeal" with which U.S. Army intelligence and later CIA personnel protected war criminals, including the infamous "Angel of Death" Joseph Mengele; his assistant, "the butcher of Lyon," Klaus Barbie; Walter Rauff, the SS mobile gas chambers supervisor; Friederich Schwend, another mass murderer; and Walter Emil Schreiber, the Nazi chief of medical science, who the CIA brought to the "global preventive medicine" division of the Air Force School of Aviation Medicine (see fig. 18.1). All of this occurred under Project "Paperclip."[1]

Scott wrote:

> [I]t has become only too obvious that the OSS, the wartime precursor to today's CIA, arranged for numbers of wanted criminals to "escape" from camps, and when necessary supplied them with new identities to protect them from justice. Murderers, far from being exempted from such protection, seem to have been among those most likely to obtain it.[1-3]

Scott explained that not by coincidence, many of these medical sadists ended up in various countries having established "links with neo-fascist elements in the military or interior ministries." All of them collaborated in "repressive operations against the Left," and many appeared to be operating as arms dealers or intelligence assets in CIA-supported operations. Barbie and Schwend, for instance, were active during the CIA-assisted overthrow of Chile's Allende government. The two negotiated arms deals with "the German *Bundesnachtrichtdienst* (BND: federal intelligence ser-

Nazi Doctors in Demand

In September 1951, after 28 months with the Project Paperclip medical staff in Frankfurt, Germany, Major General Walter Emil Schreiber was brought to the United States for a six-month stint at the Air Force School of Aviation Medicine in Texas.

As Nazi chief of medical science, "Doctor" Schreiber was directly responsible for some of the most ghoulish medical experiments the Nazis conducted on concentration

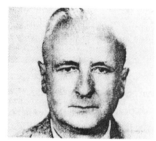

Credit: U.S. Air Force.

Walter Emil Schreiber.

camp inmates. According to massive evidence revealed during the Nuremberg Trials, some of the experiments cleared or reviewed by Schreiber included:

• Supervising Dr. Karl Gebhardt, later hanged for his crimes, who had operated on young Polish girls using gas gangrene.

• Injecting humans and mice interchangeably with transfers from each other of deadly typhus virus, to produce a live vaccine. Others were injected with infectious epidemic jaundice.

• Sterilizing male prisoners by surgery, X-ray, and drugs.

• Submerging victims in tanks of ice water to measure shock levels.

• Locking prisoners in low-pressure chambers to simulate flight at altitudes of up to 68,000 feet, which invariably resulted in the collapse of their lungs.

• Exposing subjects to heavy doses of incendiary phosphorus material.

With grotesque irony, Schreiber's role in Texas was consultant to the "global preventive medicine" division.

In March 1952, after Schreiber's presence in the U.S. had been discovered by columnist Drew Pearson, his continuing work for the American military was defended by Air Force General Robert Eaton: "Doctor Schreiber was hired by the Air Force because of his extensive experience in the fields of epidemiology and military preventive medicine, coupled with his peculiar knowledge of public health and sanitation problems in certain geographical areas. He has collaborated in the preparation of a treatise on the epidemiology of air travel and has been able to furnish the Air Force with valuable information."

Apparently, due to the embarrassment and controversy resulting from public exposure of their collaboration with

Schreiber, Project Paperclip officers generously found similar work for him in Argentina and flew him there on May 22, 1952.

Another of the hundreds of Nazi war criminals with whom the U.S. joined forces was Major General Kurt Blome. Some of the Nuremberg charges against him included:

• Wholesale practice of euthanasia by injecting intravenous undiluted lethal phenol.

• Executions of tubercular Polish prisoners.

• Various uses of biological warfare, his specialty. He admitted to U.S. Army interrogators in July 1945 that he had conducted experiments on his victims with plague vaccine, on orders of the notorious mass murderer, Heinrich Himmler.

Incredibly, Blome was acquitted by the Nuremberg tribunal, though the prosecutors had gathered a great deal of evidence about his activities. Just two months after his acquittal, he was contacted by four employees of the Army Chemical Corps at Camp Detrick for a discussion about biological warfare. Blome cooperated and also volunteered the names of other German biological warfare specialists.

In August 1951 he signed a "Project 63" contract as the camp doctor at the U.S. Army occupation force European Command Intelligence Center at Oberusal. A subsequent Defense Department contractual document shows the following 'entry under the heading of Qualifications. "Professor of medicin [sic] with emphasis on research of tuberculosis and cancer and biological warfare."

One of the lesser known Nazi doctors, Hubertus Strughold, a Luftwaffe member, was reportedly knowledgeable about the deadly low-pressure chamber experiments on concentration camp inmates. Though it is not known whether he came to the U.S. as part of Paperclip or 63, he worked for the U.S. Air Force for many years and is still living. Today at Brooks Air Force Base near San Antonio, Texas is the Hubertus Strughold Aeromedical Library, named after the man they fondly call "the father of aerospace medicine."   •

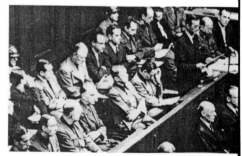

Credit: National Archives.

Nazi doctors before Nuremberg War Crimes Tribunal; standing at right is Kurt Blome; to his right is Karl Gebhardt.

Source: Preston, Jr. W. The Real Treason. *Covert Action Information Bulletin* (Winter) 1986;25:26.

vice), itself a descendant of the Gehlen intelligence network [commonly referred to as the "Gehlen Org"] which in 1945 passed from the leadership of the Nazi SS to that of American intelligence, and eventually the CIA." Later it was determined that both Barbie and Schwend were on the U.S. payroll, and worked, after World War II, for U.S. Army Counter Intelligence.[1] The organization, I recalled, for whom Henry Kissinger also worked to uncover such Nazis.[1,4]

Kissinger, Bolling, and Paperclip

By this time, I was hardly surprised to learn that General Alexander Bolling, for whom Kissinger translated, played a leading role in Project Paperclip and the Joint Intelligence Committee (JIC). This information came from Linda Hunt's meticulously documented exposé, *Secret Agenda: Nazi Scientists, The United States Government, and Project Paperclip 1945 to 1990.*

The JIC, Hunt explained, was involved in Project Paperclip from its inception, and was the "key military intelligence agency" involved in administering "a combined CIA-military intelligence project" that employed former Nazi scientists to investigate numerous mind-control techniques and drugs. It was code-named "Bluebird," later renamed "Artichoke," and paved the way for the CIA's infamous project MK-ULTRA.[5]

Moreover, according to Hunt's extensive documentation obtained through the FOIA, Bolling, in 1948, became "director of intelligence and godfather to the JIOA [the Joint Intelligence Objectives Agency] that ran Project Paperclip." At the same time, Bolling also served as a high ranking member of the Inter-American Defense Board (IADB), a Washington-based group that served to deliver Schreiber, Mengele, and Barbie to safe havens in South America where they continued to work on CIA projects.[5]

Barbie's history is best known:

> Condemned to death by the French for genocidal murders in Lyon, Barbie was concealed and protected for four years in Germany by the U.S. Army's Counter Intelligence Corps (CIC), which was using him as an informant to spy on—ironically—the French. After the Communists were dropped from General De Gaulle's cabinet, the Nazi Barbie was reassigned to spy on the "American Houses" set up by the U.S. State Department, which were, according to Barbie's American handler, "stocked with all kinds of leftwing literature." Barbie's reports may thus have helped fuel the attack on this program five years later by Joe McCarthy, whose charges against the State Department were based on documents leaked to him by a source in Army intelligence.[6,7]

Later, when a 1983 Justice Department investigation of Barbie by Allan A. Ryan revealed evidence of what Scott called, "a conscious, coordinated cover-up," it was noted that officials at the highest levels of the United States government had directed a misinformation campaign. The effort was apparently designed to dispel the impression that CIC ever had an interest in Barbie. In addition, Ryan's investigation revealed contradicting internal memos regarding the government's search for Barbie, and the mistranslation of press statements and internal memos about "Barbie" into "interagency communications about a nonexistent "Barbier."[8]

Scott noted that this behavior was easily recognized by FBI and CIA observers as a method of withholding files about "Barbier" when pressed to disclose intelligence on Barbie under the Freedom of Information Act. As another example, the Berkeley professor recalled that following the assassination of John F. Kennedy, "the CIA told the FBI it had no CIA-generated material on Lee Harvey Oswald in its files. This was true in the sense that all such documents had referred to a mythical "Lee Henry Oswald."[9]

The Merk Net

Besides disclosing Barbie's ties to the CIA, Ryan's official investigation report connected Nazi and Army intelligence to the "Gehlen Org" and "the Merk net."[1]

The Merk net, was a network of CIC informants so named for its leader Kurt Merk. The Gehlen Org had tried to recruit Merk as its "chief of counterintelligence operations."

Scott wrote that by March 1948 "CIC had established liaison with the CIA in Europe, because of the latter's interest in the Merk net." But American intelligence interest in Reinhard Gehlen "the Nazi chief of intelligence on the Soviet front," went back even further to 1945. This was just three months prior to the creation of the Office of Policy Coordination (OPC), the earliest name given the CIA undercover operations division.[1]

Scott questioned:

Could Mengele . . . a doctor with a penchant for lethal experiments on human guinea pigs—could even Mengele have been saved as a result of a secret deal between [Allen Welsh] Dulles [director of American intelligence] and the SS? Such a hypothesis would once have been almost unthinkable. But we have since been told that his colleague in the Auschwitz human experiments, Walter Schreiber, was shielded by the Americans from a Polish conviction *in absentia*, so that he could help guide the postwar researches of the U.S. Air Force in bacteriological warfare. . . .[1,10]

Given the provision of false documents and slight name changes to protect German intelligence assets, I now wondered whether there was any connection between "Merk" and "Merck." My suspicions were fueled even more by Scott's revelation that in 1960, Barbie and other high-ranking Nazi officials, including Alfons Sassen and Friedrich Schwend, had dug into their war chest to establish a CIA front company known as "Estrella." Ostensibly, Estrella dealt in "quinquina bark." The company exported the bark, "as agents for the German drug firm Boehringer, which grew rich on quinine contracts to the U.S. Army during the Vietnam War."[11] And although public registry records are nonexistent, at least one Bolivian arms dealer still remembers Estrella also dealt in the weapons trade.[11]

In essence, fortunes were being made through drugs and arms sales by the secret organization for which General Bolling and Henry Kissinger worked to draft ex-Nazi's into military and industrial leadership positions, and American intelligence posts. Some even pioneered the Merck directed biological weapons industry.

Nazis in the Navy and Viruses From the Sky

Besides the involvement of Nazis in bacteriological weapons experiments conducted by the Air Force, General Bolling's JIOA imported several BW experts into the United States for the Navy as well.

Erich Traub, for instance, "in charge of biological warfare for the Reich Research Institute on the secluded island of Riems, where his biological warfare research specialty was viral and bacteriological diseases," and his assistant Anne Burger, went to work for the Navy in 1951 under Project Paperclip. Assigned to the Naval Medical Research Institute laboratory in Bethesda, their work "included conducting experiments on animals to determine the lethal doses of more than forty strains of highly infectious viruses."[5,12] Within ten years, the Navy's Biomedical Research Laboratory (NBRL), along with Litton Bionetics, had become a chief supplier of "cell cultures for cancer research studies to NCI investigators" throughout the world.

By the early 1960s, the NBRL, became closely associated with the University of California, where Peter Duesberg was working on NCI projects. Naval studies, directed by Dr. Mark A. Chatigny and "Biohazards Control and Containment Segment" chief, Dr. Alfred Hellman, also associated with the Atomic Energy Commission, sought to identify the effects of "viral aerosols" on animals and humans. Their principal NCI grant objective was to:

> evaluate the effect of selected stress situations . . . on induction of viral disease or cancerous trauma, and to evaluate the role airborne particle size might play in such interactions.[13]

At the same time, another Navy study was underway to determine "the fundamental biology of tumor cells, and the interaction between tumor cells and viruses" that cause cancer. This study, begun October 1, 1962, relied on the expertise of Dr. Walter Nelson-Rees—described by Strecker as the keeper of America's cell lines. The Navy–University of California collaborative effort was officiated by the NCI's "Solid Tumor Virus Segment" Vice Chairman, James T. Duff, who, along with Robert J. Huebner, the segment's chairman, worked closely with Duesberg on his studies to determine the structure and regulating mechanisms of cancer viruses (see figs. 8.3 and 18.2).

Following this decade of progress, a 1971 NCI report, shown in fig. 18.2, summarized this study group's proposed course of action:

> Continue to develop cell reagents as substrates for human carcinogenesis; attempt to isolate and characterize viral agents from human tumor cells; continue a reference laboratory . . . of cells in culture; study oncogenic viral antigens during embryogenesis [development of the human embryo], and continue basic research in the biology of tumor viruses.[13]

Though by this time I had grown accustomed to shocking new evidence, I still balked on finding these documents linking Hitler's biological weapons chief to the NCI's finest.

The Gehlen Org

The Gehlen Org, the German intelligence agency run by Reinhard Gehlen, was even more powerful than the Merk net. The Org superseded even the Nazi SS because of its prewar connections with the Abwehr or German military intelligence. In fact, Gehlen's organization is largely credited for giving rise to the CIA.

After Hitler, Gehlen served Allen Welsh Dulles, whose "Operation Sunshine" brought Nazis into the U.S. spy service. According to Scott:

> What ultimately persuaded Truman in 1947 to authorize an operational CIA, was in fact partly the need to find an institutional home for the postwar Gehlen Org. In 1948 Dulles . . . helped write the memo persuading Truman to take on the Gehlen Org, on Gehlen's own terms.[1]

The Sovereign Military Order of Malta

How had Dulles acquired so much power as to persuade the nation's chief executive to form the CIA—a successful bid to shield Gehlen and the entire German intelligence network from harm's way? Gehlen was a ranking official in the Sovereign Military Order of Malta (SMOM), which maintained inconceivable financial and political influence.[14]

Figure 18.2 Navy Studies on Responses to Viral Aerosols

Naval Biological Laboratory (FS-57)

Title: Studies of Environmental and Physiological Factors Influencing Virus-Host with Action

Contractor's Project Directors: Dr. R. L. Dimmick
Mr. M. A. Chatigny

Project Officers: Dr. A. Hellman
Dr. A. K. Fowler
Mr. W. E. Barkley

Objectives: This contract has four objectives, they are:

1. Virus laboratory hazards evaluation. The objective of this section of the proposal is to evaluate the extent of possible hazards involved in biochemical and biophysical procedures used in virus-tissue culture laboratories.

2. Studies on environmental effects on physical and biological characteristics of viral aerosols. The objective of this section of the proposal is to provide survival data of both "model" and oncogenic viruses as related to environmental parameters (e.g. temperature, RH, RH changes, and trace chemicals - decontaminants) for use in Section 1, and to evaluate the importance of end-spectrum (0.1 to 0.5 um) (5 to 15 um) particles on virus-host interaction considering both the hazard to humans and animals and the potential for cross contamination.

3. Host-virus interactions. The objective of this section is to evaluate the effect of selected stress situations (physiological as by hormonal imbalance, immunological as by concurrent infection or biochemical, as by exposure to injurious chemical vapors of aerosols) on induction of viral disease or cancerous trauma, and to evaluate the role airborne particle size might play in such interactions.

4. Evaluation of disinfectants and decontamination procedures for selected viruses. The objective of this section is to conduct studies of the decontamination efficiency of selected disinfectants on the viruses selected from Section 2 with the purpose of recommending optimal procedures.

Date Contract Initiated: March 1, 1971

Souce: NCI staff. *The Special Virus Cancer Program: Progress Report #8.* Office of the Associate Scientific Director for Viral Oncology (OASDVO). J. B. Moloney, Ed., Washington, D. C.: U. S. Government Printing Office, 1971, pp. 224.

Francoise Hervet, the pseudonym of a researcher who spent many years investigating the SMOM explained:

> Representing initially the most powerful and reactionary segments of the European aristocracy, for nearly a thousand years beginning with the early crusades of the Twelfth Century, it has organized, funded, and led military operations against states and ideas deemed threatening to its power. It is probably safe to say that the several thousand Knights of SMOM, principally in Europe, North, Central and South America, comprise the largest most consistently powerful and reactionary membership of any organization in the world today. . . .

> To be a Knight, one must not only be from wealthy, aristocratic lineage, one must also have a psychological worldview which is attracted to the "crusader mentality" of these "warrior monks." Participating in SMOM—including its initiation ceremonies and feudal ritual dress—members embrace a certain caste/class mentality; they are sociologically and psychologically predisposed to function as the "shock troops" of Catholic reaction. And this is precisely the historical role the Knights have played in the war against Islam, against the protestant "heresy," and against the Soviet "Evil Empire."

> The Catholic Right and the Knights of Malta, in particular Baron Franz von Papan, played a critical role in Hitler's assumption of power and the launching of the Third Reich's Twentieth Century Crusade.[14]

Hervet further explained that the "SMOM's influence in Germany survived World War II intact." On November 17, 1948, Gehlen received the Grand Cross of Merit award, one of the organization's highest honors. Subsequently, he was installed by American intelligence officials as "the first chief of West Germany's equivalent of the CIA, the *Bundesnachtrichtdienst*, under West German Chancellor Adenauer." Adenauer had received "the Magistral Grand Cross personally from SMOM Grand Master Prince Chigi."[14]

Gehlen's brother, in the meantime, "had already been in Rome serving as Secretary to Thun Hohenstein. Conveniently for Reinhard, who was [then] negotiating with American intelligence for the preservation of his Nazi colleagues, Thun Hohenstein was Chairman of one of SMOM's grand magistral charities, the Institute for Associated Emigrations." Hohenstein, thus arranged for "two thousand SMOM passports to be printed for political refugees."[14]

Meanwhile, throughout the war, another SMOM member, Joseph J. Larkin, the vice president of the Rockefeller-owned Chase Manhattan Bank, had managed to keep the financial institution open in Nazi-occupied Paris. Larkin "had received the Order of the Grand Cross of the Knights of

Malta from Pope Piux XI in 1928. He was an ardent supporter of General Franco and, by extension, Hilter."[14]

More Financial Interests and Intelligence Ties

Somehow I wasn't surprised to learn that financial motives, besides ideological, were at the heart of SMOM and the Nazi–American alliance.

Scott critically reviewed two books by authors with wartime intelligence backgrounds. One by Ladislas Farago, entitled, *Aftermath: Bormann and the Fourth Reich* (New York: Avon Books, 1975), and the other by William Stevenson, *The Bormann Brotherhood* (New York: Harcourt, Brace, Jovanovich, 1973), and gleaned enlightening facts about the financial assets of the Nazi bureaucracy and Martin Bormann, Hitler's deputy and party chief. The books, Scott wrote:

> . . . point to the role of the extensive postwar assets collected or plundered by the SS and Bormann. This came from three sources: the proceeds from the SS forgery of British pound notes ("Operation Bernhard"), the looting of Jews and other Nazi victims, and, most significantly, the corporate contributions to a special fund set up to guarantee the survival of German multinationals abroad after the impending collapse of Hitler. Soon after the war, OSS found the extensive documentation of a meeting in Strasbourg on August 10, 1944 to establish this fund, between representatives of the SS, Party, and firms like Krupp, I. G. Farben and Messerschmidt.

> But as the Cold War encouraged the U.S. to see the German corporate presence in Latin America in a more friendly light, the role of these firms in providing new careers for war criminals abroad was ignored. In fact, it was the key to the postwar status of the *Kameraden*.[15]

After the war, documented evidence revealed that perhaps as many as 2,000 Nazi officials, many of them doctors and scientists, made their way into corporations operating in Latin America and the United States with the help of American intelligence. The infamous "Rat Line," the underground railway leading from Germany to Italy, served as the main conduit for Nazi travelers. Operated by the Austrian office of the CIC, Army intelligence, thus, maintained intimate ties to the *Kameradenwerk* set up by Barbie with assistance from the Vatican and the SMOM.

The most prominent Nazis known to have escaped by this route included Barbie himself who escaped to Bolivia (with Croatians); Friederich Schwend to Peru (with Croatians); Walter Rauff to Chile (with Croatians); Alfons Sassen to Ecuador; and Otto Skorzeny, Hans-Ulrich Rudel, and

Heinrich Müller, all to Argentina. The *Kameraden* "maintained close political, social, and business ties. By most accounts, Josef Mengele was its leading representative in Paraguay"[1,16]

> . . . Otto Skorzeny (acquitted of his criminal charges by the intervention of western intelligence) became a sales representative of Krupp. Hans Ulrich Rudel (never charged, but an unrepentant Nazi ideologue in the post war era) became a sales representative of Siemens. Walter Rauff (designer of the gas ovens at Auschwitz found his first employment in Latin America with a subsidiary of I. G. Farben (an employer of slave labor at Auschwitz) Franz Paul Stangl, chief of the Treblinka extermination camp, found postwar employment in Latin America with Volkswagen, as did Eichmann with Mercedes-Benz. And so on.[1,17]

Following Barbie's escape, the CIC provided Barbie with a package of false documents, funds, and references for his new identity as "Klaus Altmann." This information was revealed by author Magnus Linklater in, *The Nazi Legacy: Klaus Barbie and the International Fascist Connection.* A photograph of Barbie showing his alias and Bolivian intelligence ID is reprinted in fig. 18.3.

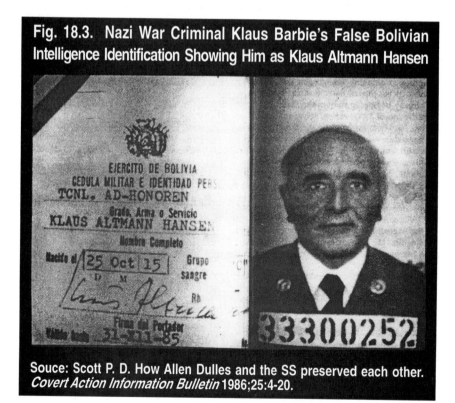

Fig. 18.3. Nazi War Criminal Klaus Barbie's False Bolivian Intelligence Identification Showing Him as Klaus Altmann Hansen

Souce: Scott P. D. How Allen Dulles and the SS preserved each other. *Covert Action Information Bulletin* 1986;25:4-20.

But U.S. intelligence played an even more decisive role in exfiltrating Nazis into the military–medical–industrial complex by protecting the proceeds of "Operation Bernhard." Western intelligence officials, Scott reported, knew enough about the British currency forging operation to protect the postwar pound. Thus, before the British government recalled the old and issued new notes, the SS profits were assured in the neighborhood of $300 million which "had been converted to genuine currency."[1]

Much of this money apparently made its way to the Vatican, and from there into Joseph Larkin's hands at the Chase Bank.[14]

The man charged with laundering the Nazi war chest was Friederich Schwend, who between 1945 and 1946 became "an important link in setting up the SS escape route to the Vatican. . . .'[1]

Indeed the Vatican did have a program underway for the exfiltration of anti-communists. This was the work of Bishop Alois Hudal of the Collegium Teutonicum, a priest close both to Pius XII and the future Paul VI as well as a public admirer of the Third Reich. After an interview in Rome with former Gestapo Chief Heinrich Müller, Hudal had begun the work of supplying Vatican documentation for such prominent fugitives as Müller, Eichmann, and perhaps Martin Bormann.[18] It was Hudal who gave . . . the necessary introductions to the International Red Cross and other "officials who, for a bribe, could smooth the fugitive's path."[19]

The combined efforts of Hudal and others, Stevenson wrote, helped hundreds of Nazis to escape.[1],[20]

Farago detailed Heinrich Müller's exodus. Driven from Merano, north of Italy, to Rome in Schwend's chauffeured Mercedes, he deposited some of the Nazi war chest at a Croatian seminary and made the historic contact with Bishop Hudal. In 1972, documents found in Schwend's possession reported that:

the bulk of the money the bishop [Hudal] needed was placed at his disposal by . . . a financier named Friederich "Freddy" Merser, partner of Friederich Schwend in Operation Bernhard. The money came from the hoard Schwend had amassed in Swiss accounts.[21]

However, Scott warned that both Farango and Stevenson withheld the most damaging evidence linking the *Kameradenwerk* and Operation Bernhard to U.S. Army intelligence. Apparently, from 1945 to 1946, while Schwend was making crucial arrangements to free hundreds of Nazi's through "the Rat Line," Schwend was working for American intelligence. U.S. documents revealed that "after passing into the hands of the 44th CIC Detachment he was used as an informant by American intelligence agencies."[11]

Corporate Collaboration

"The real treason," however, according to William Preston, Jr., a professor of history at New York's John Jay College of Criminal Justice, was that for years before World War II, and after, "a secret, conspiratorial alliance between various American corporations and their Nazi collaborators . . . betrayed and subverted U.S. national interests." Preston, who headed the Fund for Open Information and Accountability, Inc., wrote:

> This link between a "fraternity" of top business executives and the country's deadliest wartime enemy, the Third Reich, this collaboration between capitalism and fascism, has been suppressed by the politically powerful, for their own political purposes. Yet the magnitude of the crime and the damage it did, harm that included injuring and killing allied and American fighting men and women, were not approximated in any other case of disloyalty for which the government has exacted retribution.[22]

Charles Higham, author of *Trading With the Enemy: An Exposure of the Nazi-American Money Plot, 1933-1949,* wrote that "the Fraternity" of subversive business leaders shared ideological and economic reasons for collaborating with the Nazis:

> Anti-semitism, sympathy for Hitler, distastes for the Roosevelt New Deal and its supposed Jewish-communist components blended with major financial, industrial, and technological alliances between German and American enterprises. During the 1930s members of the Fraternity supported the Black Legion, a Klan type fascist organization based in Michigan; financed the American Liberty League's hate campaign against FDR; plotted a "bizarre conspiracy" to replace Roosevelt with General Smedley D. Butler; and initiated red-baiting propaganda that anticipated the House Un-American Activities Committee's worst excesses.
>
> . . . But a much more dangerous set of activities developed during the late years of the decade and continued throughout the war. These included: sharing patents; the secret shipment of oil and aircraft production data, photographs, and blueprints of military and naval bases, and enough material on weapons to give the Germans a "clear picture of American armaments" as well as of Alaskan and Northwest defense systems; sending oil to Spain and Vichy France that was reshipped to the Nazis; refueling German tankers and U-boats; supplying tetraethyl lead (an essential for aviation gasoline) to Germany and Japan; manufacturing in subsidiary companies abroad an array of communications and electronic equipment that aided the German development of artillery fuses, rocket bombs, and radio technology; maintaining crucial radio links to enemy nations in Latin America for intelligence transmissions . . . cooperating closely in financial matters through the Chase Bank in Paris and The Bank for International Settlements in Basel, Switzerland.

All this and more took place in a business-as-usual atmosphere that sought to conserve and strengthen the corporations' own worldwide marketing preeminence and postwar position in the defeated nations. It reflected not only the prewar economic arrangement, but the continued intimacy among elites now temporarily estranged by the variers of international politics but still seeing eye-to-eye on matters of corporate profit and survival.[22,23]

Hervet further revealed that before the war ended, Gehlen Org–Rockefeller banking intermediate Joseph Larkin, was "encouraged" to deposit General Franco's money as well as transfer the Third Reich's bank account to the Chase Bank in Paris. This was done even though "the Reichsbank was under the personal control of Hilter."[24]

In addition, Hervet's long list of SMOM members was especially disturbing:

> After the appointment of Knight of Malta William Casey as head of the Central Intelligence Agency, and another Knight, James Buckley, as head of the U.S. propaganda against Eastern Europe at Radio Free Europe/Radio Liberty, several historians noted with interest President Reagan's call during the summer of 1982 for a "crusade" against the "Evil Empire" in Eastern Europe.
>
> In addition to Casey, and James Buckley, its current members, or Knights, after the feudal fashion, include Lee Iacocca, John McCone, William Buckley, Alexander Haig, Alexandre de Marenches (the chief of French Intelligence under Giscard d'Estaing, himself a Knight of SMOM), Otto von Hapsburg, and various leaders of the fascist P-2 Maxonic lodge in Italy.[24]

Others included:

• Paul-Louis Weiller: Grand Cross of Merit SMOM, a close friend of Richard Nixon, member of the board of directors of Renault and several other French industrial corporations, former administrateur of Air France, whose son married the cousin of Spanish King Juan-Carlos.

• Eric von Kuehnelt-Leddihn: Munich correspondent of William Buckley's *National Review*.

• Admiral James D. Watkins: Chief of naval operations during the Reagan administration.

• Thomas Bolan: law partner of Roy Cohn. Bolan is also counsel to the Human Life Foundation of which former CIA officer and Managing Editor of *National Review*, Priscilla Buckley (William's sister) is a Director.

• Jeremiah Denton: Long-time U.S. Senator from Alabama; former rear admiral, captured by the Vietnamese while murdering people. POW 1965–1973, consultant to Pat Robertson of Christian Broadcasting Network, 1978–1980.

• Pete Domenici: Long-time U.S. Senator from New Mexico.

• William A. Schreyer: Long-time president and chairman of Merrill Lynch.

• Bernard Dorin: French attache to Ottawa 1957–1959, Ambassador to Haiti 1972-1974, and Ambassador to South Africa from 1978 until at least 1981.

• Prescott Bush, Jr.: Brother of George Bush past president and CIA director.

• Clare Boothe Luce: Board of directors of the *Washington Times* and the Nicaraguan Freedom Fund (NFF), one of many front groups for Rev. Sun Myung Moon's Unification Church which channeled $350,000 to the AMERICARES foundation in Connecticut.

• J. Peter Grace, chairman of Radio Free Europe Radio Liberty Fund— a CIA front infested with Nazi collaborators; chairman of the American Institute for Free Labor Development (AIFLD), another CIA-funded organization; and President of W. R. Grace, a major American chemical company, who along with Dow Chemical company, employed convicted Nazi war criminal Otto Ambros. The State Department acknowledged Grace's help in bringing Nazi war criminals to the U.S. through Project Paperclip.

• Myron C. Taylor: President Truman's envoy to the Vatican.

• James Jesus Angleton: former chief of counterintelligence for the CIA; liaison to the Warren Commission following the Kennedy assassination.

• John Farrell: Past president of U.S. Steel.[24]

Rockefeller, Nazis and Eugenics

While perusing the internet, I came upon a most relevant article concerning The Rockefeller Foundation's support for "eugenics"—the movement aimed at killing or sterilizing people whose heredity, according to author Anton Chaitkin, "made them a public burden."[25]

The Rockefeller Foundation, Chaitkin chronicled, became the prime promoter of depopulation activities by the United Nations. Moreover, evidence showed "the foundation and its corporate, medical, and political associates organized the racial mass murder program of Nazi Germany."

Oil monopolist John D. Rockefeller, Chaitkin recalled, created the Rockefeller Foundation in 1909, and by 1929 had invested "$300 million worth of the family's controlling interest in the Standard Oil Company of New Jersey," now called Exxon, into the Foundation's account.

According to Chaitkin, this money created the field of "Psychiatric Genetics," and funded the Kaiser Wilhelm Institute for Psychiatry and the Kaiser Wilhelm Institute for Anthropology, Eugenics and Human Heredity. The Rockefellers' chief executive in charge of these institutions "was the fascist Swiss psychiatrist Ernst Rudin, assisted by his proteges Otmar Verschuer and Franz J. Kallmann."[25]

In 1932, Chaitkin recounted, the British-led eugenics movement designated the Rockefellers' Dr. Rudin as the president of the worldwide Eugenics Federation.

Only a few months later Hitler rose to power and "the Rockefeller-Rudin apparatus became a section of the Nazi state." Rudin then headed the "Racial Hygiene Society."[25]

Rudin and his staff, "as part of the Task Force of Heredity Experts chaired by SS chief Heinrich Himmler, drew up the sterilization law." In the United States, this law was described as a "model law," and was adopted in July 1933 as published in the September 1933 *Eugenical News* (USA) with Hitler's signature attached.

Rudin's protege Verschuer and his assistant, Auschwitz medical chief, Josef Mengele, jointly authored reports for special courts to reinforce Rudin's "racial purity law against cohabitation of Aryans and non-Aryans." They also produced films to help sell their racial cleansing ideas.

"Under the Nazis," Chaitkin noted, "the German chemical company I.G. Farben and Rockefeller's Standard Oil of New Jersey were effectively a single firm, merged in hundreds of cartel arrangements. I.G. Farben was led, up until 1937, by the Warburg family, Rockefeller's partner in banking and in the design of Nazi German eugenics."

During the war, I.G. Farben built a huge factory at Auschwitz to capitalize on Standard Oil/I.G. Farben patents to make gasoline from coal with the help of concentration camp slave labor. The SS was then assigned to select and guard the inmates deemed fit for I.G. Farben's workforce. Those judged unfit were killed.

Moreover, Chaitkin reported additional Rockefeller-linked Nazi atrocities:

In 1936, Rockefeller's Dr. Franz Kallmann interrupted his study of hereditary degeneracy and emigrated to America because he was half-Jewish. Kallmann went to New York and established the Medical Genetics Department of the New York State Psychiatric Institute. The Scottish Rite of Freemasonry published Kallman's study of over 1,000 cases of schizophrenia, which tried to prove its hereditary basis. In the book, Kallmann thanked his longtime boss and mentor Rudin.

Kallmann's book, published in 1938 in the USA and Nazi Germany, was used by the T4 unit as a rationalization to begin in 1939 the murder of mental patients and various "defective" people, perhaps most of them children. Gas and lethal injections were used to kill 250,000 under this program, in which the staffs for a broader murder program were desensitized and trained.[25]

Chaitkin detailed additional links between Rockefeller interests and the horrific medical experiments conducted by Josef Mengele at Auschwitz.

In 1943, Josef Mengele's superior, the director of Rockefeller's Kaiser Wilhelm Institute for Anthropology, Eugenics and Human Heredity in Berlin, Otmar Verschuer, secured funds for genetic experiments from the German Research Council. In a progress report Verschuer wrote for the Council he stated, "My co-researcher in this research is my assistant, the anthropologist and physician, Mengele. . . . With the permission of the Reichsfuehrer SS Himmler, anthropological research is being undertaken on the various racial groups in the concentration camps and blood samples will be sent to my laboratory for investigation."

Mengele and Verschuer were especially interested in studying twins during their "special protein" investigations that required daily blood drawings. Needles were stabbed into people's eyes for eye color experiments. Others were injected with foreign blood and infectious agents. Limbs and organs were commonly removed, occasionally without anesthetics. Women were sterilized, men were castrated, and sexes were surgically altered. Thousands were butchered and their heads, eyeballs, limbs, and organs were delivered to Mengele, Verschuer, and the Rockefeller contingent at the Kaiser Wilhelm Institute.

Later, in 1946, Verschuer, according to Chaitkin, requested assistance from the Bureau of Human Heredity in London to keep his "scientific research" going. A year later, the Bureau moved to Copenhagen, and its new Danish facility was built with Rockefeller money. It was here that the first International Congress in Human Genetics convened. A decade later Verschuer became a member of the American Eugenics Society—an organizational clone of Rockefeller's Population Council.

According to Chaitkin, Dr. Kallmann directed the American Eugenics Society from 1954 to 1965. He helped rescue Verschuer by testifying at his denazification hearings. And it was Kallmann who created the American Society of Human Genetics, organizers of the "Human Genome Project," currently a $3 billion effort to map the genetics of humanity along with each race's special disease susceptibilities.

During the 1950s, "the Rockefellers reorganized the U.S. eugenics movement in their own family offices, with spinoff population-control and abortion groups," and the Eugenics Society's address changed to the Society for the Study of Social Biology, its current name. Moreover, "with support from the Rockefellers, the Eugenics Society (England) set up a sub-committee called the International Planned Parenthood Federation, which for 12 years had no other address than the Eugenics Society."[25]

In conclusion, Chaitkin observed, "the Rockefeller Foundation had long financed the eugenics movement in England," and is "the private international apparatus which has set the world up for a global holocaust under the UN flag."

Chapter 19
The CIA in Africa

AMONG the COINTELPRO strategies proposed during the Nixon era and carried out by the CIA to help resolve the "Negro Question"—the challenge posed by black militants that Kissinger and Hoover feared was African based and communist inspired—was the encouragement of "cultural nationalism" and "black capitalism."[1-7]

The CIA during the Nixon, Ford, Carter, and Reagan administrations played "with the fires of a revolutionary black consciousness" to expand America's political and economic power in Africa.[6] Under Kissinger's direction, the CIA organized the State Department, the U.S. Information Agency, the Ford and Rockefeller Foundations, and other organizations to combat black militarism. According to CIA observers, the American intelligence community sought to influence the policies of newly independent African states "by creating and subsidizing an American elite of Afro-oriented black leaders whose positions in the civil rights movement were invaluable," though often unconscious, cover for the CIA's principle aim—"to emasculate black radicalism in Africa, and eventually at home."[8]

Meanwhile, the Nixon administration quietly expanded contacts with South Africa's white governments. This resulted in what Robert Smith, Deputy Assistant Secretary of State for African Affairs, called "a number of concrete developments, ranging from major new economic undertakings, such as . . . [the] Azores agreement with Portugal [located off the Northwestern coast of Africa] to the authorization of previously forbidden sales of jet aircraft to Portugal and South Africa."[9]

This new, more "right-wing U.S. policy" had been established by Henry Kissinger in his "secret policy memorandum of 1969." The effort resulted in a CIA–South African armed forces collaborated attack on Angola in the early 1970s.[9] The organizational chain of command for the Angola operation is seen in fig. 19.1.

The censored and "bewildering" memorandum from the National Security Council meeting between Nixon, Kissinger, and their staff was finally deciphered in 1983 by researchers at the Center for National Security Studies in their report, *The Consequences of "Pre-publication Review": A Case Study of CIA Censorship of the CIA and the Cult of Intelligence.*[10]

Fig. 19.1. Organizational Chain of Command of the CIA's Covert Military Operation in Zaire/Angola

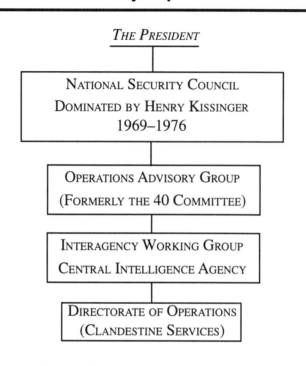

THE PRESIDENT

NATIONAL SECURITY COUNCIL
DOMINATED BY HENRY KISSINGER
1969–1976

OPERATIONS ADVISORY GROUP
(FORMERLY THE 40 COMMITTEE)

INTERAGENCY WORKING GROUP
CENTRAL INTELLIGENCE AGENCY

DIRECTORATE OF OPERATIONS
(CLANDESTINE SERVICES)

AFRICA DIVISION

HORN & CENTRAL
BRANCH

ANGOLA TASK FORCE

KINSHASA STATION:
("A temporary office
responsible from
headquarters for planning,
supervision and operation of
the Angola paramilitary
operation, August
1975–June 1976.")

EAST ASIA DIVISION
(VIETNAM OPERATIONS)
EUROPEAN DIVISION
NEAR-EAST DIVISION
SOVIET BLOCK DIVISION
LATIN AMERICAN DIV.
DOMESTIC CONTACTS DIV.
FOREIGN RESOURCES DIV.
TECHNICAL SERVICES DIV.
SPECIAL OPERATIONS GRP.
DIVISION "D"
COVERT ACTION STAFF
COUNTERINTEL. STAFF
FOREIGN INTEL. STAFF

Adapted from John Stockwell's *In Search of Enemies*. New York: W.W. Norton & Company, Inc., 1978, p. 262. Mr. Stockwell was the Chief of the CIA's Angola Task Force during the late 1960s and early 1970s.

The center's report stated that most bewildering of all examples of intelligence censorship was a series of items concerning Africa. The National Security Council in December 1969, apparently censored certain passages including one that, once restored, read:

> The purpose of this session was to decide what American policy should be toward the governments of southern Africa.

> A few lines down, the censors cut in midsentence: "There was sharp disagreement within the government on how hard a line the United States should take with the . . ." Restored, it goes on: ". . . white-minority regimes of South Africa, Rhodesia, and the Portuguese colonies in Africa."

> Then two words were cut from this sentence: "Henry Kissinger talked about the kind of general posture the United States could maintain toward the _____ _____ and outlined the specific policy options open to the President." The missing words turn out to be: "white regimes."

> Finally, the censors cut a reference to the fact that Kissinger had sent a National Security Study Memorandum (NSSM 39) to departments interested in southern Africa. NSSM 39 was in fact published and widely discussed in 1974. It took the view that the various movements for majority rule in southern Africa were unlikely to succeed soon.[10]

All of this led the security studies investigators to conclude:

> To the extent that those censored passages on Africa point anywhere, it is toward a discussion of policy. The Kissinger-Nixon policy was founded on the belief that the Portuguese would hold on to their African colonies indefinitely. Within a few years that premise was shattered, and the whole policy had to be reappraised.[10]

As a result of their findings, the researchers asked, "Is there any serious argument of security that the American public should not have been allowed, five years afterward, to reflect on the wisdom of the policy and the way it was made? What has it got to do with CIA 'secrets'?"[10]

One answer, recalling Gallo's speculation that "Portuguese sailors" had carried the AIDS virus from Africa to Asia, might be that the secrecy surrounding African affairs helped conceal Project MKNAOMI and possibly Kissinger's genocidal directives. Gallo's "Portuguese sailers" then, could plausibly have been undercover agents for the CIA.

Kissinger's Appeal

By the end of Ford's presidency, in response to increasing congressional pressure, Kissinger finally revealed some of his secret intelligence community undertakings. He appealed to a Senate Committee on Government Operations for continued support for the CIA. To accomplish this, he pleaded for trust and "sounder" relations between the executive and legislative branches of government. Kissinger said:

> The present relationship has reached a point where the ability of the United States to conduct a coherent foreign policy is being eroded. This is certainly true in the intelligence field. One has only to look at the recent leakage—indeed, official publication—of highly classified material and the levying of unsubstantiated charges and personal attacks against the executive to see the point the relationship has reached and the harm we are doing to ourselves.

> Fundamental changes are taking place in the world at an unprecedented rate. New centers of power are emerging, altering relationships among older power centers. Growing economic interdependence makes each of us vulnerable to financial and industrial troubles in countries formerly quite remote from us. . . .

> I am aware of the benefits of a certain amount of dynamic tension between the branches of our government. Indeed, the Founding Fathers designed this into the Constitution with the principle of the separation of powers. But there is an adverse impact on the public mind in this country and on our national image abroad when this beneficial tension deteriorates into confrontation. We have recently seen this happen. This is why I hope this committee and the Congress as a whole, with the help and suggestions from the executive, can construct an oversight mechanism for U.S. intelligence that can bring an end to the strife, distrust, and confusion that have accompanied the investigations of the past year.[11]

Kissinger was referring to the Church committee's investigations into the CIA's stockpiling of biological weapons, leaks about covert intelligence operations in Zaire and Angola, as well as the continued fallout over the agency's established role in the Watergate break-ins. He continued:

> I look to the development of means by which Congress can participate more fully in the guidance and review of the intelligence activities of this government and by which the executive can direct and conduct those activities with the confidence of being in step with Congress in this vital area of our foreign affairs.[11]

Superficially, Congress was being asked to rationalize CIA activities in Angola in terms of the country's strategic location adjacent the shipping lanes of the South Atlantic. Giant tankers brought oil from the Middle East around the horn of Africa to the United States.

Moreover, Kissinger argued:

Our foreign policy must cope with complex problems of nuclear and conventional arms races [As Nixon noted, Africa held "one fourth of the World's known uranium ore reserves."[12]]; traditional and ideological disputes which can trigger wider wars and sweeping economic dislocations; emerging new nations which can become the arena for great-power contests; environmental pollution, food shortages, and energy maldistribution which affect the lives of hundreds of millions; and financial shifts which can threaten the *global economic order*. In the face of these great challenges *our goals are to foster the growth of a rationally ordered world* in which states of diverse views and objectives can cooperate for the common benefit. We seek a world based on justice and the promotion of human dignity.[11] [Emphasis added]

Yet, despite this rationale, John Stockwell, the former chief of the CIA's Angola Task Force and the author of *In Search of Enemies: A CIA Story*, argued that Angola, the focus of Kissinger's covert military operation, had little importance to America's national security.[4] Angola, he wrote, was merely Kissinger's folly in seeking an opportunity to challenge the Soviets. Though Stockwell failed to acknowledge the lucrative defense contracts Kissinger was generating for his benefactors, he noted that the foreign affairs secretary had conspicuously "overruled his advisors and refused to seek diplomatic solutions" in the region. "The question was, would the American people, so recently traumatized by Vietnam," have tolerated "even a modest involvement in another remote, confusing, Third World civil war?"[4]

Covert Operations in Africa

"Covert action" was the game plan ordered by Kissinger for Angola, and carried out by the CIA in other African nations as well. All of this, occurred at the time the Vietnam War was winding down and Nixon's "war on cancer" was heating up.[1-4]

Sub-Saharan Africa, in particular, became the target of numerous clandestine activities designed to influence black-ruled "governments, events, organizations or persons in support of U.S. foreign policy conducted in such a way that the involvement of the U.S. Government" was not apparent.[1-5]

Among the organizations used to conceal intelligence operations and position agents in various parts of Africa were PUSH (People to Save Humanity), AFRICARE, CARE, the Peace Corps, The Rockefeller and Ford Foundations, the WHO, the World Bank, the CDC, and USAID. In addition, NASA was engaged in Central West Africa, allegedly for famine relief, and The National Academy of Sciences was enrolled "to provide scientific advisory services covering a spectrum of disciplines."[13]

Philip Agee, co-author of *Dirty Work-2: The CIA in Africa*,[6] and an ex-operative who served in Africa until 1969, explained that, "Secret services—the CIA and those of the other pro-Western powers"—provided money, equipment, instructions, and information to "indigenous agents" so as to enable them to take action wherein they hoped the hand of the secret service would not show. I learned from Agee that the official designation of covert action had changed to "special activities" or "special actions." An example familiar to me was the Army's biological weapons handling division termed "special operations."

Agee wrote that these secret military operations in Africa, particularly in Zaire and Angola, continued throughout the 1970s and beyond:

> Covert action has often been described as governmental intervention in the wide gray area between polite correct diplomacy and outright military action. . .
>
> In the mid-1970s, public revulsion in America to the CIA's political interventions, assassination operations,[7] and other dirty work produced hope in some that covert action, at least in peacetime, would be reduced or even renounced altogether. And the early concern over human rights in the Carter administration added to this hope because gross violations of human rights normally result from the CIA's clandestine interventions.
>
> It took just one year for these hopes to be dashed, confirming the belief of many that such hopes were not realistic from the start. In January 1978, one year after taking office, President Carter promulgated an executive order that tightened control over the CIA's covert action operations but at the same time provided exceptions that would allow the President to order the CIA to do everything it had done in the past except political assassinations of heads of state. [Unfortunately, this wasn't the case for lesser heads, that continued to roll.][6]

In fact, just seven months following Carter's executive order, *Africa Diary* carried a report broadcast over Uganda Radio entitled, "CIA Accused of Plot to Assassinate Amin." The article quoted a military spokesman as saying: "It's a shame that a country of the stature of the U.S. should allow its agencies to indulge in such evil schemes and then turn around and pose as a promolgater of peace and champion of human rights." The report referred to a statement broadcast by NBC radio "in which the former CIA director William Colby was quoted as saying the intelligence agency had tried since 1972 to kill the Uganda leader. Mr Colby also said, according to Uganda radio, that it was up to Ugandans to assassinate President Amin and that a million dollars had been placed at the disposal of Ugandans to carry out the mission by any means including poison."[14]

Indeed, the covert actions practiced by the CIA, Agee explained, continually violated "principles of international law, the United Nations charter, and local laws," as well as contradicted the "flowing rhetoric about nonintervention in the internal affairs of other nations."

Agee concluded that "for Africans and others on the receiving end" of America's covert action, any debate "may well seem irrelevant, for the fact is that these operations have never stopped."[6]

"Human Investments" in Sub-Saharan Africa

A key player in administering CIA operations in Sub-Saharan Africa was Frank C. Carlucci III. Carlucci, while advancing through the ranks of military intelligence, became the point man for CIA-infested "health care" programs in various parts of Africa.[9]

Before becoming deputy director of the CIA in 1978, deputy secretary of defense in 1980, and national security adviser during the Iran-contra scandal, Carlucci served as chief "political officer," in the African Congo's American Embassy during the early 1960s. There, according to observers, he "became the brains of the Embassy," and "wrote from Leopoldville a daily political analysis, a true calendar of 'destabilization' . . . for the management of the Department of State." Later, under Nixon, he was promoted to the position of deputy of the Department of Health, Education and Welfare. From here, Carlucci administered covert CIA operations through the DHEW front.[15]

In one instance, on February 15, 1975, following the protested arrival of American health officials to Portugal, Carlucci defended, "There are rumors [of covert operations]. . . . One of them concerns the visit of a group of doctors. The first time I heard of them was in the Portuguese press. Now they are tourists. Does Portugal want tourists to come or not? This has nothing to do with American aid to this country in the domain of health."[16]

Nonetheless, three weeks later, Portuguese specialists protested:

> "Considering the offer of the U.S. to build hospitals in Lisbon, Porto, and a city of the south . . . and the offer to send technicians to help in the domain of health and others; considering that these offers originate from the Agency for International Development, an organization well known as an instrument of the CIA; considering that those loans and grants . . . serve as cover for the enemy of the Portuguese people . . . we call the attention of the government to

the real dangers that this type of support hides, and whose consequences have been revealed in Chile, Santo Domingo, Bolivia, Guatemala and in so many other martyred countries."[16]

On February 28, 1975 while the rumors spread that the CIA had decided to make "human investments" in Portugal, Frank Carlucci, to prove America's "good faith" and desire to "respect the wishes of the Portuguese people," signed two agreements: one for a credit of $1 million for "technicians to come study the improvement of communications and the health services," and the other a grant of $750,000 to Portugal through AID.[16] Other examples of various USAID, WHO, and NATO supported vaccination, population control, and "material and child health" programs, along with selected program descriptions, appear in fig. 10.4. These documents were published in 1975 by the Department of State in their *Report on the Health, Population and Nutrition Activities of the Agency for International Development for Fiscal Years 1973 and 1974*. These programs afforded CIA agents access to virtually every country in Africa.[18]

The Zaire–Angola War Continues

By 1974, Angola's neighboring state, Zaire, had been effectively persuaded to initiate "defense operations" against its enemies in Angola. Apparently, both Zaire and Zambia (which shares Zaire's southern and Angola's eastern borders) needed little coaxing. They both, allegedly, "feared the prospect of a Soviet-backed government on their flanks," and communist control over the commercially important Benguela railroad. Zaire's President Mobutu[17] "was especially afraid of the Soviets." During the late 1960s and early 1970s, he had courted "the Chinese at the expense of both the Soviets and the Americans."[4]

By the spring of 1975, Stockwell wrote, "Zaire's internal problems had mounted until Mobutu's regime was threatened" by civil upheaval. Following fifteen years of independence, Zairian agriculture had not returned to prerevolution levels despite the doubling of the population. By then, more than $700 million had been invested in Zaire by Western institutions. The economy was stagnant, "in part owing to the conspicuous arrogance and corruption of the governing elite" who had been substantially supported by NATO allies—particularly the United States and West Germany.[2,4]

In 1975, world copper prices plummeted undermining Zaire's economy. Concurrently, fighting in Angola closed the Benguela railroad. This forced Zaire to export its goods through Zambia, Rhodesia, and South

Africa. At this important point in Zaire's short history, Mobutu turned on Western imperialists:

> Desperately seeking a scapegoat, Mobutu had turned on the United States, accusing its Kinshasa embassy of fomenting a coup against him. In June 1975, he expelled the American ambassador and arrested most of the CIA's Zairian agents, placing some of them under death sentences.⁴

Following years of financial support, Mobutu turned on his American financiers, and claimed the CIA was involved in a plot to assassinate him.[19]

The precedent for presidential assassinations had been set not long before. In October 1975, Sidney Gottlieb, the same man who had frantically shredded Project MKNAOMI documents on the eve of the Church committee hearings into the CIA's illegal storage and intended use of biological weapons, told Congressional investigators "that the CIA had intended in 1961 to poison the Congolese premier, Patrice Lumumba—Mobutu's arch rival.[21] The CIA assassination attempt was preempted, however, by others who Gottlieb alleged got to Lumumba first.

Gottlieb was a very knowledgeable witness. In 1961 he headed the CIA's chemical division, "which had made up the unused lethal dose and dispatched it to the Congo (now Zaire) for Lumumba's murder."[20,22]

Kissinger naturally denied Mobutu's allegation of a CIA coup when *CBS Evening News* anchorman Walter Cronkite asked for his reaction:

CHRONKITE: A story that has just crossed our desk from Zaire, that the U. S. Ambassador has been declared persona non grata, at least has been asked to leave the country, presumably over the allegation that Americans were involved in a plot against President Mobutu's life. Have you any reaction to that?

KISSINGER: Well, these allegations are totally unfounded, and we regret that this decision has been taken. We do consider Zaire one of the key countries of Africa with which we would like to maintain cordial relations. And the action was based on totally wrong information that fell into the hands of the Government of Zaire, probably as a result of forgery.

CHRONKITE: As a result of what, sir?

KISSINGER: It must have been forgery, because we had absolutely no connection with any plot, nor did we know there was a plot.[20]

Kissinger then directed the interview to a safer topic.

Within five months of this broadcast, however, the National Security Council director once again needed to defend his Central African policies. This time, standing before Congress, Kissinger pleaded for additional support for military operations in Zaire.[23] With or without Mobutu's support, he obviously intended to hold this Central African turf.

Kissinger explained:

"There are two significant programs proposed for Africa. Stability in the Horn of Africa has wider geopolitical meaning. To help maintain that stability we propose $12.6 million in grant aid and $10 million in credits for Ethiopia, a strategically located nation"[23] [a country in the northeastern part of the continent far removed from the Horn].

Kissinger, then President Ford's foreign policy adviser, continued:

"Zaire would receive $19 million in credits to help modernize its forces and meet its legitimate defense needs in view of increased threats to its security, particularly that posed by the instability in Angola. Our aid would help meet a defense force need recommended by a U.S. military team after careful observation and consultation with the Zaire military."[23]

Additionally, Kissinger revealed before the House Committee on International Relations that America's share of NATO's African defense budget was $68.5 million. Yet, even this was far less than the $100 million the CIA received to wage covert war in Angola.[23,24]

History of Central African Aggression

Aside from the Vietnam War, the Angola conflict became America's largest military operation since WWII. In *CIA: 40 Inglorious Years*, author P. K. Goswami summarized the events leading up to the aggression:

The Angolan people won their independence after long years of intense struggle led by MPLA, the Popular Movement for the Liberation of Angola. On November 11, 1975 the People's Republic of Angola was proclaimed, and most nations recognized its independence. However, the victory of the progressive forces dedicated to the struggle against colonialist holdovers, South African racism, and imperialist forays, was seen as a challenge in Pretoria and especially in Washington.

The US administration immediately took an openly hostile stand and tried to bring down the new popular government by force, coordinating its efforts with South Africa. The CIA received some 100 million dollars to assist National Union for the Complete Independence of Angola (UNITA) and National Front for the Liberation of Angola (FNLA), counter-revolutionary groups led by CIA puppets Jonas Savimbi and Holden Roberto. US Air Force transport planes airlifted weapons and ammunition to the UNITA and FNLA base in Zaire. US military advisers and instructors appeared in the counter-revolutionary units. American mercenaries took part in military action against Angolans.[24]

According to John Prados, the author of *The Presidents' Secret Wars: CIA and Pentagon Covert Operations From World War II Through*

IRANSCAM, Angola was viewed as a cold war necessity. Nathaniel Davis, the newly appointed assistant secretary of state for African Affairs was assigned by Kissinger to study the region's political and military challenges. "Davis, according to his own account, had already advised Kissinger against covert support to Savimbi, who was soliciting arms everywhere," explained Prados. "UNITA had been receiving some from the Chinese since 1974, and had had ties to Mao Tsetung for a decade before that." Davis warned Kissinger that the United States would have to confront "probable disclosure," and argued that "at most we would be in a position to commit limited resources, and buy marginal influence."[25]

Consequently, the interagency group chaired by Davis recommended nonintervention; instead, they urged diplomatic efforts in the hope that the three factions might reach a political settlement.[25] This reflected a "basic understanding that Angola was an African, and not a cold war problem." Military intervention, Prados wrote, promised to strain already tense relations across Africa, particularly in so far as Portugal was concerned. Intervention offered only limited benefits and "potentially contributed to increased involvement by the Soviet Union and other foreign powers."[25]

But Kissinger intervened to gag the Davis group's counsel. Prados documented:

> According to the Pike committee, which studied the Angola covert operation in some detail, the Davis group's recommendation was removed from their report "at the direction of National Security Council aides" and presented to the NSC as merely one policy option, the others being to do nothing or to make a substantial intervention. The June 13 report of the interagency group was thus used to frame a stark choice for President Ford, who [Kissinger persuaded to select] . . . the intervention option.

> Action then returned to the 40 Committee, dominated in 1975, as before by Henry Kissinger. Meeting on July 14, the Special Group directed the CIA to propose a covert action program within forty eight hours. OPERATION FEATURE was the result. Although the evidence is not yet clear, it appears that the top leadership at Langley may have opposed this intervention—the CIA came back to warn of the risk of exposure as well as to estimate a $100 million price tag for the effort, an amount that was not available in the DCI's contingency fund. Nevertheless, the 40 Committee gave the go-ahead and on July 17 President Ford approved an expenditure of $14 million. The CIA, which had advised against Track II in Chile and the Kurdish operation, was again given marching orders, for which it was lukewarm. That a plan was proposed at all was used by Kissinger, in 1976 Senate testimony, to argue that "the CIA recommended the operation and supported it."[25]

In the end, the intervention played out as its opponents had predicted. As in Vietnam, despite massive allied investments, the Western intruders faired poorly. The situation required reinforcements, and South Africa's regular troops were lured in.

Back home, the CIA's action in Angola resulted in waves of protest. With Southeast Asian wounds still stinging, the American public demanded an end to Kissinger's secret war in Central Africa. By 1976, public outrage forced the U.S. Congress to enact the Clark Amendment designed to ban covert and open aid to UNITA and FNLA.

The Clark Amendment, however, did little to stop the regional aggression. Support for the counterrevolutionaries continued as Kissinger effectively shamed Congress for passing the restrictive amendment. He then politically overpowered his adversaries and continued to direct destabilization efforts in Angola with support from racist South Africa.

Later, in a concerted effort to vindicate himself and rebuild political support for his Angolan initiatives, in February 1976, Kissinger unveiled the CIA operation in Zaire.[26] He recalled the region's aggressive history and excused his decision to deploy covert forces in the area this way:

> The outcome in Angola will have repercussions throughout Africa. The confidence of countries neighboring Angola—Zambia and Zaire—as well as other African countries, in the will and power of the United States will be severely shaken if they see that the Soviet Union and Cuba are unopposed in their attempt to impose a regime of their choice on Angola. . . .

> The means we have chosen have been limited and explained to Congress.

> Our immediate objective was to provide leverage for diplomatic efforts to bring about a just and peaceful solution. They were not conceived unilaterally by the United States; they represented support to friends who requested our financial assistance.

> We chose covert means because we wanted to keep our visibility to a minimum; we wanted the greatest possible opportunity for an African solution. We felt that overt assistance would elaborate a formal doctrine justifying great-power intervention. . . .

> *The Angola situation is of a type in which diplomacy without leverage is impotent, yet direct military confrontation would involve unnecessary risks. Thus it is precisely one of those gray areas where covert methods are crucial if we are to have any prospect of influencing certain events of potentially global importance.*

> We chose a covert form of response with the greatest reluctance. But in doing so, we were determined to adhere to the highest standard of executive-legislative consultation. Eight congressional committees were briefed on 24 sepa-

rate occasions. We sought in these briefings to determine the wishes of Congress. While we do not claim that every member approved our actions, we had no indication of basic opposition.

Between July and December 1975 we discussed the Angolan situation on numerous occasions with members of the foreign relations committees and the appropriations committees of both Houses and the committees of both Houses that have CIA oversight responsibilities. The two committees investigating CIA activities—*the Church Committee* and the Pike Committee—were also briefed. Altogether more than two dozen Senators, about 150 Congressmen, and over 100 staff members of both Houses were informed. . . . [emphasis added]

So the Church Committee, I realized, was briefed that the Zaire–Angola arena was a "gray area" targeted for covert military operations, and thus, a likely proving ground for the CIA's preferred "gray area" arsenal. In this case—biological weapons. Kissinger had effectively incriminated himself and Congress as well. The Church Committee's investigation of the illegal storage and, according to Colby, anticipated use of biological weapons, concealed Project: MKNAOMI's apparent application in Central Africa.

Subsequent Administrations' Policy in Zaire

Stephen Weissman, a U.S.–African relations critic and political science scholar, gathered additional details about the Zaire–Angola conflict. Weissman, who in 1978, was an associate professor at the University of Texas in Dallas, and who later joined the staff of the U.S. House Foreign Affairs Committee, Africa Subcommittee, noted how this region represented important NATO interests, though he admitted the actual Russian threat in the region was minimal.[26]

Weissman chronicled events in the region beginning in March 1977, when an estimated 800 to 1,500 armed, "leftish Katangan exiles returned to their home province from neighboring Angola and nearly toppled the Mobutu Government."

As the poorly paid and politically demoralized 60,000 man Zairian army proved to be ineffective, the regime was forced to call upon 1,200 Moroccan troops, 80 French military advisers, about 50 Egyptian pilots and mechanics, French transport planes, and Belgian and Chinese arms. Although the new U.S. [Carter] Administration was reluctant to lead the counterrevolution (no arms or advisers were dispatched), it did provide tangible aid: $15 million of combat support equipment. . . . And President Carter's request for $32.5 million in military aid for Zaire in Fiscal Year 1978—half the total for Africa—indicated a continuing commitment to the Mobutu regime.[27]

Furthermore, there is evidence of CIA covert action planning in the days before Mobutu was able to clinch his French and Moroccan personnel support. In an open letter of resignation to the CIA Director, Angola Task Force Chief Stockwell charged:

> Yes, I know you are attempting to generate token support to help Zaire meet its crisis—that you are seeking out the same French mercenaries the CIA sent into Angola in early 1976. These are the men who took the CIA money and fled the first time they encountered heavy shelling.[27]

By June 1977, Mobutu's foreign supporters had contained the Kantangan threat as the exiles retreated to fight a guerrilla rather than conventional war. "Old problems of political fragmentation also prevented the Kantangans from gaining the active support of similarly disposed forces in other areas" of Zaire, Weissman acknowledged. Still the Mobutu regime's military humiliation and demonstrated political weakness suggested that its days were numbered. Most "academic experts and many diplomats expected a military or military-civilian coup" to unseat Mobutu in the near future. The new government was expected "to have, or take account of, anti-U.S. and anti-CIA sentiment" if the U.S. persevered in its close association with Mobutu.[26]

Nonetheless, Western and U.S. intervention on behalf of Mobutu intensified as did the political cleavages in Africa. While a few, small, conservative, and French-speaking, African governments encouraged Western intervention, many leading countries, not all of them "leftist," criticized such incursion. For example, the official newspaper of "moderate" Zambia stated:

> The almost obscene haste with which the west has rushed to pour arms into Zaire reinforces the argument of many Africans that behind every attempted or successful coup on this continent is the hand of a foreign power. . . . Although Cyrus Vance and others have not come out and said so bluntly, there is little doubt that they are hoping for a full-scale confrontation between Zaire and Angola. It gives them an opportunity to make amends for alleged betrayal of the anti-MPLA forces during the civil war. It is to be hoped that President Carter puts a halt to this political adventurism before he is saddled with his own Vietnam. If he and his administration hope to come out of such a confrontation with their image in Africa unscathed, they need to do some rethinking.[28]

Significant reservations were expressed by Nigeria, Tanzania, and Algeria. The Angolan war raised the possibility of future counteraction in Rhodesia and Southwest Africa as well.

The primary rationale for United States involvement, however, continued. Weissman explained:

> It was clear that behind such official slogans as 'friendship,' 'historic ties,' and 'territorial integrity,' lurked the fear of a 'pro-Soviet' regime in the geographic center of Africa. Yet there was no evidence that the anti-Mobutu Katangans were Soviet-influenced. Indeed the populist flavor of their propaganda was more reminiscent of Lumumbism than of even Angolan Marxism. Ironically, U.S. support of 'anti-Communist' Zaire probably contributed to the Katangan invasion itself. According to an informed American official, the U.S. did not examine very closely Angolan charges that Mobutu was permitting exile attacks on Northern Angola. Mobutu's assurances that he had 'cut back' support of the Angolan exiles were simply accepted. However the sequence of events suggests that Angola allowed the Katangans to return to Zaire in response to these incursions.[26]

The crisis in Zaire had, Weissman wrote, "dramatized the long term risks for U.S. interests of two decades of U.S.–CIA intervention" in the region:

> By contributing to inter-African polarization and Cold War tension, the U.S. was increasing the chances for a great power proxy war in Central and Southern Africa and diverting its attention from the new, multilateral issues of Third World interdependence that were becoming more and more urgent.[26]

The long term "instrumental goals" of U.S. anti-Communist efforts in Zaire and Angola were, Weissman continued, "political visibility, 'development,' and African acceptance." With this in mind, the political scholar questioned:

> . . . with increasing consciousness of America's economic, political and military interdependence with the Third World, they are also becoming terminal objectives. . . . Has U.S. involvement with its Zairian and Angolan friends generally improved American relations with Africa, or has it tended to complicate them?[26]

In 1979, the CIA secretly brought UNITA's Jonas Savimbi to Washington where he met with then former presidential adviser on national security, Henry Kissinger, and several high-level U.S. officials. This was evidence that Kissinger continued to play a vital role in developing African foreign policy long after he was officially retired from this responsibility.

During his election campaign, Ronald Reagan openly supported UNITA. He hailed Savimbi as a leader who "controls more than half of

Angola," then added, "I don't see why we shouldn't provide them with weapons."[25]

On the eve of Ronald Reagan's inauguration, William Casey, soon to become CIA Director, and Richard Allen, subsequently Presidential assistant on national security, met with UNITA representatives and assured them of U.S. support. After his inauguration, Ronald Reagan firmly demanded that Congress overrule the Clark Amendment.[25]

Then, in March 1981, Savimbi was again brought to Washington—this time on an official visit. That same month, Alexander Haig, then secretary of state, discussed the need to aid UNITA with NATO representatives in London. Not long after, in December 1981, Savimbi was received by the State Department officially as the "national liberation leader of Angola."[25]

Such were the methods employed by America's shadow government and its secret militia, the CIA, in initiating political ties, instilling Western loyalists, and establishing an economic New World Order based on "diplomatic leverage" that was wholly immoral and often lethal.

Now I knew, that besides desiring population control in this politically volatile region of the world, Kissinger had directed covert military operations there, and had apparently even discussed with CIA director William Colby (and possibly the Church committee as well) the likelihood of using illegally developed and stockpiled biological weapons in Zaire/Angola. This may have been the information they withheld for "national security" reasons. It thus occurred to me that the AIDS-like virus development option Kissinger ordered for Project: MKNAOMI would have been the ideal untraceable weapons for achieving his goal to "keep our visibility to a minimum" while "influencing certain events of potentially global importance" in this "gray area" of CIA operation.

Later, with Bill Colby's untimely and suspicious drowning in the Spring of 1996, allegedly the result of, like Hoover, a heart attack, it also occurred to me that Kissinger and his benefactors may have been secretly grateful to have a chief Project: MKNAOMI administrator, and potentially devastating congressional witness, forever silenced.

Chapter 20
OTRAG: Links to Nazis, NATO, NASA, the NCI, and AIDS

FOR years preceding the end of the cold war, the KGB gathered evidence, that Russian officials ultimately reported, suggesting an American origin of AIDS. Officials alleged that the AIDS virus had been a Pentagon invention—a germ unleashed for political purposes in Zaire.[1] Comics, as shown in fig. 20.1, even satirized the allegation.

In response, the CIA waged a counterintelligence campaign against all such foreign and domestic accounts of the origin of HIV. Fort Detrick public relations director Norman Covert wrote that the Soviets spread their "disinformation" in an effort to diffuse blame for "the death of nearly 80 persons near Sverdlosk in 1979 due to accidental exposures to a biological weapon."[2] That incident was "deflected for more than a decade by disinformation programs emanating from the KGB," he wrote. "Such disinformation programs included the charge that AIDS resulted from a 'cruel experiment at Fort Detrick, which went awry. . . .'" The U.S. Army spokesman further alleged "the AIDS charge was disavowed in 1987 by then Soviet President Mikhail Gorbachev, who apologized to President Ronald Reagan for the accusation."[2]

Among the government documents I discovered, while visiting the BPL in search of the Rockefeller Commission report, was a *Moscow World Service* radio broadcast alleging a Pentagon link to the development of AIDS. I realized that Covert was mistaken. Gorbachev had not laid the AIDS allegation to rest in 1987. In the Spring of 1988, a high-ranking Soviet press official, Boris Belitskiy, offered the latest Soviet position regarding Pentagon involvement in the creation of HIV:[1]

BELITSKIY: Several U.S. Administration officials, such as USIA [CIA] Director Charles Wick, have accused the Soviet Union of having invented this theory for propaganda purposes. But actually it is not Soviet scientists at all who first came up with this theory. It was first reported in Western journals by Western scientists, such as Dr. John Seale, a specialist on venereal diseases at two big London hospitals and one of the first scientists to point to the viral nature of AIDS.[1]

The host then asked if there had been any new evidence to support Seale's contention. The offical replied:

BELITSKIY: Just recently a Soviet journalist in Algeria, Aleksandr Zhukov, managed to interview a European physician at the Moustapha Hospital there, who made some relevant disclosures on the subject. In the early seventies, this physician and immunologist was working for the West German OTRAG (Orbital Transport and Missiles, Ltd.) Corporation in Zaire. His laboratory had been given the assignment to cultivate viruses ordinarily affecting only animals but constituting a potential danger to man. They were particularly interested in certain unknown viruses isolated from the African green monkey, and capable of such rapid replication that they could completely destabilize the immune system. These viruses, however, were quite harmless for human beings and the lab's assignment was to develop a mutant virus that would be a human killer.

Fig. 20.1. Soviet Cartoon Depicting an American Origin of the AIDS Virus

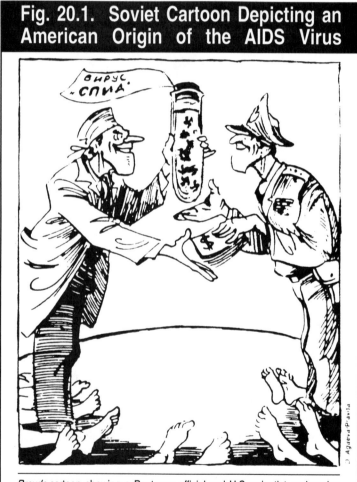

Pravda cartoon showing a Pentagon official and U.S. scientist exchanging money for a vial of "AIDS virus." U.S. diplomats protested vigorously about the slur. Courtesy of *Covert Action Information Bulletin* 1987 (Summer);28:37.

HOST: Did they succeed?

BELITSKIY: To a large extent, yes. But when they inoculated the inhabitants of several jungle villages with such a mutant virus on the pretext of giving shots against cholera, this did not produce the immediate results required of the lab. Now, it is well-known that people infected with the AIDS virus can live for several years without developing the disease but at the same time the result was summed up as proving the unsuitability of the virus as a biological warfare agent. The lab was ordered to wind up the project and turn the results over to certain U.S. researchers who had been following this work with keen interest, to such an extent that some of the researchers believed they were in reality working not for the West German OTRAG Corporation but for the Pentagon. In fact, two U.S. assistants had been with the lab throughout the work on this project. Several years after the lab had turned over its findings to the Americans, back came the news of the first AIDS cases in San Francisco. The researcher believes that the Pentagon had tested the mutant virus on convicts in California.[1]

"Interesting." I remarked to Jackie that evening during dinner when she inquired how my work was going. "OTRAG's alleged work in the early 1970s was essentially identical to the work Gallo and his colleagues published at that time."

"What incentive could Belitskiy have had to make up such a story?" Jackie asked.

"I can't imagine," I replied, "it seems to me he had more to lose than gain by the report." By then, I realized, the Russians were looking for American aid to support parastroika. "But I'd love to learn more about OTRAG," I added.

A week later my speaking schedule directed me to Bloomington, IL. Jackie, now beginning her last trimester, and Alena were traveling along in our motorhome heading to Florida by way of Illinois.

Arriving early, I had a couple of free days to search the Illinois State University library for more information about OTRAG. By good fortune, I quickly came across a couple of reports. One revealed "the complete text of a secret contract" between the government of Zaire and the little known West German OTRAG Corporation. Published in the fall of 1977 in *Race and Class*, the journal of the Institute on Race Relations and the Transnational Institute in London, the contract disclosed that 29,000 square miles of Southeast Zaire had been leased to OTRAG by Mobutu. The agreement gave the company "complete sovereignty and control over the area."[3]

The company was ostensibly in the business of developing "cheap satellite-launching missiles for private industry, but the application of its technology to military purposes—purposes forbidden by the West German government since World War II—was quickly apparent."[3]

I found several other articles that appeared in African and European newspapers suggesting links between OTRAG and the West German government, the CIA, and the South African government. Little, however, was confirmed. This led the Informationsdienst Südliches Afrika [German Information Service of South Africa] to conduct their own investigation. Soon thereafter, they published their shocking findings:[3]

> We have traced OTRAG and its supporters back to those Nazi scientists who worked on the V1 and V2 rockets during World War II, and who later continued their activity in the United States, France, and Argentina. For example, Dr. Kurt H. Debus, at present Chairman of the Board of OTRAG, once worked at the Peenemünde V2 program and later, until 1975, worked as director of the Cape Canaveral space program.
>
> Richard Gompertz, OTRAG's technical director and a U.S. citizen, once was a specialist on V2 engines and later presided over NASA's Chrysler space division.
>
> Lutz Thilo Kayser, OTRAG's founder and manager, when young was quite close to the Nazi rocket industry, often called "Dadieu's young man," a reference to Armin Dadieu, his mentor, who served as prominent SS officer and as Göring's special representative for a research program on storing uranium. While working for OTRAG, Kayser also acted as a contact for the West German government, a special advisor to the Minister of Research and Technology on matters concerning OTRAG. He was also on the ad hoc committee on the Apollo program transport systems.[3]
>
> *Financing by the German Federal Government*
>
> According to its own definition, OTRAG is a private company financed by private funds. Indeed, during a Lusaka press conference Chancellor Helmut Schmidt insisted upon this: "The government has no shares in OTRAG nor does it have any other finger in the pie." The real facts are rather different.
>
> OTRAG is chartered as a transcription company, which means that shareholdings are credited by the government . . . that is, OTRAG is subsidized by the government. . . .
>
> Kayser's business group was given many strange government orders. For example, in 1976 its technology research group received DM 764,000 for scientific investigations of coal gas. . . .
>
> *A Colonial Treaty*
>
> The contract between OTRAG and the government of Zaire, involving the "unlimited use" of nearly 30,000 square miles, made OTRAG sovereign over territories once inhabited by 760,000 people. OTRAG is authorized to conduct any excavation and construction it chooses, including air fields, energy

plants, communication systems, and manufacturing plants. All movement of people into and within the OTRAG territory is only with the permission of OTRAG. The state of Zaire is obliged to keep everyone else out and away. The same applies to the air space over the granted territory. OTRAG is absolved from any responsibility for and damage caused by the construction or transport of missiles. Its people enjoy complete immunity from the laws of Zaire in the granted territory. These exclusive rights are granted until the year 2000.[3]

War Preparations

The governments and the press in Angola, Tanzania, Zambia, and Mozambique have expressed worries about the development of offensive military weapons using OTRAG missiles in Zaire. The Soviet Union, the German Democratic Republic, Yugoslavia, and Cuba have all denounced the OTRAG project as a means by which West Germany may circumvent the restrictions against certain weapons laid down in the 1954 Brussels Treaty. The *London Evening Standard* quoted U.S. military officials as suspecting the West Germans and France of the secret development of missile forces on OTRAG territory to prohibit an invasion of South Africa. In March 1978 an article in *Penthouse* by Tad Szulc said, based on secret service sources, that OTRAG was an extension of West Germany's arms companies Dornier and Messerschmidt—developing and testing cruise missiles and middle-range rockets on OTRAG territory. France and the U.S., the article said, were also participating in the project. . . .[3]

Despite all this, the West German government continued to insist that OTRAG was a peaceful project. A question in Parliament by Representative Norbert Gansel "whether the Federal Government was able honestly to deny that OTRAG missiles are being used for military purposes" was given this false response: "According to our own investigations, the missiles, still in a state of development, are not fit for military purposes. However, in an interview with the magazine *Der Spiegel*, OTRAG chief Lutz Kayser admitted that "of course everything could be used militarily. . . ."[3]

The history of OTRAG underlines the close contact between the company and the Ministry of Defense in Bonn. Chairman Debus would not name the three high NASA officials who inspected and praised OTRAG's concept. . . . A CIA agent told a British journalist that the Boeing Company had provided OTRAG with Cruise missile technology. . . .[3]

In another article about OTRAG published in *New Scientist*, Farooq Hussain, a research student at the Department of War Studies, at King's College, London, reported that the "private West German company" had offered "cut-price satellite launches—from a private range in Zaire that is half the size of England—to any country or commercial organization able to afford it."[4]

Hussain heartily criticized the earlier report by former *New York Times* correspondent Tad Szulc published in *Penthouse*. Szulc alleged that West Germany [along with the United States] was "supplying small arms to Zaire, having secret projects to develop nuclear weapons, and of hiding the funding for the Zaire project."

Hussain, however, confirmed that OTRAG's initial research was "sponsored by the West German government" and "carried out at Deutsche Forschungs-und Versuchs-Anstalt für Luft und Raumfahrt, the Federal Rocket Research Institute at Lampholthausen, near Stuttgart. This project was led by Eugen Sanger and Wolf Pilz, two wartime scientists from the Nazi rocket facility at Prenemude. They were joined by a brilliant young engineer, Lutz Kayser."

> Following Sanger's death in 1970, his widow helped Kayser form a company which continued work on the low cost launcher at Lampholthausen under government contracts worth £7 million. But by 1974 the West German government [allegedly] decided to devote its rocket research efforts solely in the direction of a joint European launcher which was based on familiar missile technology. Kayser, determined to continue with his project, formed OTRAG, but he continued to make use of the facilities at Lampholthausen for rocket motor test burns. Kayser recruited the former director of the V-2 programme, Dr. Kurt Debus, who was also the director of Kennedy Space Center at Cape Canaveral, Florida until 1975.
>
> Under the terms of the UN Space Treaty an individual or private company cannot place satellites in orbit without the sponsorship of a government. This problem was resolved in part by the signing of an agreement between OTRAG and Zaire. . . .
>
> The OTRAG agreement with Zaire—which was never [as] secret as *Penthouse* claimed—has rightly caused uproar. The terms are reminiscent of the deal made by Cecil Rhodes with King Lobengula. The size of territory—100,000 sq. km—was [allegedly] determined for launch safety precautions and is in a thinly populated part of the Shaba province. . . .[4]

It suddenly struck me that Hussain's Department of War Studies affiliation might have biased his prose. First, it occurred to me that an area that included 760,000 African natives might be called something other than "thinly populated." Then, it seemed odd that the Shaba province, the center of covert CIA military operations in the region, might be determined the safest launch site. The area was as close to a war zone as one could get without being in the middle of it.

Hussain continued:

> . . . OTRAG has use of this area of Zaire rent free until the firm becomes profitable. After that the Zaire government receives 25 million Zaires annually—and retrospectively from 1976—paid into any bank designated by President Mobutu Sese Seko. But this is not inflation-proof, and Zaire's inflation is currently running at around 70 percent.
>
> OTRAG promises to launch a Zaire military reconnaissance satellite for free—although it doesn't say when. Zaire does have the option of the first satellite launch, but it loses all the rent due up to that point, unless it pays for the launch in foreign exchange. This is made easier by providing Zaire launch facilities at a 20 per cent discount.
>
> Zaire cannot withdraw from its contract with OTRAG until the year 2000, but OTRAG can withdraw at any time.
>
> By 1981 OTRAG intends to begin operating at around 10 launches per year. . . .[4]

Hussain went on to deride OTRAG for having little hope of attracting customers. "The value of reconnaissance satellites for Third World countries is extremely doubtful," he claimed, "because the data received requires experienced technicians and large computer facilities to interpret."

NATO's Yellow Press?

Either Hussain wasn't keeping up with realities in his area of special studies, or he was moved to produce disinformation for NATO, I realized.

OTRAG's project seemed to fit the Western allies need exactly. During my research I had stumbled on a North Atlantic Assembly report by Christian Brumter, Head of Studies at the University of Paris. Brumter reviewed NATO's space and upper atmospheric objectives.[5] He noted that cooperation between Germany and the United States was discussed first in 1960 and "again in 1969, on the basis of a study by the Economic Committee which, after having recognized the exploration of outer space as one of the common goals which can help relieve world tensions, regretted that 'the current national space programmes are duplicative and extremely costly.' This clearly raised the problem of the relations in this field between the United States and some European countries."[5]

In 1971, the NATO Assembly (see civil and military structure in fig. 20.2 and commanders in fig. 20.3) recommended that Alliance member counties:

> • Continue or undertake European action in the space field in view of the creation of a single European space body.

• Continue the development and perfection of launchers capable of placing in orbit satellites weighing more than 600 kg and which would guarantee European independence in the telecommunications field by harnessing the scientific and industrial efforts of European industry. . . .

• Continue to improve space cooperation in the INTELSAT programmes and through technical and commercial agreements at the bilateral or multilateral level, especially in the post-Apollo programme.[5]

And regarding "meteorological questions" intended to be answered through satellite technology as in the case of ERTS, in 1962 "NATO's program of space research for peaceful purposes, recommended that a long-range weather forecast system be established by NATO. . . ." And the Assembly "also requested that 'in accordance with NATO's policy of good neighbor relations, information be made available to the neighboring friendly nations, not only in Europe but also in Africa."[5]

So, in 1975, when USAID called for NASA to develop these systems, and Zaire was chosen as the central site for satellite launching and data collection, NATO's program had been on the drawing board for over a decade. And OTRAG's program evolved virtually simultaneously with NATO's.

This knowledge, combined with the fact that OTRAG's space program served all the needs articulated by Kissinger's State Department, made me think that Hussain and not Szulc was purposely spreading disinformation.

Additional evidence for this conclusion came from U.S. Representative W. Tapley Bennett, Jr. who stood before the U.N. General Assembly on October 18, 1976. The congressman, then, defined OTRAG's market and indirectly linked OTRAG to German–American efforts to develop space programs for USAID, NASA, and NATO. He noted:

The year 1976 has been an active and successful year both in outer space and in the U.N. Committee of the Peaceful Uses of Outer Space. . . .

During the past year, the United States has continued to participate cooperatively with other nations in the exploration of outer space. We have, for example launched Helios-2, built by the Federal Republic of Germany, the second scientific satellite to investigate the properties of interplanetary space close to the Sun. In January we launched the CTS [Communications Technology Satellite], an experimental high-powered communications satellite developed jointly with Canada.

Fig. 20.2. NATOs Military Structure and Command Centers

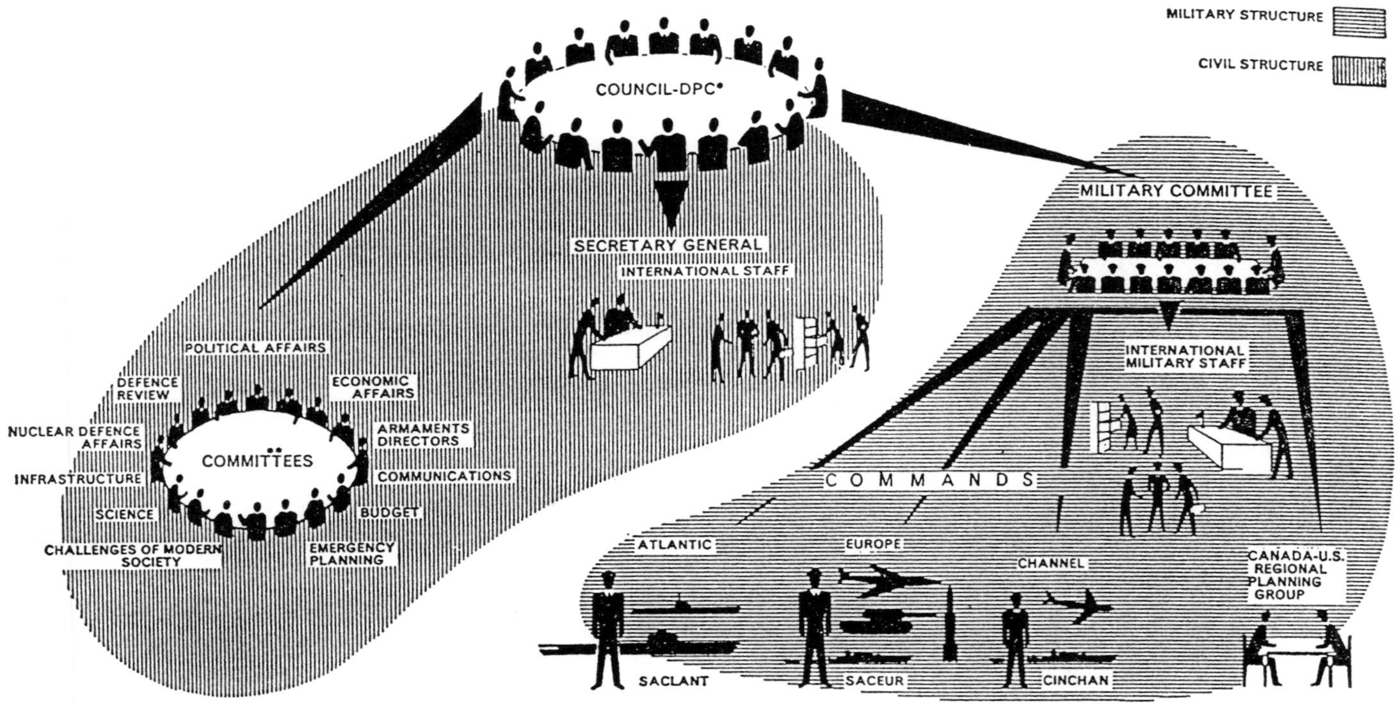

MILITARY STRUCTURE

CIVIL STRUCTURE

COUNCIL-DPC*

SECRETARY GENERAL
INTERNATIONAL STAFF

MILITARY COMMITTEE

INTERNATIONAL MILITARY STAFF

COMMANDS

ATLANTIC

EUROPE

CHANNEL

CANADA-U.S. REGIONAL PLANNING GROUP

SACLANT

SACEUR

CINCHAN

COMMITTEES

POLITICAL AFFAIRS

ECONOMIC AFFAIRS

ARMAMENTS DIRECTORS

COMMUNICATIONS

BUDGET

EMERGENCY PLANNING

DEFENCE REVIEW

NUCLEAR DEFENCE AFFAIRS

INFRASTRUCTURE

SCIENCE

CHALLENGES OF MODERN SOCIETY

Fig. 20.3. Major NATO Commanders

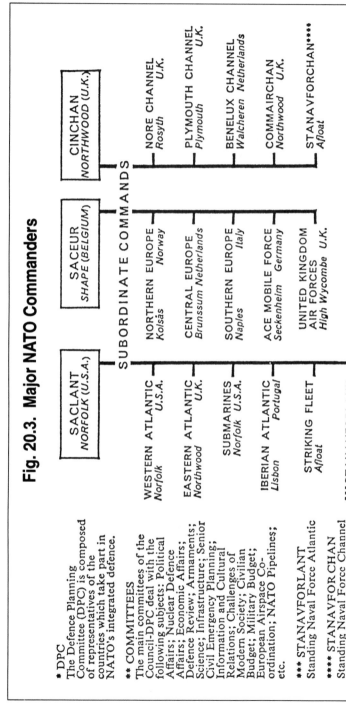

SACLANT
NORFOLK (U.S.A.)

SACEUR
SHAPE (BELGIUM)

CINCHAN
NORTHWOOD (U.K.)

SUBORDINATE COMMANDS

WESTERN ATLANTIC   U.S.A.
Norfolk

EASTERN ATLANTIC   U.K.
Northwood

SUBMARINES   Norfolk U.S.A.

IBERIAN ATLANTIC   Portugal
Lisbon

STRIKING FLEET
Afloat

***STANAVFORLANT
Afloat

NORTHERN EUROPE   Norway
Kolsås

CENTRAL EUROPE   Netherlands
Brunssum

SOUTHERN EUROPE   Italy
Naples

ACE MOBILE FORCE   Germany
Seckenheim

UNITED KINGDOM   U.K.
AIR FORCES
High Wycombe

NORE CHANNEL   U.K.
Rosyth

PLYMOUTH CHANNEL   U.K.
Plymouth

BENELUX CHANNEL   Netherlands
Walcheren

COMMAIRCHAN   U.K.
Northwood

STANAVFORCHAN****
Afloat

* DPC
The Defence Planning Committee (DPC) is composed of representatives of the countries which take part in NATO's integrated defence.

** COMMITTEES
The main committees of the Council-DPC deal with the following subjects: Political Affairs; Nuclear Defence Affairs; Economic Affairs; Defence Review; Armaments; Science; Infrastructure; Senior Civil Emergency Planning; Information and Cultural Relations; Challenges of Modern Society; Civilian Budget; Military Budget; European Airspace Co-ordination; NATO Pipelines; etc.

*** STANAVFORLANT
Standing Naval Force Atlantic

**** STANAVFORCHAN
Standing Naval Force Channel (Mine Counter Measures).

The military structure and command centers of The North Atlantic Treaty Organization. NATO is governed by the North Atlantic Council composed of representatives from member nations. Its "Science Committee" is responsible for overseeing the development and deployment of chemical weapons. NATO allegedly does not use biological weapons. However, while OTRAG was setting up a missile base in Southeastern Zaire, NATO forces were being summoned into action in the same area (Shaba region) by President Carter. Source: *Department of State Bulletin* July, 1978, pp. 1-12.

In cooperation with the Agency for International Development [USAID], using the ATS-6 satellite [Applications Technology Satellite], NASA is currently conducting demonstrations of the applications of space-age technology for the benefit of developing countries. These demonstrations will be seen in 27 countries in Asia, the Middle East, Africa, and Latin America.[6]

And regarding the Zaire project, Bennett said:

This year the Scientific and Technical Subcommittee has again noted that the Landsat system continues to provide the international community with data and experience in the new field of remote sensing by satellite. . . .

The Economic Commission for Africa has just endorsed a comprehensive training and station development program for Africa, and the European Space Agency has formulated a plan for rationalizing Landsat data acquisition and use in Europe . . . Zaire will be acquiring data on a regional basis.[6]

The fact is, the Helios-2 project that Bennett alleged was built by "the Federal Republic of Germany," was actually developed by the OTRAG-linked Messerschmitt-Bölkow-Blohm company from Munich. According to Messerschmitt literature, their company built . . . HELIOS A & B, [the] German/American solar probes."[7]

In summary, OTRAG had arrived at the right place at the right time to succeed financially and in every other way in serving NATO's interests. The evidence showed that USAID maintained connections to NASA and NATO, and all three had acted on Kissinger's behest in Zaire at the time OTRAG leased a sizable share of the country. Run by ex-Nazi's—Debus who had directed Cape Kennedy, Gompertz who presided over NASA's Chrysler space division, OTRAG's founder, Lutz Kayser, whose ties to NASA and NATO leaders on both sides of the Atlantic and connections to America's top military–industrial firms were both evident and unsettling.

Moreover, this knowledge fueled my suspicion that OTRAG was related to Litton Bionetics in a way Beletskiy had not mentioned. Kayser, as an Apollo space program consultant with, like Kissinger, ties to Boeing, may have purchased military hardware from Litton Industries as he had from Boeing. Being a major military contractor, it seemed logical that Litton Industries might have supplied satellite technology along with reagents for biological weapons research to OTRAG.

Given OTRAG's link to Messerschmitt, I thought, which after World War II had contributed greatly to the fund administered by Martin Bormann, Hitler's Deputy and Third Reich Party chief, Kayser was likely part of the Kameradenwerk, and possibly even a member of the SMOM. In either case, he was undoubtedly among the 900 or so Nazi scientists drafted by Army intelligence under Project Paperclip.[8]

Later, I discussed these findings with Jackie:

"Could OTRAG have been a NATO or CIA front?" she asked.

I decided to search for the answers.

Major Covert Connections

I began my search for additional evidence connecting the CIA to OTRAG by reviewing what I knew about the latter. Kayser had leased 29,000 square miles of eastern Zaire to do any kind of military experiments—anything they wanted with the territory 760,000 African villagers called home. Next, I considered the place and time—1975, at the height of the CIA's paramilitary operations in that exact region. OTRAG, I realized, could have served as a front for several covert CIA and NATO operations including military and satellite surveillance over MPLA forces in Angola; tactical nuclear weapons buildup; scientific efforts to help Gallo and his Litton Bionetics colleagues develop and test the immune-altering viruses ordered by Kissinger through the DOD for MKNAOMI, helping Hilleman at Merck and Manaker at the NCI develop and test experimental cancer vaccines for populations at high risk for viral infections; bringing new technology to Zaire as the Western allies promised; and enhancing NATO and NASA communications systems through the development of ERTS.

During my next U of I library excursion, I learned that a year before Debus left his directorship of Cape Canaveral to head OTRAG's experimental military base in Zaire, Horst Ehmke, the Minister of the Federal Republic of Germany for Research and Technology paid the United States a visit. A joint statement issued simultaneously in Washington and Bonn noted that from March 2 to 8, 1974, Ehmke had met with American officials "to discuss common interests in the programs and plans of both countries in science and technology research and development. Among the notables were:

. . . the Honorable Roy L. Ash, Director, Office of Management and Budget [and Litton, Industries Inc., President]; the Honorable Edward M. Kennedy, U.S. Senator [and then NATO, Vice President]; the Honorable William J. Casey, Under Secretary of State for Economic Affairs [and future CIA Director]; . . . the Honorable H. Guyford Stever, Director, National Science Foundation; the Honorable James C. Fletcher, Administrator, National Aeronautics and Space Administration; the Honorable Helmut Sonnenfeldt, Counselor of the Department of State [and Kissinger NSC appointee].[9]

Ehmke, the release said, also visited "the gaseous diffusion enrichment facility at Oak Ridge and the research and development facilities of the Oak Ridge National Laboratories," the site of numerous horrific chemical weapons experiments, cancer virus research studies, and related international conferences.[13] Here, "besides traditional fields of cooperation in nuclear energy development and in space research and technology," the German–American contingent considered other areas "particularly appropriate" for joint investments. Biomedical research and technology was among the most pressing.[9]

Obviously then, Roy Ash had lobbied for Litton firms to play a major role in the German–American "exchange." So Litton Bionetics was likely an industrial intermediary in the OTRAG–Nazi connection.

This made perfect sense. Kissinger was Ash's alternate for the NSC directorship following his service to General Bolling and Rockefeller. The former directed Project Paperclip to take advantage of the Nazis' most advanced aerospace and biological weapons developers. Rockefeller's bank received much of the Nazi war chest. So it made sense Debus and company might be called upon to take charge of Kissinger's most urgent Third World exercise.

"You can't create a new order with the old Germans, with Hitler and all that," argued Klaus Barbie's colleague Alfredo Mingolla in 1982. The fanatical Nazi and admitted CIA agent assigned to infiltrate Reverend Moon's Unification Church added, "You have to find something modern."[10] Viral weapons and "Star Wars" certainly fit the bill.

Nazi researchers, I realized, were perfect for OTRAG's assignments. Besides their brilliance in chemical engineering, aerospace, and germ warfare, they established the field of seroepidemiology. They examined all human blood types to determine varying susceptibilities to different diseases. The purpose was, of course, to develop a super-human race; freedom from the mundane illnesses that attacked those of lesser purity. OTRAG's assignment to develop monkey viruses that were "capable of such rapid replication that they could completely destabilize the [human] immune system," as Belitskiy charged, seemed perfectly suited for Nazi research. I also realized that the Marburg and Ebola fast-acting viruses did just that.

I tried to fathom the relationship between Gallo's work and OTRAG's based on Belitskiy's report.[1,11] Recalling that before 1969 only American organizations stockpiled simian monkey virus "reagents" for later distribution, I knew the WHO's "reference centre" in San Antonio, the NIH, and the NCI were the original monkey virus suppliers for those qualified to study them.[12] So most likely, I realized, in the early 1970s, OTRAG would have needed to get their simian virus testing reagents—their antibodies, cell lines, and other standard viral research requirements from an American source. Most likely from Gallo or some other NCI source, I thought, not only because he was their top gun in retrovirology, but also because he was heavily funded by the Department of Defense through Litton Bionetics.[13]

Indeed Belitskiy's report made the most sense. With it came the realization that Gallo's biological weapons consortium—Litton Bionetics and the NCI, Merck, and the NYUMC—would have most probably desired a laboratory operating in a remote area of Central Africa where monkeys were plentiful and populations were expendable. I already knew they maintained laboratories in Central Africa. And upon realizing Gallo's group or Bionetics would have needed to supply OTRAG's researchers with essential experimental reagents, I reckoned, maybe OTRAG was a subcontractor for Gallo or Litton, and, if lucky, I'd find a paper trail here as well.

"It all really does seem to fit," I said to Jackie the evening before we left for our road-trip to Florida.

"Will you be going back to the library again tomorrow?"

"Yeah. Just for a few hours. I need to see if I can find more information about the one organization I know least about—Litton Bionetics."

Litton Industries, Inc. and Bionetics

Early the next morning, I began my investigation of Litton Bionetics in the corporate microfiche files of the library. Having reread Belitskiy's broadcast along with the Informationsdienst Südliches Afrika report several times, I realized "based on secret service sources . . . OTRAG was an extension of West Germany's arms companies Dornier and Messerschmidt."[3] So while I was searching the reference literature on Litton, looking for ties to OTRAG, I decided to investigate these other companies as well to see if their operations paralleled OTRAG's or Litton's. Direct evidence, I realized, given that OTRAG was to have remained top secret, would probably be classified and, therefore, unavailable in the reference literature.

My Litton Industries search was quickly rewarded. Within a few hours, I held several annual reports the corporation had filed with the Securities and Exchange Commission.[14-16] The information included financial statements and moderately detailed corporate operations reports for the years 1976–1978, the period during which OTRAG was receiving the most media attention.

I immediately learned that Litton Industries, Inc., a Delaware Corporation with its central office in Roy Ash's home town of Beverly Hills, California, was highly diversified. Incorporated first in 1953 under the name Electro Dynamics Corporation, a year later its name changed to Litton Industries, Inc. "The Company," their 1978 report stated, "ranks as a major industrial corporation, serving worldwide markets for commercial, consumer, industrial and defense related products. [It] produces or provides a wide variety of highly competitive products and services which are classified into six major business segments." These included, in order of their percentage of $3,653,209,000 in total 1978 sales: 25% Business Systems & Equipment, 20% Electronic & Electrical Products, 17% Industrial Systems & Services, 16% Marine Engineering & Production, 14% Advanced Electronic Systems, and 8% Paper, Printing & Publishing. As fiscal year 1979 began, the company employed "over 90,000 people, 25 percent of them outside the United States, principally in West Germany, Canada, France, Italy, and the United Kingdom." Yet, despite its apparent success, the company recorded a "net loss" that year "of $90.8 million, or $2.66 per share, including a $172.9 million after-tax loss" from a "settlement agreement" with the Navy.

In terms of West German connections, Triumph-Adler—Litton's West German subsidiary—the report noted, was responsible for a major increase in corporate earnings. "In anticipation of future market growth, Triumph-Adler acquired Diehl Data Systems of West Germany in April, expanding its business and technological base" in several fields including multistation minicomputers for administrative, technical, scientific and medical applications."[16] Litton's German subsidiary Hellige in particular was hailed for having "achieved its fifth consecutive year of outstanding performance as sales of its electronic medical systems grew by more than 15 percent."[15] Other relevant parts of their 1976–1978 reports included:

In June, [1976] Litton Bionetics won the fourth renewal of its contract to manage the operations of the National Cancer Institute's Frederick (Md.) Cancer Research Center. More than 750 scientists and support personnel are engaged in intensive basic and applied research at FCRC on the causes, diagnosis, treatment and prevention of human cancer.

"Holy smoke!" I broke the silence of the library. The revelation that Bionetics managed and operated the entire FCRC for the NCI stunned me.

A major thrust in immunologic control of cancer at FCRC recognizes that cancer is not autonomous in its development and growth, and that natural host mechanisms exist. Research approaches have developed new insights into the cell types involved in tumor destruction, as well as the mechanisms of tumor recognition and killing on the cellular and subcellular levels. The program's scientists believe this work could lead to practical immunotherapeutic approaches to cancer.[14]

Litton Bionetics further expanded its activities in the rapidly growing U.S. and European markets for biosafety testing. . . . New business came from commercial and industrial firms moving to comply with the new U.S. Toxic Substances Control Act which will soon require the testing of 70,000 industrial chemicals already on the market—as well as the 1,000 or so new ones introduced each year—to keep cancer- and mutation-causing agents out of the environment.

The division's in vitro assays primarily involve Ames-type testing procedures where a specially bred strain of bacteria is exposed to test chemicals in a culture dish. This bacterial mutates at a very rapid rate, making it possible to identify potential carcinogens and mutagens at a relatively inexpensive cost in most cases. . . .

Earlier in the year [1978], Bionetics was awarded a five-year renewal of its contract to manage and operate the Frederick (Md.) Cancer Research Center for the National Cancer Institute, and also began marketing the first product it has developed for clinical testing laboratories—a new test for infectious mononucleosis.[16] [Emphasis added]

Infectious mono, I recalled from my pathology training, was caused by the Epstein-Barr virus (EBV), which is also associated with Burkitt's lymphoma and nasopharyngeal carcinoma. All three diseases along with EBV were exactly what Gallo's senior Dr. Manaker at the NCI and several other researchers were avidly studying in Central West Africa during the early 1970s,[17] I recalled.

I quickly looked up infectious mononucleosis in a medical reference book. Indeed, the infection was most commonly found in that part of Africa. "A survey in Ghana, Africa, found a seroconversion rate of 85% by age 2." Burkitt's lymphoma also "occurs predominantly in Africa," the text noted, "and virtually all African children with BL have very high titers to EBV. . . . Nasopharyngeal carinoma occurs frequently in southern China and northern Africa. Again, there are high titers of antibodies to EBV almost universally, and the genome is found in the tumor cells."[18]

Bionetics was operating in Bethesda *and* Africa at the same time OTRAG was there? There's got to be more proof!

I considered that almost a decade after Manaker and others at the NCI and Merck received federal funding to study EBV, BL, and nasopharyngeal cancer, Litton Bionetics was marketing a test kit based on their research. This was the third time I discovered that taxpayer supported NCI grants had funded pharmaceutical developments from which private concerns were now capitalizing. It seemed most plausible the same had been done with the AIDS test.

To confirm my suspicions, I placed a call to the Frederick Cancer Research Center from a nearby phonebooth. I was told by an administrator that Bionetics Research Lab *had* been involved in developing an AIDS test and that it had sold the product to a private concern. Soon thereafter, Litton also sold Bionetics Research Labs to Medpath—among the largest medical laboratories in the United States. Litton Bionetics, I was also informed, was still involved in administering funds for the NCI.

It now seemed even more plausible that Litton Bionetics, having managed Fort Detrick's major cancer virus research for so many years, might have managed OTRAG's "mutant virus" program and the CIA's Project MKNAOMI as well.

More West German Aerospace Business

Besides Triumph-Adler and Diehl Data Systems, Litton's SEC reports noted other connections to West German companies in the aerospace industry.

Litton's Advanced Electronic Systems division billed itself as "the world's leading supplier of aircraft inertial navigation systems (INS) and a major producer of U.S. Cruise missile guidance hardware." In 1977, the company had outfitted "West Germany's Alpha close-air-support jets with Doppler radar navigation systems,"[15] and acknowledged LITEF, the Freiburg, West Germany based military contractor for having "increased its business volume by more than 20 percent." The purchase was pursuant a combat aircraft guidance system that a consortium of British, German, and Italian companies were building for various customers. Then the division disclosed its sales to NATO of missile guidance and satellite reconnaissance technology. Data Systems, another Litton Industries subdivision, the report said:

> gained major follow-on business on its NATO Integrated Command System/ Telegraphic Automatic Relay Equipment (NICS/TARE) contract, which calls for the integration of computers, teletypes, videodisplays and other peripheral units into a communications network linking NATO members in Europe and North America. Deliveries begin in calender 1979 and the system becomes operational in the 1980s, when current processing methods will be unable to keep up with the projected number of transmissions.[15]

In addition, the company boasted sales to Amecom which:

> . . . began production on a major contract for an airborne system that senses sources of enemy ground based radiation, determines the signals' direction and locates potential anti-aircraft artillery or missile threats. Designated TEREC (Tactical Electronic Reconnaissance), it will be the first operational tactical reconnaissance system deployed in quantity by the U.S. Air Force.[15]

Such technology, I realized, would have served OTRAG's needs exactly.

Realizing that tactical reconnaissance was exactly what Kissinger had urged CIA forces in Zaire to deploy against the MPLA in Angola,[19] recognizing that aerial surveillance was what USAID had requested from NASA to help with "agriculture" and "water management" in Central Africa,[20] knowing that the Federal Republic of Germany was a partner in Skylab wherein "one of Skylab's most significant payload components was its Earth Resources Experiment package (EREP), a complement to ERTS-1, the Earth Resources Technology Satellite launched in 1972, and the State Department acknowledged that plans for similar stations are under way in Africa,"[21] and knowing that the United States and Germany were reducing NATO costs by coordinating their military and scientific programs to reduce duplication of efforts; it seemed most plausible that Litton divisions had supplied OTRAG with a mix of aerospace hardware, software, and germ warfare products needed to carry out the multiple military missions Kissinger defined as urgently needed in Central Africa.

My next step was to research back issues of the *Wall Street Journal* and *Aviation Week*. I thought, for sure, Litton would have announced these large business dealings and perhaps provided additional intelligence.

Litton Industries in the News

Knowing that OTRAG had been developing its prototype launch vehicles that peaked NASA's interest in 1976, and was likely to be in full swing by 1980, I directed my *Wall Street Journal* search to this period.[22-27]

Indeed, I found the *Wall Street Journal* had announced virtually all of these transactions between Litton Industries and its West German customers and affiliates.

Among the first entries I came on was one that cheered "a $32.9 million Air Force contract for electronic reconnaissance sensor equipment."[24] This order, I realized, may have supplied the military equipment needed for the USAID and NATO satellite reconnaissance effort developing at that exact time in Zaire.

Then a couple months later, the *Wall Street Journal* announced NATO's purchase of $11.3 million of "computerized communications systems from Litton Data Systems"—a group intimately connected with the Litton division, that included their West German Hellige Company and Litton Bionetics.[14,25]

I also learned that this $11.3 million NATO contract had followed a much larger $40 million award for a "communication system" to supplement a "NATO computerized Satcom system." A requisition most likely destined for Zaire because of the unique nature and timing of the purchase.[26]

Undoubtedly, then, a mass of circumstantial evidence indicated that the Litton organization was in the satellite reconnaissance business, and linked to OTRAG through its West German Hellige Division, Litton Bionetics, as well as NATO purchasing.[26]

Moreover, just as I had suspected, the satellite reconnaissance systems administered by USAID and NASA for allegedly "humanitarian" and "agricultural" purposes had actually been designed, purchased, and directed by NATO officials.[27]

I photocopied all the incriminating evidence in haste, not wanting to hit the road too late, and then returned to the motorhome to share my findings with Jackie.

"Since Litton Bionetics was subcontracting for the Special Operations Division of the Army and the CIA during Kissinger's Project MKNAOMI, the allegations that OTRAG was subcontracting for the Pentagon were apparently accurate. The results of their biological weapons development program, then, could have easily been tested in the same region of Zaire that OTRAG operated," I explained.

"So you think they intentionally released the new viruses in Zaire?" she asked.

"Well it's certain the deliberate release in that region could have served, besides population control, three CIA Kissinger-directed programs," I replied. "The covert military Operation FEATURE, Project MKNAOMI, and COINTELPRO.

"Isaacson was right," I concluded, as we headed south. "Kissinger was devilishly brilliant."

A Twisted Web

Later that week, I digested the articles I had photocopied. I learned that Tad Szulc's allegation that OTRAG was an extension of West Germany's arms companies Dornier and Messerschmidt was apparently accurate. Besides testimony by an unnamed CIA official who stated that "the Boeing Company had provided OTRAG with Cruise missile technology,"[3] my search of *Aviation Week* revealed a number of confirming details. The first fact: Boeing owned a 12% share of Messerschmitt-Boelkow which it sold to Siemens Corporation in July 1978.[28]

Moreover, besides being engaged in all facets of the aerospace industry, both Messerschmitt and Dornier maintained medical research and technology subsidiaries, making OTRAG a suitable acquisition if not secret military affiliate.

Also during the period that I searched the financial and aerospace literature, the West-German-based Teledyne Corporation purchased increasing amounts of Litton Industries stock so that by 1978 it owned 27 percent of the company.[29] Meanwhile, another German-owned company—Grummann Aerospace—was Litton's fiercest competitor for American defense contracts and had worked as Teledyne's chief subcontractor building navigational computers and data processing systems.[30] Apparently, Teledyne grew tired of losing revenue to Grummann and invested more heavily in Litton Industries, which Grummann had battled to secure the $1 billion NATO radar-reconnaissance work up for bid in 1977.[31] All this underscored, for me, the twisted web of NATO's dealings with the allied German–American military–medical–industrial complex.

Fraudulent Claims

In my search for Litton Industries announcements in the *Wall Street Journal*, I ran across numerous articles in 1978 that focused on the company's criminal activities. One such article detailed a Supreme Court decision to have the company reimburse the Navy for hundreds of millions of dollars in fraudulent charges. On Tuesday, October 3, 1978, a Washington correspondent explained:

> Litton Systems, Inc., a subsidiary of Litton Industries Inc., lost its Supreme Court bid for dismissal of an indictment charging Litton with filing a fraudulent claim on a Navy submarine project.[32]

> The indictment of Litton stemmed from a $30 million claim filed against the Navy in 1972 by Litton's Ingalls nuclear shipbuilding division. . . .[33]

Then in a second court action, Litton agreed to settle a dispute that required congressional committee review.[34] The staff reporter wrote:

> The Navy and Litton Industries, Inc. settled a $1.09 billion shipbuilding contract claims dispute with an agreement that saddles Litton with a $200 million loss and the Navy with $447 million in additional payments.

> The settlement, which must be reviewed by Congress, resolves a nine-year dispute between the company and the Navy over a contract to build five amphibious assault ships called LHAs.

> **"Loss" for Fiscal Year**

> Charles Thornton, Litton's chairman, said: "The settlement will result in a substantial loss for the current fiscal year," in which record earnings had been expected previously. In the nine months ended April 30, Litton earned $53.8 million on sales of $2.7 billion, almost equal to the $55.9 million it earned on sales of $3.4 billion in fiscal 1977.

> He said the company will take a pre-tax loss of $333 million this year, which works out to an after-tax loss of $174 million. The loss is composed of the $200 million called for in the settlement, plus $133 million start-up costs at the Pascagoula, Miss., shipyard of Litton's Ingalls shipbuilding division.

> Besides the dispute over the LHA program, the agreement also covers contracts for 30 DD963-class destroyers the company is building for the Navy at Pascagoula. The estimated costs of these contracts at completion is $4.73 billion.

> Under the settlement, Litton waives all claims against the Navy under the LHA contract, signed in 1969, and the destroyer contract, signed in 1970. Litton will also withdraw two suits filed against the Navy under the LHA contract and pending in the federal court of claims. . . ."[34]

I instantly realized, that the period in which the contested contracts were signed, between 1969 and 1970, was just after Nixon gave Kissinger the NSC directorship he had been considering for Litton's president, Roy Ash. Instead, I recalled, Roy Ash was given the chairmanship of the President's Advisory Council on Executive Organizations—his title: "Assistant to the President of the United States"—and his company, Litton Industries, Inc., was then awarded well over $5 billion in military contracts along with the privilege of developing AIDS-like viruses for a New World Order.[33-38]

Chapter 21
Marburg, Ebola, and Chilling Propaganda in *The Hot Zone*

IN late March, we made our way back from sunny Florida to New England. Again my seminar schedule gave us three leisure days, which I spent exploring the libraries of the University of North Carolina, Chapel Hill. The ladies spent the time admiring the blossom-bedecked town at its spring peak. Though their assignment was less confining, I assure you mine was far more engaging.

My first day's assignment was to track down the Marburg virus along with Ebola Zaire and Ebola Sudan. All were relative newcomers to the virology scene. All were believed to be HIV relatives if only for their decade of common emergence. Marburg had struck three vaccine production facilities almost simultaneously in 1967. Two outbreaks occurred in two West German cities and another in Yugoslavia. Oddly, the virus then disappeared until 1975, when it once again reared its ugly head in of all places South Africa. Then, less than two years later, two larger outbreaks erupted in southern Sudan and northern Zaire (see map fig. 21.1).

I thought it curious that the European outbreaks occurred virtually simultaneously in 1967 and then eight years later in South Africa. I knew that to be about the time Gallo and his colleagues at the NCI, Litton Bionetics, Merck and allegedly OTRAG began experimenting with similar viruses to produce an assortment of potential bioweapons. Moreover, the Sudan and Zaire outbreak areas were literally war zones, and South Africa was not too far off geographically and militarily. So I began my search for Marburg's origin with these factors in mind.

In Search of Marburg

A MEDLAR search at the UNC medical library immediately led me to an abstract in the October 1977 issue of *Tropical Diseases Bulletin*. The text discussed three papers that described the "isolation and characterization" of the Marburg virus from the blood of a Zairian patient who "became ill during a large outbreak of hemorrhagic fever in northern Zaire and southern Sudan in the second half of 1976. Material from Zaire was originally

Fig. 21.1. Map of Central West Africa

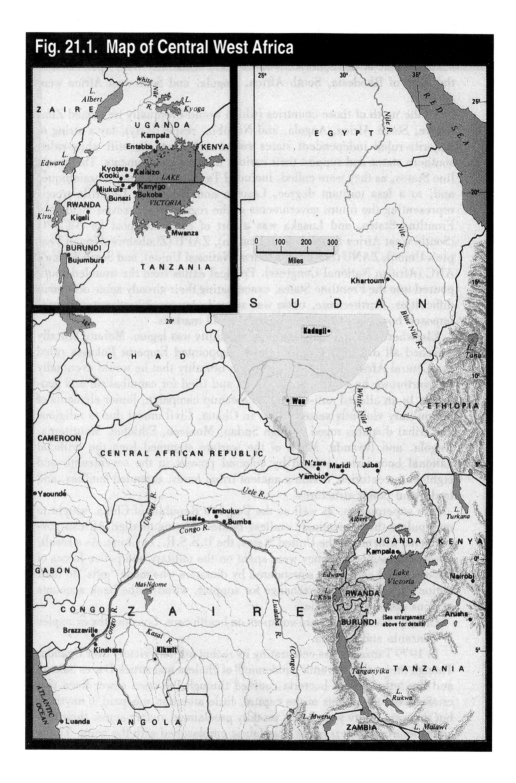

sent to Antwerp [Belgium] and from there specimens were dispatched to Porton Down and Atlanta."[1]

Porton Down was England's biowarfare laboratory, and Antwerp was close to where Gallo had presented his research before NATO on the "entry of foreign nucleic acids into cells" in 1970. Antwerp was, therefore, likely to have been another Western alliance BW research lab.[2]

The *Tropical Diseases Bulletin* reported that the three viruses—Marburg, Ebola Zaire and Ebola Sudan—were "morphologically indistinguishable," although antibody studies confirmed distinct differences between the strains that broke out in Germany and Yugoslavia in 1967, and those that hit the Ebola river valley in 1976. Thus, the Sudan and Zaire strains were named Ebola to distinguish them from the original Marburg virus.[1]

Another reference I reviewed that morning was *Marburg Virus* by Rudolph Siegert who was affiliated with the Hygiene Institute of the Philipps University in Marburg (Lahn), Germany.[3]

Siegert, caught up in the mystery of Marburg, explained:

> In Europe no new diseases have been observed in many decades. Thus a mysterious hemorrhagic fever which broke out simultaneously in Germany and Yugoslavia in 1967 stimulated considerable interest; it posed a demanding challenge for clinicians, microbiologists, epidemiologists, and the public health service.

> The disease appeared in mid-August and affected 31 persons in Marburg/Lahn, Frankfurt/Main, and Belgrade. Seven cases ended in death. At first, only employees of the Behringwerke, the Paul Ehrlich Institute and the Institute for Sera and Vaccines Torlak became ill. . . . The common source of the infections was soon traced to certain shipments of monkeys *(Cercopithecus aethiops)* from Uganda. . . . There can be no doubt that the pathogen responsible for the "Marburg monkey disease" fulfills the morphologic and biologic criteria for a virus. This is indicated by its cell-dependent replication, as well as its complex structure and helical symmetry. The genetic material is RNA.[3]

Siegert agreed with most authors, that the structural pattern of the "Marburg virus" exhibited many features similar to a group of viruses known as rhabdoviruses. These included the culprits responsible for rabies and vesicular stomatitis. A more technical name for the Marburg virus was coined from the monkeys who passed it to the victims in Marburg—*Rhabdovirus simiae*.[3]

The Marburg virus expert described the horrifying clinical features of the disease and then focused on several specific cases. In one instance, a nurse who had no contact with a victim's blood became infected. Siegert thus concluded it seemed "likely that she acquired the infection by way of contaminated air or contact with excreta."[4]

Reporting on the epidemiology of the European outbreak, Siegert noted that although all the infected monkeys had died or been slaughtered, the killer germ had been identified from cell cultures obtained and frozen before the monkeys were incinerated. At least ten infected monkeys were believed to have been responsible for the twenty cases among Marburg veterinarians and animal caretakers. Frankfurt's cases were traced to two more monkeys from "*the same animal catching station in Uganda*," and those in Belgrade were infected by one more.

Siegert continued:

> Four shipments were determined as possible sources; they had arrived in Europe between July 20th and August 10th, 1967, and comprised a total of 500-600 animals. Their distribution to the affected institutions was quite various. Frankfurt received only 10 per cent, and this small number in two batches. It is hardly likely that all the monkeys were infectious from the start; in that case an increased mortality would be expected, which was reported only from Belgrade. Presumably the infection spread during the course of three weeks in the groups of monkeys kept in quarantine for 25 days in Belgrade and in Marburg for up to 29 days. The animals probably became contagious five to eight days after exposure. Even if we assume this minimal time, the first monkeys must have acquired the infection before their arrival. . . . In cases involving several monkeys in separate cages in the same room, aerogenic transmission is suspected. . . .[4]

Human cases of Marburg disease, Siegert explained, had only been reported in Germany and in Yugoslavia, "although *numerous shipments of monkeys from the same dealer were sent simultaneously from Uganda to the USA, Italy, Japan, Sweden, and Switzerland.* [Emphasis added]" This prompted a Central African investigation wherein no evidence was found that the disease had occurred in animals or natives there. Thus most experts concluded that "the reservoir of the Marburg virus" though not found in *Cercopithecus aethiops* or other animals, must be "in the native habitat of the monkeys in Africa."[4]

So the virus did not make its home in monkeys. It resided somewhere in the local habitat of Central Africa. How interesting, I thought, knowing Uganda was just across the border from OTRAG's base. I wonder if OTRAG or Litton Bionetics rhabdovirus experiments might have infected the monkeys that were later sent to labs in Europe. Odd that Siegert didn't mention the name of the "monkey dealer." He documented everything else meticulously. Obviously it had to have been a large facility to simultaneously ship 500-600 animals.

A Bogus "United States Antigen"

What Siegert documented next was even more remarkable. The CDC apparently sabotaged international efforts to locate the source of the outbreak. Siegert wrote:

> Monkeys themselves did not seem to be the probable natural reservoir of the virus, since in spite of their widespread use in experiments, transmission of this hemorrhagic fever in laboratories has not been otherwise observed. The fact that all infections of monkeys proved lethal under experimental conditions, even after minimal dosages, also supports this contention. For this reason it came as a great surprise when [CDC] seroepidemiologic studies indicated a wide distribution of the Marburg virus, not only among monkeys from Central Africa, but also among those from Asia.[4]

These findings, Siegert explained at length, were highly "inconsistent." Blood studies using guinea-pig-derived antibody, run by the "Special [Virus] Studies Laboratory" of the CDC in 1968, "indicated that of 129 African green monkeys from Ethiopia, Kenya, and Uganda, 50 per cent reacted positively." Furthermore, "no differences were found between animals imported into the USA and those studied immediately following capture. The same percentage of antibody carriers was also determined in a limited number of chimpanzees, gorillas, and orangutans." according to the CDC researchers.

But numerous other international studies failed to show this high presence of Marburg virus in the blood samples of various monkey species.[4]

Moreover, Dr. Seymour Kalter, director of the Southwest Foundation for Research—America's premier simian monkey lab—questioned the inconsistency Siegert observed. It didn't seem possible, he explained, with such high titers of antibody against Marburg infection demonstrated by the CDC, "that neither illness nor excessive mortality was observed." During experiments, monkeys exposed with *Rhabdovirus simiae* developed antibodies and died shortly after. Kalter, Siegert, and others therefore questioned: "With such widespread contamination it is . . . difficult to imagine why no cases have occurred until now involving humans having close contact with monkeys."[4]

The explanation ultimately focused on "the specificity of the antigen used" to detect the antibodies diagnostic for Marburg infection. To study the problem, Kalter and another group of researchers compared the CDC's guinea-pig-derived antigen with those developed from monkeys infected with the Marburg virus. The results proved that the "United States antigen probably contained a second component not specific for Marburg virus. . . ." Thus, the CDC's research methods and materials were faulted for producing falsely positive test results. Siegert wrote:

> The authors are convinced that the Marburg virus is absent among the two species [of monkeys] studied in South Africa, or occurs at most only to a limited extent. [Other researchers] point out the possibility that the antibodies might not only have been directed against the Marburg virus *but simultaneously against a less pathogenic related virus which circulated in Uganda at the same time.*[4] [Emphasis added]

In other words, the CDC developed a testing procedure that led the international scientific community astray. The allegedly innocent mistake prompted researchers to conclude the Marburg agent commonly infected monkeys throughout the world. Thus, scientists were beguiled, and the issue remained confused during the first critical years of the investigation when interest in the outbreak peaked.

Even more suspect was the fact that the CDC's testing reagent—the "United States antigen"—contained a Marburg-like, "less pathogenic related virus" that had been circulating in Uganda at the same time the deadly germ infected the monkeys destined for Europe. Meaning? The CDC had manipulated a different, but related, less deadly virus from Uganda to produce the bogus "United States antigen." Thus, using Strecker's metaphor again, the CDC had dressed a quadriplegic infant in a disguise. Except this time, when it arrived at the party, party goers saw through the disguise and knew the CDC had dressed and delivered the baby.

These findings were reinforced, Siegert wrote, when researchers finally developed an optimally effective and specific antigen to detect the Marburg virus. With this preparation, no antibody was found "in any of 136 monkeys from Uganda and South Africa, or in 25 serum samples which had been found positive by other teams" using the CDC's "United States antigen."[4]

"For this reason," Siegert concluded, "it seems inappropriate to refer to the Marburg virus as a simian virus so long as its origin remains unclear. Determination of the virus reservoir is one of the most important tasks yet to be accomplished. It is not impossible that a unique chance event is involved. . . . For this reason the risk of future outbreaks cannot yet be determined. . . ."[4]

The WHO on Marburg

Another text I found that morning at UNC's medical library was a 1977 WHO publication written by Dr. I. H. Simpson from the Department of Medical Microbiology at the London School of Hygiene and Tropical Medicine.[5] Simpson had led one of the WHO-dispatched teams to the Ebola region of Zaire during the 1976 outbreak.

Although Simpson's text lacked the depth of Siegert's, he did provide a few more interesting details about the obscure origins and virus reservoirs of Marburg, and the possible infection routes through intact skin and the air.[5]

Simpson also described the "alarming" case-fatality rate that occurred during the Ebola outbreaks:

> Between July and November 1976, two very extensive and almost simultaneous epidemics of a similar disease occurred about 1000 km apart in Southern Sudan and northern Zaire. Secondary and tertiary person-to-person spread of the infection was a distinct feature of these outbreaks, particularly among hospital staff. In some cases in Sudan as many as eight "generations" of infection were found, but this was unusual. There are believed to have been over 300 cases, with 151 deaths, in Sudan, and in Zaire some 237 cases, with 211 fatalities, have been documented; the actual numbers may be greater. In one Sudanese hospital 76 members of a staff of 230 were infected and 41 died. Throughout the Zaire epidemic and during the earlier stages of the Sudanese outbreak the case-fatality rate was of the order of almost 90%, leading to fear and panic in the local populations. These alarming figures emphasize the tremendous public health importance of this disease.[5]

> The outbreak in Sudan is thought to have begun in the first week of July 1976, with the illness of a cloth-room storekeeper in a cotton factory in Nzara (Western Equatorial Province). Two weeks later a second storekeeper also became ill, followed a further two weeks later by another cotton factory employee. One of his contacts introduced the disease to Maridi, some distance east of Nzara. The source of the original infection has still not been determined. The infection spread swiftly but only through close and prolonged household contact with an active case. Health personnel in particular were involved through contact with patients' blood, and Maridi hospital acted as an amplifier of the disease. When good nursing techniques, supplemented by the use of protective clothing, were introduced the number of contact infections fell dramatically.

> In Zaire, the first recognized case occurred during the first week of September 1976 and is thought to have originated at a small mission hospital in Yambuku, just north of Yandonage, Equateur Region. It is thought that parenteral [through the skin] injections may have played a role in transmission. Patients

infected in the hospital environment probably then carried the infection back to their villages, setting up new pockets of infection in their homes. The source of the infection in Zaire remains unknown, but it may have been introduced to Yambuku by a patient presenting at the outpatient clinic with a nonspecific febrile illness.[5]

Besides acknowledging the similarity of Marburg viruses to "the Rhabdoviridae," Siegert also mentioned the possibility that the germs, given their large size and unmistakable appearance, could have evolved from "a whole roster of plant viruses."[4] I recalled that because of their large size, plant viruses were among the first viruses studied and manipulated by NCI researchers,[6] including Robert Gallo's team.[7] Thus, it seemed even more plausible that the "natural reservoir" of the Ebola and Marburg viruses was, in NCI laboratories.

The Walter Royal Davis Library

Fortunately, as it turned out, UNC's medical library did not hold the vast majority of references the computer provided. Several were history texts and the rest were government documents. To retrieve these, a kindly librarian told me, I needed to visit the Walter Royal Davis Library a few blocks away. So I packed my gear and headed over to the campus's main library.

A dimly lit upper floor of Davis housed the German history books. After several minutes of perusing its stacks, I came upon two texts about Marburg, both in German. With my rusting memory of conversational German, I plowed through the books in search of clues. They were either nonexistent or I missed them.

I rode the elevator back to the first floor confident that Davis held more for me than dead ends. The government documents department was my next hope.

My first objective was to locate a five-volume set entitled, *Virology*. The texts were written by a task force from the National Institute for Allergies and Infectious Diseases (NIAID) and published by USDHEW in 1979. I presented the citation to a librarian who said she would retrieve the books in the library's basement. She turned, left, and five minutes later returned with *Virology*.

"Are you going to be doing more research in this department?" she asked.

"Very possibly; over the next two days," I said.

"Then you may as well get a pass to the basement so you can access your references yourself."

Twist my arm, I thought, knowing that special treasures always appeared whenever I roamed such places.

"See the fellow at the end of the counter. He'll issue you a pass."

I took her advice. Then I claimed an empty desk and began to read *Virology.*

The sections dealing with Marburg and Ebola basically reviewed what I had already learned.

Several parts of *Virology,* though, were very interesting. I learned one most important fact—researchers preferred working with simian monkey (SV40) viruses because they were "the most malleable and best characterized," which made them easier "to clone and propagate" specific fragments of foreign DNA in mammalian cells.[8]

Evolution of the Species

Virology also explained that during the late 1960s, researchers advanced a new theory of evolution. Some believed that evolution of species was not so much based on "survival of the fittest." Viruses were thought to play a more important role. Researchers proposed that foreign DNA transmitted to plant and animal hosts by viruses caused organisms to evolve.[9]

Thus, viruses were not only believed to hold the key to vaccine development and disease prevention, but to human evolution as well. Many researchers claimed that through "future research on viral evolution," a genetically superior race of humans may be synthetically evolved. In the task force's jargon: "Further exploration of the molecular paleontology of endogenous retroviruses could help elucidate the processes of speciation."[6]

Retroviruses, the report continued, were particularly important in this regard. Studies on the "evolution of viruses," had allegedly provided new evidence in support of the theory "that man originated in Asia rather than in Africa."[10] Taking particular pride in this evidence, the authors then commented that, "accommodations between host and [viral] parasite[s] are alleged to have played a major role in the political and economic development of civilizations."[10]

The Hot Zone

Early that evening, I caught up with my family for dinner. Jackie and Alena had spent part of the day shopping, and had bought Daddy a gift—*The Hot*

Zone, by Richard Preston.[11] I had heard about this allegedly true account of the famous Hazleton monkey house outbreak of the dreaded Reston (Ebola-like) virus as I was finishing up work on *Deadly Innocence*. I just hadn't gotten around to reading it since it seemed off the subject of AIDS. Now, however, the time seemed perfect. So that night in a motel room, as the girls watched television and then drifted off to sleep, I started and finished *The Hot Zone*.

For a "nonfiction" book, the Random House publication had remained on the *New York Times* best-seller list far longer than even most works of fiction. Preston, the author of an earlier book entitled *American Steel*—about "the Nucor Corporation and its project to build a revolutionary steel mill"—won several awards for his writing, including the prestigious American Institute of Physics Award, and the McDermott Award in the Arts from M.I.T. How this investigative journalist with no medical background had gone from revealing revolutionary steel industry accomplishments to viral epidemics struck me as suspicious—especially since I knew the steel industry had been targeted, by Bobby Kennedy, for investigation because of widespread corruption, and had in its ranks SMOM Nazi-linked industrialists, including John Farrell, the past president of U.S. Steel.

My suspicions, soon grew feverish. *The Hot Zone*, I realized, omitted almost all of the relevant scientific facts. Preston completely overlooked the extraordinary research environments in which the AIDS, Marburg, Ebola, and Reston viruses emerged. He gave no hint of the covert military operations that had permeated Central Africa at the time of the major Ebola outbreaks in 1976. He wrote nothing of the political forces effecting African development and population control at the time. He failed to mention the numerous USAID-sponsored immunization programs and widespread vaccine experiments that ran throughout the AIDS belt and the sixteen Central West African countries. Apparently he felt this was immaterial for his "terrifying true story."

Indeed, *The Hot Zone* was a labor of devout censorship. The only logical explanation for Preston's treatise is that the CIA and military–medical–industrial complex had persuaded the author to produce a marvelous piece of yellow press, and acquired Random House to publish it.

Preston and patrons of *The Hot Zone* clearly wanted people to know that the world might soon be plagued by viruses far more deadly than AIDS and to be prepared for the worst. What frightened me most about that realization was the probability that those who fanned such fears would make good on their threats.

Viral Propaganda

The Hot Zone's main thesis would be laughable were it not for its seriousness. Through exceptionally gruesome prose, Preston advanced the notion that new human-immune-system ravaging germs most likely emerged from bat guano on the floor of Kitum cave in Southwestern Kenya during the mid-1970s. The viruses were then, allegedly, picked up by neighboring monkeys and delivered around the world by African animal traders.

Preston lost his credibility in the *The Hot Zone*'s opening chapter when he discussed the initial outbreak of the deadly Marburg virus (Ebola strain). Here he alleged the virus claimed its first victim—Charles Monet, a Frenchman, whose job, Preston claimed, was "to take care of the sugar factory's water pumping machinery." In nauseating detail, Preston described Monet's alleged sojourn. Monet then died at "Nairobi Hospital," but not before vomiting into the "eyes and mouth" of Dr. Shem Musoke, who nine days later allegedly "broke with the infection" too.

Terrifying? Yes. True story? Hardly.

By Simpson's scientific and more accurate account, Ebola's first victim was "a cloth-room storekeeper in a cotton factory in Nzara (Western Equatorial Province). Two weeks later, a second storekeeper also became ill, followed a further two weeks later by another cotton factory employee."[5]

Giving Preston the benefit of doubt, had he made a mistake, had he thought the Zaire outbreak was Ebola's first, then he should have described events emanating from Yambuku's and not Nairobi's hospital.

Marburg, Preston continued:

> . . . is an African organism, but it has a German name. Viruses are named for the place where they are first discovered. Marburg is an old city in central Germany, surrounded by forests and meadows, where factories nestle in green valleys. The virus erupted there in 1967, in a factory called the Behring Works, which produced vaccines using kidney cells from African green monkeys. The Behring Works regularly imported monkeys from Uganda. The virus came to Germany hidden somewhere in a series of air shipments of monkeys totaling five or six hundred animals. As few as two or three of the animals were incubating the virus.[11]

"They were probably not even visibly sick," Preston speculated. "At any rate, [meaning, 'I'm not sure, but let's continue with this allegedly true account anyway'] shortly after they arrived . . . the virus began to spread among them, and a few of them crashed and bled out. Soon afterward, the Marburg agent jumped species and suddenly emerged in the human population of the city. This is an example of virus amplification."[11]

Propaganda is a more accurate description of this example, I thought, realizing it was highly unlikely that quality European vaccine producers would rely on careless "monkey traders" to supply their animals. As I realized earlier that day, and Preston later noted,[18] the supplier undoubtedly would have maintained a large quarantined monkey facility in order to be exporting so many expensive monkeys around the world at one time.

Given the bizarre nature and extreme virulence of the germ, it was far more likely, then, that DOD or NCI biological weapons contractors like Litton Bionetics or OTRAG had slipped up somehow and European vaccine workers paid the price. As Gallo and numerous others published,[13] and the Army's director of defense Research and Engineering explained, cancer-causing monkey viruses were being manipulated at the exact time, and for the first time in history, simultaneously in Uganda, Bethesda, New York, and elsewhere. At this time, "new infective microorganisms" that differed from "any known disease-causing organisms" were being produced by the billions. Many were likely to have escaped accidentally.[14]

Fort Detrick's accident record, for instance, was appalling. I recalled that during the 1969 congressional hearings on chemical and biological warfare, senators learned that at Fort Detrick, some 3,300 accidents were recorded between 1954 and 1962. "Half of these in laboratories involving the infection of more than 500 men. . . . There was even one case of a worker who caught plague."[15]

Even physician Robin Cook's fictional account of the source of these viruses in *Outbreak* noted a military origin and purpose.[17] Preston's account, therefore, seemed an insult to medical intelligence and common sense.

Explaining that the Hazleton monkey house was generally considered a safe haven for monkey immigrants, much of Preston's book detailed the hysteria that ensued when a "honker from Zaire" resembling Ebola broke out among one floor of African monkeys "from the Phillipines."[18]

"What was it doing near Washington?" one of Preston's characters questioned. "How in the hell had it gotten here? What would it do? . . . I'm onto something really hot."[19]

Preston explained that an unidentified African monkey dealer had sold the hot monkeys to a Philippine wholesaler who dealt with the U.S. military. To his credit, Preston explained that the U.S. Army Medical Research Institute of Infectious Diseases at Fort Detrick was the Hazleton monkey house's chief customer. The operation, he noted, was owned and operated by Hazleton Research Products, a division of (Dow) Corning, Inc.

What he failed to mention was that besides monkeys, Hazleton Research Products sold monkey *viruses* to military scientists. The NCI's retrovirus chief Robert Gallo was one of their customers.[20] Hazleton supplied Rausher leukemia viruses for Gallo's group at Litton Bionetics, and there is evidence that Hazleton obtained monkeys from Litton Bionetics.[13] The CIA's Project MKNAOMI was, apparently, another end user.[20]

Twisted Truth and Tall Tales

For all its deception, *The Hot Zone* chronicled some important events associated with the famous Ebola virus outbreaks. In each chapter, however, Preston managed to either twist the truth or tell tall tales.

Enter Preston's hero, Eugene Johnson. "Those people who work with Ebola are crazy. To mess around with Ebola is an easy way to die. Better to work with something safer, such as anthrax."[21] Mr. Johnson, was apparently one such crazy person. According to Preston, he was "a civilian biohazard expert who was running the Ebola research program at the Institute." When ever, I thought, would the U.S. Army hire a civilian to run one of its most important, top-secret research projects?

My suspicions intensified when I read that Johnson had "virtually ransacked Africa looking for these life forms, but despite his searches he had never found them in their natural hiding places. . . To find the hidden reservoir of Ebola was one of Johnson's great ambitions."[21]

I found it difficult to believe that some slightly looney civilian was going to spend his hard-earned cash and years of work ravaging through the rain forests of Africa to capture a virus that if touched or breathed might kill him in days.

Preston continued:

Whatever these Ebola proteins do, they seem to target the immune system for special attack. In this they are like HIV, which also destroys the immune system, but unlike the onset of HIV, the attack by Ebola is explosive. As Ebola sweeps through you, your immune system fails, and you seem to lose your ability to respond to the viral attack. Your body becomes a city under siege, with its gates thrown open and hostile armies pouring in, making camp in the public squares and setting everything on fire; and from the moment Ebola enters your bloodstream, the war is already lost; you are almost certainly doomed. You can't fight off Ebola the way you fight off a cold. Ebola does in ten days what it takes AIDS ten years to accomplish. . . . In Zaire during the 1976 outbreak, grieving relatives kissed and embraced the dead or prepared the body for burial, and then, three to fourteen days later, they broke with Ebola.[21]

"The virus," Preston wrote, "erupted simultaneously in fifty-five villages surrounding the hospital." This, of course, would have been virtually impossible without the help of a mass vaccination or dissemination program. Otherwise, as Simpson described,[5] the virus would have begun to spread slowly: first from one individual to a few others, then perhaps to many more in a couple of villages; then to several others wiping the first ones out. Despite evidence that Ebola can spread through the air,[3,5] aerosolized spread could not reconcile large *simultaneous* outbreaks in "fifty-five villages" unless Mark Chatigny and Alfred Hellman, the NCI's experts in viral aerosols, dropped them from airplanes.

> First it killed people who had received injections, and then it moved through families, killing family members, particularly women, who in Africa prepare the dead for burial. It swept through the Yambuku Hospital's nursing staff, killing most of the nurses, and then it hit the Belgian nuns. The first nun to break with Ebola was a midwife who had delivered a stillborn child. . . .[22]

The nun's blood was "flown to a national laboratory in [Antwerp] Belgium," wrote Preston, without mentioning they co-hosted NATO's bioweapons conference in 1970,[23] was one of only four labs that in 1977 reported to maintain "optimum biocontainment facilities." Fort Detrick was not listed, nor was Gallo's lab at the NCI or Bionetics. Only the "Special Pathogens Branch" of the CDC, the "Special Pathogens Unit" at Porton Down, Moscow's Institute of Poliomyelitis and Virus Encephalitides, and Antwerp's Institute de Médecine Tropicale Prince Léopold were listed.[1]

What ever would have possessed the American and British labs to share the word "Special" in their titles? Given the use of the term in the CIA and the military denoted "secret" or "covert," I would have thought they might have avoided the inference.[24]

The "Maximum Leader of Zaire"

According to Preston, not long after the nun's blood was shipped to Europe, the CDC's Special Pathogens Branch director, Dr. Karl M. Johnson (not to be confused with the eccentric "civilian" Eugene Johnson mentioned earlier), "telephoned a friend of his at the English lab, Porton Down" to request a sample of this especially rare blood. And when news of the horrendous outbreak was received at WHO offices in Geneva, the place "went into a full-scale alert. People who were there at the time said that you could feel fear in the hallways, and the director looked like a visibly shaken man. . . ."[25]

By this time, President Mobutu Sese Seko, whom Preston described as the "maximum leader of Zaire," sent his army to the Bumba Zone.

> He stationed soldiers around Ngaliema Hospital with orders to let no one enter or leave except doctors. Much of the medical staff was now under quarantine inside the hospital, but the soldiers made sure that the quarantine was enforced. President Mobutu also ordered army units to seal off Bumba Zone with roadblocks and to shoot anyone trying to come out. Bumba's main link with the outside world was the Congo River. Captains of riverboats had heard about the virus by this time, and they refused to stop their boats anywhere along the length of the river in Bumba, even though people beseeched them from the banks. Then all radio contact with Bumba was lost. No one knew what was happening upriver, who was dying, what the virus was doing. Bumba had dropped off the face of the earth into the silent heart of darkness.[25]

The WHO then made contact with Dr. Johnson who then "became the chief of an international WHO team" that gathered in the capital city of Kinshasa.

Following the orientation, Preston recounted how some of the team flew on to the Bumba region in "President Mobutu's private plane." The prize-winning author described the aircraft as a "C-130 Buffalo troop-transport, an American-made military aircraft that belonged to the Zairean Air Force." He even detailed the plane's interior, noting it had been "equipped with leopard-skin seats, folding beds, and a wet bar, a sort of flying presidential palace that ordinarily took the president and his family on vacations to Switzerland, but now it carried the WHO team into the hot zone, following the Congo River north by east."[26] Given Preston's love for fine detail, I thought it odd he failed to mention Mobutu's plane, along with most of Zaire's military hardware, was a gift from Dr. Kissinger; delivered courtesy of the CIA.[27]

But the most important factor missed in *The Hot Zone* was the turbulent and bizarre relationship between Zaire's supreme dictator and America's premier imperialist, shortly preceding the 1976 Ebola outbreak.

I recalled that in June 1975, after decades of accepting more than $2 billion in aid from Western allies,[28] Mobutu expelled the American ambassador and arrested most of the CIA's Zairian agents, placing some of them under death sentences.[29] My *Africa Diary* search showed that preceding this action, the "maximum leader of Zaire" had "criticized the U.S. for following a passive and sometimes negative policy towards Africa. American leaders," he insinuated, "spoke of all continents in their major speeches except Africa. South Africa's policy of granting independence to small tribes under its control was criminal, he said, because it ensured that the free territories would depend completely on South Africa economically."[30]

Far worse than his open criticism of Western imperialists, however, was Mobutu's legislative response. In February 1975, he issued orders to nationalize all foreign-owned companies. The *Africa Diary* reported:

> Extensive measures of nationalisation, restriction of imports, establishment of agricultural brigades and cooperatives, a ban on religious instruction in schools and the destruction of all faculties of theology are among decisions made recently by the Political Bureau of the MPR. All places connected with the life of President Mobutu Sese Soko have been proclaimed "places of meditation."[31]

"President Mobutu," Azap News Agency reported, had "also declared war on the country's Bourgeoise. . . . Speaking at the opening session of the National Assembly, the President accused functionaries who had used their positions to grow [rich and influence the nation's] commerce. 'It is not tolerable that the 300 colonial families that pillaged Zaire and who we fought should be replaced by 300 Zaire families,' he said."[31]

Then, in a move that would have surely and irrevocably irked the ardent Papal supporters of the SMOM, Mobutu "complained that the walls of schools were decorated with photographs of Pope Paul and crosses while they did not have photographs of the President."

> "Zaire citizens must first know of the man who sacrifices night and day for their happiness before knowing of the Pope and other strangers." He also described Christian religious ceremonies such as Christmas and Ascension Day "as a form of [spiritual] alienation repugnant to the public of Zaire."[31]

Mobutu later denied he wanted "to create a devine [aura] around the presidency by banning religious education."[31] He also denied that the decisions taken by the government were communist inspired. He did announce, though, that he had recently visited China and Russia and that these countries along with North Korea would soon begin "construction of munitions and agricultural machinery plants in Zaire."[31]

Six months later, the CIA was blamed for a failed assassination attempt on Mobutu's life.[32] A year later, Ebola broke out in Nzara along Zaire's northern border. Four months later, the Ebola valley was hit.

Is there any doubt why Mobutu suddenly reestablished ties with Washington, expelled the Soviet and Cuban diplomats from Zaire, and recanted on many of his social taboos?

Chapter 22
The Special Virus Cancer Program

THE next morning, figuring I had learned as much about Marburg as the experts (not including Preston) chose to reveal, I decided to look for the few *Congressional Record* citations I couldn't find in other libraries. This time, with the Davis Library "basement pass" in hand, I approached a tall weighty fellow standing behind the government document librarian's desk.

"Hi. I'm looking for these *Congressional Record* references," I said, pointing to a few computer printouts.

"The *Congressional Record*s are in the basement," he replied in a mildly inconvenienced tone. Then with a stuffy air of library science about him, he added, "I'll have to go down to get you a few at a time."

"I have my own pass," I proudly displayed. "How 'bout if you just show me where to look?"

"Fine. Follow me," he conceded.

I negotiated the department's swinging gate, passed through a set of open doors, and skipped down a flight of stairs in hot pursuit of my guide. As I entered the huge documents room, the librarian, who had gained about ten yards on me, pointed ahead and said, "The *Congressional Record*s are over there."

Then, something very strange happened. Customarily, at least out of courtesy, I would have followed the man. But suddenly I felt myself entering what I can only describe as a "twilight zone." It was as if time and everything else stood still. My intuition told me to turn right. Without hesitating or missing a step I simply obeyed leaving my guide behind.

I had heard of uncommon intuitive leaps that led scientists to make important discoveries. I often used the example of Einstein who explained his theory of relativity ($E=MC^2$) as a breakthrough that came to him during twilight sleep. I suppose, in retrospect, this experience was like that for me—somewhat of an intuitive breakthrough—except I wasn't sleeping.

Instinctively, I was being drawn in another direction; like metal to a distant magnet. I simply went with the force. Concerned my behavior, which must have seemed rude and impulsive, would further inconvenience the librarian, I blurted, "You don't mind if I have a look over here?"

That, along with my abrupt departure, obviously startled him. Stumbling for words, he replied, "You're not going to find anything over there."

Then when he realized my course was set, he half obligingly advised, "That's not how you conduct research. You're likely to miss what it is you're looking for."

"I appreciate that," I said, but clearly paid no heed. I just continued along my merry way down the isle to the source of my beguilement.

The librarian, forced to concede, said, "I'll get your *Congressional Records*." We parted, him leaving me to prove myself wrong.

I wandered auspiciously for about fifteen yards. A voice inside said, "Turn left." I obeyed and then began to slow. My neck suddenly cranked to the left. Instantly and intently my eyes began scanning the unmarked shelves for something I knew would be there. I just wasn't sure what it was. Momentously, my focus turned knee high, and roamed title by title for a treasure. Then, suddenly, there it was. A faded red-covered book with white letters bleeding through. The words *Special Virus Cancer Program* touched my soul.

I grabbed the title in total disbelief. Completely amazed at what had just happened, all I could say was, *"Wow! This is just what I'm looking for!"*

Seconds later, the librarian walked up carrying three volumes of *Congressional Record*'s. "Here's what you wanted," he said as he laid the texts down on a desk. "I'm glad you found what you wanted." Then he turned and walked away.

Still dazed as he disappeared from sight, I returned, "Thanks a lot, I really appreciate your help."

For months, I had read dozens of authors acknowledging the NIH's "Special Virus Cancer Program." Now, here was the book on it (see fig. 22.1).[1] The text, covered the period from 1970 to 1971—the critical period during which I knew Gallo and company had created numerous AIDS-like retroviruses. I thumbed through the 383-page NCI "Progress Report #8" and realized it detailed virtually all the important investigations conducted in support of Nixon's "war on cancer." It identified all the contracting agencies; summarized their grant proposals; and provided the names, addresses, and even telephone numbers of the project directors, officers, and study consultants for the entire operation.

More incredibly, as I turned the pages toward the end of the book, my thumb caught on page 273. There in black and white read "Progress Report on Investigation of Carcinogenesis with Selected Virus Preparations in the Newborn Monkey—Submitted By Bionetics Research Laboratories, Inc.,

A Division of Litton Industries." In it was a summary of "The Inoculation Program," wherein between 1962 and 1971, "a total of 2,274 primates have been inoculated" on behalf of "over 70 investigators in 50 different laboratories throughout the world." Here was documented evidence that Litton Bionetics had not only been involved in the development of AIDS-like, Marburg-like, and Ebola-like viruses, but had been inoculating simian monkeys with these mutant horrors as early as 1962, and had shipped the infected monkeys dead and alive, whole and in parts, to labs around the world—including the ones in which the Marburg and Reston outbreaks occurred.[2]

Without further ado, I raced back upstairs to photocopy what on gross examination appeared to be the essential parts of the DHEW publication. Then, I did the same with its shelf-mate "Progress Report #9."[3] After about an hour of photocopying, I found a chair, sat back, and began to read the volumes from cover to cover. The task ultimately consumed the remaining part of my stay at UNC.

The Special Virus Cancer Program

The Special Virus Cancer Program was introduced by the Program Staff of the Viral Oncology, Etiology Area of the NCI. The finishing touches to the manuscript were added October 24 through 27, 1971, at "the Annual Joint Working Conference, SVCP at the Hershey Medical Center, Hershey, PA.," a location half-way between Bethesda and New York City, and at the same time, I noted, was fairly close to West Point—Merck-town, U.S.A.

The NCI staff explained:

The Viral Oncology Area is responsible for planning and conducting the Institute's program of coordinated research on viruses as etiological agents of cancer. Scientists within this Area not only provide the broad operational management for intramural and collaborative research but also conduct comprehensive investigations on specific animal oncogenic viruses and their interaction with host cells and apply this information to search for viruses which may be etiologically related to the initiation and continuation of human cancer.

Contract supported research is conducted within the Viral Oncology Program under the Special Virus Cancer Program (SVCP) whose primary objectives are: (1) to determine whether viruses comparable to those known to induce cancers of laboratory and domestic animals are causative agents of human cancer, and (2) to develop therapeutic and preventive measures for control of human cancers when such causative agents are found. A detailed history of events leading to the development of the SVCP may be found in previous Annual Reports of the NCI.

Briefly, in 1964, the Congress of the United States provided funds to the NCI for an intensified program in virus-leukemia research because many scientists were convinced that an effort to identify viruses or to detect virus expression in human tumors would contribute to the determination of the etiology of cancer. Using a new planning approach (Convergence Technique), an overall program aimed on the premise that one virus is an indispensable element for the induction (directly or indirectly) of at least one kind of human cancer and that the virus or viral genome persists in the diseased individual. In 1968, the program was enlarged to encompass all types of cancer. The Program plan is reviewed regularly by the Director, NIH; the Director, NCI; the National Cancer Advisory Council; the Scientific Directorate, NCI; and the Etiology Program Management Group, NCI.

During the past seven years, the Institute has developed an effective management program which has made rapid, substantial progress in understanding cancer induction by viruses. The funding level for this Program in fiscal year 1971 has been about $35 million.[4]

The staff proceeded through a lengthy description of the SVCP's organization and management, which they summarized graphically in an organizational chart and list of managers (see fig. 22.2). This was followed by a list of 105 "Consultants to the Special Virus Cancer Program—Fiscal Year 1971." Several doctors whose names I immediately recognized were: David Baltimore, MIT; Mark Chatigny, Naval Biological Laboratories; Leon Dmochowski, M.D., Anderson Hospital and Tumor Institute; Peter Duesberg, University of California, Berkeley; Sidney Farber, Children's Cancer Research Foundation, Boston; Peter Gerone, Fort Detrick, Maryland; Richard Herberling and Seymour Kalter, Southwest Foundation for Research; Maurice Hilleman, Merck Institute for Therapeutic Research; John Landon; Bionetics Research Laboratories; Brian MacMahon, one of my professors at Harvard University; Albert Sabin, Weizman Institute, Rehovot, Israel; and Howard Temin, McArdle Research Laboratory, University of Wisconsin; and last, but not least Erling Jensen of Hazleton Research Laboratories.[5]

SVCP Highlights

Next, "Progress Highlights" of their scientific activities were presented. The majority of highlights focused on Type C viruses which, of course, Gallo's group had manipulated by the dozens. The NCI staff reported

Fig. 22.1. Special Virus Cancer Program Book Cover

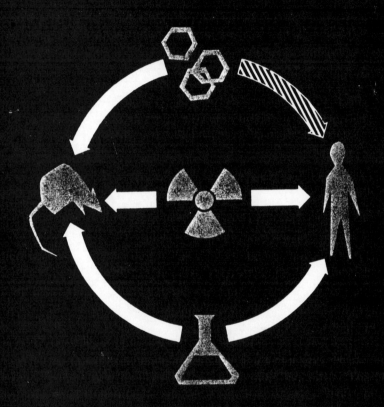

This book was removed by NCI administrators from the Fort Detrick library's catalog. It was discovered by the author serendipitously in the basement of the University of North Carolina Davis Library.

Fig. 22.2. Organizational Chart and Program Managers of the NCI's Special Virus Cancer Program

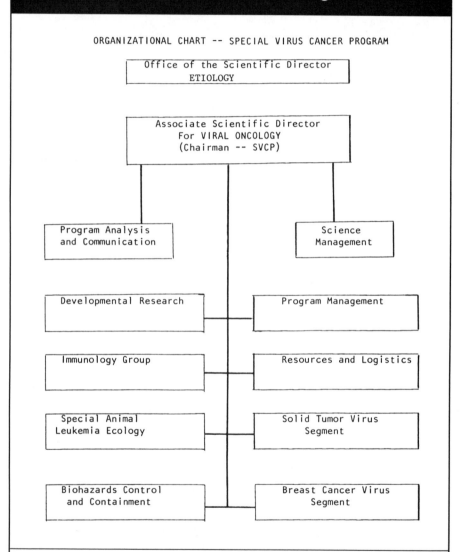

ORGANIZATIONAL CHART -- SPECIAL VIRUS CANCER PROGRAM

Office of the Scientific Director
ETIOLOGY

Associate Scientific Director
For VIRAL ONCOLOGY
(Chairman -- SVCP)

Program Analysis
and Communication

Science
Management

Developmental Research

Program Management

Immunology Group

Resources and Logistics

Special Animal
Leukemia Ecology

Solid Tumor Virus
Segment

Biohazards Control
and Containment

Breast Cancer Virus
Segment

Source: NCI staff. *The Special Virus Cancer Program: Progress Report #8*. Office of the Associate Scientific Director for Viral Oncology (OASDVO). J. B. Moloney, Ed., Washington, D. C.: U. S. Government Printing Office, 1971, pp. 11-14.

PROGRAM MANAGEMENT PERSONNEL

Science Management Team

Dr. J. B. Moloney, Associate Scientific Director for Viral Oncology, NCI
Mr. L. R. Carrese, Deputy Associate Director for Program, NCI
Dr. L. R. Sibal, Associate for Program Coordination, Viral Oncology, NCI
Dr. D. J. Rubin, Scientific Coordinator for Extramural Research, VO, NCI

Administrative Officer, Assistant Administrative Officers and Contract Specialists

Mr. John P. Patterson
        Mr. Nick Olimpio
        Mr. Robert Velthuis
        Mr. J. Thomas Lewin
        Mr. Maurice Fortin
        Mr. Thomas Porter
        Mr. Fred Shaw
        Mr. John Gibbons

Program Segments and Membership

Developmental Research Segment

Dr. Robert Manaker, Chairman
Dr. Jack Gruber, Vice Chairman and Executive Secretary
        Dr. Samuel Dales, Public Health Res Inst., N.Y.C.
        Dr. Paul Gerber, DBS, NIH
        Dr. Anthony Girardi, Wistar Institute
        Dr. Timothy O'Connor, NCI
        Dr. Alan Rabson, NCI
        Dr. Bernard Roizman, University of Chicago
        Dr. Duard Walker, University of Wisconsin
        Dr. Virginia Dunkel, NCI

Special Animal Leukemia Ecology Segment

Dr. Michael Chirigos, Chairman
Dr. John Glynn, Vice Chairman
Dr. George Burton, Executive Secretary
        Dr. Friedrich Deinhardt, Presbyterian St. Luke's Hospital
        Dr. Bernice Eddy, DBS, NIH
        Dr. Charles Rickard, Cornell University
        Dr. William Moloney, Peter Bent Brigham Hospital
        Dr. Mearl Stanton, NCI
        Dr. Peter Vogt, University of Washington
        Dr. David Yohn, Ohio State University
        Dr. Hans Sjogren, Pacific Northwest Research Foundation

12

Solid Tumor Virus Segment

Dr. Robert J. Huebner, Chairman
Dr. James Duff, Vice Chairman
Mrs. Harriet Striecher, Executive Secretary
   Dr. Charles Boone, NCI
   Dr. Maurice Green, St. Louis University
   Dr. Leonard Hayflick, Stanford University
   Dr. Karl Hellstrom, University of Washington
   Dr. Edwin Lennette, Calif. Dept. of Public Health
   Dr. Joseph Melnick, Baylor University
   Dr. Herbert Rapp, NCI
   Dr. Wallace Rowe, NIAID, NIH
   Dr. Hans Meier, Jackson Laboratories

Immunology Group

Dr. Paul Levine
Dr. Herbert Rapp Co-Chairmen
Dr. Ernest Plata, Executive Secretary
   Dr. Charles Boone, NCI
   Dr. Berton Zbar, NCI
   Dr. Tibor Borsos, NCI
   Dr. Ronald Herberman, NCI
   Dr. Maurice Hilleman, Merck Institute
   Dr. Barry Bloom, Einstein College of Medicine
   Dr. Arthur Brown, University of Tennessee
   Dr. George Santos, Johns Hopkins University

Resources and Logistics Segment

Dr. Robert Holdenried, Chairman
Dr. George Todaro, Vice Chairman
Dr. Roy Kinard, Executive Secretary
   Dr. James Duff, NCI
   Dr. K. Arnold Fowler, NCI
   Dr. Adi Gazdar, NCI
   Dr. Paul Levine, NCI
   Miss Marie Purdy, NCI

13

Biohazards Control and Containment Segment

Dr. Alfred Hellman, Chairman
Mr. Emmitt Barkley, Vice Chairman
        Mr. Mark Chatigny, Naval Biological Laboratory
        Dr. Peter Gerone, Fort Detrick
        Dr. Seymour Kalter, Southwest Foundation
        Dr. Maurice Mufson, Hektoen Institute for Medical Research
        Dr. William Payne, Div. of Environmental Health Sciences, NIH
        Dr. Briggs Phillips, Becton-Dickinson
        Dr. Arnold Wedum, Fort Detrick
        Dr. Richard Griesemer, Ohio State University
        Dr. Simon Sulkin, U. of Texas Southwestern Medical School
        Dr. George Michaelsen, University of Minnesota

Human Leukemia Therapy Segment

Dr. Seymour Perry, Chairman
Dr. Edward Henderson, Vice Chairman

Breast Cancer Virus Studies Segment

Dr. W. Ray Bryan, Chairman
Dr. Robert Depue, Vice Chairman
Dr. H. J. Clausen, Executive Secretary
        Dr. Louis R. Sibal, NCI
        Dr. Ernest Plata, NCI
        Dr. Harish Chopra, NCI
        Dr. J. R. Fraumeni, NCI
        Dr. Richard Bates, NCI
        Dr. E. Vollmer, NCI
        Dr. M. Black, New York Medical College, N.Y.C.
        Dr. M. Brennan, Michigan Cancer Foundation
        Dr. K. DeOme, University of California, Berkeley
        Dr. W. Feller, Georgetown University
        Dr. R. Gilden, Flow Laboratories
        Dr. D. Moore, Institute for Medical Research

Program Management Segment

Dr. J. B. Moloney, Chairman
Dr. L. R. Sibal, Executive Secretary
        Dr. W. Ray Bryan, NCI   Dr. Robert Manaker, NCI
        Dr. A. J. Dalton, NCI   Dr. Deward Waggoner, NCI
        Dr. James Duff, NCI   Dr. Robert Holdenried, NCI
        Dr. Michael Chirigos, NCI   Dr. George Todaro, NCI
        Dr. Robert Huebner, NCI

14

"There are now over 100 viruses which are known to cause virtually all kinds of cancer in every major group of animals including nonhuman primates."

Viruses of one (Type C) are known to cause leukemias, lymphomas, and sarcomas in chickens, mice, and cats. Particles, which closely resemble Type C viruses, can be found in human patients affected with these same kinds of cancers.

. . . By using techniques developed from animal tumor virus studies, every effort is being made to determine whether these viruses cause human malignancies. . . . Some important new discoveries that have been made are: (1) Certain oncogenic viruses are unable to produce malignancies unless a "helper" virus is present [such as EBV], thus suggesting that an interplay exists between two viruses. (2) Certain tumor-inducing chemicals, irradiation, (carcinogens) may act as cofactors in activating latent, oncogenic viruses within cells. [This dovetailed what Peter Duesberg had argued with regard to AIDS.6] (3) Certain tumor viruses contain unique enzymes which are required in the replication of viruses in cells [exactly what Gallo and coworkers from Litton Bionetics had been studying with the reverse transcriptase enzyme]. These and other important developments will be discussed further in this report.5

Type C Particles

When the Special Virus Cancer Program was initiated, highest priority was given to the search for human leukemia viruses resembling the Type C viruses causing chicken and mouse leukemias. Since that time, many Type C viruses, the total is now about 85, have been found in a variety of tumors from many species of two vertebrate classes. All of these species continue to be studied intensively under the broader scope of the Special Virus Cancer Program. Several of the Type C viruses are established as the causative agents in leukemias, lymphomas, and sarcomas of chickens, mice, cats and hamsters. Many of these can infect and produce malignancies in other species (e.g. a sarcoma virus of the cat produces tumors in marmoset monkeys). Furthermore, some of these viruses can cause malignant transformation to occur in animal and human cells grown in the laboratory (e.g. cat leukemia and sarcoma viruses alter embryonic human cells). Type C virus particles have been found in association with malignancies of a spectrum of animal species including nonhuman primates, rats, cattle, wooley monkeys, gibbons, and man. . . .5

After reading this, I reflected on "Gallo's Research Anthology" (see fig. 6.8). I recalled he not only received credit for discovering the first two types of human leukemia viruses, HTLV-I and II, but he published manipulating Type C monkey viruses—he extracted the viruses' nucleic acids, infused their empty envelopes with chicken and cat leukemia/sarcoma RNA, grew the mutants in human WBC cultures, then prompted them to infect human T-lymphocytes and produce the leukemias, sarcomas, general wasting, and essentially all the symptoms of AIDS (see fig. 6.5).7

Creating More AIDS-like Viruses

Under the report's next heading, "Reactions between Type C viruses causing leukemias and sarcomas (solid tumors)," the NCI staff explained how and why they created more AIDS-like viruses:

> When inoculated into appropriate cell cultures, Type C sarcoma viruses of chickens, mice and cats produce foci [cancerous growths] of altered cells. This fundamental discovery provides a readily visible indicator reaction for the detection of sarcoma viruses. On the other hand, leukemia viruses grown in tissue culture do not cause foci or other detectable changes. The finding that leukemia viruses can either inhibit or enhance focus formation by sarcoma viruses of the same species has led to the development of methods for the detection and quantitation of leukemia viruses indirectly.
>
> Certain of the chicken, cat and mouse sarcoma viruses are "defective" in that they do not produce foci in cell cultures or tumors in animals in the absence of a co-infecting, "helper" leukemia virus. [Amazingly, the researchers called carcinogenic viruses "defective" if they were unable to produce cancers without the help of other factors including chemicals, radiation, and here leukemia viruses.] Further, in the presence of a defective sarcoma virus the helper action of leukemia viruses can be used as a specific indicator for their detection and quantitation. It is now believed that defective sarcoma virus–leukemia virus interactions may be more widespread in nature than originally thought and that similar systems may be found in man. A mouse leukemia virus which has been adapted to grow in human cells is now available to search for defective human sarcoma viruses, if they exist.[8]

In other words, humans would eventually be inoculated with mouse leukemia viruses in an effort to locate inactive human sarcoma viruses. Like the BLV experiments Strecker described in cows, here humans were to become the "mixers" for mutant leukemia and sarcoma viruses.

Here, in almost lay terms, the NCI staff described their greatest accomplishment in 1971 was to produce AIDS-like viruses for pre-cancer diagnosis. In continuing this effort, they reported an "alternative approach" had been developed for the detection of possible human leukemia viruses:

> A defective mouse sarcoma virus and its leukemia virus helper can be made to form tight functional aggregates, which behave as one virus. Using a mixture of mouse sarcoma virus and cat leukemia virus, a hybrid aggregate which could be grown continuously in cat cells was produced. [Again, this is exactly what Gallo reported.[7]] Because the aggregate is defective, it requires the simultaneous presence of a cat leukemia virus for producing altered foci in cat

cells. Thus, a focus forming sarcoma virus of the mouse, artificially changed to one possessing infectivity for cat cells, can now be used in cultures for the detection of cat leukemia viruses.

This hybrid virus, as well as the cat leukemia virus, will also grow in human embryonic cells in tissue culture. If sufficient amounts of the Type C particles found in association with human leukemia can be obtained, the possibility exists that the cat-adapted mouse sarcoma virus can be hybridized with the human agent to produce an indicator system for the detection of human leukemia viruses.[8] Fig. 22.3 presents a graphic description of this work.

Litton's Group in Uganda

The NCI staff went on to explain how Type C virus particles can get into the genes of normal cells and cause them to develop cancer. Then they discussed in great detail, the enzyme that represented "a dramatic breakthrough" in the investigation of cancer. Without naming Gallo, they discussed his explicit area of expertise—RNA-dependent DNA polymerase—and explained, as Gallo had in numerous publications, the "biochemical pathways of tumor virus infection and replication."

> Intensive investigations have now revealed polymerase activity in cells of patients with acute lymphoblastic leukemia; more preliminary evidence has shown the enzyme is in cells of sarcomas, Burkitt's lymphoma and breast cancer. Since the RNA-dependent DNA polymerase is apparently always present in the RNA tumor viruses of animals, its discovery in the human tumor cells offers good supportive evidence that viruses are associated with cancers in man. The RNA-dependent DNA polymerase of human leukemia cells is inhibited by a drug, n-dementhyl rifampicin [which Gallo had received from another documented Nazi employer and biological weapons contractor, Dow Chemical Company, and which he subsequently studied and reported on,[9] and] which also inhibits the enzyme activity found in the Type C RNA tumor viruses of animals. Studies are underway [principally in Gallo's lab] to explore the action of this drug and the various modifications of it. These investigations could provide new approaches to the treatment of malignancies in man.[8]

Following a shorter review of Type B viruses thought to be associated with breast cancer, and Herpes-type viruses "associated with some forms of chronic leukemia, lymphoma and postnasal carcinoma . . ." the NCI staff focused on EBV. Their program, they said, had studied the significance of Epstein-Barr viruses extracted from Burkitt's lymphomas and postnasal carcinomas "through the International Agency for Research on Cancer (IARC) in the West Nile District of Uganda." This, of course, was close to where Preston noted AIDS, Marburg, Ebola, and Reston viruses were be-

Fig. 22.3. A Technique Devised by NCI Researchers Including Robert Gallo as an Alternative Approach for the Detection of Possible Human Leukemia Viruses

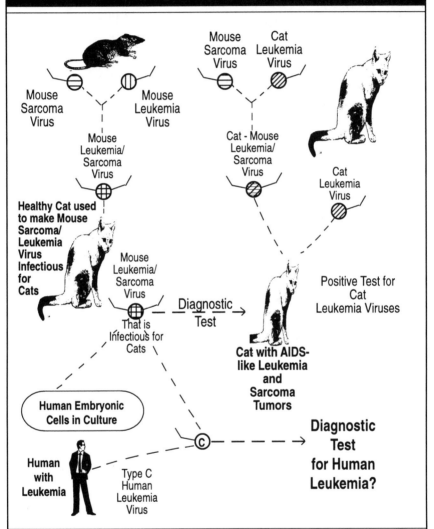

A bizarre series of cancer research experiments in which numerous leukemia and sarcoma viruses from cats and mice were mixed to produce a variety of mutants. One such virus infectious for cats was cultured in human embryonic cells to develop a diagnostic test for human leukemia. Source: NCI staff. *The Special Virus Cancer Program: Progress Report #8.* Office of the Associate Scientific Director for Viral Oncology (OASDVO). J. B. Moloney, Ed., Washington, DC.: U.S. Government Printing Office, 1971, p. 22.

lieved to have originated. The purpose of the NCI/NARC collaborative effort was "to determine the feasibility of further studies on EBV in relation to Burkitt's tumor. . . ." Also mentioned was the fact that "EBV infection has been associated with the development of infectious mononucleosis in young adults, a disease with the attributes of a self-limiting leukemia."[10]

Now it all seemed to fit. Gallo's group at Litton Bionetics, unlike any other, had performed the core services needed during the SVCP for the NCI to achieve its principle goals. Not only had Litton Bionetics been contracted to "manage the operations of the [entire] National Cancer Institute's Frederick (Md.) Cancer Research Center, including more than 750 scientists and support personnel,"[11] but here was evidence they ran the show in the West Nile District of Uganda as well. Reflecting on what I had just read about Litton Bionetics being the world's principal supplier of monkeys during the 1960s and early 1970s (see the first four grant summaries in fig. 22.5),[2] they obviously maintained a facility in this area—close to where OTRAG operated. Thus, I realized, the unnamed animal supplier who sent Marburg-infected monkeys to Europe was *undoubtedly* Litton Bionetics.

Moreover, I knew Gallo had worked with EBV to make his retroviruses grow faster. I was certain he knew his cell lines needed to be free of EBV lest they continue to mass produce retroviruses.[12] But here was the most damning evidence that the entire French–American fracas was a farce—truly a distraction. This document proved that Gallo's group was intimately involved in EBV studies simultaneously in Bethesda and Uganda, which would also explain how Litton Bionetics ended up with the patent on the mononucleosis blood test.[13]

Into the Future With OTRAG and Gallo

Next, the report provided their "projections" of how their research would be developed or expanded into the future. "Human studies," they wrote, would be expanded   "to identify viruses or detect virus expressions in human tumors . . . [and] to search for candidate viruses or subviral products which induce human malignancies. . . ." Such studies were desired:

> (1) To identify and isolate candidate viruses or subviral products in leukemias, lymphomas and sarcomas.
>
> (2) To identify and isolate candidate viruses or subviral products in breast, lung and other carcinomas.
>
> (3) To develop methods for the detection of high cancer risk groups, i.e., individual susceptibility of predisposition to transformation by human viruses.

(4) To develop suitable reagents for mass diagnostic screening for candidate viruses.

(5) To characterize, biologically and biochemically, presumptive viral agents.

(6) To increase emphasis on understanding the relationship of environmental agents (e.g. chemical carcinogens) as cofactors in viral carcinogenesis. This represents a major expansion of effort requiring combined efforts of the Viral Oncology and Chemical Carcinogenesis Areas.[14]

This later function was one Litton Bionetics's chief revenue producing specialties.

The SVCP's projections regarding future "Molecular Studies," which again was Dr. Gallo's forte, and their "Immunological Studies" in which Hilleman, Krugman, and Poeisz majored were summarized next (see fig. 22.4).

Next, the SVCP "Summary Reports" reviewed progress which had been made in every working group. In this section, the staff disclosed the principal researchers directing each group and area of investigation.

Under another heading "Other Research Developments" in the Viral Leukemia and Lymphoma Branch, the staff described a variety of viral experiments, including those using Epstein-Barr, cat leukemia/sarcoma, and monkey leukemia/lymphoma/sarcoma viruses. Here they announced a major breakthrough:

> Herpes saimiri is a DNA containing virus indigenous to the squirrel monkey. Recent studies have shown that this virus will induce acute lymphocytic leukemias as well as lymphomas and reticulum cell sarcomas in owl monkeys and marmosets. This is the first demonstration that a virus produces leukemia and lymphomas in primates and may serve as an important model for human leukemia and lymphoma.[15]

This disclosure obviously foreshadowed the announcement made almost ten years later by Gallo that he had discovered HTLV-I, a leukemia virus he identified as the cause of T-cell leukemia in Japan.

I thus wondered whether HTLV-I had been developed by Gallo and company during the early 1970s as part of the SVCP. HTLV-I, like HIV and the Marburg viruses, may have then been accidentally released or *deployed* to initiate the Japanese epidemic for which Gallo could later claim the discovery of its etiologic agent. This would put a new spin on what Shilts described as "something of a backward scientific affair," I realized.[16] In fact, the entire HTLV-I saga, in light of this evidence, was reasonably a possible pilot study or model for the AIDS epidemic a decade later.

Fig. 22.4. A Description of the Molecular and Immunological Studies Conducted During the NCI's Special Virus Cancer Program

Molecular Studies

In recent months rapid major advances have been made in the field of molecular biology. These findings have direct application to the study of the relationship of viruses to tumors. There is evidence that the genetic material (RNA) of the tumor viruses can direct the synthesis of new DNA. The demonstration that RNA tumor viruses contain enzymes (polymerase, ligase) which may be required for viral infection, interaction with host cell genome, and viral replication has provided the basis for the development of new, extremely sensitive methods for the detection of oncogenic viruses or their "fingerprints." Indeed, knowledge of the fundamental molecular events which occur during virus infection and subsequent cell transformation provides the first truly rational approach to therapy. Enzyme activities analogous to those of RNA tumor viruses have recently been found in cells of human leukemics. This offers strong supportive evidence that viruses are associated with cancers in man.

a. **Basic studies**

The Program is prepared to broaden its activities for identifying and characterizing the spectrum of enzymes (and other mediators) required by tumor viruses for replication and transformation.

b. **Applied studies**

As knowledge of the fundamental molecular events in virus-cell interactions is developed, the Program will apply this information to the study of human cancer as follows:

(1) To identify and characterize similar enzymes or enzymatic activities within normal and malignant human cells.

(2) To develop highly sensitive methods for the detection of virus or virus activity in human cells.

(3) To develop a rational basis for therapy or prevention by exploring various approaches to blocking of viral replication and/or tumorigenesis at the cellular and subcellular levels. The therapy could be directed at any or all of the stages of cell transformation beginning with cell infection by a tumor virus.

Ultimately these studies will require an exhaustive effort to develop drugs, anti-enzymes, gene repressors or inhibitors effective at the molecular level.

3. Immunological Studies

    Immunologic research has provided extremely sensitive techniques for detection and characterization of tumor viruses, viral antigens, and changes in surface membranes of tumor cells. Indeed, such efforts have contributed to an understanding of the role of immunological mechanisms in host-tumor and host-virus interactions which provide an approach to the prevention and treatment of cancer.

    a. Basic studies. Investigations of selected model systems, representing tumors induced by Type C, Type B, and Herpes-type viruses, will be extended to further identify, characterize and determine the viruses, viral antigens, and membrane antigens of tumor cells. This includes development and application of improved techniques with the sensitivity and specificity required to detect cellular alterations induced by tumor viruses alone or as the result of interaction with other environmental agents (e.g. chemicals, irradiation). Efforts will be increased to develop similar immunological methods and diagnostic reagents for application to human cancer. Research will be intensified and expanded:

        (1) To study cellular and humoral immune mechanisms and to determine their relative significance in host recognition of and response to tumor and/or tumor viruses.

        (2) To develop methods to enhance host response to tumor or virus antigens.

    Increasing emphasis will be directed toward research on spontaneous or naturally occurring tumors in model systems relevant to human cancer. These studies would provide the basis for a rational approach to prevention (vaccines) and treatment (immunotherapy) of cancer.

    b. Applied studies. Basic research will provide the framework for identification and characterization of viruses, viral antigens, and cell membrane alterations in human cancers. Immunological methods and reagents will be developed and applied:

29

417

(1) To relate candidate human viruses to known oncogenic agents.

(2) To identify and characterize interspecies viral antigens which are present in known mammalian tumors, and therefore, could provide the basis for a formidable probe to detect human tumor viruses or viral antigens.

(3) To launch large-scale seroepidemiological surveys which will define high risk populations.

(4) To determine the presence of cross-reacting antigens in various human tumors.

Clinical studies will be directed toward understanding and manipulation of immune mechanisms in human cancer as a basis for:

(1) Development of vaccines from identified and fully-characterized human tumor virus (es).

(2) Determination of the role of host immune responses in tumor recognition and rejection.

(3) Application of (1) and (2) in the prevention and control of human cancer.

As research progresses, increased emphasis on application will be as follows:

(1) Immunodiagnosis and seroepidemiology
(2) Clinical studies on the role of immune mechanisms in human cancer
(3) Immunotherapy
(4) Vaccines (conventional or other)

Ultimately, these studies would be organized to coordinate and integrate the application of appropriate biochemical, immunological, and genetic methods of detection, prevention, and control of various types of human cancer.

4. Test Systems

In vitro and in vivo (animal) test systems will be carefully selected to evaluate the work outlined in the previous research areas; specifically: (a) to determine the oncogenic potential of candidate human viruses; (b) to develop bioassay systems for testing viral, and viral/chemical carcinogens; (c) to begin vaccine (conventional or other) testing and immunization programs; (d) to begin therapy testing programs; and (e) to explore special animal tumor systems with particular relevance to human cancer.

30

Source: NCI staff. *The Special Virus Cancer Program: Progress Report #8.* Office of the Associate Scientific Director for Viral Oncology (OASDVO). J. B. Moloney, Ed., Washington, D. C.: U. S. Government Printing Office, 1971, pp. 28-30.

A Cat Owner's Nightmare

Another paragraph dealt with cat owners and AIDS-like diseases in cats. Having studied feline leukemia/sarcoma viruses, the staff reported, "About one and one-half years ago, a nationwide effort was initiated to obtain cancerous cats (primarily leukemias and sarcomas) from cat breeders and owners." The NCI put out a nationwide call "for materials and cancerous purebred cats with pedigrees." Letters were "sent to cat owners soliciting cats with veterinarian-diagnosed cancers."[15]

The authors wrote, "The procurement effort not only obtains valuable research material but reassures the cat owners and other concerned citizens of NCI's active program for the evaluation of the unlikely hazard of this disease to human health."[15]

How ironic, I thought, the NCI was spending hundreds of millions of taxpayer dollars to prove that animals, including cats and monkeys, were potential reservoirs for cancer viruses at the same time they assured people that it was safe to handle these animals. Then, even more bizarre, was the fact that as pet owners supplied the NCI with experimental cat viruses, the researchers engineered them to cause cancer in humans.

Apparently, I realized, cancer virus-infected animals posed less of a risk to the public's health than did the NCI.

Filling in the Missing Pieces

The staff continued to describe dozens of studies in which "special viruses" were bioengineered in order to identify more viruses, develop a better understanding of cancers, and produce potential experimental vaccines. A list of 120 contracts given to a couple dozen SVCP contractors was provided in this section.[17] Their "TABLE II" included each contractor's name, telephone number, and project title. "Contract Summaries" followed this list. Fig. 22.5 provides selected reports from this section including those of: Bionetics Research Laboratories, Inc.;[18] Merck and Company, Inc.;[19] Public Health Research Institute of the City of New York;[20] the University of California;[21] and Hazleton Research Labs (also spelled "Hazelton" in the same government document).[22]

These SVCP contract summary reports filled in many of the gaps in the knowledge I had concerning the relationships between the various suspects and their activities. For instance, Gallo's boss, Robert Manaker was commonly cited as the chief of the Viral Biology Branch and Chairman of the

Etiology Area for the entire SVCP. Dr. Roy Kinard served as vice chairman until March 2, 1971, and Dr. Jack Gruber, who reviewed the vast majority of contracts carried the title of executive secretary under Manaker.[23] Manaker and Gruber administered the Merck and Company, Inc. project entitled, "Research on Oncogenic and Potentially Oncogenic Viruses, Large-scale Virus Production and Vaccine Development" directed by Maurice Hilleman. Manaker was the principal "Project Officer" on the contract as well as the "Segment Chairman."[19] He was also the NCI's project officer for Hazleton Laboratories "Studies on the Etiology of Canine Cancer."

Surely Preston would love to see this, I thought facetiously, as I read that Hazleton not only supplied the NCI with viruses, but they conducted virtually the same experiments that Gallo had performed on monkeys using dogs. Their summary report in fig. 22.5 showed they innoculated dogs, "kittens," and mice with leukemia and sarcoma viruses in a failed attempt to develop vaccines for "immunotherapeutic" control of "naturally occurring" cancers in humans.[22]

A Bionetics contract summary disclosed that Dr. John Landon served as the director of Litton Bionetics along with David Valerio and Robert Ting. Ting had co-authored numerous Gallo research publications. The SVCP report noted that Gallo served as an NCI "Project Officer" overseeing several Bionetics contracts, and that Gruber and Kinard shared this responsibility with Gallo[18] (see also fig. 22.5).

This report confirmed that Bionetics and Merck had co-investigated African green monkeys, and both had challenged them with the Australia antigen associated with hepatitis B transmission. Both companies were involved in the research that led to the development of Merck's infamous hepatitis B vaccine, most plausibly responsible for spreading AIDS throughout the world.[19]

While reading the SVCP progress reports, many of my grimmest suspicions proved to be true. For instance, the Merck and Company contract gave for its "proposed course":

> The investigators will devote initial efforts to developing methods for propagation, purification, concentration and specific quantitation of candidate viruses suspected or shown to cause cancer in man. At the present time, investigations will be focused upon herpes-type (DNA) viruses and "B" and "C" type (RNA) particles [that is, the viruses known to cause lymphomas, leukemias, sarcomas, general immune suppression and wasting—all commonly associated with AIDS]. Parallel studies to evolve live attenuated and killed

virus vaccines in appropriate animal model systems will be conducted. Particular attention will be given to developing and applying optimal methods for viral attenuation, viral inactivation, viral quantitation, vaccine safety assessment, and vaccine potency assay.[19]

Thus, in 1971, Merck's research agenda (NIH contract 71-2059)[19] completely overlapped Bionetics work (contract NIH contract 71-2025)[18]—a highly incriminating fact which might best explain both the rapid spread of HIV following Merck vaccine trials, as well as the simultaneous AIDS outbreaks in Central Africa and New York City.

Additionally incriminating in this regard was another Bionetics contract that called for the company to supply "Support Services for the Special Virus Cancer Program" (NIH contract 69-2160).[24] The Litton group was paid not only to supply monkeys and biochemical testing reagents to other research groups, including those at Merck, but also to compare and manipulate AIDS-like viruses in Africa and America simultaneously.[24] Begun on June 27, 1969, and completed within a year, their work evaluated EBV levels in blood taken from "American patients with Burkitt's lymphoma and age- and sex-matched patients with acute lymphocytic leukemia, African Burkitt lymphoma, and nonmalignant diseases." At the same time, in the same study, to complete the Bionetics contract, NCI officer Bassin and his co-worker Dr. Pienta were "to rescue and isolate" viruses from "undifferentiated sarcomas" from human patients "by co-cultivation, hybridization, and other techniques."[24]

Just as I theorized, had OTRAG assisted in the development or testing of AIDS-like viruses, they would have received their experimental reagents and animals from Litton Bionetics.

Adjacent this Bionetics research report was one coded NIH 71-2149. Here $75,000 a year went to the Massachusetts Institute of Technology (MIT) for essentially identical "Studies on RNA-Dependent DNA Polymerase" on which Gallo's teams had reported. The project director, David Baltimore, the researcher Strecker had accurately cited as a pioneer of the work Gallo made famous, and NCI officer/Bionetics overseer George Todaro, performed this series of studies to identify the genetic codes in cancer viruses that enabled them to cause human tumors. This work, the progress report stated, had been given the "highest priority in the SVCP" (see fig. 22.6).

Another contract of interest was "The Production of Simian Viruses and Homologous Antisera" (NIH 69-93) directed by Seymour Kalter from the Southwest Foundation for Research and Education. (see final contract in fig. 22.5). Here, the summary revealed, Kalter's group served as quality control experts for the NCI's chief monkey virus suppliers, principally Litton Bionetics. In addition, Kalter was responsible for diagnosing the "viral isolates that may emerge from studies done. . . ." In other words, as new forms of mutant monkey viruses emerged from Bionetics and other labs, Kalter diagnosed what kind of bugs they were, and what they might be expected to do in monkeys and man.

I suddenly realized where the phrase "emerging viruses" came from.

In summary, I realized this SVCP report documented three frightening facts: (1) the Litton and Merck network of researchers undoubtedly produced an array of AIDS-like viruses under these contracts alone; (2) such work was ongoing at the time Merck hepatitis B vaccine studies were being conducted in New York and Africa under Krugman and Hilleman, these men shared their information and resources; and, most alarming, (3) Robert Gallo's affiliates at Litton Bionetics supplied the experimental viruses and monkeys—both infected and uninfected—to NCI and Merck researchers in Bethesda, Central Africa, New York, and Pennsylvania. Therefore, had either one infected monkey, or a bit of monkey-virus-contaminated material, been used to develop one batch of experimental hepatitis B vaccine, in any one of their labs, this alone might explain the origin of AIDS and the epidemic's simultaneous emergence in New York and Central Africa during the late 1970s.

BIONETICS RESEARCH LABORATORIES (NIH-69-2160)

Title: Support Services for the Special Virus Cancer Program.

Contractor's Project Director: Dr. Robert C. Y. Ting

Project Officer (NCI): Dr. George Todaro

Objectives: To provide a laboratory that will collect, process and test specimens from human and animal sources suspected of containing virus associated antigens or antibodies, and to provide other virology, immunology or cell culture services as required.

Major Findings: Services and resources provided in close collaboration with NCI investigators during the past year include: (1) biochemical studies of cell growth regulation with Dr. Todaro; (2) attempts to isolate a human cancer virus with Dr. Bassin; (3) tests for EBV antigens for Dr. Levine; (4) immunological tests of leukemia patients, including studies of twins, for Dr. Levine; (5) CF tests for gs antigens for Dr. Hellman; (6) membrane antigen preparation from human tissue for Dr. Herberman; (7) collection of familial cancer sera and histories for Dr. Fraumeni; (8) tissue and serum bank for Dr. Levine et al; (9) American Burkitt registry and follow-up; and (10) data processing with Dr. Waggoner.

When abortively transformed cells containing SV40 genome were re-infected with SV40, they had a lower rate of transformation than cells without the genome; thus, the presence of SV40 did not confer immunity.

Fetal thymus cells of dogs were cocultivated with irradiated human sarcoma cells. The dog cells showed degeneration and transformation (chromosome analysis now being done).

Rhesus cell cultures infected with Mason-Pfizer virus showed evidence of transformation and caused regressing tumors when subsequently inoculated into newborn rhesus monkeys.

Cellular immunity studies of leukemia patients, using lymphocyte cytotoxicity and cytotoxicity inhibition tests, suggest that cells of such patients possess leukemia-associated antigens and that a widespread antigen system may be operative in human and animal tumors.

Significance to Biomedical Research and the Program of the Institute: This contract laboratory provides an opportunity for a systematic,

326

large-scale effort to detect viruses and/or viral antigens in human tumor materials (particularly leukemias and sarcomas), using tissue culture, immunological, biochemical and EM techniques. This is a major objective of the SVCP.

Proposed Course: It is proposed that this contract will continue to supply the necessary supportive services required to meet the needs of the SVCP.

Date Contract Initiated: June 27, 1969

Current Contract Level: $800,000

327

Date Contract Initiated: March 1, 1971

BIONETICS RESEARCH LABS., INC. (NIH 69-2160)

Title: Support Services for SVCP

Contractor's Project Director: Dr. Robert Ting

Project Officers (NCI):   Dr. George Todaro
                          Dr. Paul Levine
                          Dr. Robert Bassin

Objectives: To provide a laboratory that will collect, process and test cancer specimens from human and animal sources suspected of containing virus associated antigens.

Major Findings: EBV studies were carried out under the supervision of Dr. Paul Levine.   One study initiated and completed during this year was a seroepidemiological study comparing EBV titers in American patients with Burkitt's lymphoma and age-and sex-matched patients with acute lymphocytic leukemia, African Burkitt lymphoma, and non-malignant diseases.   The African Burkitt sera were significantly higher than the American Burkitt sera ($P < 0.005$).   The role of EBV in human lymphoma was evaluated by immunological techniques detecting humoral and cellular immunity to the virus.   The importance of careful clinical evaluation was emphasized by a study of twenty American patients with Burkitt's lymphoma and age and sex matched controls.   Treatment and prognosis correlated with EBV titers in both lymphoma and leukemia patients, indicating that seroepidemiological studies which include single samples on a patient may be misleading.   The studies clearly demonstrated that American patients with Burkitt's lymphoma, although their histopathology is indistinguishable from African patients, have different immune patterns to EBV.

Five individuals with low titers to EBV who were identified on an earlier study of Hodgkins disease were followed over a three year period.   Half the patients developed high titers while the other half maintained low titers.

A study of leukemia in identical twins was initiated to determine whether an antigen could be detected in the cells of a leukemia twin which would not be identified in his normal HLA identical twin.   Leukemia-associated antigens were detected in four of the seven families studied to date using the lymphocyte cytotoxicity test.   In the animal system, this test is positive only when the lymphocytes are presensitized by an antigen, so that the reactivity of the family members against

187

the leukemic patient's cells but not against the normal twin's cells suggest that an environmental agent, perhaps a virus, is present.

Sera from 43/102 (42%) of breast cancer patients had antibodies to BeLev antigens. Sera from 29% of patient's with sarcomas had detectable antibodies, whereas, 13% of patients with benign breast diseases and 3.6% of normal blood bank donors reacted.

Significance to Biomedical Research and the Program of the Institute: Provides opportunity for systematic, large-scale effort to detect viruses or viral antigens in human or animal materials using tissue culture, immunological, biochemical and EM techniques. This is a major objective of the SVCP.

Proposed Course: Although this contract will continue to supply necessary supportive services to SVCP, the workscope has recently been divided into three major areas, each being co-directed by a senior investigator at Bionetics and an NCI project officer. Drs. Rein and Todaro will attempt to isolate, characterize, and purify the factor(s) in serum which overcome contract inhibition and regulate the growth of normal and transformed 3T3 cells in culture. Drs. Pienta and Bassin will attempt to rescue and isolate a viral genome in undifferentiated sarcomas from untreated patients by co-cultivation, hybridization, and other techniques. Drs. Levine and Ting will continue studies to detect tumor specific antigens in patients with leukemia, lymphoma and breast cancer. In the leukemia studies, special emphasis will be placed on testing patients who have an identical twin; in the lymphoma studies, the serums of patients in selected disease groups will be tested for antibodies to EBV.

Date Contract Initiated: June 27, 1969

188

426

BIONETICS RESEARCH LABORATORIES, INC. (NIH-71-2025)

Title: Investigations of Viral Carcinogenesis in Primates

Contractor's Project Directors: Dr. John Landon
                                Dr. David Valerio
                                Dr. Robert Ting

Project Officers (NCI): Dr. Roy Kinard
                        Dr. Jack Gruber
                        Dr. Robert Gallo

Objectives: (1) Evaluation of long-term oncogenic effects of human and
animal viral inocula in primates of various species, especially newborn
macaques; (2) maintenance of monkey breeding colonies and laboratories
necessary for inoculation, care and monitoring of monkeys; and (3)
biochemical studies of transfer RNA under conditions of neoplastic transformation and studies on the significance of RNA-dependent DNA polymerase in
human leukemic tissues.

Major Findings: This contractor continues to produce over 300 excellent
newborn monkeys per year. This is made possible by diligent attention to
reproductive physiological states of female and male breeders. Semen
evaluation, artifical insemination, vaginal cytology and ovulatory drugs
are used or tried as needed.

Inoculated and control infants are hand-fed and kept in modified germ-free
isolators. They are removed from isolators at about 8 weeks of age and
placed in filtered air cages for months or years of observation. The holding
area now contains approximately 1200 animals up to 5 years old. Approximately
300 are culled every year at a rate of about 25 per month. This is necessary
to make room for young animals inoculated with new or improved virus preparations.

During the past year macaques were inoculated at birth or in utero with the
Mason-Pfizer monkey mammary virus, Epstein-Barr virus, Herpesvirus saimiri,
and Marek's disease virus. EB virus was given with immunostimulation and
immunosuppression (ALS, prednisone, imuran). Australia antigen was given
to newborn African green monkeys.

The breeding and holding colonies were surveyed for antibody to EBV. All
breeders were positive and their offspring contain maternal antibody for
several months. Colony-born offspring that have lost maternal antibody
and are sero-negative will be surveyed periodically for conversion to the
EB positive state.

An RNA-dependent DNA polymerase similar to that associated with RNA tumor
viruses was detected in human leukemic cells but not in normal cells stimulat
by phytohemagglutinin. The enzyme was isolated, purified and concentrated
200-fold, making possible its further characterization and study in relation
to the leukemic process in man.

Significance to Biomedical Research and to the Program of the Institute:
Inasmuch as tests for the biological activity of candidate human viruses will
not be tested in the human species, it is imperative that another system
be developed for these determinations and, subsequently for the evaluation
of vaccines or other measures of control. The close phylogenetic relationship of the lower primates to man justifies utilization of these animals for
these purposes. Further study of altered transfer RNA and polymerase
enzymes would determine their significance in neoplastic change and provide
a basis for selection of therapeutic agents.

Proposed Course: Continuation with increased emphasis on monitoring and
intensive care of inoculated animals to determine if active infection occurs,
effects of infection, and degree of immunosuppression when used. Further
studies of human neoplasms at a molecular level will continue.

Date Contract Initiated: February 12, 1962.

BIONETICS RESEARCH LABORATORIES, INC. (NIH 71-2025)

Title: Investigations of Viral Carcinogenesis in Primates

Contractor's Project Director: Dr. Harvey Rabin

Project Officers (NCI): Dr. Roy Kinard
Dr. Jack Gruber
Dr. Gary Pearson

Objectives: (1) Evaluation of long-term oncogenic effects of human and animal viral inocula in primates of various species, especially newborn macaques; (2) maintenance of monkey breeding colonies and laboratories necessary for inoculation, care and monitoring of monkeys; and (3) biochemical studies of transfer RNA under conditions of neoplastic transformation and studies on the significance of RNA-dependent DNA polymerase in human leukemic tissues.

Major Findings: This contractor continues to produce over 300 excellent newborn monkeys per year. This is made possible by diligent attention to reproductive physiological states of female and male breeders. Semen evaluation, artifical insemination, vaginal cytology and ovulatory drugs are used or tried as needed.

Inoculated and control infants are hand-fed and kept in modified germ-free isolators. They are removed from isolators at about 8 weeks of age and placed in filtered air cages for months or years of observation. The holding area now contains approximately 1200 animals up to 5 years old. Approximately 300 are culled every year at a rate of about 25 per month. This is necessary to make room for young animals inoculated with new or improved virus preparations.

New importance is being given to the New World species of monkeys, including squirrel, marmoset, and spider monkeys. Animals currently on study are being actively culled to reflect this change.

Special emphasis has been placed on virological studies characterizing the Mason-Pfizer monkey virus (M-PMV). Seven sublines established from chronically M-PMV-infected rhesus foreskin cultures were shown to be releasing moderately high titers of infectious M-PMV, and in addition seemed to have undergone in vitro transformation. Inoculation of cells of these sublines into newborn rhesus monkeys produced palpable masses at the sites of inoculation. Biopsies performed on these masses and on the regional lymph nodes of the same animals revealed the presence of proliferating virus character-istic of M-PMV by both electron microscopic and cell culture

195

analysis. Proliferating M-PMV was found in the lymph nodes of monkeys inoculated with cell-free M-PMV preparations.

Chromatographic examination of transfer RNA's (tRNA's) from control and virus-transformed rat and mouse embryo cells demonstrated differences in phenyl-alanyl-tRNA's and aspartyl-tRNA's. No differences were noted in the elution profiles of seryl-, tyrosyl-, leucyl-, asparaginyl-, or glutaminyl-tRNA.

The effects of 11 rifamycin derivatives on viral reverse transcriptase and on DNA polymerases from human normal and leukemic blood lymphocytes were evaluated. Compound 143-483, 3-formyl rifamycin SV: octyl oxime showed the greatest potency and inhibited all DNA polymerases from both viral and cellular origins.

The contractor also engaged in collaborative studies involving the oncornavirus, RD-114, from a human sarcoma, isolated by Drs. McAllister, Gardiner, and Huebner. The virus is being produced and supplied by Dr. Gilden of Flow Laboratories. Another virus, a human papovavirus associated with progressive multifocal leukoencephalopathy, is being supplied by Dr. Duard Walker for inoculation into newborn monkeys.

Significance to Biomedical Research and to the Program of the Institute: Inasmuch as tests for the biological activity of candidate human viruses will not be tested in the human species, it is imperative that another system be developed for these determinations and. subsequently for the evaluation of vaccines or other measures of control. The close phylogenetic relation-ship of the lower primates to man justifies utilization of these animals for these purposes. Further study of altered transfer RNA and polymerase enzymes would determine their significance in neoplastic change and provide a basis for selection of therapeutic agents.

Proposed Course: The previously mentioned studies will be continued and expanded. Particular attention will be given to research on animals inoculated with candidate human cancer viruses, and investigations will be carried forward into the nature of neoplastic changes and their possible control at the cellular level. Collaborative efforts with other researchers within the SVCP will continue.

Date Contract Initiated: February 12, 1962

Current Annual Level: $2,153,850

Merck and Company, Inc. (NIH-71-2059)

Title: Study of Viruses in Human and Animal Neoplasia.

Contractor's Project Director: Dr. Maurice R. Hilleman

Project Officers (NCI): Dr. Robert A. Manaker
Dr. Jack Gruber

Objectives: To perform investigations designed to develop vaccines or other agents effective for the prophylaxis and therapy of human neoplasia of suspected viral etiology.

Major Findings: This is a new contract.

Significance to Biomedical Research and the Program of the Institute:
Current data support the concept that a virus or viruses are the essential element in most animal tumors studied and that viruses are probably the necessary etiological component in human neoplasia, though expression may be greatly influenced and modified by host and environmental factors. If viruses are the essential element in human cancer, then prophylaxis by vaccines to prevent or minimize infection should provide a rational approach to cancer prevention. This could be accomplished by utilization of live or killed virus vaccines or possibly by vaccines of purified virion subunits.

Vaccines would obviously provide their greatest benefit in preventing infection with oncogenic viruses transmitted horizontally after birth. However, even the possible vertical transmission of hypothetical neoplastic agents does not rule out a potential benefit from vaccines. Nononcogenic viruses may function as essential cofactors in expression of neoplasia, and immunity against such secondary agents might prevent expression of the neoplastic state. Additionally, antibody or cellular immunity may be enhanced by vaccination with homologous virus in virus-dependent cancer. Obviously this research investigation is of fundamental importance to the goals of SVCP and can make unique contributions to the total program.

Proposed Course: The investigators will devote initial efforts to developing methods for propagation, purification, concentration and specific quantitation of candidate viruses suspected or shown to cause cancer in man. At the present time, investigations will be focused upon herpes-type (DNA) viruses and "B" and "C" type (RNA) particles. Parallel studies to evolve live attenuated and killed virus vaccines in appropriate animal model systems will be conducted. Particular attention will be given to developing and applying optimal methods for viral attenuation, viral inactivation, viral quantitation, vaccine safety assessment, and vaccine potency assay.

Date Contract Initiated: March 1, 1971

MERCK AND COMPANY, INC. (NIH-71-2059)

Title: Oncogenic Virus Research and Vaccine Development

Contractor's Project Director: Dr. Maurice Hilleman

Project Officers (NCI): Dr. Robert A. Manaker
                         Mr. J. Thomas Lewin

Objectives: To conduct investigations designed to develop vaccines or
other agents effective for the prophylaxis and therapy for human neoplasia
of suspected viral etiology.

Major Findings: Multiple construction and renovation projects have been
involved in the expansion and reorientation for this program. Remodeling
of a laboratory, physically separated from the animal tumor virus area,
was recently completed and is in use for Herpes simplex type 2 vaccine
work. Two rooms (440 sq. ft.) in Bldg. #43 were remodeled and equipped
and are in use for the germ-free derivation of kittens for the SPF cat
colony breeding nucleus. Plans were completed for the renovation of
half of Bldg. #65 (5,940 sq. ft.) for housing an SPF cat colony and
for housing experimental cats. The construction and equipping of the
new biohazard containment building #26B (12,096 sq. ft.) for laboratory
work is progressing on schedule. The projected completion date is
September, 1972.

Tumor-specific cellular vaccine development: The preparation and assay
of tumor cell vaccines for protective efficacy in the hamster model
system was continued at a lower priority level. Testing of adenovirus
31 tumor cell fractions prepared by mechanical disruption of the cells
and fractionation by differential centrifugation was completed.
None of the vaccines (crude cell homogenate, nuclear fraction-$\omega^2 t = 10^7$
pellet, membrane fraction-$\omega^2 t = 5 \times 10^9$ pellet, particulate fraction-$\omega^2 t =$
10^{11} pellet, cell sap-$\omega^2 t = 10^{11}$ supernate) protected hamsters against
development of tumors when they were challenged by inoculation of viable
homologous tumor cells. Work on the preparation of two other types of
tumor cell antigens was continued. Cell membranes were prepared from a
adenovirus 12 tumor cells by hypotonic extraction and were solubilized
by sonication. The solubilized material was fractionated on Sephadex G200

139

columns and the desired fraction concentrated by the Diaflo membrane technique. The first batch of test and control antigens is on test for protective efficacy in hamsters. Preparation of additional batches of antigen for assay is in progress. Technology is still being developed for the preparation of adenovirus 7 tumor cell membranes by flow sonication and flow zonal centrifugation.

Investigation of the host immunologic response to nonprotective tumor cell vaccines is being conducted in hamster-tumor model systems. The first series of experiments was designed to test the effect of inoculation of known nonprotective vaccines before, simultaneously with, or after immunization with a known effective vaccine (5×10^6 γ-irradiated tumor cells). Most of the experiments in this series are on test. Final results with one of the nonprotective vaccines, SV_{40} tumor cell ghosts prepared by hypertonic extraction, showed that this vaccine did not interfere with the ability of the host to reject viable homologous tumor cells after vaccination with 5×10^6 γ-irradiated SV_{40} tumor cells.

Attempts to render nonprotective SV_{40} tumor cell vaccines effective by the administration of poly I:C before, simultaneously with, or after vaccine, single or multiple doses, or by different routes were not successful in the hamster model system.

Studies on the role of fetal antigens in tumor immunology are being conducted in the SV_{40}-hamster model system. In the first series of experiment, γ-irradiated, 9-12 day gestation fetal cells of multiparous origin did not protect adult male or female hamsters against tumor development when challenged with 5000 homologous tumor cells. Experiments are in progress wherein the vaccines were prepared from primaparous 10-day gestation embryos and are being tested in the SV_{40} virus-newborn hamster model system and in the adult hamster-tumor cell challenge system with a 2500 cell challenge dose.

Virus vaccine development: This project is still in the initial stages. The work in progress is concerned primarily with basic needs such as virus propagation, virus concentration and purification, preparation of specific antisera, and establishment of routine assay procedures.

The KT (Kawakami-Theilen) strain of feline leukemia virus (FLV) was routinely propagated in roller bottle (1 liter/bottle) suspension cultures of the virus-shedding FL74c cell line. Ten liter lots of culture fluid were concentrated (1000x) and purified by flow zonal centrifugation and isopynic centrifugation on sucrose gradients. Modifications in technology are still being made to increase the purity of the concentrated virus. Virus yields of 10^{13} virus particles/ml were readily achieved.

In order to provide an adequate supply of healthy cats for future experimental work, establishment of a specific pathogen-free cat colony was proposed. The first step, the germ-free derivation of the breeding has been in progress for two months. All eight isolators are occupied by kittens (16 females, 7 males) ranging from 1 to 8 weeks in age.

Significance to Biomedical Research and the Program of the Institute:

If viruses are an essential element in the genesis of some human cancers, prophylaxis by vaccines to prevent or minimize infection should provide a rational approach to cancer prevention. This could be accomplished by living or killed virus vaccines or possibly by vaccines of purified virion sub-units. Although greatest benefit could be derived by prevention of infections transmitted horizontally after birth, a potential benefit from vaccines may be derived where viruses are transmitted vertically but do not express their full antigenic complement. Nononcogenic viruses may function as essential co-factors in expression of neoplasia, and immunity against such secondary agents might prevent expression of the neoplastic state. In addition, vaccination with homologous virus in a virus-dependent cancer may enhance specific humoral antibody or cellular immunity. This research project is of fundamental importance to total program.

Proposed Course: Efforts to prepare tumor-specific cellular antigens for immunoprophylaxis of cancer and to study the immunologic response to such antigens will continue. Tests with poly I:C for adjuvant effect on ineffective cellular vaccines will be completed. Work towards development of a feline leukemia-sarcoma virus vaccine and a herpesvirus type 2 vaccine will be continued as rapidly as possible. If no problems arise, the germfree derivation of kittens for the SPF cat colony should be completed in several months.

Date Contract Initiated: March 1, 1971

Current Annual Level: $1,016,000

HAZELTON LABORATORIES, INC. (NIH-69-2079)

Title: Studies on the Etiology of Canine Cancer

Contractor's Project Director: Dr. Erling M. Jensen

Project Officers (NCI): Dr. Michael A. Chirigos
Dr. Robert A. Manaker

Objectives: To determine whether any canine cancer is caused by viruses and whether there is any possible etiological relationship between canine and human cancers.

Major Findings: A common antigen in several specific canine sarcomas was detected by immunofluorescence tests with sera from the tumor-bearing and other sarcomatous dogs. Successful transplantation of a canine mammary carcinoma was achieved by inoculation of beagles in utero. If continuous passage proves possible, the tumor will provide a valuable system for studies on viral etiology, therapy, and possibly hormonal influence on tumor development. Cells of a canine osteosarcoma inoculated into kittens in utero were recovered after birth of the animals and placed in culture. Attempts are underway to determine whether this procedure activated virus production.

A convenient, quantitative infectivity focus assay for feline virus was developed for studies using feline leukemia viruses in attempts to recover defective viruses from canine tumors. Treatment with BUdR and IUdR was introduced in attempts to induce virus release from canine tumor cells. Exposure of XC rat cells, which have been routinely used to titer murine leukemia viruses, to BUdR activated virus production. Two viruses appear to be present.

Studies were initiated to evaluate the effect of combined chemotherapy and nonspecific immune stimulators on spontaneous lymphosarcoma in dogs. In some preliminary tests, streptonigrin was used to determine its inhibitory effect on dog cells infected with feline leukemia virus. Even at toxic drug levels, the reproduction of the virus was not eliminated. Focal areas of morphological change were observed in the canine cells exposed to streptomycin.

Significance to Biomedical Research and the Program of the Institute:
Study of canine neoplasms for evidence of viral associations is important in several respects. Since humans are in close contact with canine pets, the possibility that they may be exposed to a canine tumor virus must be investigated. In contrast to the cat and mouse, viruses are not regularly shed by canine tumor cells. An analogous situation exists in the human. The dog provides an excellent experimental animal to determine the presence of covert viral infections contributing to neoplastic transformations. If such viral relationships to cancer in the dog can be firmly established, the dog will provide opportunity to study the mechanisms for transmission of infection, virus-host relationships, and evaluation of control measures. In this respect, the dog would be one of the best models for human cancer.

Proposed Course: Redirection of the effort in this laboratory is being considered to utilize the facilities for more intensive study on tumor viruses, a more concentrated effort on viral relationships to canine mammary carcinoma, and evaluation of immunotherapeutic approaches to control of naturally occurring neoplasms.

Date Contract Initiated: May 26, 1969

Current Annual Level: $400,000

PUBLIC HEALTH RESEARCH INSTITUTE OF THE CITY OF NEW YORK, INC.
(NCI-E-72-2028)

Title: Study of Cell Surface Alterations Induced by RNA and DNA
Viruses.

Contractor's Project Director: Dr. Thomas Benjamin

Project Officers (NCI): Dr. George Todaro
                         Dr. Roy Kinard

Objectives: To investigate the relationship between cell surface
alterations induced by RNA viruses and those induced by DNA viruses
using several oncorna viruses and non-transforming mutants of
polyoma virus.

Major Findings: Eight cell lines including 3T3, 3T12 and sarcoma
virus transformed lines, have been transferred from Dr. Todaro's
laboratory successfully and are being checked for possible selection
of variants. This contract is new and no other results have been
obtained.

Significance to Biomedical Research and the Program of the Institute:
The long range goal of the research program of this laboratory is
an understanding of how oncogenic viruses overcome cellular growth
controls. Ultimately, an understanding of the mechanism of neoplastic
transformation by viruses will depend on progress in two areas:
(1) the identification and characterization of those viral gene
functions which are essential to the transformation process, and
(2) the determination of how and where these essential viral genes
interact with the cell and with factors which normally operate
in regulating cell growth. The proposed contract will allow
Dr. Benjamin to continue and extend his impressive work on this
problem and will foster collaboration with other NCI and SVCP workers.

Proposed Course: Continuation to achieve the objectives described.

Date Contract Initiated: December 3, 1971

Current Contract Level: $36,800

324

CALIFORNIA, UNIVERSITY OF (NIH-NCI-E-70-2048)

Title: Comparative Leukemia and Sarcoma Viral Studies

Contractor's Project Director: Dr. Leo K. Bustad

Project Officer (NCI): Dr. Robert J. Huebner

Objectives: To further study the two simian Type C viruses (woolly monkey sarcoma and gibbon lymphosarcoma) which were first isolated in this laboratory.

Major Findings: (1) Woolly Monkey Fibrosarcoma (SSV): (a) SSV-infected bonnet monkey cells, cultivated in roller bottles, are yielding significant amounts of SSV virus. Several other cell lines of human, bovine, and simian origin also support SSV replication. (b) Bovine cells infected with woolly monkey sarcoma virus were inoculated into the autochthonous host at 10- to 14-day intervals as viable and freeze-thawed disrupted cells. Serum samples taken prior to inoculation and 6 weeks later were tested for antibody against the woolly monkey sarcoma virus by immunodiffusion. A positive precipitin band developed with a serum sample taken 6 weeks post-inoculation. (c) Radioimmune precipitation assays using SSV replicated in bovine thymus cultures were positive for bovine anti-SSV antisera but negative for bovine anti-FeSV antisera, indicating that SSV-infected cultures are free of FeSV antigens and that SSV and FeSV do not possess common envelope antigens. (d) Cellular and cell-free materials from tissue culture were inoculated subcutaneously into two newborn cotton-topped marmosets. Nodules (7 to 13 mm diameter) developed at the site of inoculation within 12 to 14 days. However, nodules regressed within 3 weeks. One nodule detected 28 days after inoculation reached 1 cm in diameter and has remained that size for 4 months. Blood samples from each animal have been examined monthly and no significant abnormalities have been noted. All inoculated monkeys are being held for continued observation.

(2) Gibbon Lymphosarcoma (SLV): (a) The cell line initiated from the gibbon tumor tissue remains the best producer of SLV, although bovine, African green monkey kidney (AGMK),

257

and human cell lines support low levels of SLV replication.
(b) Transmission of the gibbon lymphosarcoma was tested in
neonatal squirrel monkeys and pigs. Three of four newborn
squirrel monkeys inoculated with gibbon lymphosarcoma tissue
culture cells had a transient enlargement of the regional
lymph node draining the site of inoculation. No signs of
neoplasia have been observed during the 4 to 5 months following challenge; regular examination of blood samples has
revealed no abnormalities. All monkeys remain under
observation. Three of eight inoculated pigs were
sacrificed 4 months after injection and found to have
slightly enlarged mesenteric lymph nodes; histopathologic
diagnosis was lymphoid hyperplasia. No other lesions were
detected. Surviving pigs have shown no signs of neoplasia
in the 7 to 9 months since inoculation and remain under
observation.

Significance to Biomedical Research and the Program of the
Institute: The finding at this laboratory of two Type C
viruses associated with tumors of different primate species
is evidence that the higher animals, including man, are
likely to be among the growing number of species harboring
oncornaviruses. Since monkeys and man are closely related
phylogenetically, the proposed studies, which are oriented
toward characterization of the primate viruses and seeking
possible relation with human tumors, are of direct relevance
in establishing the etiology of human cancer.

Proposed Course: (1) Characterize in greater detail the
molecular components of the woolly monkey fibrosarcoma and
gibbon lymphosarcoma viruses by analysis of enzymes,
structural proteins and nucleic acid. (2) Determine the
in vitro and in vivo biological activities of woolly monkey
and gibbon lymphosarcoma viruses. (3) Initiate serologic
studies for the detection of antigenic components in
spontaneous tumors of simian and human origin that may be
common to know simian RNA Type-C viruses. (4) Continue
efforts to isolate oncogenic agents from spontaneous tumors
of primates and complete limited studies on canine systems.
(5) Complete studies on humoral antibody response in cats
to the leukemia-sarcoma virus complex.

Date Contract Initiated: November 16, 1969

Current Contract Level: $550,000

258

Title: The Production of Simian Viruses and Homologous Antisera

Contractor's Project Director: Dr. Seymour S. Kalter

Project Officer (NCI): Dr. James T. Duff

Objectives: To determine the quality of simian virus reference reagents (seed material and antisera) packaged for NCI by another contractor. In addition, the laboratory serves as a diagnostic laboratory in a limited capacity for viral isolates that may emerge from studies done by other SVCP contractors.

Major Findings: The simian foamyvirus (FV) reagents were extensively tested and an attempt was made to determine whether a relationship exists between the Mason-Pfizer monkey virus and the foamyviruses. Assistance was given NCI personnel in the identification of Herpesvirus saimiri, a woolly monkey virus and in the study of other viruses isolated from primate neoplastic tissues.

All seven FV types grew at least on one of a variety of cell lines indicating viability of the ampouled stocks. Secondary rabbit kidney cell cultures supported the growth of all seven types and working pools are in preparation on these cells. The Baboon Submaxillary Lymph Node cell (SMLN) culture has proven most useful in working with all the types except 5. This is a diploid culture now in its 10th subpassage. Cytopathology on these cells is rapid (6-8 days), reaching a maximum in two weeks and is easy to read because of the uniformity in appearance of the cell sheet. Working pools of types 1, 2, 4, 6 and 7 have been prepared on SMLN cells with titers of 2.0-3.0 logs/0.1 ml. Vero cells were next most susceptible to foamyvirus infection, producing CPE with FV 1, 2, 3, 6 and 7.

Cross neutralization testing indicated an unanticipated FV 2-7 cross reaction and FV 6 and 7 appear to be "mislabelled."

There appears to be no serologic relationship between M-PMV and FV 1, 2, 3, 4, 6, 7.

Significance to Biomedical Research and the Program of the Institute: These reagents will be useful to investigators in characterizing viruses isolated from neoplastic diseases (natural or induced) that occur in primates, and for monitoring primate colonies.

Proposed Course: Certify the packaged simian virus reagents and serve as a diagnostic laboratory for viral isolates referred to SWFRE by NCI.

Date Contract Initiated: June 15, 1966

Source: NCI staff. *The Special Virus Cancer Program: Progress Report #8.* Office of the Associate Scientific Director for Viral Oncology (OASDVO). J. B. Moloney, Ed., Washington, D. C.: U. S. Government Printing Office, 1970 and 1971. Page numbers are as shown.

MASSACHUSETTS INSTITUTE OF TECHNOLOGY (NCI-E-71-2149)

Title: Studies of Leukemia Virus DNA Polymerase.

Contractor's Project Director: Dr. David Baltimore

Project Officers (NCI):   Dr. George Todaro
                           Dr. Roy Kinard

Objectives: To characterize the enzyme, its product, its mechanism of reaction, and formation of viral RNA during infection.

Major Findings: Using polyribionucleotides as templates, complementary primer was necessary to initiate DNA synthesis. Using poly(A) as a template for the DNA polymerase, the amount of poly(dT) synthesis was proportional to the amount of added template. The best primers were oligodeoxyribonucleotides such as oligo(dT) as a primer for poly(A). Polyribonucleotides were in general much better templates than polyribodeoxynucleotides.

The endogenous reaction involves the copying of the 60S-70S RNA found in the virion. The initial reaction product formed when the virion DNA polymerase copies the endogenous viral RNA consists of small pieces of DNA attached to the 60S-70S RNA. The DNA can be released from the bulk RNA by procedures which disrupt hydrogen bonds. The density of the product is not that of a free DNA but that of a covalently-bonded DNA-RNA hybrid. This finding, which was made both with mouse leukemia virus and avian myeloblastosis virus, indicates that the primer for the endogenous reaction is an RNA molecule.

The globin messenger RNA or, more strictly, the 10S RNA from rabbit reticulocytes polyribosomes, was the best template for the DNA polymerase found. Synthesis of DNA amounting to 30-80% of the added template was observed with this RNA. Actinomycin D inhibited the reaction to about 50% indicating that half of the reaction involved copying of RNA and the other half the copying of the complementary DNA into a double-stranded DNA. In order to investigate the nature of the reaction product they studied its size and its ability to hybridize specifically with 10S RNA. They were able to demonstrate that the product was completely complementary to 10S RNA and was not complementary to other RNA's found in reticulocytes and elsewhere. This RNA may be of utility in many aspects of molecular cell biology and a number of experiments have been initiated using it.

Significance to Biomedical Research and the Program of the Institute: The characterization of the enzyme that produces DNA from the tumor viruses genetic material (RNA) has the highest priority in the SVCP. It may provide much more sensitive techniques for finding cancer virus genetic information in human tumors.

Proposed Course: Continuation with slight decrease in budget.

Date Contract Initiated: May 1, 1971

Current Contract Level: $75,000

MASSACHUSETTS INSTITUTE OF TECHNOLOGY (NIH 71-2149)

Title: Studies on RNA-Dependent DNA Polymerase

Contractor's Project Director: Dr. David Baltimore

Project Officer (NCI):   Dr. George Todaro

Objectives: To characterize DNA polymerase and its product, to study its mechanism of reaction and formation of viral RNA during infection.

Major Findings: None reported yet, this is a new contract.

Significance to Biomedical Research and its Program of the Institute: The objectives above have highest priority in the SVCP.   The results may provide very sensitive techniques for finding cancer virus genetic information in human tumors.

Proposed Course: Continuation with addition of EM capability.

Date Contract Initiated: May 1, 1971   189

Massachusetts Institute of Technology study summary (NIH) 71-2149. Document shows retrovirus pioneer David Baltimore, in cooperation with NCI chief George Todaro, performed similar studies to those performed by Robert Gallo's teams in Bethesda and Uganda. Todaro, Vice Chairman of Resources and Logistics for the Special Virus Cancer Program, was also the NCI officer who oversaw several AIDS-like virus studies conducted by Bionetics in the early 1970s. Source: NCI staff. *The Special Virus Cancer Program: Progress Report #8.* Office of the Associate Scientific Director for Viral Oncology (OASDVO). J. B. Moloney, Ed., Washington, D. C.: U. S. Government Printing Office, 1970, pp. 188-189, and 1971 pp. 214-215; 322-323.

Chapter 23
The Man-Made Origin
of Marburg and Ebola

THE following week, I flew into Baltimore–Washington International airport. Jackie made plans for me to drive from BWI to Pittsburgh for my next seminar. The main purpose for the road trip was so that I could spend a couple of days in Frederick, Maryland, exploring Fort Detrick and the NCI library.

Arriving on the morning of April 4, 1995, I stopped to photograph its mildly intimidating gate (see fig. 23.1); then I drove right past an unsecured checkpoint. As I circled the complex, the Fort teamed with activity as construction crews and researchers bustled about. Several new buildings were going up, including the library annex. The NCI certainly appears to be immune to the real estate recession, I mused.

The NCI's new library seemed modest compared to all the others I had visited in the previous months. The floor area, about 2,000 square feet, supported the typical library fixtures.

I immediately approached two librarians who were conversing quietly at their station behind the main checkout counter. "Excuse me," I said politely, "I wonder if you have a series of NCI publications dating to the early 1970s entitled the "Special Virus Cancer Program Progress Reports?"

"Have you tried the computer?" quipped the senior staffer.

"Thanks a lot. I'll do just that." Please forgive my ignorance, I thought.

I turned, took three steps back to an open monitor and keyboard, and in the subject field entered the words "SPECIAL VIRUS CANCER PROGRAM (SVCP)." The computer immediately provided a list of SPECIAL VIRUS CANCER PROGRAM "Special Technical Publications." All right! I thought, excited by the possibility of finding something new. Quickly highlighting the first entry, I pressed the Enter key. To my absolute amazement, the computer responded:

Your search for the TITLE: SPECIAL VIRUS CANCER PROGRAM (SVCP), Special Technical Publication is not used in this library's catalog.

"What!" I can't believe that, I thought. The publication documenting the earliest efforts in the NCI's "war on cancer" is not here. No way.

I returned to the previous field, selected the second listing—SPECIAL VIRUS CANCER PROGRAM "Special Technical Publication American Society for Tx," and pressed Enter. The computer, without pause, returned:

Your search for the TITLE: SPECIAL VIRUS CANCER PROGRAM (SVCP), Special Technical Publication is not used in this library's catalog.

"Oh, come on!"

I repeated the effort seven times; going down the list of SVCP Special Technical Publications that had obviously been written by the NCI staff. They were all apparently removed from the NCI "library's catalog."

Then I called the senior librarian over to the computer and demonstrated the problem.

"I guess we just don't have any of them," she defended, "but if you think the books are something we should have, you can fill out a special requisition form, and we'll get them."

"Thanks, but I'm only going to be in town for a couple of days," I said.

I walked away, amazed that these documents—perhaps the most important and revealing in the history of the NCI—had been apparently pulled from the library's shelves.

Fig. 23.1. Entrance Gate to Fort Detrick, Home of the NCI

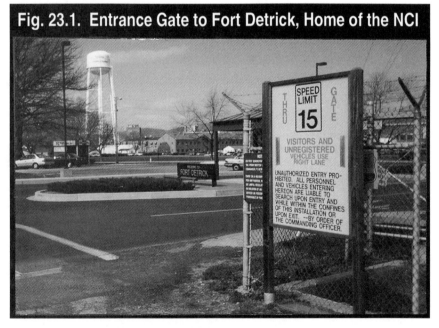

Bridging the Blood Barrier

Other revealing documents had not been made classified, and my trip to Fort Detrick was ultimately worth the effort. As I searched shelf by shelf and title by title, I found four final pieces of the origin of AIDS, Ebola, and Marburg puzzles.

The first was published in *Research Animals in Medicine*.[1] The National Heart and Lung Institute of the NIH had invited New York University School of Medicine researcher Dr. J. Moor-Jankowski to present a paper entitled "Blood Groups of Apes and Monkeys: Human and Simian Types." During her presentation, she acknowledged that she and Dr. Alexander S. Weiner from NYUMC had helped establish the Laboratory for Experimental Medicine and Surgery in Primates in New York. Together, they gained "access to animals [simian monkeys] maintained by the U.S. Air Force and by some of the primate centers," most exclusively Litton Bionetics. [1-4]

The NYUMC researcher described the research that set the stage for the use of monkey blood for human vaccine trials. Then she called attention to Dr. Weiner's ground breaking simian monkey experiments, which led to his "epoch-making discovery of the RH factor." Her work with Weiner was explained this way:

> In 1962, Dr. Weiner and the author joined forces for a long-term study of blood groups of nonhuman primates. The results obtained during the first phase of our research program led us to establish the concept of human-type, simian-type and cross-immune-type blood groups in primates including man. The definition of these three categories, at which we arrived in 1964, has been most conducive for planning and advancement of further research.[1]

Their work had paved the way for human and monkey blood typing, and cross-matching experiments designed to give researchers and physicians advice on which monkey blood types might be compatible with which human blood types.

She concluded:

> The information accumulated through our work during the last decade has resulted, among others, in the increased use of primate animals in experimental surgery requiring blood transfusion and priming of the heart-lung machine. All chimpanzees and baboons used as organ donors for human patients throughout the world since 1964, as well as most of the primate animals used in cross-circulation of patients in hepatic failure, have been tested in our laboratory.[1]

Though these researchers' efforts are not suspect—since they had nothing to do with the viral experiments conducted by their NYUMC colleagues and other bioweapons contractors at Merck, the NCI, and Litton Bionetics—their work established the precedent upon which all other researchers depended. Once human and monkey blood was successfully typed, interspecies blood mixing and transfusions, organ transplants, and *cross-species vaccine research* could proceed without fear of massive allergic reactions. That is, the barrier presented by the host's natural immune system—the rejection of foreign proteins—could be bridged. Wiener's and Moor-Jankowski's efforts opened the way for an avalanche of monkey–man vaccine experiments in which numerous deadly viruses were created, tested, and apparently deployed in unsuspecting and uninformed subjects.

Hard for most people to imagine, this was confirmed during an interchange with a member of her audience. Dr. Stormont asked:

> You were talking about the complete interchange of blood between chimpanzees and man. Have you heard of any recent experiment where lower animal species' blood has been used to transfuse man? For an example, Dr. Wiener and Dr. Unger had one patient, an aged lady, who had autoimmune hemolytic disease. Finally she couldn't tolerate human blood and had developed antibodies for practically every antigen system known in man. As a last resort, they asked me to ship them some cattle blood from a healthy animal immediately. I sent them some and they transfused her with the blood. It kept her alive eight weeks beyond her expected death time.[1]

To which Moor-Jankowski innocently replied, "I haven't heard of this, which is quite interesting because I work so closely with Dr. Wiener. In light of what is being done now with nonhuman primates, I think this should be published."

More Litton Bionetics–Hazleton Monkey Business

When I linked Moor-Jankowski's source of simian monkeys to information on monkey suppliers provided by Drs. Fine and Arthur during a 1980 Cold Spring Harbor symposium, it became even more obvious that Litton Bionetics, Inc. was the principal exporter of monkeys throughout the world for military and industrial research. Fig. 23.2 was prepared by Fine and Arthur. It showed that Davis and Hazleton* Labs needed to import their monkeys, whereas only "LBI" maintained "colony-born" chimpanzees in Uganda.[4]

Gallo contributed an article in the same Cold Spring Harbor report wherein the NCI lab chief and several coauthors listed a series of their monkey virus experiments (see figs. 23.3 and 23.4). Fig. 23.2 showed

---

* same firm and government grant [SVCP 69-2079] as "Hazelton" misspelled in several publications.

Gallo's group used four major monkey suppliers: three American and one African. The three domestic suppliers that imported various monkey species from LBI included Hazleton Labs, Davis (California Primate Research Center), and the Mason Research Institute (of Worcester, Massachusetts). Apparently only Litton Bionetics, Inc. maintained a monkey facility in Northwest Uganda and did not need to import their monkeys.[4,7]

Most incriminating is the fact that the specific rare species of monkeys—*Cercopithecus aethiops* and *Macacus mulatta*—that Litton Bionetics, Inc. exported and other animal suppliers imported, were the Marburg virus carriers to Europe during the first outbreak of the hemorrhagic fever in 1967, and the Davis AIDS-like virus outbreaks in 1969, 1976, and 1978 respectively. The Reston and Philadelphia outbreaks of Ebola-like viruses in 1989 and 1990 were associated with monkeys that had either originated at Litton Bionetics, or had contacted colony born Litton monkeys when the animals were housed in KLM's Amsterdam facility awaiting transport to New York.[12]

Landon's Ugandan Rhabdovirus Experiments

The next to last puzzle piece fell into place on reviewing a NCI Monograph entitled, *The National Cancer Program and International Cancer Research.*[3] Here, a 1974 article by John Higginson and Calum Muir reviewed the "Epidemiologic Program of the International Agency for Research on Cancer (IARC)" and the "geographic distribution of some Agency programs." They graphically displayed their findings in a figure that I had seen months earlier. This time, however, when I saw the map (see fig. 8.2), I noted that the most intense viral research activity in Uganda covered areas specifically investigated by Litton Bionetics, Inc. (LBI). LBI and Merck investigators had studied herpes-type virus infections in the area,[5,6] both had also studied hepatitis and possible liver cancer viruses there,[5,6] and LBI had conducted extensive carcinogen tests on more than 140 substances, many apparently on monkeys in Uganda also.[2, 5, 8-10]

After viewing the map, I returned to the lengthy addendum LBI provided in the 1971 "SVCP Progress Report #8," wherein they disclosed numerous studies they had conducted with Rhabdoviruses on monkeys and other animals. Rhabdoviruses, I recalled, were considered by many experts as the germ from which Marburg and Ebola viruses most likely evolved.[13] These viruses the LBI report showed had been manipulated, mutated, or mixed with other deadly viruses, including sarcoma and leukemia viruses.[7]

Fig. 23.2. Varieties of Litton Bionetics, Inc. Colony Born Monkeys Exported From Uganda to Hazleton, Davis, and Mason Labs

Demonstration of IPA Specificity Based on Serum Absorption with Various Retroviruses

Animal	Species	Description	Colony	Serum unabsorbed/absorbed with	IPA reactivity[a] to					
					GALV	MMC-1	BaEV	MPMV	SMRV	MMTV
B1596	M. mulatta	Burkitt's lymphoma and MPMV-inoculated female (colony-born)	LBI/MRI[b]	unabsorbed	–	–	+	+2	+	–
				MPMV	–	–	–	–	–	–
				MMC-1	–	–	+	+2	+	–
				MMTV	–	–	+	+2	+	–
B1414	M. mulatta	HSV-2 and MPMV-inoculated female (colony-born)	LBI/MRI[c]	unabsorbed	+	+	+	+3	+	+
				MPMV	–	–	–	–	–	–
				MMC-1	–	–	+	+3	+	–
				MMTV	–	–	+	+3	+	–
B6931	M. mulatta	normal male breeder (colony-born)	LBI	unabsorbed	–	–	+	+2	+2	–
				MPMV	–	–	–	–	–	–
				MMC-1	–	–	–	+2	+	–
				MMTV	–	–	+	+2	+2	–
Mmu8008 and Mmu7492	M. mulatta	normal female breeders (imported)	Davis	unabsorbed	–	+2	–	+	–	–
				MMC-1	–	–	–	+	–	–
				MPMV	–	+2	–	–	–	–
Mra16149	M. radiata	normal female breeder (imported)	Davis	unabsorbed	–	–	+2	+2	+2	–
				MPMV	–	–	–	–	–	–
				SMRV	–	–	–	–	–	–
				BaEV	–	–	–	–	–	–
				MMTV	–	–	+2	+2	+2	–
44	C. aethiops	normal male (imported)	Hazelton Labs	unabsorbed	–	+	–	–	+	–
				MMC-1	–	–	–	–	+	–
45	C. aethiops	normal female (imported)		unabsorbed	+	+	–	–	–	–
				SMRV	–	–	–	–	+	–
				GALV	+	–	–	–	–	–
				MPMV	–	–	–	–	+	–

Values expressed in IPA are based on a scale of +1 to +4 ranging from weak to strongly positive reactions, respectively. Negative indicates no reaction.
[b] Animal born and inoculated at Litton Bionetics, Inc. (LBI) with Burkitt's lymphoma, transferred to Mason Research Institute (MRI) at 6 years of age, and inoculated with MPMV.
[c] Animal born and inoculated at LBI with herpes simplex type II, transferred to MRI at 6 years of age, and inoculated with MPMV.

Note: The name "Hazelton" is misspelled. The correct spelling is noted in the caption. Source: Fine DL and Arthur LO. Prevalence of natural immunity to Type-D and Type-C Retroviruses in primates. In: Viruses in Naturally Occuring Cancers: Book B. Myron Essex, George Todaro and Harald zur Hausen, eds., Cold Spring Harbor Laboratory, 1980, Vol. 7, pp. 793-813

LBI Rhabdovirus studies began in 1965. At that time the LBI group leader, Dr. John Landon, took minced tissue containing Rhabdoviruses along with numerous hybrids (Hybrid Rhabdoviruses were made by cross-breeding them with simian sarcoma and leukemia viruses to form mutant strains called "Rhabdomyosarcoma or Rhabdomyosarcoma L") and inoculated them into dozens of monkeys. Most died or were transferred.

Obviously if they survived Landon's experiments they had developed antibodies and immunity to the Rhabdoviruses. These monkeys, then, were considered valuable for the production of vaccines. Most of these were then transferred to various vaccine production facilities internationally. Consequently, the timing was perfect for the initial Marburg virus outbreaks in Marburg, Frankfort, and Belgrade in 1967 at the Behringwerke, the Paul Ehrlich Institute, and the Institute for Sera and Vaccines, respectively—all vaccine production facilities.[7, 13]

Fig. 23.5 contains the Rhabdovirus monkey experiments, among numerous others, conducted by Landon and company at LBI between 1965 and 1970. Details regarding the broad array of inoculated materials and viruses used by LBI and NCI researchers on monkeys are provided.

Considering the "MK" in MKNAOMI

The LBI addendum also provided a possible link to the CIA biological weapons testing Project MKNAOMI. In this, "Summary of Studies," the first entry was titled "BFKMRS, 10/65-3/66." It was further explained that the code letters "BFKMRS" represented Drs. Bryan, Falk, Kotin, Manaker, Rausher, and Sevenson. The next coded section was "MK-SVLP 2/66-3/67."

Earlier, the "SVCP Progress Report #8" explained that "SVLP" represented the "Special Virus Leukemia Project." More important, the letters MK before SVLP indicated Drs. Manaker and Kotin. Manaker, I recalled, was the chief, of the Viral Biology Branch and chairman of the Etiology Area for the entire SVCP. Kotin's identity, however, required investigation. I learned from a search of the NCI library's database that Kotin was considered an expert in the field of biohazard control and laboratory safety and design.[14-16] Together, Manaker and Kotin maintained formidable multidisciplinary knowledge—virtually all the knowledge needed to set up a safe biological weapons testing lab and direct a multidisciplinary team of scientists in special operations research. The MK in the CIA's MKNAOMI,

Fig. 23.3. Human Tissues and Cell Lines Examined By Dr. Robert Gallo for Simian Monkey Sarcoma Viruses

Human Tissues and Cell Lines Examined for
SiSV(SSAV)-related DNA Fragment

Source of specimen	Number tested	Results
Normal donors		
placenta	4	4+
spleen	1	+
kidney	1	+
lung	1	+
brain	1	+
tonsil	1	+
blood cells (buffy coat)	1	+
Neoplastic tissues		
blood cells AML	10	10+
blood cells CML	9	9+
blood cells ALL	1	+
placenta from AML	2	2+
spleen CML	6	6+
Cell lines		
B lymphoblasts	4	4+
rhabdomyosarcoma (A204)	1	+
promyelocytic leukemia (HL-60)	1	+
promyelocytic leukemia (HL-60)		
+BaEV	1	+
+ SSAV	1	+
+DMSO	1	+
osteogenic sarcoma (HOS)	1	+
CML undifferentiated blasts (K562)	1	+
T-cell leukemia (CEF)	1	+
A204 + BaEV	1	+
A204 + SSAV	1	+
normal trophoblasts	1	+
Total examined 53		
Total positive 53		

DNA fragment of 12 kb from BamHI digestion.

Fig. 23.4. Experiments Conducted by Dr. Robert Gallo During the 1970s to "Probe" Human and Animal Genes for Signs of Simian Monkey Sarcoma Virus Infection

Specificity of SiSV(SSAV) RNA among Various
Type-C Viral RNA Probes in Detection of Virus-related
Sequences in Human DNA

Source of viral RNA	Host	Presence (+)/absence (-)
Primate		
SiSV(SSAV) 71AP1	marmoset	+
SSAV M55	rat	+
SiSV(SSAV) A204	human	+
SiSV(SC185)	marmoset	+
GALV (Hall's Island)	bat	–
GALV (San Francisco)	bat	–
BaEV M7	dog	–
Cat		
RD114	human	–
FeLV (Rickard strain)	cat	–
FeSV (MSTF)	mink	–
Mouse		
R-MuLV (ecotropic)	mouse	–
SC185 (amphotropic)	mouse	–
BALB-V2 (xenotropic)	rat	–
KSV(K-MuLV)	rat	±

Aliquots of 30 μg of human cell DNA digested with BamHI were fractionated on 0.8% agarose gels, transferred to nitrocellulose sheets according to the method of Southern (1975), hybridized to the various [^{125}I]RNA probes indicated above, and then subjected to autoradiography.

The two preceding figures were prepared by Dr. Robert Gallo and coworkers from the NCI and Litton Bionetics. Fig. 23.3 lists the human tissues and cell lines examined for simian monkey sarcoma viruses. Fig. 23.4 shows subsequent work in which numerous "Type-C" RNA retroviruses were injected into human cells to probe for the presence of simian monkey sarcoma DNA (provirus strand) in the human chromosome. This work was ongoing well before the first AIDS cases were identified. Source: Gallo RC, Wong-Staal F, Marhkam PD, Ruscetti R, Kalyanaraman VS, Ceccherini-Nelli L, Favera RD, Josephs S, Miller NR and Reitz, Jr MS. Recent studies with infectious primate retroviruses: Hybridization to primate DNA and some biological effects on fresh human blood leukocytes by simian sarcoma virus and Gibbon ape leukemia virus. In: *Viruses in Naturally Occurring Cancers: Book B*. Myron Essex, George Todaro and Harald zur Hausen, eds., Cold Spring Harbor, NY: Cold Spring Harbor Laboratory, 1980, Vol. 7, pp. 793-813.

was therefore, very possibly, a code identifying principal investigators Manaker and Kotin.

I still had no idea who or what "NAOMI" might be.

The Man-Made Origin of AIDS, Ebola, and Marburg

Finally, I stumbled on expert testimony that the only time a simian monkey virus presents a danger to humans is when it has contaminated a vaccine and then is injected during a vaccination, and that the Marburg and Ebola hemorrhagic viruses were man-made. These statements came from two of the world's leading experts in simian monkey virology—Drs. Seymour Kalter and Robert Whitney.[17]

Kalter, the doctor charged with diagnosing new viruses emerging from NCI-supported laboratories, and whose research was instrumental in determining that the search for the Marburg agent had been clouded by the CDC's bogus "United States antigen," made his irreverent comments during a Frederick Cancer Research Center symposium. His testimony was entered into the official record entitled, *Biohazards and Zoonotic Problems of Primate Procurement, Quarantine and Research: Proceedings of a Cancer Research Safety Symposium.* The event, held on March 19, 1975, soon after the second Marburg virus outbreak in South Africa, brought America's leading laboratory animal science directors together to discuss the issue. Participants included Alfred Hellman from the NCI's Office Biohazard and Environmental Control Branch; Peter Gerone from Tulane University's Delta Regional Primate Research Center; Elizabeth Muchmore—a colleague of Krugman and Moor-Jankowski—from the Laboratory for Experimental Medicine and Surgery in Primates at the New York University Medical Center; David Valerio from Hazleton Laboratories; and Robert Whitney, a veterinarian from the Division of Research Services of the NIH.

Whitney prompted Kalter's comments following his presentation on "Important Primate Diseases (Biohazards and Zoonoses)." Whitney stated that:

> Simian hemorrhagic fever is a sporadically occurring viral disease that has caused high mortality in large colonies of rhesus monkeys. The agent is a small RNA virus [as opposed to the much larger Marburg and Ebola viruses] that multiplies within the cytoplasm. . . . This, as well as many other diseases, dictates the need for separation of species of nonhuman primates.[17]

Fig. 23.5. Summary Report of Monkey Inoculation Studies Conducted by Litton Bionetics and NCI Researchers in Northwest Uganda.

FORMAT OF THE REPORT

This review is divided into five types of studies plus an Addendum. The studies are:

A. Major Studies
B. Special Studies
C. Other Active Studies
D. Long-term Holding Studies
E. Terminated Studies

A major study is the product of an ad hoc committee formed within the Special Virus Leukemia Program to investigate areas of significance. These are major group or collaborative efforts with emphasis on inoculation of human material and subsequent long-term holding. These studies extend from August 1964 to May 1967.

The special studies program was formally initiated in June 1969, although procedures of this type had been employed since September 1968. With the shift in emphasis from gross tumor development to more sophisticated procedures involving inoculation and detection, a new type of program was developed. The objectives were to provide for experimental manipulation, close observation and monitoring of a limited number of selected animals. These studies proceed according to more formal protocols which involve greater varieties of inoculation procedures, possible animal preconditioning such as immunosuppression, or surgical manipulation, delayed hypersensitivity and more extensive and diverse monitoring.

Section C consists of current studies not of a special nature. These are programs with specified time limits for review, evaluation and subsequent implementing of decisions. Many of these may be considered preliminary investigations into previously undefined areas.

Section D includes those animals being maintained for extended time periods. The rationale is based on known long latent periods in primary animal tumor systems. In most of these, the inocula were human leukemic or tumor materials inoculated between 1962 and 1965.

Section E lists all completed studies.

The Addendum contains reports on two uninoculated groups:

1. Spontaneous neoplasia in the primate breeding colony;
2. Incidence of neoplasia in animals experimentally manipulated elsewhere and held at Bionetics.

Under Sections A through E, the studies are arranged alphabetically by investigator. Various codes are used to make the tables containing the information more meaningful. Origin of material is a capital letter (key 1.a) and is associated with the disease type, which is also coded (key 1.b). Information relative to source--the type of material used--is coded by numeral (key 1.c). The number inoculated and the number dead or

278

transferred are real numbers. The dates present in the tabulations refer to the time the animals were placed on study.

1. Material inoculated

   a. Origin

A	avian
B	bovine
C	chemical
E	equine
F	feline
G	guinea pig
H	human
M	murine
O	ovine
R	rabbit
S	simian

   b. Diagnosis

A12S40	Adenovirus 12 + SV-40
A2S40	Adenovirus 2 + SV-40
Ad2P	Adenovirus 2 + parainfluenza
Ad 7	Adenovirus 7
AL	Acute leukemia
ALL	Acute lymphocytic leukemia
ALL I	Acute lymphocytic leukemia + influenza
ALL PI	Acute lymphocytic leukemia + parainfluenza
AM BL	American Burkitt's lymphoma
AML	Acute myelogenous leukemia
AM MOL	Acute myelogenous leukemia + monocytic leukemia
AMOL	Acute monocytic leukemia
Arbo	Arthropod-borne virus
AT MON	Atypical monocytosis
Au Ag	Australia antigen
Bac Agt	Bacterial agent
BL	Burkitt's lymphoma
BOL	Bovine leukemia
CA	Condyloma acuminatum
CCHy	Congenital cerebral hyperplasia
CF	Control familial
C-H	Chediak-Higashi
Chondr	Chondrosarcoma
CLL	Chronic lymphocytic leukemia
CML	Chronic myelogenous leukemia
CMV	Cytomegalovirus
CSCL	Congenital stem cell leukemia
DC	Disease control
D Enc	Dawson's encephalitis
Echo 9	Echovirus 9
EL	Erythroid leukemia

279

452

Eosinp	Eosinophilia
Fibro	Fibrosarcoma
GB	Glioblastoma
H-1	H-1 virus
Herp/G	H. genitalis
Herp/S	H. simplex
HD	Hodgkin's disease
HV	Herpesvirus
I	Influenza
IM	Infectious mononucleosis
Kuru	Kuru
L	Leukemia
Liposar	Liposarcoma
L lymph	Lymphocytic leukemia
LRL	Leukemoid reaction of the liver
LS	Lymphosarcoma
Lymph	Lymphoma
Mamm T	Mammary tumor
Mening	Meningitis
MH	Malignant histiocytosis
Misc L	Miscellaneous leukemia
Misc V	Miscellaneous virus
ML	Malignant lymphoma
MM	Multiple myeloma
MSV	Moloney sarcoma virus
MSV AV	Moloney sarcoma virus + arbovirus
MSV L	Moloney sarcoma virus + leukemia
MSV MT	Moloney sarcoma virus + monkey tumor
Osteo S	Osteosarcoma
P	Papilloma
PI	Parainfluenza
PIA C	Pia mater control cell culture
Plyctm	Polycythemia
PPLO	Mycoplasma
R	Rubella
Rau Vi	Rauscher virus
RCS	Reticulum cell sarcoma
Reo 1	Reovirus 1
Reo 3	Reovirus 3
● Rhabd L	Rhabdomyosarcoma + leukemia
Rhabdo	Rhabdomyosarcoma
RTC	Rous transformed cells
S	Sarcoma
S20S40	SV-20 + SV-40
SA 7	Simian agent 7
SCL	Stem cell leukemia
Sq S	Squamous cell sarcoma
SV-5	Simian virus 5
SV-20	Simian virus 20
SV-40	Simian virus 40
T	Thrombocytopenia

280

● = Possible Marburg predecessor

```
            Trn Ce    Transformed cells
            Undiag    Undiagnosed
            W Tumr    Wilm's tumor
            Yaba      Yabavirus

        c.  Source--coded as follows.

            1          tissue culture
            2          blood
            3          plasma/serum
            4          tissue mince
            5          buffy coat
            6          chemical
            7          ascites
            8          milk
            9          spinal fluid
            10         bone marrow
            11         culture

    2.  Number of animals inoculated.
    3.  Number of animals dead or transferred.
```

Fig. 23.6. Bionetics Summary Report of Studies Code Named According to Researchers' Last Names Including MK-SVLP (Manaker/Kotin–Special Virus Leukemia Program)

SUMMARY OF STUDIES*

A. Major Studies

1. BFKMRS, 10/65-3/66

    This study was established under the Special Virus Leukemia Program of the NCI to investigate human leukemic materials, human papilloma and infectious mononucleosis in conjunction with the co-carcinogens benzo[a]pyrene and benzanthracene. The program was a product of the study group that included Drs. Bryan, Falk, Kotin, Manaker, Rauscher and Stevenson. This study has recently been terminated and the remaining animals are in the process of being transferred.

Inoculum	Source	No. inoculated	Dead or transferred
H P	1	11	6
H L	1	15	3
H IM	1	11	3
Control		9	2

*Some studies summarized are in the process of being terminated and this may not be reflected in the total numbers. This is due to lag times in finalization of reports on selected studies.

2. Fink-Malmgren-Rauscher, 8/64 - 9/65

This program was designed to investigate the ability of fresh human leukemic materials, as well as cultured and manipulated cell products, to induce similar neoplasia in the newborn monkey.

Inoculum	Source	No. inoculated	Dead or transferred
H AML	2	6	5
H ALL	2	11	9
H EL	2	5	5
H CML	2	2	1

3. Irradiation Study, 2/67 - 5/67

The major emphasis of this study was to determine the suppressive effects of radiation upon primates and the subsequent enhancement or creation of a more favorable environment for neoplastic alteration. The program was under the direction of Drs. Reisinger and Bowser, with Drs. Rauscher, Landon, Stewart, Moloney, Perry and Hart collaborating.

Inoculum	Source	No. inoculated	Dead or transferred
H BL+Irr.*	1	16	2
H BL+Irr.+ BSA		8	5
H L+Irr.	2	8	2
H S+Irr.	3	4	3
M S+Irr.	4	3	2
S LE1,2+Irr.	1	4	2
A S-R+Irr.	1	5	1
Irr.		35	12
Irr.+BSA		17	3

*Irradiation

4. MK-SVLP, 2/66 - 3/67

This study was initiated by Drs. Manaker and Kotin in collaboration with an ad hoc committee of the SVLP. The prime objective was the induction of neoplasia in primates using Burkitt and other lymphoma material in conjunction with the co-carcinogens benzanthracene and benzo[a]pyrene.

Inoculum	Source	No. inoculated	Dead or transferred
H BL	1	105	11
H Lymph	1	33	5
H L	1	18	3
H Sq S	1	13	0
Control		6	1

5. Perry-Rauscher, 7/66-10/68

This program was initiated by Dr. Rauscher in collaboration with Dr. Perry of NCI and Dr. Landon of Bionetics. Fresh whole blood from leukemic patients was inoculated directly into monkeys using multiple sites and volumes as large as possible.

Inoculum	Source	No. inoculated	Dead or transferred
H CML	2	26	6
H AML	2	12	0
H LS	2	4	0
H ALL	2	18	0
H CLL	2	6	0
H RCS	2	1	0
H HD	2	3	1
H AT MON	2	2	1
H ML	2	2	0
H C-H	2	4	2
H BL	2	1	0
H Lymph	2	1	0

6. PSG-Melnick, 9/65-1/68

This study was a product of the Primate Study Group headed by Dr. J. Melnick. The primary objective was the investigation of the possible oncogenicity of selected human prototype viruses in primates in conjunction with the use of co-carcinogens. This study is in the process of being terminated with the remaining animals being transferred to Dr. Melnick.

Inoculum	Source	No. inoculated	Dead or transferred
H Reo 1	1	9	6
H Reo 3 + BL	1	15	15
H CMV	1	12	5
H P	1	1	1
H Herp/S	1	12	7
H Ad2P	1	12	1
H&S A2S40	1	12	1
H R	1	12	2
H Echo 9	1	12	5
C	1	1	0

B. Special Studies (active)

		Inoculum	Source	No. Inoc.	Dead or Transferred
1.	Ablashi, 10/70	S; H. saimiri	1	22	9
2.	Bryan-Jensen, 1/69	S; Mamm T	1	20	8
3.	Levine, 6/69	H; BL	1	38	8
4.	Melendez, 3/70	S; H. saimiri	1	16	5
5.	Pearson, 3/71	H; BL	1	16	0
6.	Rickard, 6/69	F; Lymph	1	11	3
7.	Theilen, 6/69	F. Fibro	1	13	0
8.	Witter, 7/70	A; HV of turkeys	1	8	0
		A; Marek's disease	1	8	0

Special Studies (terminated)

		Inoculum	Source	No. Inoc.	Dead or Transferred
1.	Dunkel, 7/70	H; BL	1	37	37
2.	Landon, 7/70	S&H; Misc V	1	26	10
3.	Landon-LaFontaine, 7/70	F; S	1	3	3
4.	Sibinovic-Ulland, 8/70	C; Dilantin	6	6	6

C. Other Active Studies

		Inoculum	Source	No. Inoc.	Dead or Transferred
1.	Adamson, 5/68	C; MCA-Cu chelate	6	37	26
2.	Blumberg-London, 3/68	H; Au Ag	3	11	7
3.	Gerber, 4/64	H; BL	3,5	16	16
		H; BL	7	2	0
		O&S; Misc V	2	12	4

D. Long-term Holding Studies

		Inoculum	Source	No. Inoc.	Dead or Transferred
1.	Feller, 7/66-11/66	H; Mamm T	8	5	0
2.	Fischinger-O'Connor, 8/69	F; Lymph	1	6	0
3.	Kelly, 6/67-4/68	C; MCA	6	3	3
		C; Benzo[a]pyrene	6	10	7
4.	Landon-O'Gara, 6/70-7/70	S; Misc L	4	5	0
5.	Landon-Rauscher-BRAF, 12/67	S&M; Rhab L	4	17	7
6.	Manaker, 8/64-10/69	H; BL	1	16	13
		H; L	2	1	1
		H; S	1	8	1
		H; Rau Vi	1	8	0
		S&M; Misc L	1	9	2
7.	Manaker-Landon, 5/67	H; ALL	1	1	0
8.	Manaker-Landon-Rauscher, 2/67	H; BL	1	8	7

		Inoculum	Source	No. Inoc.	Dead or Transferred
9.	Manaker-Rauscher, 6/66-7/67	H; RCS	1	1	0
		H; BL	1	3	0
10.	Manaker-Stevens, 6/67-12/68	H; BL	1	11	2
		H&S; BL + Malaria	1,2	12	0
		H&S; BL + Reo + Malaria	2	3	0
		S; Malaria	2	19	14
11.	Melnick, 12/63-6/68	H; AL	3	6	6
		H; IM	1	13	9
		H; ALL	1	21	15
		H; P	4	5	5
		H; Herp/G	1	44	1
		H; Reo 1	1	3	3
		H; Ad2P	1	4	1
		H; Herp/S	1	4	1
		H&S; Adeno+SV-40	1	3	2
12.	Moloney, 4/62-2/69	M; L lymph	1	12	8
		H; ALL	1	23	21
		H; CLL	3	5	5
		H; AMOL	3	1	1
		Control		23	13
		H; CSCL	3	3	2
		H; AML	3	20	15
		H; LS	1	4	1
		H; HD	3	1	0
		H; SCL	1	7	4
		H; CF	3	5	2
		H; CML	1	20	16
		H; MM	3	1	1
		H; P	1	1	1
		H; BL	7	14	5
		M; S	4	2	2
		H; RCS	3	2	2
		M; MSV	4	1	1
13.	Moloney-Reisinger-Bowser, 5/67	M; MSV	4	4	2
14.	Moore, 9/69	H; BL	1	2	0
15.	O'Connor, 4/65-9/67	H&M; ALL PI	1	3	3
		H&M; ALL I	1	3	3
		H; Rhabdo	1	3	0
16.	Old, 9/67-12/69	H; Osteo S	1	3	0
		S; Osteo S	1	2	0
17.	Rauscher-Landon, ● 12/66-2/70	S; Rhabdo	1	2	2
		H; ML	1	4	3
		H; BL	7	13	0
		S; Mening	4	2	2
		M; AL	3	4	3
		H; HD	1	1	0

285

		Inoculum	Source	No. Inoc.	Dead or Transferred
18.	Rauscher-Reisinger-Bowser, 4/67-5/67	H; BL	1	14	6
		Irradiation		1	1
		H; CML	2	1	0
19.	Sarma-Huebner, 9/69	F; Fibro	1	3	0
20.	Shachat-Moloney, 8/65-11/66	M&S; MSV MT	1	2	2
		M; Rhabdo	1	10	8
21.	Stewart, 4/62-6/68	H; ALL	1	56	24
		H; AML	1	6	6
		A; S	4	32	23
		H; GB	1	2	2
		H; BL	1	51	31
		H; CML	1	2	2
		H; HD	1	9	9
		H; Liposar	1	4	4
		H; D Enc	1	3	3
		H; Undiag	1	2	2
		S; SV-5	1	3	3

E. Terminated Studies

		Inoculum	Source	No. Inoc.	Dead or Transferred
1.	Aisenberg-Zamecnik, 5/64-6/64	H; HD	2	8	5
2.	Blumberg-Moloney, 6/66-10/66	● M; Rhabdo	4	1	1
		M; MSV L	1	2	2
3.	Chirigos, 5/66-3/69	C; pI:C	6	8	7
		M; S	1	6	6
		M; Arbo	1	2	2
		M; MSV AV	1	2	2
		M; MSV	1	2	1
4.	Cohen, 3/68-1/69	H; AL	2	6	5
		H; BL	1	3	3
		R; ALS	3	7	6
		Control		2	2
		H; AML	2	2	0
		H; CLL	2	2	0
		H; EL	2	2	0
5.	Dreyer, 9/64	H; ML	1	2	2
6.	Gajdusek, 1/67	H; D Enc	4	4	3
7.	Gajdusek-Gibbs, 4/66-5/66	H; Kuru	4	8	4
8.	Gazdar-Moloney, 7/69-8/69	F; Fibro	4	3	0
9.	Grace, 2/64-8/64	H; MyL	1	1	1
		H; AML	1	10	8
		H; ALL	1	2	1
10.	Grace-Horoscewicz, 5/67	H; BL	1	6	5
11.	Gross, 5/62-4/63	M; L lymph	4	12	7

		Inoculum	Source	No. Inoc.	Dead or Transferred
12.	Howard-Notkins, 5/67-1/68	H; Gamma globulin	3	16	16
13.	Huebner-Coates, 8/64-3/68	H; Ad 7	1	3	3
		H; Ad 12	1	6	4
		A; S	1	3	2
		M; S	1	4	3
		S&H; A12S40	1	2	0
14.	Johnson-Hull, 8/65-3/67	S; SV-20	1	4	3
		S; SA 7	1	10	10
15.	Kinard-Rauscher, 3/67-9/67	A; S	3	18	18
16.	Koprowski-Jensen, 4/66-6/66				
17.	Landon, 7/65-5/70	H; Ad 7	1	2	2
		B; Non-inf	2	14	9
		Control		16	14
	●	S; Rhabdo	1	7	7
		S; Rhabdo	4	18 *	9
18.	Landon-Darrow-Stewart, 1/68	S; CCHy	9	2	2
19.	Landon-Rauscher, 2/68-7/68	S; Plyctm	2	8	6
20.	Landon-Valerio, 8/67	S; LRL	4	2	2
21.	Manaker-Landon-Darrow, 6/68-7/68	Skin graft		6	6
22.	Manaker-O'Connor, 3/66	H; BL	1	2	2
23.	Moloney-Herbert, 4/67	M; L	4	2	2
		M; L lymph	4	3	3
24.	Moloney-Manaker, 4/67	CF		2	2
		H; BL	1	2	0
25.	Moloney-Stewart, 5/63-7/63	H; DC	1	2	2
		H; ALL	1	1	1
		H; CLL	1	1	1
26.	Morgan, 3/65	H; CA	4	3	3
27.	Morris, 9/65-5/66	S; SV-20	1	7	7
		S; S20S40	1	1	1
28.	Morton, 6/68-9/69	H; Osteo S	1	12	6
		H; Liposar	1	15	9
		Control		8	6
		H; Trn Ce	1	4	2
		H; Chondr	1	1	0
		E; ALS	3	4	3
		S; Bact Agt	4	1	0
29.	Nadel-Rauscher, 1/65-2/65	G; SCL	5	3	3

287

Then, most incredibly, Whitney noted that simian monkey viruses would only cause disease in humans if they were transmitted, just as I had concluded earlier (see pages 130-134), by vaccines:

There are viruses which naturally occur in apes and monkeys which are apparently nonpathogenic, but might cause disease in human beings by being transmitted in biologics [vaccines] manufactured from nonhuman primate [monkey] tissues. An example of this is the SV-40 virus from macaque kidney cells. It must have been administered to thousands of humans in polio virus vaccine. Fortunately, there were no undesirable effects [recorded or reported] in man, but it causes sarcoma in newborn hamsters. The term SV-40 refers to simian virus 40 of the simian-virus series *introduced by Hull and his collaborators in 1956.* This series [Whitney showed a slide for the group] is a list of the many simian viruses recovered from monkey kidneys or stools in the course of research work on poliomyelitits and other diseases. Most of these viruses are "orphan" which means that they are simply viruses which seem to have no pathogenic effects.[17]

Rhesus monkeys, cynomolgus monkeys (M. fascicularis), and chimpanzees have been used extensively in the study of poliovirus infections and development of vaccines. *Inoculation of the agents by parenteral route is necessary to establish infection in rhesus and cynomolgus monkeys. . . .*[17] [Emphasis added.]

Following brief statements about polio and rabies, Whitney explored the 1975 Marburg virus outbreak:

Marburg Virus Disease is also known as "green monkey disease" and "vervet monkey disease." It was first reported in humans in Europe in 1967. A total of 31 human cases occurred in the outbreaks, and death resulted in seven cases. Twenty-five of these cases occurred in humans who were working in laboratories that utilized green monkey tissue for vaccine production. No cases were reported in personnel working with the live monkeys. Apparently, all the monkeys were sacrificed. Whether the animals were sick or if they had lesions was never determined as necropsies were not performed nor were detailed records maintained. [This was obviously quite suspicious given the panic that ensued and the immediate WHO and CDC intervention.] Studies on these human cases and on additional monkeys demonstrated that the disease was caused by an . . . extremely large, cylindrically shaped [virus]. . . .

This disease was not reported again since the European outbreaks, either in man or nonhuman primates, until February 1975. Three non-laboratory associated cases in man were reported from South Africa. There is no specific therapy and no vaccine for this deadly disease. It is the most recent and impressive example of the potential public health threat to man from nonhuman primates.[17]

Kalter apparently took exception to Whitney's last remark, but Gerone voiced his concern first. "In the latest morbidity-mortality report that crossed my desk on Monday, Marburg virus disease seems ready to come to a head again."

Obviously, the CDC had warned the medical research establishment to prepare for future Ebola outbreaks, which occurred in Sudan and Zaire about eighteen months later.

Kalter, the senior monkey expert had heard enough. Obviously annoyed at the dearth of scientific evidence, he immediately shot back, "The information is very, very meager."[17]

Then with uncustomary rambling, he explained:

> Three cases seem to be involved. Two of these involve a young man and young lady traveling around Africa, where they evidently picked up the disease. The epidemiology of their cases is not known. Their contact with monkeys as monkey handlers is nil; however, they did associate with monkeys at farms and homes. The third case involved a nurse, and it followed the same pattern as established in Germany and Yugoslavia, where the secondary cases are as much of a problem as the primary cases. The young man died, the two ladies (the companion and nurse) are evidently recovering. I simply have to hold off on any comments regarding the epidemiology until we know more about it. But monkeys have not been excluded [or, for that matter, he obviously thought, included] definitely.[17]

Then, doing what he said he had to "hold off"—apparently he couldn't help commenting: "For the sake of completeness, we might mention one or two other points that are important to the total picture. I'll address myself principally to some of the viral diseases. We just referred to Marburg. I believe simian-hemorrhagic fever is important. It appears to be a man-made disease."

Undoubtedly, Kalter's words stunned many in the audience. Without pause, he had in essence insinuated the simian-hemorrhagic fever RNA had been experimentally transfused into the larger Marburg cylinder, and now was infecting humans.

Having said what he feared best not be said, he quickly added as an off-the-cuff example, "Tattooing has been important in the epidemiology of outbreaks of tuberculosis in the States, Soviet Union, and in England." He then changed tacks again and rambled on at length about a variety of viruses, monkeys, and dreaded diseases.

Hellman's Rebuttal

Few words were said following Kalter's heretical remarks. His wasn't a hard act to follow by any means, but most of the audience sat speechless.

The tentative silence was finally broken by Alfred Hellman from the NCI. In an obvious effort to break the tension and fortify the institute's politically correct theory of Marburg's evolution from the ape, Hellman said:

> In regards to what Sy Kalter was saying about the RNA tumor viruses, reports have appeared in recent newspaper articles, for example, *The [N.Y.] Times*, on the isolation of a virus from a woman with myelogenous leukemia. Thus far, the immunology and some of the hybridization biochemistry data on this virus would suggest that it has some relation, if not a lot of relation, with the Wooly and Gibbon agents which cause a malignancy in these animals. Apparently at least from the data . . ., it appears that the Gibbon ape lymphosarcoma virus probably is transmissible horizontally. I believe one should be aware of this and concerned about the possible relationship of these agents with that isolated from a human.

Why might Hellman have defended the establishment's untenable theory that Marburg and other monkey viruses could readily transmit their infections "horizontally" to humans?

As mentioned earlier, the "Special Virus Cancer Program Progress Report #8" identified Hellman as the the chairman of the NCI's section on Biohazards Control and Containment. He was also executive project officer for the NCI in their effort to test the "Aerosol Properties of Potentially Oncogenic Viruses" with the Navy. Hellman, oversaw the Naval Biomedical Research Lab studies in which viruses were spread through the air in an effort to study "virus-host interaction considering both the hazard to humans and animals and the potential for cross contamination."[8] These studies, similar to what had been conducted on the USS Coral Sea and the USS F. D. Bailey in 1950, were apparently a follow-up to the studies conducted by the Special Operations Division of the Army in cooperation with the Navy and the CIA.[18] This time, in 1971, instead of exposing unwitting servicemen to aerosols containing relatively mild, *Serratia marcescens* and *Bacillus globigii* bacteria, humans and animals were exposed to carcinogenic viruses. In these reports, Hellman and his colleagues wisely chose to keep the identity of their human and animal test subjects classified.[8]

Chapter 24
Ebola Kikwit and the
Sloan/Hot Zone/Plague Connection

WHILE typing these final words, *New York Times* medical reporter Lawrence Altman broke the story about the 1995 Ebola outbreak in Kikwit, Zaire—an area about 200 miles north of the still militarized Angolan border.[1]

For several months prior to this medical emergency, as Gerone and Hellman said had been done in the Spring of 1975, the media foretold of Ebola's likely return. *The Coming Plague* by *Newsday*'s health and science writer Laurie Garrett had joined *The Hot Zone* as the talk of the town. As Preston and Garrett toured the television talk-show circuit, the film *Outbreak* was trouncing its competitors at the box office. At the same time the networks were replaying versions of *The Andromeda Strain*. Then on Monday May 8, just two days before Altman's article appeared, CBS aired its highly publicized made-for-television movie *Virus*, another spin-off from Robin Cook's novel *Outbreak*.

Like the media, I too had warned friends and colleagues for months about the coming plague. Unlike the media's fairy tale, though, my prediction was based on the knowledge that the authorities had created and maintained stockpiles of such viruses for allegedly scientific purposes. I also knew that it made good business sense to re-release a proven money-maker.

In late 1994, my suspicions were further provoked when I received an invitation to attend my alma mater's "6th Annual Public Health Rounds." The Harvard program, "Patterns of Disease Evolution: Preparing for the Next Pandemic," warned that, "Global changes in climate, the environment, economic patterns and migration have contributed to the spread of AIDS, Lyme disease, Ebola and pneumonic plague." To my knowledge "global changes in climate" had nothing to do with "emerging viruses," while the other factors held little consequence as compared to the SVCP.

Given all the disinformation from the media as well as academic sources, it was only reasonable to conclude Ebola would likely come again.

The 1995 Ebola Outbreak

Officials at Zaire's health ministry allegedly traced Ebola's sudden reemergence to a "surgical patient" at a Kikwit hospital. Beginning April 10, the virus quickly spread to and from the hospital's staff. Among the first victims were three Italian nuns who served as nurses. One traveled to Mosango for care and died there, but not before infecting at least ten more medical staff. The virus ultimately reached several other areas, including Zaire's capital city Kinshasa.[1-3]

Teams of experts were immediately dispatched from the WHO, the CDC, and the Institute Pasteur, according to Dr. James W. LeDuc, a hemorrhagic fever specialist at the WHO. Tissue samples from the victims, LeDuc said, were initially sent to the Tropical Disease Institute in Antwerp, Belgium, but had to be forwarded to the CDC, through the Belgian Embassy, because scientists there, unlike the 1970s, were no longer working on hemorrhagic viruses.

Capitalizing on the opportunity to editorialize, LeDuc said, "It just shows the deteriorating capacity of the world to diagnose these diseases." Altman apparently agreed. The *New York Times* reported that LeDuc's view was shared by "a number of leading experts who, in recent years, have called attention to the threat from new and emerging viruses, like Ebola, and deplored the ability of laboratories to detect them."[1]

"At the CDC," Altman wrote, "where the blood samples arrived mid-Tuesday," Dr. Clarence J. Peters, an expert in hemorrhagic fever viruses, said in an interview, "We're still in the stage of trying to read tea leaves from third hand overseas reports. . . . We don't know how long it will take to get an answer. It's like planting a garden, sometimes everything comes up quickly, other times it takes longer."

This was a fast-growing garden however. The "mystery virus" was identified by television news reporters as Ebola, oddly, even before such reports were officially confirmed.

That night, Ted Kopel opened his special ABC News *Nightline* report this way:

KOPEL: We are, it turns out, reasonably flexible about plagues. All things considered, Americans have adjusted remarkably well to the plague that has been among us for the nearly fifteen years now. It is the worst in the world these days. But, because we've become reasonably informed about how it is passed on and how to avoid it, AIDS doesn't provoke a great deal of hysteria anymore. In fact, it barely arouses much interest. Just to keep things in perspective, the Ebola virus . . . only exists in this country in our fevered imaginations. We have watched Dustin Hoffman pretend to deal with a pretend outbreak in a pretend movie, and that has made us more receptive than we might otherwise be to a genuine outbreak that is killing people horribly and very quickly in Zaire. It is an important story, and we're not above using a couple of movie clips to engage your interest in it. But what is most important . . . is to keep what's happening in perspective.

Ebola is without question a biological Satan. . . . The second part of the virus nightmare is that it could travel even further. Someone carrying the virus might get on a plane, leave Zaire, and in a matter of hours carry it across the world.[2]

Having grabbed America's attention, media moguls used Richard Preston and CDC spokespersons, including Ruth Berkelman, their Deputy Director of Infectious Disease, and Don Francis who was on the "front line of the battle against the 1976 Ebola epidemic in the Sudan" to knock home their point—increased funding was "vitally" needed by the CDC to protect the public against Ebola and other new "emerging" viruses.

The Hot Zone author, Preston argued:

PRESTON: There are things going on in the tropical rain forests that we don't understand very well. And new viruses, and new agents, new organisms that are infectious are emerging and attempting, as it were, to break into the human species and to spread widely. I think probably the best example of this, of course, is the AIDS virus itself.[2]

"Politics may matter as much as biology; especially in a place like Zaire—a country whose leader is widely seen as corrupt, whose military steals what it wants; whose medical system is crippled by an economy in collapse. Disastrous conditions for ordinary people; ideal conditions for extraordinary viruses," ABC news reported.

Newsday's Laurie Garrett was interviewed next. Garrett had written a highly detailed account of research conducted in the aftermath of the Marburg and Ebola outbreaks in her book *The Coming Plague*. Though she reviewed Siegert's work regarding the first time this new hemorrhagic fever virus broke out in Europe, she wrote that "investigators hit pay dirt when they determined that all the monkeys came from three shipments of wild animals transported from Uganda to Belgrade, then on to Marburg and Frankfurt." This, I noted, was somewhat misleading as Siegert noted four suspected monkey shipments from a single dealer, that is, Litton Bionetics.[4]

Moreover, Garrett, had gone so far as to note that German scientists immediately turned to Dr. Jordi Casals, director of the Rockefeller Foundation's arbovirus laboratory at Yale, for assistance in identifying this bizarre Marburg agent. Casals, one of only two hemorrhagic disease experts throughout the world, Garrett recalled, was asked "to screen patient blood samples against all the viruses in his Rockefeller facility." Between 1951 and 1971, she wrote, "the Rockefeller Foundation's Virus Program" had "operated facilities in eight countries through which over sixty viruses" were allegedly "discovered."[4]

Yet, despite Garrett's detailed knowledge of such key researchers, their activities, and those of their affiliated institutions, rather than stating what the mass of circumstantial and scientific evidence showed—Ebola was apparently man-made—Garrett blamed the Kikwit outbreak on social factors and insterility. She stated the virus's reservoir was unknown:

GARRETT: It can be no coincidence that this has occurred now in Zaire. This is a virus that takes advantage of social disruption, of the lack of proper medical equipment—of syringes, so that people reuse syringes that are contaminated and inject the virus directly into their patients.

One of the key lessons that we have to learn from this outbreak right now. . . . We don't know where Ebola lurks—where it exists, when it doesn't appear [until] suddenly in 1976 and 1979. We don't know what animal carries it or insect. We don't know how the original human being who brings the virus into a village or a setting got it, and from where. And unless we know the natural ecology of this organism, we can never predict when it will appear again; where it will appear again. What we can do, however, is deal with the amplifying effect, which in the case of Ebola every single time has involved a hospital—a substandard facility—with shortages of syringes; with recycled syringes being used over and over again on the same people; improper sterile technique. That's an amplifier. It takes that one individual who's infected who got it from some animal, that we don't know, out in the rain forest, brought it into that hospital setting and the hospital becomes this amplification system to magnify it into an epidemic. That's what we need to attack. We as human beings spread these things around. It's our incompetence, our idiocy, our inequities all over the world that are responsible for these things. And if we don't confront those issues, this is only one of many outbreaks, many epidemics we will see and that will accelerate with time.

KOPEL: But Dr. Berkelman, that's where we run into the crossover between the medical problem and the political problem. Because it's not always that easy, for example, for the World Health Organization to move into a country and say, 'Here's what you've got to do in your hospitals.' Or even if a million new hypodermics are sent into a country like Zaire, likely as not they'll end up on the black market rather than ending up in the hospitals that Ms. Garrett was talking about.[2]

Evading the question of political corruption and incompetence, Berkelman—like a well-trained media spokesperson—replied:

BERKELMAN: Yes, but at the same time the world has grown pretty complacent about infectious diseases. We do have some diseases that are targeted. But for the last few decades, we really have said, 'Well, we've conquered smallpox, and we're dealing with some of the others. And we really have not done what we could do, and we need do more. . . . And we have been working at CDC to deal with the emerging infections that we have become complacent about; not only in the United States, but in other developed countries and developing countries. And the World Health Organization even right now is considering a resolution to say it's time that we really deal with the issue of these infectious diseases. That we haven't conquered them; that they're going to continue to evolve, and we have to deal with not only what is coming, but what may reemerge and what may continue to be causing problems. . . ."[2]

What a coincidence, I thought, that the WHO was just now 'considering a resolution' to commit millions more to their infectious disease efforts. The outbreak, for that measure, was certainly well timed.

Kopel then asked Francis, "To what degree should this outbreak of Ebola be a wake-up call to the world at large?"

Francis responded as did Berkelman by lobbying for additional funding:

FRANCIS: I think it should be a very strong wake-up call to back up what Dr. Berkelman said. Despite all of the screams from Gingrich et al. to slice government funding, we should be damn glad that Dr. Berkelman and her colleagues at the CDC have a team going off to Zaire, and have a group of experts who can help the world. We have got to have a commitment to prevention, by and large, and frankly, for my twenty-five years working in this field, I have yet to see the United States truly have a commitment to prevention, and doing things in a logical way. We get very excited about short-term situations and then forget it.[2]

Thus, the 1995 Ebola outbreak was exploited by CDC officials and the media. Indeed, Americans got "very excited" about prospects of bleeding, "from all open orifices—from the mouth, nose, eyes, what have you."[2] The threat was then used to justify the alleged need for massive infusions of cash into CDC coffers.

The following week, *Newsweek's,* cover story quoted Francis and Stephen Morse, a virologist at Rockefeller University. Writers for the magazine asked rhetorically:

What needs to be done on the domestic front? The Centers for Disease Control in Atlanta is this absolutely crackerjack government agency. It's one of the very few agencies in the federal government that really works. But they have terrible funding problems and are spread really thin. And they don't have any political constituency. There's no political-action group there hammering away at Congress to give them the money they need to do their job. . . . It's important because we are linked now, biologically, to the rest of the world. If Congress cuts the budget of the CDC, Congress is going to cut the throat of the American people.[5]

The same financial concerns were echoed in *USA Today.* The "heroes," "disease busters," "disease cowboys"—those "front line scientists of the CDC" the cover story contended, "should have their own airplanes"; yet are in dire fiscal straights. Their numbers "are shrinking, labs are deteriorating and administrators worry about the day when two Ebola-like emergencies happen at the same time, and they find themselves short of heroes."[6]

"If Ebola showed up in other parts of Africa now we'd be in trouble," said Dr. James Hughes, head of the CDC division of infectious disease. "Or if there was a Lassa fever outbreak tomorrow in West Africa, we'd be unable to respond. These things don't tend to occur simultaneously, but someday they will."[6]

"At first glance," Kim Painter of *USA Today* wrote, "CDC seemed fairly prosperous, an agency of 6,500 full-time employees, with an annual budget of more than $2 billion." But "only six people at CDC" were qualified to work in their BSL 4 lab—"one of only two maximum-safety labs in the country and six in the world." Which meant, Painter quickly noted, "that while the Ebola work goes on, virtually everything else screeches to a halt."[6]

Finally, Don Francis complained about the frugal atmosphere in which he conducted the 1976 Ebola investigation in Sudan. "It's all low-budget stuff," he said. "I think it's a shame. With an outbreak like this, they (CDC officials) should have their own damned airplanes. . . . If we need to send 40 experts over to Zaire we should be able to do it."[6]

"Still," Painter lamented, those at the CDC weren't expecting "such largesse" anytime soon:

> In fact, they're hoping they won't lose some of the money Congress has already promised for this year.
>
> A pending bill at one point cut out $47 million the agency was promised for a new lab building. It also cut about half of the $5.3 million it was promised to invigorate its system for monitoring emerging infectious disease the CDC says needs $100 million to $125 million.
>
> In the latest version of the bill, the money for the lab building and the emerging disease program is intact.[6]

"We just haven't learned our lessons very well," said Dr. Joe McCormick, a CDC physician who had joined Francis's 1976 Ebola expedition. Defending the need to spend $150 million more a year to finance ten more virology labs and fifteen surveillance clinics proposed for the outskirts of rain forests and large tropical cities, McCormick warned, "We're going to pay now or pay later."[5]

Exploiting a tragic Ebola outbreak to further CDC special interests followed the precedent of turning tragedies into political expedients long established by the government and healthcare NGOs. The CDC ultimately got its money. McCormick's advice, I feared, was more malignant however. Given the facts, I concluded his presage was like extortion—"pay now or pay later"—akin to a ransom notice for ongoing genocide.

As Garrett disclosed, the concept of "fifteen surveillance clinics" as a defense against the coming plagues was "the brainchild of Stephen Morse . . . at Rockefeller University." He had discussed the matter with ardent biowarfare protester and Nobel laureate Joshua Lederberg "in 1988 while planning the historic 1989 "Emerging Viruses" conference. The Program for Monitoring Emerging Viruses (ProMED), in essence, resurrected "the old Rockefeller Foundation international network of tropical laboratories," that had been previously administered by the CDC and the foundation.[4]

On May 11, 1995, Dr. Brian Mahy, a virologist at the CDC whose team had confirmed the outbreak was caused by Ebola, revealed to Dr. Lawrence Altman of the *New York Times*, that the strain of the Kikwit virus was "nearly identical to the one that caused the first known epidemic, in the Ebola region of Zaire in 1976." Altman reported that the surprise was shared by numerous experts who "had expected greater differences because viral strains from different locales tend to vary."[7]

Indeed it was hard to believe that Ebola Zaire, which had differentiated itself genetically from its predecessor, Ebola Sudan, over the course of five months and 500 miles, had emerged almost twenty years later, over the same distance, virtually unaltered. Some believe that modern technology may have helped, that is, refrigeration.

Filing for "Bankruptcy"

A week after Ebola Kikwit monopolized the headlines, on May 16, 1995, Dow Corning announced it was filing for Chapter 11 bankruptcy. The move was precipitated by a $4.2 billion class-action suit brought against the company on behalf of 400,000 women who reported ill health effects following the placement of breast implants manufactured by the company.

"Ironically," one wire service reported, "while the courts have handed down multimillion-dollar awards based on the presumption of a health hazard, major scientific studies now being completed have pointed to the opposite conclusion: that there is no evidence that breast implants are harmful."[8]

The media had gotten this information from Dow Corning's president, Richard A. Hazleton who argued the need for placing liability in such matters on the shoulders of the American taxpayer. To do otherwise, he claimed, would endanger health companies' research and development potential.

Hazleton further charged that the American economy and justice system had been corrupted by "junk science. . . . Having successfully attacked silicone breast implants," he lamented, "plaintiff's attorneys now have their sights set on another health care product: Norplant™."[9]

To help free American corporate "litigation targets" from attack by what he called "Litigation, Incorporated," Hazleton advanced a series of congressional recommendations for which he pledged to lobby. These included:

- The exclusion of biomaterials suppliers from litigation brought against medical device manufacturers. . . .
- A cap on punitive damages.

- The elimination of joint and several liability were the company with the deepest pockets pays the most, regardless of their degree of liability.

- Greater adherence to the *Daubert* principles which require judges to act as "gatekeepers" with respect to the admissibility of scientific evidence in the courtroom.

- And . . . a tightening of requirements when it comes to expert witnesses' credentials—simply being a medical doctor does not qualify you to testify about diseases unrelated to your field.

- Limiting the grounds for claims in accordance with generally accepted medical illnesses and their causes. Most of the claims against Dow Corning are for diseases that are not even recognized in medical text books. They also happen to be ailments that primarily affect women during, and shortly after, child-bearing age—surprise!—the same group most likely to have breast implants.[9]

Noting the identical spelling of Hazleton's name with that of the NCI and USAMRIID contractor in charge of the "Reston monkey house," I immediately placed a call to Virginia to determine if there was any relationship between the two. To my astonishment, the receptionist answered, "Good afternoon, this is Corning–Hazleton Biotechnologies, how can I help you."

I asked to speak with someone from the public relations department, and once connected requested information on the subject of Mr. Hazleton's identity and bankruptcy efforts. I was then directed to dial a toll free number to speak with someone from "client services." Here, another receptionist answered, "Medpath. Good afternoon." Now I realized that Medpath, the large laboratory conglomerate that had purchased Litton Bionetics labs, was now, at least administratively, directing traffic for Hazleton under the Dow Corning umbrella. A final call to Midland, MI, Dow Corning's home office, resolved my suspicion. Richard A. Hazleton, the C.E.O. of the company, Barbara Meussig, the media relations manager informed me, "has no connection to Corning–Hazleton."

The Media's Role

On Tuesday evening September 7, 1993, the *CBS Evening News* aired a special "Reality Check" segment. Dan Rather reported that the U.S. government spends between $2.5 and $3 billion of taxpayer money every year on public relations campaigns. The administration directs 10,858 federal public affairs workers to generate a barrage of press releases that target the media and daily influence world news. In essence, Rather reported, "critics say too much taxpayer money is being spent by the government to say nice things about itself."[11]

The previous year during another *CBS News* report on "Watergate: The Secret Story," Rather admitted publicly that much of what the news media broadcasts is censured by political bigwigs. Through the CIA, FBI, and FCC, the *CBS News* anchorman reported, politically correct positions are guarded and counterintelligence campaigns are continuously waged and won. Rather noted, for instance, that during the Nixon administration, the CIA "had ways of influencing a lot of [media] people on the beat, either through their editors or publishers or through granting of favors, all the ways that guys, politicians from county courthouses and city halls and state legislatures do it, but in very sophisticated ways. . . ."[12,13]

Likewise, in *Keeping America Uninformed*, author Donna Demac traced the demise of America's free press largely to the FBI and CIA again during this same period in history. Demac wrote:

> Richard Nixon, for example, for whom journalists were a persistent headache, eventually had intelligence agents wiretapping reporters' telephone lines, opening their mail, and raiding press offices. Such measures were believed to have ended when Nixon left office. [However,] . . . the Reagan administration also authorized the FBI and CIA to search newsrooms and institute a stream of ad hoc restrictions. It was primarily interested . . . in designing laws and regulations that would outlast the administration and reposition the media as a subordinated source of information about the actions of government.[14]

According to the Church Committee, by February 1976, fifty American journalists were working for the CIA. Carl Bernstein wrote for *Rolling Stone* that according to CIA documents, "more than 400 American journalists . . . in the past 25 years have secretly carried out assignments for the CIA." Such efforts, wrote Bernstein, contributed to the distortion of news at home as well as abroad.

The authors of *Covert Action Information Bulletin* added:

The CIA has at various times owned or subsidized more than 50 newspapers, news services, radio stations, periodicals and other communications entities, sometimes in the U.S. but mostly overseas. Another dozen foreign-based news organizations, not CIA-financed, were infiltrated by paid CIA agents. Nearly a dozen American publishing houses, including some of the most prominent names in the industry, have printed at least a score of the more than 250 English-language books financed or produced by the CIA since the early 1950s, in many cases without being aware of the Agency involvement. A substantial number of the bogus news stories planted abroad were published as genuine in the United States, a phenomenon the CIA calls "blowback," "replay," or "domestic fallout."[15]

Other times news stories and headlines are tweaked, or distorted, just enough for "damage control." Such was the case when *USA Today* carried a special report entitled "Doctor ties gulf war illness to anti-chemical pills." The brief report on page 6 came as Pentagon officials openly denied a common cause for "Gulf War Syndrome"—the headaches, chronic fatigue, nausea, and other symptoms that as many as 50,000 Desert Storm veterans experienced in the aftermath of the war. A brief one line disclosure by the principle investigator, Scottish scientist Goran Jamal, noted the most likely cause of the syndrome "were vaccinations" and not "pills."[16]

Days later an esteemed American cancer researcher, Dr. Garth Nicolson, chairman of the Department of Tumor Biology at the University of Texas, M. D. Anderson Cancer Center made headlines, in the *National Enquirer*, for a different reason.[17] For months he had tried to gain media attention regarding his discovery that more than half of "Chronic Fatigue-Immune Dysfunction Syndrome" (CFIDS) patients were infected by a variant of a common germ known as *Mycoplasma fermentans*. His letter to the editor of the *Journal of the American Medical Association*, and a lengthy article in the *Journal of Occupational & Environmental Medicine*, included the discovery that about 80 percent of these people were helped by taking an inexpensive antibiotic—Doxycycline.[18,19] More astonishing, however, was his finding that the microbe's strength and insidious behavior was associated with a special gene *identical* to the one that codes for HIV's outer envelope.[19] His conclusion? The organism was undoubtedly developed in a lab and most likely transmitted, once again, accidentally or intentionally through the vaccines administered to the soldiers.[17]

Within days, however, major television networks responded by broadcasting alternative conclusions reached by other scientists, incredibly, from the University of Texas, where Nicolson was suddenly being pressured to leave his tenured post. Their studies, funded suspiciously by Ross Perot, showed that chickens injected with the chemicals given to Gulf War soldiers to prevent infections were weakened by the drug interactions.[20]

"What does it all mean?" asked investigative reporter Bill Schaap, a long-time CIA observer:

> It is not rhetoric to claim that "though control" is [here]. . . . COINTELPRO and Operation CHAOS are alive and well. The government wants, on the one hand, a blank check to spread its disinformation, and on the other, vast powers to prevent anyone from accusing it of doing so. Clearly, truth is the first casualty of cold wars as well as hot wars.[21]

Sloan/Hot Zone/Plague Connections

Shortly after the Ebola outbreak in Kikwit, Jackie gave birth to a beautiful, seven-pound-thirteen-ounce baby girl. Eight weeks later we drove to New York to introduce Aria Katriel to friends and relatives in Manhattan. Here I happened to read a *New York Times* article entitled "Grants by Foundations Help Technology Books Make It to the Shelves." The story revealed *The Hot Zone*'s author, Richard Preston, had received a generous grant from the Sloan Foundation "though the book did not fit into the Sloan technology series."[22] How interesting, I thought.

Years before I had read Paul Starr's book, *The Social Transformation of American Medicine: The Rise of a Sovereign Profession and the Making of a Vast Industry.* Starr noted the important role the media and private foundations played in marketing cancer research. He wrote:

> In the late forties, a new force began to be felt that greatly spurred the expansion of the NIH. This was the emergence of a private, lay lobby for medical research. Its chief architects, Mary Lasker and Florence Mahoney, brought money and influence to a cause of ready-made appeal. Mrs. Mahoney's husband owned the Cox newspaper chain, and Mrs. Lasker and her husband, who had made a fortune in advertising, had recently taken a major role in reorganizing the American Society for the Control of Cancer. The Lasker group had led the organization which they renamed the American Cancer Society, to introduce modern advertising techniques and to devote the proceeds to cancer research. Mass fund raising for medical research had already been turned into a high art by . . . 1937.
>
> This "noble conspiracy," also known as "Mary and her little lambs," believed that the doctors and research scientists were too accustomed to thinking small. . . . NIH discovered that the way to open wide the public's purse was to call attention to one disease at a time.[23]

"Why would the Sloan Foundation provide major funding for a work that didn't fit their agenda?" I asked Jackie, as my intuition drew on Starr's revelations.

A search through Sloan Foundation's annual reports, on file in Manhattan's New York Public Library, revealed nine ghastly and incriminating reasons that, most incredibly, tied all the elements of my investigation together. The Sloan Foundation: (1) supported black educational initiatives consistent with the COINTELPRO Black Nationalist Hate Group campaign;[24] (2) administered mass-media-public-persuasion experiments completely consistent with the CIA's Project MKULTRA—efforts to develop brainwashing technologies and drugs to affect large populations;[25] (3) funded much of the earliest cancer research involving the genetic engineering of mutant viruses;[26] (4) began major funding of the National Academy of Sciences, Cold Spring Harbor Laboratory (for "neuroscience" and molecular genetics research), the Salk Institute (for viral research), and the Scientists' Institute for Public Information between 1968 and 1970;[27] (5) funded population control studies by Planned Parenthood-World Population, New York, N.Y.;[24](6) funded the Community Blood Council of Greater New York, Inc., the "council of doctors" who established the infamous New York City Blood Bank;[28] (7) maintained Laurence S. Rockefeller, the director of the Community Blood Council of Greater New York and the president of the Rockefeller Brothers Fund, as chairman of the board of the Memorial Sloan-Kettering Cancer Center, and a trustee for the Foundation;[29,30] (8) gave in excess of $20,000 annually to the Council on Foreign Relations;[27] and (9) maintained among its "marketable securities," 16,505 shares of Chase Manhattan Bank stock (in 1967, which it apparently sold by 1970 probably to avoid conflict of interest charges) along with 24,400–53,000 shares issued by Merck & Co., Inc. (which it maintained at least until 1973, the end of the investigated period).[31]

"This is like the icing on the cake," I said to Jackie after relaying the information. "No wonder they funded *The Hot Zone*"

I later learned that Laurie Garrett was also "subsidized by the Alfred P. Sloan Foundation" during her writing of *The Coming Plague*.[4]

Background on Sloan

Alfred P. Sloan, for many years the chief executive officer of General Motors Corporation, began The Sloan Foundation in 1934. In its early years, the foundation's work focused on its founder's personal conviction that "ignorance of the principles of capitalism and free enterprise was both a danger and an opportunity." The Massachusetts Institute of Technology, Sloan's *alma mater*, was the principal recipient of foundation support during the first ten years.[25]

As the Second World War was winding down, Sloan joined the board of directors of New York City's Memorial Hospital for Cancer and Allied Diseases. Soon thereafter, Sloan founded the Sloan-Kettering Institute for Cancer Research to administer the hospital's research activities. Then, in 1945, Sloan persuaded his General Motors colleague Charles F. Kettering to lend his name to the Institute.[25]

> For the next thirty-four years, the Sloan Foundation maintained a special relationship with "Sloan-Kettering," as it is popularly known. General support grants were made each year, as well as frequent grants for particular projects. . . . Today, Sloan-Kettering (the official name is now Memorial Sloan-Kettering Cancer Center) is the largest private institution in the world for the treatment of cancer and for cancer-centered research and training. Its operating budget in 1980 was $183 million, of which $44 million was spent on research and training.[25]

Their 1967–1973 annual reports document the foundation's activities and orientation. Besides the organization's heavy investment in genetic engineering and cancer research, between 1969 and 1979, four particular programs were implemented and completed:

> one to increase the number of minority students in medicine and management; one to support experimental work in educational technology; one to establish the new discipline of neuroscience; and one to increase the number of minority students in engineering.[25]

By the early 1980s, the foundation's principal scientific focus, under the neuroscience umbrella, became mass persuasion technologies. The "program in cognitive science," was a pure research program "focused on problems of understanding human mental processes." Financial aid during this program went to support "highly interdisciplinary research in psychology, linguistics, neuroscience, philosophy, anthropology, and computer science." Discoveries made during this program laid the foundation for later work that focused on "management education," or "public management," as it was called. Explained in *The Greenwood Encyclopedia of American Institutions*, the foundation's concept of "public" management involved "the analysis of public problems and the management of government" in an effort to solve those problems.[25]

Apparently, this work was initiated as the foundation's response to Nixon administration "national security" concerns. The rising tide of racial violence and antiwar protests weighed heavy on the minds of foundation leaders. As Kissinger took control of the NSC, the CIA, the FBI, and COINTELPRO, Sloan Foundation activities reflected such adjustments. Everett Case, then the foundation's president, articulated the seriousness of the times and the need for the foundation to respond accordingly in a report published in the spring of 1968. Case wrote:

the multiplication and growth of many of our besetting social problems seem all too reminiscent of the behavior of the cancerous cell. Who would have predicted at the beginning of this decade that racism would infect and inflame the minds of even a vocal minority of the Negroes who, in this country, have been its principal victims? Who would have foretold the rise in resort to violence not only among the swelling ranks of the criminals but also as a means of social protest and even as a weapon of dissent?[24]

Case's next paragraphs were most enlightening:

More effective techniques for the control of population growth are at hand. The genetic code has been deciphered, and the elements of DNA can now be made synthetically. So, too, the hundreds of young scientists who have earned Sloan fellowships in basic research have made important contributions to our understanding of both the macrocosm and the microcosm.

It is different when one leaves the laboratory or the field experiment, and the disciplined minds they attract, for the sprawling, clamorous, and slippery problems which confront, say, the President of the United States or the Mayor of New York City. It is easy to ascribe outbreaks of urban violence to the intolerable conditions of the ghettos. It is easy to ascribe those conditions to the neglect or apathy of the landlords, to the massive immigration of unskilled and disadvantaged Negroes from the South, to the cupidity of the real estate operators and the building trades, or to the ineptitude and corruption of city officials. It is much harder to get at the *root* causes of such phenomena, and even more difficult to discover and apply effective cures.

. . . Some such observation applies as well to those who see our salvation simply in terms of a return to the "old-fashioned morality." It is not that the younger generation (and moral confusion is not limited to them) have found anything better than the golden rule or the New Testament's "Second Commandment"; indeed, many of them are seeking new ways of applying these precepts more effectively. In the canyons and ghettos of megalopolis, however, the simple injunction to "love thy neighbor as thyself" too often seems meaningless or irrelevant. Moreover, the new knowledge and new technology which we owe to science can not only change our environment in ways that bewilder and confuse, but can themselves become instruments of exploitation. By the same token, they may convert the stuff of moral and legal controversy into an academic exercise. . . .

[S]cience . . .whatever its problems, including the apprehension of a popular revulsion against its untoward consequences, it is clear that science is an enterprise too dynamic to be "turned off" if we would, and too fundamental to our security and our economy to be abandoned if we could. Certainly the search for the causes and possible cures of cancer must be accelerated, not brought to a halt. Together with technology, engineering and management, moreover, science has an indispensable role to play in any effective assault society may launch upon the stubborn complexities of our urban problems.[24]

The Sloan Foundation, thus, implemented grant programs consistent with the COINTELPRO Black Nationalist Hate Group's campaign to dissuade black America against violent revolution, and refined their resources for "public management." Undoubtedly, they fulfilled their founder's goal to take advantage of people's "ignorance of the principles of capitalism and free enterprise," and the military–medical–industrial opportunities that presented themselves in genetic engineering, cancer research, and population control.

Chapter 25
Smoking Guns
and Conclusions

On June 27, 1983, before the AIDS virus was even officially discovered, the French newspaper, *Libération*, carried the headline "Institut Pasteur, Sick With Gay Cancer" alleging the Institut Pasteur Production (IPP), 45 percent of which was owned by the "Institut Pasteur," had received and used "AIDS contaminated" American blood serum to manufacture hepatitis B vaccines that were given to sexually promiscuous gays, as well as exported to foreign countries.[1] The article noted that IPP was Merck, Sharp, & Dohme's (MSD) strongest competitor in the burgeoning Asian hepatitis B vaccine market.

Thus, the possibility that MSD, perhaps through the CIA, arranged for HIV-tainted American blood serum shipments to the IPP, which may have spread AIDS to Europe and Asia, crossed my mind.

Such a consideration would seem unreasonable were it not for the fact that the CIA had commonly conducted industrial espionage operations against French firms on behalf of American companies.[2] As past CIA Director R. James Woolsy remarked, "With the end of the Cold War, the CIA must enter the era of economic espionage." In the language of espionage, a French columnist explained, this meant that "the CIA will henceforth do many services for American enterprises which take the trouble to ask it for 'help' in both counterespionage and espionage itself."[3]

The Hilleman Interview

Soon after the galleys of *Emerging Viruses* arrived in a select few reviewers' hands, I received an urgent message from Dr. Watson, at the Medical–Legal Foundation, instructing me to obtain a copy of *The Health Century* by Edward Shorter, Ph.D.[4]

Shorter, a medical historian at the University of Toronto, was commissioned by the NIH to write a one hundred year summary of the Institutes' "medical miracles." He was given carte blanche access to all department heads, researchers, and Institute officials. According to Shorter, "tapes of the interviews" were "deposited in the History of Medicine Division of the National Library of Medicine." The resulting book, published by Doubleday, contained information that was refreshingly frank and even embarrassing.[5]

In his seventh chapter, Shorter traced the NIH's early cancer research efforts to James Ewing, at New York's Memorial Hospital, later part of the Memorial Sloan-Kettering Cancer Center, who "suggested to colleagues that they try mustard gas on various cancers." In 1942, Ewing's recommendation was taken up by Yale University scientists Louis Goodman and Alfred Gilman, who studied "what mustard gas did to white cells." Their research gave rise to the modern day use of alkylating agents which stop cancer cells from multiplying along with every other cell in the body.[4]

The first cancer virus, Shorter reported, was discovered by two women, Bernice Eddy, a doctor of bacteriology, and Sarah Stewart, a cancer researcher. Eddy's story went back to her discovery, in 1954, of live monkey viruses in the "supposedly inactivated" polio vaccines developed by Jonas Salk. "This discovery had not been well received at the NIH," Shorter wrote, and Eddy, considered a "whistle-blower," was demoted. Later, unbeknownst to her superiors, she teamed up with Sarah Stewart to discover the SE polyoma virus. The "SE" refers to *S*tewart and *E*ddy. "The polyoma was particularly important," Shorter said, "because, up to that time, scientists had thought of viruses as causing cancer mainly in birds." The polyoma virus caused cancers in every animal receiving it.[4]

Unfortunately, Eddy and Stewart never received the recognition they deserved. Their male counterparts largely censored, and then took credit for, the women's findings. Allegedly independent of Bernice Eddy's discovery, Shorter reported, a virologist named Laurella McClelland, working under Maurice Hilleman at Merck's vaccine division, noted "something funny" going on in the Rhesus monkey kidney cells being used to test Merck's polio vaccines. The company, at the time, produced both the Salk inactivated polio vaccine and Sabin's live virus vaccine. The latter was being field tested in the Soviet Union and in Europe at the time of Stewart's polyoma virus discovery. Both vaccines, produced in Rhesus monkey kidney cells, were so badly contaminated with strange viruses, that Hilleman requested African green monkeys be imported to safety test both the vaccines and the rhesus cells. McClelland reported the frightening results of these tests to her boss. "For some reason," wrote Shorter, "the viruses the rhesus monkeys were carrying didn't destroy their own kidneys, but they destroyed those of the greens." This led to Hilleman's discovery of SV40.[4]

Not long after I read this, Dr. John Martin sent me a copy of Shorter's audiotaped interview with Hilleman.[5] During the session, Shorter asked, "Tell me, how did you find SV40 in the polio vaccine?"[6]

"Well that was a Merck thing." Hilleman replied. "I can tell you very briefly. . . . I came to Merck [in 1957 from the OSRD—the Defense

Department's Office of Scientific Research and Development—then, a scientific intelligence contributor to the WRS and later the CIA] and I was going to develop vaccines, and we had wild viruses . . . you remember those wild monkey kidney viruses. And I finally gave up. I said you can't develop vaccines with these damn monkeys . . . If I can't do something [about them], I'm going to quit."

So Hilleman called Washington, D.C. zoo director, Bill Mann for help. "These lousy monkeys are picking [the viruses] up while being stored in the airports, in transport, at these off loading places." Hilleman said.

Mann told Hilleman his problem was "very simple." Hilleman recalled that Mann advised him to "go ahead, get your monkeys out of West Africa. Get the African green. Bring them into Madrid. Unload them there. There are no other traffic through there for animals. Fly them into Philadelphia and pick them up. Or fly them into New York and pick them up right off the airplane."

"So," Hilleman continued, "I brought African greens in. I didn't know we were importing AIDS virus at the time."

One might have expected shock from Hilleman's listeners. Shorter was joined by a film producer and crew from WGBH, Boston's famous PBS production center. Instead, laughter filled the room.

"Oh, now we know," said a woman heartily.

"What Merck won't do to develop a vaccine," Shorter chided between fits of laughter, obviously clueless why Hilleman was dead serious.

"Yeah, right," the woman replied as Hilleman continued.

"We brought in those monkeys . . .this was the solution. Because these monkeys didn't have the wild viruses."

"Why didn't the greens have the wild viruses since they came from Africa?" Shorter questioned, gathering his wits.

"Because they weren't being infected in these group holding things with all these other 40 different [monkey] viruses," Hilleman answered.

"But they had the ones they brought from the jungle, though?"

"Yeah, they had those, but there were relatively few. What you do is if you have gang housing then you're going to have an epidemic transmission of infection in a confined space."

"Oh, so that's it," Shorter replied, suddenly getting the picture.

Hilleman continued. "So anyway, the greens came in, and now we had these, and then we're taking our seed stocks to clean them up, and God, now I'm discovering new viruses. So, I said, 'Judas Priest!'"

Merck's vaccine director, who admitted to Shorter retaining military and NIH ties while working for Merck, continued to explain how he came to announce this discovery before an international gathering of scientists. The Copenhagen conference was sponsored by Sabin's benefactor—the Sister Kenny Foundation—the counterpart to the March of Dimes Foundation that supported Salk.

Prior to the meeting, Hilleman had wondered what he would talk about. He decided a presentation on "something that's gonna attract attention. . . . I know what I'm gonna do," he enticed Shorter, "I'm going to talk about, the detection of non-detectable viruses. . . . So I thought gee that damn SV40. I mean, I mean that," Hilleman stuttered awkwardly for the first time, "that damn vacuolating agent that we have, I'm going to pick that particular one. So I picked it, and quick worked it up, and I thought, boy now, that virus has got to be in the vaccines. And it's got to be in Sabin's vaccine. So I tested it, and sure enough it was in there."

"I'll be damned," Shorter said with a sigh, the seriousness of Hilleman's admissions finally sinking in.

"So now. . . . I go ahead,"

"So you just took stocks of Sabin's vaccine off the shelf here at Merck," Shorter interrupted.

"Yeah, it was made at Merck."

"You were making it for Sabin at this point?"

"Yeah, it was made before I came."

"Yeah, but at this point Sabin was just doing these massive field trials?" Shorter asked for clarification.

"Uh huh. In Russia and so forth," Hilleman replied.

In the meantime, Merck's vaccine chief said, "we had taken this virus and put it into hamsters." The hamsters grew tumors, just as Eddy's had. "So the joke of the day was that we would win the Olympics because the Russians would be loaded down with tumors." Shorter footnoted that "Sabin had field-tested his oral polio vaccine extensively in the Soviet Union."[4]

Consequently, just prior to delivering his lecture, Hilleman decided to break the news to Albert Sabin, after which Sabin rebutted, "This is just another obfuscation that is going to upset vaccines."

"I said, 'well you know, you're absolutely right,'" Hilleman continued, "but we have a new era here, an era of detection. And the important thing is to get rid of these viruses."

Shorter interrupted, "Well, why did he call it an obfuscation if it was a virus that was contaminating the vaccine?"

"Well now, because there were 40 different viruses in these vaccines anyway that we were inactivating, and ah."

"But you weren't inactivating the [SV40] . . . "

"No, that's right." Hilleman under pressure explained. "But yellow fever vaccine had leukemia virus in it, and you know this is in the days of very crude science. So anyway I went down and talked to him.

"He said, 'Why are you concerned about it?'"

"I said, I have a feeling down in my bones that this virus is different . . I don't know how to tell you this, but I've been around vaccines for a long time. I just think this virus may have some long-term effects."

Sabin asked what kind?

"I said cancer."

Shorter then asked why the press didn't pick up on the controversy.

A confused Hilleman replied with sudden memory loss, "Well I guess it did. I guess it did. I don't remember very well. We had no press release on it. Obviously you don't go out, this was a scientific affair within the scientific community."

Changing the subject, he then said, "But anyway, the next thing you know we had run out activation curves on these things. We knew it was in our seed stock for making vaccine. . . . We'd run it down and it would all be killed, you see. But," Hilleman chuckled, "when we were able technologically to grow more virus, then we found it wasn't being inactivated. That virus, you see, has one in 10,000 particles [that] is not inactivated by formaldehyde. Which was a very strange phenomenon. . . . It was good science at the time because that's what you did. You didn't worry about these wild viruses."

Later, Shorter asked when SV40 and the respiratory adenoviruses, another Hilleman discovery, were "first identified to be tumorigenic in mammals?"

Hilleman replied, "I think the SV40 and the adeno's, gee, they were sort of contemporary. I think they were contemporary. . . . "

"Is that right?" Shorter replied a bit surprised.

Indeed, Hilleman explained, the SV40 virus was in "the same family, you know, that causes progressive multifocal leukoencephalopathy. All of us carry it. You get immunosuppressed and you come down with this head disease."

"This is projected as AIDS?"

"JC virus," Hilleman returned, apparently referring to the encephalitis virus infection that remains latent until the immune system collapses.

Minutes later Shorter asked why Hilleman didn't continue his SV40 cancer research.

"I couldn't go ahead and form an SV40 cancer lab and ultimately go on into molecular biology [as Gallo and others had done]. I had to go into other things."

"Well why is that?" queried Shorter.

"Because I had to go on to develop vaccines for Merck."

A moment of silence later, followed by audience laughter, Shorter wryly chided, "Just what Merck wants to hear of course, that you were driven by the compassion for commercialism away from revolutionary science."

"No. No. No. No. . . . " Hilleman missed the joke, "Now, now, now look, now don't get the wrong idea," he defended. "Don't quote me wrong. Because in the real world, all of these, these basic [Hilleman paused to gather his thoughts] background things. Now that SV40 discovery for example, if that had been a human carcinogenic agent that could have been like the discovery of AIDS virus, you know, for iatrogenic spread of cancer."

"Because it had already been injected into 10 million people," Shorter said with a nervous burst of laughter.

"That's absolutely right," Hilleman replied not realizing he had contradicted and incriminated himself. Only minutes earlier he had told Shorter how SV40 had, as Bernice Eddy avowed, been carcinogenic to humans. "If you stop it. And we did stop it. Absolutely." Hilleman lied, defending, "That brought vaccines to a halt for polio until that was cleaned up."

It was never cleaned up entirely. Minutes later, Hilleman recalled his human cancer research that included, "the basic research with SV40." And later, when they worked on cancer immunology, he proudly described "taking a person's tumor, grinding it up, and putting it back into him," using "our SV40 hamster model."[6]

Shortly after Hilleman formally presented his SV40 findings in Copenhagen, Yale researchers with an electron microscope determined that SV40 and the SE polyoma were very similar viruses.

"Nothing about the monkey virus causing cancer had yet surfaced in either the lay press or scientific literature although insiders were aware. Alan Rabson, a former senior administrator at the NCI, attended the conference and told Shorter, "Everyone in the grapevine knew."[4]

Members of "the grapevine," recognizing that millions of children had received both polio vaccines, were now frantic. "Everyone was very excited" at the NIH, Rabson said. Hilleman believed the inactivation process used to produce Salk's polio vaccine had been successful.[7] He was wrong. Live SV40 remained. Recipients maintained traces of SV40 antibodies in their blood. Those who had received Sabin's vaccine, however, lacked SV40 antibodies. Luckily, the virus was substantially inactivated in the process of digestion.[8] "The Russians, supposed to show up at the Olympics dragging with tumors, were safe!"[9] wrote Shorter sarcastically.

Finally, on July 26, 1961, the *New York Times* reported that Parke-Davis, another vaccine manufacturer, and Merck decided to pull the plug on their Salk vaccines, "until they can eliminate a monkey virus." There was still no mention of cancer. The article, adjacent another about overdue library books, was buried on page 33. The cancer connection was suppressed until February 1962, when the *Times* finally reported it on page 27.[10]

"Was this silence merely the incompetence of the press in the face of a complex scientific question," Shorter asked, "or was there a deliberate effort to keep a lid on the story?" In December 1986, an elderly Sabin replied, "I think to release certain information prematurely," he said, "is not a public service. There's too much scaring the public unnecessarily. Oh, your children were injected with a cancer virus and all that. That's not very good."[4]

One needs to recall "how badly the whole public health system had been burned by the Cutter incident five years previously," Shorter considered in an effort to understand Sabin's attitude. In 1955, the first lots of improperly inactivated Salk polio vaccine was processed and shipped by the Cutter Laboratories in Berkeley, California. "Live polio virus was being injected into children," wrote the medical historian. "The gratitude of the public turned to horror as the Cutter vaccine gave polio to almost 80 recipients; these children in turn went on to spread the disease to another 120 playmates and relatives; three quarters of the victims were paralyzed and 11 died."[12]

It was Bernice Eddy whose lab tests showed the Cutter vaccine had been inadequately treated. Eventually she lost her labs pursuing and espousing the truth. Her treatment scandalized the scientific community, and resulted in a U.S. Senate investigation during which she warned legislators that unless the vaccine contamination problem was addressed, slow monkey viruses would surely deliver human cancer epidemics around the world.[13]

Unfortunately, senators and the media were unimpressed. The date was October 15, 1971—four days before President Nixon's helicopter touched down on Fort Detrick's parade field in celebration of the transition from America's top biological weapons testing center into the Frederick Cancer Research Facility of the National Cancer Institute. It was to be the leading facility in the fight against what he called, "America's No. 1 enemy—Cancer!"[14]

When asked if Nixon's war on cancer had been won or lost, Hilleman said "it never produced anything really because the science wasn't there, it wasn't right. But it produced the money that eventually allowed for the breakthroughs.[6]

What type of breakthroughs? "As far as I'm concerned," Hilleman explained, "when the onco[cancer]viruses were discovered, and you have to credit Bob Huebner [Peter Duesberg's NCI–University of California supervisor, see fig. 8.3] for the oncogenes, that concept, (and I think he should get the Nobel prize for it, but he won't) but that was the beginning of the modern era of cancer etiology. From that came the business of activation of normal host genes, that there are genes that have to do with replication of cells, and if you activate them, screw them up some way, or carry them from cell to cell, you can produce cancer. Now that to me was the beginning of the modern cancer era. Now you understand things at a genetic level. And that is what is great."[6]

Hilleman never revealed to Shorter Merck's participation in the NCI's Special Virus Cancer Program. Or that by 1965 the rampent biohazard and containment problems were to be largely solved by Dow Chemical Company through an NCI contract. The "Research and Development of Biohazards Containment Facilities," contract, seen in fig. 25.1, showed that Bionetic's Kensington, Maryland operation had been among the first to be given site visits by Dow consultants. A mere one percent of the entire Special Virus Cancer Program budget went towards preventing cross contamination and viral outbreaks from reoccurring (see fig. 25.2).[15]

More Live Vaccine Contaminants

Apparently, SV40 was not the only virus allowed to contaminate American made vaccines. Using a combination of advanced tissue culture methods and genetic probes, Dr. W. John Martin, Professor of Pathology at the University of Southern California, assayed blood samples from patients with chronic fatigue syndrome and related nervous disorders. This work led to his discovery of unique cell-destroying viruses that were not recognized by the immune system. Termed "stealth viruses," the germs were able to cause persistent infections because they were missing specific genes which, if expressed, would evoke effective antiviral immunity.[16,17]

In March of 1995, Martin communicated to FDA officials that some stealth viruses clearly originated from African green monkey simian cytomegaloviruses—a type of herpesviruses that are known to infect man,

Fig. 25.1. Dow Chemical Company's Special Virus Cancer Program Biohazard and Containment Contract Summary

The Dow Chemical Company (PH43-65-1045)

Title: Research and Development of Biohazards Containment Facilities

Contractor's Project Director: Mr. Cyril B. Henke

Project Officer (NCI): Mr. W. Emmett Barkley

Objectives:

The objectives of this contract are to evaluate possible hazards to
personnel conducting research in the virus-cancer field, study the
state-of-the-art of agent control and containment from the standpoint
of personnel protection and increasing the validity of experimental
studies; assist in the planning, construction and evaluation performance
of new concepts for facilities and programs involving hazardous agents.

More specifically, the current contract effort is being directed to the
following program areas:

1.   Applied research and development studies on biohazards control
and containment.

2.   The continued implementation and further development of an
environmental monitoring program for Building 41.

3.   The continued evaluation of the performance of environmental
control features incorporated in Building 41 and into the prototype
laboratory units.

4.   Related operational activities in Building 41.

5.   Consultation for the Special Virus Cancer Program with special
emphasis on providing assistance to NCI contractors through a site
visit program.

Significance to Biomedical Research and the Program of the Institute:

The data collected in this program indicates that the facility systems
and operational procedures are very effective in maintaining low
contamination levels and minimizing cross contamination within the
facility. Dow personnel continue to provide operational engineering
analysis support to the NCI virus containment facility to improve
the operation and maintenance of the primary and secondary barrier
systems.

A theoretical analysis has been completed in which equations were
developed to describe the removal of airborne contaminants from a room
utilizing various combinations of air filtration, building ventilation
systems and air recirculation devices. It has been concluded that
while such devices are impractical for controlling room air pressures,
they are highly effective in improving room air quality. A significant

part of the work effort during this contract period has been given to the NCI safety and environmental control site visit and consultation program. Site visits have been made to the following facilities:

Bionetics, Kensington, Maryland
Microbiological Associates, Bethesda, Maryland
University Laboratories, Highland Park, New Jersey
Flow Laboratories, Rockville, Maryland
Albert Einstein College of Medicine, Bronx, New York

Proposed Course of the Project: Experiments are being prepared to: 1) obtain comparative data between theory and operation of air recirculation unit(s) within a typical research laboratory, 2) determine the unit size required to obtain an equivalent high air change rate and 3) determine how unit location and air distribution can most effectively minimize high concentrations of contaminants at specific locations within the laboratory.

Date Contract Initiated: June 25, 1965

223

Source: NCI staff. *The Special Virus Cancer Program: Progress Report #8*. Office of the Associate Scientific Director for Viral Oncology (OASDVO). J. B. Moloney, Ed., Washington, D. C.: U. S. Government Printing Office, 1971, pp. 222-223

Fig. 25.2. Annual Funding Levels for Viral Oncology Segments of the NCI's Special Virus Cancer Program

TABLE I
ANALYSIS OF CONTRACTS BY SEGMENTS IN
VIRAL ONCOLOGY

SEGMENT	NO. OF CONTRACTS	ANNUAL LEVEL[1]	(PERCENT)
TOTAL	120[2]	$31,590,401	(100)
Developmental Research	24	10,119,281	(32)
Immunology Group	8	956,709	(4)
Special Animal Ecology	17	4,068,618	(13)
Program Resources & Logistics	24	2,354,772	(7)
Biohazards Control & Containment	5	388,796	(1)
Program Management	11	2,979,100	(9)
Solid Tumor Virus	23	9,603,320	(30)
Breast Cancer Virus	8	1,119,805	(4)

[1] Funds obligated by Viral Oncology during Fiscal Year 1971.'

[2] The total includes non-recurring contracts funded during FY 1971.
See TABLE III for individual contracts involved.

Source: NCI staff. *The Special Virus Cancer Program: Progress Report #8.* Office of the Associate Scientific Director for Viral Oncology (OASDVO). J. B. Moloney, Ed., Washington, D. C.: U. S. Government Printing Office, 1971, pg. 63.

monkeys, and other animals. Along with a complete account of his research, he sent the FDA an article published in July 1995 that said, "The potential introduction of pathogenic viral variants into humans through the use of African green monkey-derived cell lines" during the production of live viral vaccines "should be evaluated."[16]

Martin easily made the vaccine connection since he had previously served, between 1976 and 1980, as the director of the Viral Oncology Branch of the FDA's Bureau of Biologics (now the Center for Biologics, Evaluation and Research). During his tenure at the bureau, he reported to his supervisors that even the contemporary polio vaccines contained foreign DNA that should raise concerns. At the time he detected this, he had not been informed of a 1972 study that showed that simian cytomegalovirus was present in the kidney cultures of all eleven African green monkeys imported for vaccine production by Lederle—the sole producer of Orimune® live polio vaccines for the United States.[18]

Instead of rewarding Martin for his expertise, FDA officials advised him to discontinue this work because, they alleged, it was outside the scope of the testing required to approve the polio vaccine. Martin recalled being told by the bureau's director, "Stop worrying about it, every time you eat an apple you ingest foreign DNA." His project was quickly terminated.[18]

After Martin published his 1995 findings, he begain to receive calls and documents from other scientists regarding what others had learned years ago about the viral contaminants in polio vaccines. Walter Kyle sent him a 1972 "Cytomegalovirus Contingency Plan" prepared by Lederle in case the Bureau of Biologics took issue with the continued production of polio vaccine in possibly contaminated monkey kidney cells. The plan was never tested, however, as the Bureau chose not to pursue the entire matter. A year later, in a letter addressed to the President of American Cyanimid, the parent company of Lederle, by a Lederle official, it was clearly understood that indeed the FDA could have, and should have acted to halt further Orimune® development until the monkey virus contamination problem had been resolved.[19]

In June 1995, Martin again formally communicated his concerns to the FDA that certain stealth viruses may have originated from simian cytomegaloviruses. He asked the FDA to help him investigate the prevalence of infection by this virus in the general population and in the concentrated polio vaccine lots. His requests were denied leaving him little option but to notify others.

In November 1995, Martin reported his findings to the Vaccine Safety Forum of the Institute of Medicine, part of the National Academy of Sciences. In spite of requests for action by many of those in attendance, FDA officials remained uncommitted. Lederle's response was that they had complied with all of the FDA's requirements. CDC representatives also said it was not their problem.

In March 1996, Martin again presented new evidence. This time, during the "Twentieth Century Plagues symposium in Los Angeles and San Francisco sponsored by California's Department of Health. Here, Martin reviewed the early developments of both the Salk and Sabin polio vaccines. Commenting on the issue of SV40 contamination, he referred to published works by Drs. Lednickey and Cristaudo, and their colleagues, identifying SV40 gene sequences in childhood choroid plexus brain tumors and in mesotheliomas—rare cancers arising from cells lining the cavity surrounding the lung.[18,19]

In other words, anyone, and particularly those who received polio vaccines prior to 1964, is at risk of carrying SV40, and spreading it to others at home or in the community. The virus is apparently circulating now throughout the human race, and may give rise to more virulent viruses over time. Moreover, the possibility of SV40 genes being transmitted congenitally from human parents to offspring cannot be ruled out.

An even more threatening situation applies to vaccine-derived stealth viruses. Martin noted that the increased incidence of chronic fatigue syndrome, attention deficit hyperactivity disorder, autism, and other behavior-linked illnesses "may be an inadvertent consequence of stealth virus vaccine contaminants."

If a vaccine program were initiated today, Martin concluded, "one would surely not import wild monkeys from Africa, create short term primary kidney cultures, add a human virus, and administer the crude gamish derived from the virally infected cells to virtually every child in the country. Nor would one want to withhold applying the many molecular biological techniques developed over the last 30 years to assess vaccine purity. Yet this is essentially the situation with live polio vaccine, and comparable arguments can be made for other human and animal viral vaccines. . . . If animal viruses have been inadvertently introduced into humans, the sooner we find out the better."[18,19]

Martin, like Hilleman, concurred with the conclusion I reached in chapter thirteen regarding the iatrogenic, that is accidental, theory on the origin of AIDS. It is certain that, at least, the building blocks for the AIDS virus came to North America the same way SV40 had come—through the importation of contaminated monkeys used for viral vaccine and other research. Not from an African green monkey bite, and not from a gay flight attendant.

The Intentional AIDS Transmission Theory

It has been theorized, and circumstantial evidence in this book supports the theory, that black Africans and American homosexuals may have been targeted for viral weapons experimentation by activists in America's military–medical–industrial complex and agents for the CIA.

According to the Church commission hearings, Henry Kissinger, and by association Elmo Zumwalt or Melvin Laird, and Sidney Gottlieb ordered or administered the development and/or stockpiling of biological weapons, including immune-system-destroying viruses functionally identical to HIV, and the deployment of systems necessary to administer these viruses to large populations. Frank Carlucci, Joseph Califano, and Alexander Haig may also have been involved.

The principal military scientists and industrialists involved in the development, study, and/or possible deployment of AIDS-like viruses, which may have included Ebola and Marburg-like rhabdoviruses, included Robert Gallo of the National Cancer Institute; John Landon and Robert Ting of Litton Bionetics; Litton Industries president Roy Ash; research affiliates of MSD, including Maurice Hilleman; and a handful of researchers at the New York University Medical Center, the New York City Blood Bank, the University of California, and the CDC. Additional institutions which may have played a role in the development of such germs during the 1960s and early 1970s include the Massachusetts Institute of Technology, the Navy's Biomedical Research Laboratory, Hazleton Laboratories, Inc., the NIAID, and the AEC.

It is likely that most of the scientists involved in developing such viruses for military contractors, the NCI, the CIA, and the Special Operations Division of the Army, believed they were serving the interests of national security, or humanity. The question of their supervisors purposes, motivations, and intent can only be fully answered through a Congressional inquiry.

With regard to the theory of *intentional* AIDS transmission for population control, undoubtedly, the motives and mechanisms existed to support this possibility. The evidence shows a channel through which experimental (mutant) viruses, viral vaccines, other reagents, and drugs flowed between the NCI and affiliated testing laboratories at Litton Bionetics and Fort Detrick, to MSD and its related research labs in New York and Central Africa, was the Drug Development Branch of the NCI. Through this channel, or another, the CIA, or a saboteur, may have delivered a single roller bottle[20,21] containing AIDS viruses to experimental vaccine producers or directly to Merck's hepatitis B (and perhaps other multicomponent) vaccines—the vaccines that appear to have played a principal role in infecting scores of human subjects in the early 1970s in New York City, Central Africa, and other regions of the world hardest hit by AIDS.[22,23]

Also, considering Merck, Sharp & Dohme's relationship with the military, and its economic competitor the Institute Pasteur Production, in contrast to previous theories on the initial international spread of AIDS from Central Africa through needlesticks or homosexual practices, covert operations by the CIA, contaminated vaccines, and even industrial espionage, may explain the rapid progress of the epidemic to African, European, South American, and eastern nations.

Given the cold war climate in the 1970s, the believed strategic importance of Central Africa, and the activities to promote military and economic dependence of several black nations—in particular the resource wealthy region of Angola and Zaire—the use of HIV and Ebola as biological weapons to affect military, economic, and "national security" objectives, including population control, must be considered. This theory is bolstered by the following facts:

• As national security advisor under Nixon, in 1969, Henry Kissinger ordered a reassessment of America's biological weapons capabilities from which the option to develop immune-system-destroying viruses was selected. Such viruses were to be used when necessary to keep U.S. military "visibility to a minimum" during a "gray" area operation intended to influence "certain events of potentially global importance." Shortly following their development, Kissinger also ordered the CIA (whose scientists developed and stockpiled numerous deadly viruses for Project MKNAOMI) to conduct covert military operations in the Zaire/Angola arena—the region of Africa hardest hit by the AIDS and Ebola epidemics.[24-26]

• The Defense Department and NCI paid Litton Bionetics (as supervised by Dr. Robert Gallo at the NCI), and other affiliated biological weapons contractors, millions of dollars during the 1960s and early 1970s to produce immune-system-depleting and cancer-causing viruses. These would include the viruses with the pathological effects of the HIVs and the hemorrhagic fever viruses Ebola and Marburg.[25-31]

• U.S. congressional documents confirm the CIA obtained dozens of biological weapons, including deadly viruses, and illegally maintained them in storage facilities on the grounds of Fort Detrick as late as 1975. Thereafter, they possibly retained private firms for such purposes despite all such actions being illegal.[26]

• CIA chiefs acknowledged their likely use of biological weapons through covert operations long after the ratification of the Geneva accord by Kissinger and Nixon, despite knowledge that all such actions were illegal.[24]

• The CIA conducted dozens of biological warfare experiments on hundreds of thousands of unsuspecting human subjects both domestically and in foreign lands.[24]

• DOD biological weapons contractors Merck and/or Litton Bionetics conducted numerous AIDS-like virus and vaccine experiments during the 1960s and early 1970s simultaneously in New York City and/or Central Africa—the two areas hardest hit by the AIDS epidemic.

• Population control was deemed a high priority foreign policy and national security objective during the late 1960s and early 1970s by then the Honorable George Bush of Texas. More recently, groups active in the Council on Foreign Relations have urged policy makers and industrialists to reduce even the size of the U.S. population to between 125 and 150 million people, "or about its size in the 1940s."[32]

The fact that the epidemic overwhelmingly and specifically struck groups that had been consistently targeted by American intelligence agencies does not necessarily give more weight to the intentional transmission theory since MSD and other military vaccine producers routinely used black Africans, prisoners, and other high risk groups for vaccine experiments.

The Accidental Alternative

It is highly plausible that the earliest AIDS, Ebola, Marburg, and Reston virus outbreaks occurred *accidentally.* The most common source of these outbreaks was not African monkeys, per se, but more specifically African primates inoculated with such viruses and subsequently exported by Litton Bionetics for vaccine production, cancer studies, and biological weapons research. The weight of evidence, then, falls on Litton—the principal military–medical–industrial "support services" provider to all NCI contractors including MSD, the NYUMC, Hazleton Laboratories, Inc., Davis Laboratories, and others. Given the number of documented laboratory outbreaks alone, in 1967, 1976, 1978, and 1989, all associated with specific monkey species supplied by Litton Bionetics, or Litton monkey cohabitants, it is reasonable to conclude that an independent investigation of the records and quarantine facilities of Litton's foreign and domestic primate research and supply centers is in order.

Another concern regarding vaccine production facilities and their products is the fact that government and industry standards disregarded simian virus contaminants. Contamination of experimental and production vaccines, including polio and others, by SV40, SFV, $SIV_{agm,}$ and possibly SIV_{cpz} in the range of 100 particles per dose, occurred routinely, very likely giving rise to viral recombinants that might have crossed species barriers as, in many cases, they had been engineered to do through human tissue culturing. All told, such methods and materials used by NCI researchers could have easily created AIDS-virus progenitors including SIV_{agm}, SIV_{cpz}, and HIV-2. Thus, the iatrogenic theory of HIV development is strongly supported.

With the North American AIDS epidemic, besides the NCI and Litton Bionetics, the Merck company and the NYUMC appear chiefly accountable. It is reasonable to propose HIV-1, HIV-2, or other progenitors, initially infecting Litton-supplied monkeys, were accidentally transmitted to MSD or NYUMC experimental vaccines that were then tested on mentally retarded children, gay volunteers, and others in New York City as early as 1970.

Though polio vaccines are also suspected of transmitting HIV-1 and other viruses, the unique epidemiology, and concurrent outbreaks of AIDS in New York City and Central Africa, appears to coincide more closely with the administration of experimental hepatitis B vaccines than with either the Salk or Sabin vaccines. The polio vaccine trials were conducted during the mid to late 1950s and early 1960s. Had HIV-1 been transmitted then, the outbreaks would have been more likely to have occured during the late 1960s or early 1970s, that is, almost a decade before the onset of clinical cases, and prior to when molecular genetics indicates HIV-1 evolved.

However, the possibility that HIV-1 evolved in Willowbrook children and/or gay men as a result of first polio *and then* hepatitis vaccine contamination cannot be ruled out. The first four lots of Merck's experimental hepatitis B vaccine may have been partially derived from the children and/or the men's blood serum, which may have included live SV40, SFV, SIV_{agm}, or other viruses—potential building blocks of HIV-1—transmitted to the human donors during polio vaccination a decade earlier. Thus, recombination of HIV-1 ancestors may have occurred in one or more of the hepatitis B serum donors. This, as an alternative to purposeful or chimpanzee mediated contamination of the Merck vaccine, could have resulted in the transmission of AIDS as well.

Another polio vaccine theory advanced by Dr. Howard B. Urnovitz, founder and chief science officer for Calypte Biomedical company in Berkeley, California is also noteworthy. Urnovitz concluded that HIV-1 may be a monkey-human hybrid since a certain number of the polio vaccine recipients possibly maintained the HIV-1 envelope in their cells as a normal gene.[33] This gene then could have recombined with any of the viruses likely to have contaminated the human vaccines in question, to produce a monkey/human hybrid on the way to becoming HIV-1.

Like Martin, Kyle, Shultz, Ellswood and Stricker, Urnovitz called for careful PCR analyses of the experimental vaccine lots in question in order to prove or disprove these hypotheses, providing the lots, allegedly in safe keeping at the FDA, have not been altered or destroyed.

Plausible Denial and Self-Incrimination

Unless the U.S. Congress orders an independent investigation, thorough genetic analyses of the suspected hepatitis B and polio vaccine lots, and look-back studies of disease among their recipients, the origin of AIDS mystery will likely remain unsolved.

Given all the facts, however, there is one thing for certain—the speculation that AIDS jumped species naturally to initially infect people, virtually simultaneously, on two far removed continents, and more oddly, in the two exact regions wherein the suspected AIDS-like virus and vaccine experiments took place, must be seriously questioned. Moreover, based on the mass of evidence compiled herein, scientists (including those at the NCI and CDC) who advocated such farfetched notions of the origin of AIDS, in contrast to their knowledge of the NCI's Special Virus Cancer Program and recombinant viral vaccine experiments, have obviously incriminated themselves.

Such self-incrimination is additionally evident considering the same core group of research institutions and researchers *falsely* alleged: (1) that HIV was widely distributed in central Africa in the early 1970s and even long before, (2) that the Marburg agent was likewise found in monkeys throughout the world, (3) that Merck's hepatitis B vaccine was vindicated as the source of HIV transmissions, (4) that American researchers required the French to discover how to keep HIV infected T-cells alive, (5) that key investigators, including Don Francis and Luc Montagnier, were unaware of Robert Gallo's AIDS-like virus experiments during the early 1970s, (6) that funding would not be withheld during the early 1980s to allow other researchers to investigate the virus suspected of causing AIDS, (7) that the AIDS-virus took several years to discover, (8) that the discovery of HIV (HTLV-III/LAV) took place during the 1980s simultaneously by Gallo and Montagnier, (9) that the discovery of HIV-2 occurred virtually simultaneously by Essex and Montagnier, (10) that the subsequent French American AIDS fracases evolved so inexplicably, (11) that the Ebola viruses represented a serious *natural* threat to humans, despite evidence and expert testimony that it was man-made, and (12) that HIV-1 cannot be the cause of AIDS as argued by Peter Duesberg.

Finally, that virtually no attention was paid by any of the suspects to the iatrogenic theory of AIDS, is additionally suspicious if not criminal.

Making a Difference

In 1982, after the national broadcast of the award winning television documentary "DPT: Vaccine Roulette," parents in the Washington, D.C. area whose children had been injured by the DPT vaccine founded Dissatisfied Parents Together (DPT) and launched what is now recognized as the consumer vaccine safety movement in the U.S. In 1985, the book *DPT: A Shot in the Dark* by Harris Coulter, Ph.D., and Barbara Loe Fisher, co-founder of Dissatisfied Parents Together, was published by Harcourt Brace Jovanovich indicting the whole cell pertussis vaccine and documenting serious flaws in America's highly politicized mass vaccination program. Media coverage of DPT vaccine associated injuries and deaths became widespread and, although most vaccine injury lawsuits were settled out of court for modest sums (with pressure being placed on plaintiff's to agree to having all court records sealed from public view as a condition of settlement), there were several well publicized multimillion dollar awards against vaccine manufacturers.[34]

These events were immediately followed by pressure placed on Congress by the vaccine manufacturers, including Lederle, Connaught and Merck, to pass an exclusive remedy federal vaccine injury compensation program that would remove all liability from drug companies who make vaccines and physicians who administer vaccines. The threat the drug companies delivered to Congress, with the help of physician organizations such as the American Academy of Pediatrics and the American Medical Association, was that they would stop producing vaccine for the nation's childhood vaccination program.

In response, in 1986, President Reagan signed the National Childhood Vaccine Injury Act. The law was to have created a non-adversarial, no-fault alternative to lawsuits for victims of mandatory vaccinations. It also: included safety provisions such as a centralized vaccine adverse event reporting system; mandatory reporting by doctors of hospitalizations, injuries and deaths following vaccinations; mandatory record keeping by doctors of vaccine lot numbers and reactions; and requirements that doctors give patients/parents vaccine benefit/risk information. Punitive damages in lawsuits against vaccine manufacturers or physicians were outlawed, except for cases where criminal negligence would be proven. However, Congress did not completely remove all liability in the court system from the vaccine manufacturers and preserved the right of vaccine victims to bring a lawsuit if they were turned down by the federal system or they considered the award to be too small.

Following the law's passage, the Departments of Justice and Health and Human Services systematically gutted the program and made it highly adversarial. Each claim was fought by taxpayer funded government lawyers and hired physician experts. Compensation was denied to three quarters of all child vaccine victims. What was to have been a fairer, less emotionally draining, and less time consuming alternative to litigation, turned into a sham. Dissatisfied Parents Together, which operates the National Vaccine Information Center (NVIC) and helped to create the law, described the program as "a drug company dream, a consumer's nightmare, a scientific travesty, and a national tragedy."

"What we have in this country," said Barbara Loe Fisher, NVIC Co-Founder and President, "is that every citizen is forced by law to use vaccines which are being poorly studied, tested, and regulated for safety, as well as unsafely administered, and no one is held accountable when a citizen, usually a child, is injured or killed by that product. No other product in America is protected from the pressures of the marketplace like that. The public has little way to exert economic pressure to force bad vaccines off the market, force improvement of existing ones, or force doctors to administer them more safely because nobody has the right to refuse to use them or hold manufacturers and negligent physicians accountable when injuries and deaths occur."

The federal government has pressured states to set up tracking systems to tag and track all children from birth to ensure that they are injected with multiple vaccines, all of which have not been adequately studied to evaluate their impact on humans at the cellular and molecular biology level.

"Nor is there informed consent in America when it comes to vaccination," said Fisher. "At its core, forcing individuals to risk injury or death without their consent is a violation of civil and human rights, the Nuremberg Code, and the Helsinki Declarations. In principal, it is also a violation of the tenets embodied in the scriptures of every major religion. If the State can tag, track down, and force American citizens against their will to risk injury and death by being injected with biologicals of unknown toxicity today, there is no limit on what freedoms the State can take away in the name of the greater good tomorrow."

To meet the challenge, NVIC has helped build a coalition of consumers, health providers, and allied organizations to educate the public to act at the local, state, and federal levels to insure the right to informed consent to any medical procedure, including vaccination, which involves the risk of injury or death. At the time of this writing, NVIC was also: calling for a congressional oversight hearing on existing vaccine laws; a congressional investigation into gross mismanagement of the mass vaccination system by federal government officials with the cooperation of the pharmaceutical industry; and FDA reforms that require government health officials involved in licensing, testing, and regulating vaccines to release information to the public on the safety and efficacy of vaccines which, as John Martin explained, government officials are prohibited by law from releasing.

"The vaccine manufacturers are being protected by outdated and highly ineffective FDA regulations," Fisher concluded. "Until the government stops protecting drug companies, the public health and safety will continue to suffer."[34]

Final Thoughts

Sean MacBride, the former foreign minister of Ireland, a 1974 Nobel Peace prize recipient, and the president of the International Peace Bureau, wrote that despite his "deep affection for, and tremendous admiration of, the United States and its people":

> I came to the conclusion that all the values that made me admire the American people were being eroded by the covert operations of the CIA and kindred secret bodies. . . .
>
> Time after time the United States has generously aided other countries threatened by famine or disaster. The survival of this great tradition is of importance, not only to Americans, but to all freedom loving people in the world.
>
> But in my view, the survival of this great democracy is now being gravely threatened by the covert criminal actions of the Central Intelligence Agency and its associate services. If the United States is to be protected from this grave danger, it is essential that the activities of this secret agency should be fully exposed to the people of the United States.
>
> . . . I am a fierce believer in the democratic system of governments. Among the democracies, the Constitution of the United States can be, and has proved to be, a bastion of civil liberty.
>
> However, democracy and the rule of law could not survive side by side with a state agency that engages in covert operations ranging from assassinations to levying mercenary armies [to directing lethal biological weapons experiments and public health policies]. Even if there is, now, an attempt being made by some to check the activities of the CIA and the other United States intelligence agencies, the whole concept of a secret government and army within a government is a menace to the democratic system.[35]

The disclosures made herein provide additional evidence that Sean MacBride's prose is accurate. "We the People of the United States," and peace-loving citizens around the world, now face a nightmarish danger. Deadly animal viruses are now multiplying in our bodies. This, at a time when we seem to have less and less influence over the system of government on which we depend for our health and safety.

One reaction is to turn away, and choose, as so many do, denial as a means of coping. Such a truth tears at the hearts of especially those who embrace the paternal role of government—those who are comforted by our military, medical, and intelligence capabilities. Living relatively comfortable lives, unscathed by the unusual cancers and bizarre plagues that have struck so many *other* families, the pain threshold for the masses is but a date with destiny.

Not so for the vast majority of Africans, and urban African Americans. This dynamic may partly explain why the vast majority of white people react to the genocidal theory of AIDS with disbelief whereas blacks largely embrace the notion.[36]

There is some consolation in knowing this general atmosphere is not unique in political history. On the brink of the American revolution, the great patriot Patrick Henry warned that it is natural to indulge in illusions:

> We are apt to shut our eyes against a painful truth, and listen to the song of that siren till she transforms us into beasts. Is this the part of wise men, engaged in a great and arduous struggle for liberty? Are we disposed to be the number of those who, having eyes, see not, and having ears, hear not, the things which so nearly concern their temporal salvation? For my part, whatever anguish of spirit it may cost, I am willing to know the whole truth; to know the worst, and to provide for it.[37]

What will it take to break the trance of complacency lulled by the siren's song? Realizing that maybe, or even probably, your relatives and friends have also died, or now suffer, from any number of cancers or immune system disorders whose skyrocketing incidence begs attention and an honest explanation. Only through lessons learned can the millions of lives lost to the present and coming plagues be reconciled.

Reconciling the origin of the world's emerging viruses is urgent. From this work comes the knowledge that those blamed for starting the AIDS epidemic were blameless, while those truly responsible continue to reap the pandemic's rewards. By understanding how the AIDS and Ebola viruses came to be, we are much closer to discovering how to pick them apart, piece by piece and gene by gene, until the part that overwhelms the human immune system is located and inactivated, or some alternative therapy is proven as effective. Hopefully this work will sound enough alarms to prevent such outbreaks from ever happening again.[38]

Finally, readers are encouraged not to mark those implicated for violent retribution, but rather, to confront their soul's similar assassins. There are elements in each of us that instill fear, cloud the mind, harm the body, weaken the will, and violate the human spirit, just as the villains do in this search for truth. The wisdom and divine guidance needed to lay such inhumanity to rest lies within.

Epilogue

In Vancouver, Canada, on July 10, 1996, at the XI International Conference on AIDS, I was privileged to become the first investigator in the history of the esteemed meeting to defend a scientific paper that concluded the human immunodeficiency viruses (HIVs), and their closest relatives, the simian immunodeficiency viruses (SIVs), most likely evolved from men's desire to play God in the name of science. The abstract, D3678, weathered the social science committee's peer review process and is reprinted in figure 26.1.[1]

Later that week, following moderate coverage by Canada's leading news sources, and total censorship by their American counterparts, I was interviewed by Vancouver's top-rated talk show host, Fanny Kiefer, on CKNW radio. Carol Punt, an independent film producer who was in the middle of developing a documentary about vaccines, and their risks, filmed the session. Following the interview Carol informed me that Dr. Gallo was scheduled to host a forum the next night in which the public was invited to ask questions. "Would you like to attend with us and ask Dr. Gallo a question or two?" Carol asked.

"How can I refuse?" I replied.

So the next evening, when Gallo was finished speaking, before a few hundred Canadians, the press, and Carol's documentary film crew, I took the microphone. I asked Gallo if he was at all concerned that his early experiments, with Litton Bionetics investigators, in which monkey viruses, like simian virus 40 (SV40), and others, recombined with numerous animal cancer viruses, like cat leukemia and chicken leukemia/sarcoma, "might have given rise to HIV or its relatives following their culture in human tissues; and that these mutants might have contaminated some live viral vaccines produced in contaminated monkeys and chimps supplied to vaccine manufacturers" through his colleagues at Litton Bionetics?

To say that Dr. Gallo became angry is an understatement. "Quite frankly, I don't know what the hell you're talking about," he said shaking his head. Many in the audience laughed.

"I'll cite your papers Dr. Gallo."

"If you can," Gallo challenged, "you've got a paper that I don't know I ever published. I'd sure like you to cite it. Would you begin?"

"Sure. I'd be happy to. *Proceedings of the National Academy of Sciences*, 1970, Gallo et al. That was an oral presentation which you gave before a NATO audience in Mol, Belgium . . . I'll be happy to show you the paper."[2]

"Okay. Stop. Stop. I mean this is beyond asinine," he said. "In Mol, Belgium—it was my first trip to Europe so I can remember—a NATO meeting did take place. NATO meetings fund all scientific meetings, all over the world, even East/West at that time, biologic meetings, scientific, chemistry meetings. All kinds of meetings—meetings about motherhood, fatherhood, everything. And what I talked about in Mol, Belgium was in the 1960s, long before gene cloning took place, before I ever worked in virology. What I talked about was cellular transfer RNA. Okay? That was Mol, Belgium. *Proceedings of the National Academy of Sciences.* And SV40, I never published a paper in my life on SV40, except the transfer RNA species in SV40 transformed [i.e., caused cancer in] hamster cells compared to non-transformed [normal] cells as a control.

"You've got pineapples, kiwis, grapes, and cherries, mixed in with some other tutie-fruitie. I don't know what in the hell you're talking about." Amidst audience laughter Gallo continued, "I'm a little bit tired about this kind of nonsense and crap."

"Excuse me," I continued, "and Gallo, Sarin et al. with Litton Bionetics researchers as your coauthors in which you combined leukemia/sarcoma complex models?"[3]

"Let me . . . OK. We created. Yes. Very smart. We did. Everything was created by us working in our laboratories," Gallo defended sarcastically. "Look, just for those with some remote . . . some little bit of understanding of this; who care about this, ahh . . . kind of idea. I've never . . . I, I've . . . I mean [I've] had a lot of things said, but never had anything quite like that one.

"There were people who thought and made postulations that . . . It was not actually directed at me. This is a good one; a new one. But that HIV could have been created in laboratory experiments. The two answers to that, that are definitive, conclusive, [are] that no scientist could have deliberately created them unless he was a super genius and ten years ahead of his time. The AIDS virus definitively existed *long* before molecular cloning. That's point one. Point two [is] we know the full sequence of the genome of HIV. It was published by our lab in 1985 with comparisons done around the same time. The genome has no homology to any known existing virus in the world except SIV discovered after it. It has nothing to do

THE MYSTERIOUS ORIGIN OF HIV: REVIEWING THE NATURAL, IATROGENIC, AND GENOCIDAL THEORIES OF AIDS

Horowitz, Leonard G.,* Strecker R, Cantwell A, Vid D, and Grossman G.
Tetrahedron, Inc., a nonprofit educational corporation, Rockport, MA 01966, U.S.A

Issue: Two-thirds of African Americans recently surveyed believe the AIDS epidemic may be genocide. Such beliefs may impair health service utilization and preventive behaviors. Moreover, reconciling the origin of HIV is additionally important for 1) sociological reasons—victims of AIDS should not be blamed for starting the epidemic, 2) scientific reasons—new therapies might be developed from a better understanding of HIV's origin; and 3) ethical reasons—the events precipitating the epidemic should never be allowed to happen again.

Project: In an effort to shed light on this most mysterious and controversial subject, a review of the literature was initiated to determine the most plausible origin of HIV-1. During a two year period, more than 2,500 documents were collected and critically analyzed. This analysis included all natural, iatrogenic, and genocidal theories of AIDS's origin as previously presented in the scientific literature and lay media.

Results: The lay media appears to be an important factor in the development of beliefs regarding the origin of AIDS. Numerous publications and broadcasts on this subject were found, most advancing the natural—African green monkey—theory of AIDS's origin. The scientific literature, however, provided no direct evidence for HIV's natural evolution from monkey to man, only circumstantial evidence. Alternatively, a growing body of evidence in the scientific literature suggested an iatrogenic origin of AIDS. Specifically, the possibility that HIV-1 and HIV-2 evolved during early laboratory investigations and vaccine trials is of growing interest. Evidence supporting the genocidal theory of AIDS which appeared in numerous lay publications, and rarely, in esteemed periodicals, was clearly circumstantial, albeit disconcerting.

Lessons Learned: The speculation that HIV naturally evolved to be horizontally transmitted from the African green monkey to man must be seriously questioned. Alternatively, more consideration should be given to a growing body of scientific evidence supporting an iatrogenic origin. Moreover, the genocidal theory of AIDS could not be ruled out.

The above abstract appeared in the scientific proceedings book as abstract # D3678 presented on July 10, 1996 during the social sciences session of the conference. The paper was defended by lead author Dr. Leonard G.Horowitz. The American news meda failed to cover the presentation despite multiple invitations.

with cats. It has nothing to do with chicken sarcoma viruses. SV40 is a DNA virus that comes from little animals that can transform cells in culture," Gallo continued condescendingly, "it has no sequences in HIV. Further, we never worked with SV40 with those viruses together, and if we did the whole thing would be irrelevant. And I think you need to begin with biology 101 *highschool* [level]. Okay?"

The forum ended and Gallo rushed off guarded by James Jennings, Executive Director for one of the largest public relations firms in the world—Hill and Knowlton of Washington, D.C.—the publicists employed by the Bush administration to incite public outrage against Sadam Hussein in support of America's entrance into the Gulf War.[4]

Later, someone handed Gallo a marketing flier describing this book with Dr. John Martin's name appearing on the cover. Dr. Martin was well known to Gallo. Not only was Martin recognized as one of the world's leading authorities in vaccine contamination analysis, but he had rented a room in Gallo's house while living on the East Coast. Moreover, only weeks earlier, Gallo had visited Martin at his University of California laboratory to learn what breakthroughs Martin and coinvestigator Zaki Salahuddin, who had previously worked for Gallo, were exploring.

Then another notable drew Gallo's attention—Dr. Garth Nicolson, who was, at the time, Gallo's counterpart at MD Anderson Cancer Research Center.[5] Both had been affiliated with Fort Detrick researchers during the "Special Virus Cancer Program," and Gallo knew Nicolson's credentials were impeccable. Dr. Nicolson's testimonial on the back of the flier (and book) raised Gallo's ire. So days later Gallo telephoned Nicolson for an explanation as to why such an esteemed scientist would hail the work of "an obvious loon."

"Bob. First of all he's no loon," Nicolson replied. "He's a Harvard grad. Second of all, have you read his book?"

"No," Gallo admitted.

"Bob, you'd better read his book. . . . Here's his number. . . . "

Minutes later my telephone rang. "This is 'Gallo,'" he announced. Indeed, I was surprised and puzzled why the world's leading AIDS researcher would contact someone who obviously needed *highschool* level biology training.

Gallo immediately apologized for slighting me publicly. He defended that he did initially believe that I was looney, but that Garth had straightened him out on the matter. He allegedly called to offer his support for my investigation into the facts surrounding the origin of AIDS. He stated that he too was a "humanitarian." He had very little to do with Litton Bionetics researchers. (See their contract on page 427.) He said their association was only a way to financially "grow my lab." He confessed virtually no association with Fort Detrick biological weapons testers.

Expecting the conversation to continue for awhile, with tape recorder readied by my phone, I asked, "Dr. Gallo, do you mind if I record this conversation?"

"For what purpose?" he asked.

"Why for publication purposes of course. I now find myself in the role of an investigative reporter."

He thought it over for a moment and then replied, "All right."

The recording began and lasted about a half hour. On tape Gallo expressed no regrets or concerns over the possibility of having contributed to the biological weapons (BW) race, or to the development of HIV. In fact, regarding the BW issue, Gallo stated, "I certainly believe that we, America, needed research on germ warfare because we know today, for example, ahh, direct conversations with people in the former Soviet Union; that there was a rather massive undertaking in potential germ warfare. So at minimum we needed it for defense purposes. That would be my philosophy, of course. . . . I mean rationally."

Additionally, he articulated four objections to my thesis that HIV might have evolved from laboratory experiments in which various animal cancer viruses were recombined with monkey viruses. I listened intently recognizing the fact that I needed to hear and study these objections carefully if I were to respectably provide a scientific defense.

Objections to the Man-made Theory

Gallo's main objections were as follows:

First, he claimed that viruses such as monkey, cat, chicken, cattle, and sheep, could not be recombined. They "lack the homology" or likeness, he claimed, needed for recombination.

"Regarding experiments that might have created the AIDS virus," he said, "why I thought you were joking, you see, or just, you know, playing around, is that when you said cat . . . or chicken sarcoma virus, cat leukemia virus, and SV40, first, . . . it is impossible for them to recombine. There has to be regions of homology for any genome to recombine. It is an impossibility to have recombination occur in the absence of homology. Those three viruses you mention have no homology, one to another. They cannot recombine."

In other words, these viruses, he said, were so different that they could not be brought together by laboratory experiments into forming new virus species. This argument I knew was false as I held documented evidence that not only had investigators under Gallo's supervision done this type of work, but that Gallo's mentors instructed him that it could and was being done.

Second, Gallo claimed that even if such animal cancer viruses had recombined, they bear no similarity (or "homology" once again) to the HIVs. "Therefore, none of them could contribute to any part of HIV," he continued, "That's why, for somebody who understands things, what you said was funny. I thought it was a joke."

It is no joke, and few others laughed. Several authorities had counseled me as to certain genetic similarities between the "type-C" animal cancer viruses, Gallo and others experimented on, and the human AIDS virus. Moreover, I had recently returned from a Florida university research lab[6] wherein the homology between common oral polio vaccine viral contaminants and HIV-1 had been studied. Some of the matches were as high as forty percent. That is, *extremely* high homology.

Third, Gallo claimed the technology did not exist to create HIV-1, at that time, in one of their labs. He stated specifically that "the sophisticated molecular genetics biotechnology needed to construct the AIDS virus, gene by gene," did not exist in any lab before 1975. Though this was true, I knew that Alexander Graham Bell did not need fiber optics to make his first telephone call. I held government documents that proved that crude and sloppy laboratory techniques were being used by Gallo's understudies during the late 1960s and early 1970s to accomplish immune-system-ravaging/cancer virus recombination.

In fact, Gallo's allegation that bioweapons developers did not have the wherewithal to develop HIV, or perform genetic engineering on viruses until the late 1970s or early 1980s is unequivocally false and misleading. Here is more evidence directly from *Biological and Toxin Weapons Today* (Oxford University Press, 1986) by Erhard Geissler with contributions by David Baltimore and Raymond Zilinskas:

> The full promise of biotechnology did not become apparent and seize the imagination of people everywhere until the first of the revolutionary genetic engineering techniques, recombinant DNA, was developed in the early 1970s. Previous to this, the improvement of genetic characteristics of micro-organisms was laborious and time-consuming since it depended on random mutation, screening and selection—a hit or miss strategy with a moderate

probability of successfully manipulating cells for planned ends. Recombinant DNA, however, allows researchers to manipulate directly the genetic material of cells in a purposeful manner to achieve predetermined goals. Genetic engineering received another boost in 1975 when scientists were able to fuse a cell. . . .[7]

David Baltimore, it should be noted, during the late 1960s, had undoubtedly led members of the National Academy of Sciences, National Research Counsel, in their offer to help the Department of Defense spend the $10 million appropriated for the development of immune-system-ravaging viruses for germ warfare.

These authors went on to report that "although HTLV-III [Gallo's name for HIV] is not considered as a potential BW agent, studies of AIDS and of its causative agent may nevertheless be interesting for designers of BW agents. AIDS induces many severe psychological reactions, especially among the major risk group, and production of 'desired psychological effects' is one of the additional characteristics of potential BW agents, as characterized by the US Army. Therefore, an agent like HTLV-III might be considered an ideal BW agent by terrorists. . . ."[7]

Also, regarding the Marburg and Ebola viruses, Lassa fever, and Legionnaire's disease, the authors reported that these agents "have been regarded by US Army scientists as among those 'putative BW agents having the highest liability for operational use.'" However, they continued, biohazard and containment technologies improved during the mid-1970s and 1980s so that the risk of studying, and mass producing, these potentially useful biological weapons was greatly reduced. They acknowledged:

> . . . the possibility offered by genetic engineering of replicating nucleic acids (including viral genomes in bacterial host cells) greatly reduces the need for safety requirements to work with these viruses. The genome of Lassa virus has already been studied [in 1983–84] by physical mapping (oligonucleotide fingerprinting) and its N gene segment has been cloned and expressed in *Escherichia coli*. Obviously, the new techniques make it feasible to develop such viruses into BW agents which can be manufactured on a larger scale.[7]

Indeed, biological weapons investigators were hard at work, from the 1960s to the present, developing and testing viruses, including AIDS and Ebola, for military operations and even "psychological warfare." Dr. Gallo would have certainly suspected this and known that biological weapons developers were five to ten years more advanced than commercial labs.

Finally, Gallo argued that "monkeys are infected with viruses. . . . We know [HIV] came from monkeys. No rational informed person could argue otherwise." I knew this was scientifically unconfirmed. In fact, when Cape Cod producer Mike Carrie, of WXTK's "Gino Montesi Show," later asked the director of the Centers for Disease Control and Prevention (CDC), Dr. David Satcher, to comment on my thesis following Gallo's refusal to do so, CDC communications officer Tammy Nunnally faxed Mike the following statement:

"Scientists are not certain how, when, or where the AIDS virus evolved and first infected humans. HIV, the virus that causes AIDS, is not a man-made virus and did not originate in laboratories in this country or other countries. It is a human virus that evolved naturally over time, as other viruses have. Attached is a cite from the *World Book Encyclopedia* which was written by one of our experts. . . ."

The citation added that, "Researchers have shown that HIV-1 and HIV-2 are more closely related to simian immunodeficiency viruses, which infect monkeys, than to each other. Thus, it has been suggested that HIV evolved from viruses that originally infected monkeys in Africa and was somehow transmitted to people. One argument against this theory is that HIV has only been found in human beings. It never has been isolated from any wild monkey or other animal species."[8]

Though Gallo admitted that the "missing link" between the SIVs and the HIVs was perplexing, the cat, chicken, monkey, or cow virus recombination theories, he reiterated, was "altogether an impossibility. I would tell you if something [like that went wrong]. I can think of more rational and possible things that could have happened *by accident* at that period of time, but that's really the wrong tree."

I balked at hearing the world's leading retrovirologist intimate he might provide a more plausible accidental theory on the origin of AIDS.

So I pressed him for more information on the plausibility of my general thesis by asking, "So there's absolutely no possibility that these types of experiments, not necessarily in your lab, presented building blocks where hybrids were being created [that might have given rise to the HIVs]?"

Surprisingly, Gallo replied, "No. I can not say no to you. I don't say no to you. I said that we don't have any virus, that we know of, that has homology to HIV-1, to say this became HIV-1, except for the monkey virus SIV, or the human [virus] HIV-2, which is essentially exactly the same as the strain of SIV. We just don't have any virus that has those sequences in it.

Fig. 26.2. Letter to Dr. Gallo From Dr. Horowitz Addressing Gallo's Objections to the Man-made Theory of AIDS's Origin

Dr. Leonard G. Horowitz — LGH

October 28, 1996

Dr. Robert C. Gallo
Director, Institute for Human Virology
725 West Lombard Street
Baltimore, MD 21201

Dear Bob:

Thank you very much for the interview you gave me on July 30, 1996. I found the discussion very interesting, and am responding herein.

First, I greatly appreciate your offer to help in determining the origin of human immunodeficiency viruses (HIVs). I understand that you must, however, limit your views partly for political expediency, and partly due to lack of any definitive knowledge.

In any case, my responses to your four specific objections to my thesis—that HIV-1, or its progenitors, could have evolved from laboratory experiments and subsequent human vaccine contaminations (i.e., hepatitis B and polio) with simian and type-C cancer viruses routinely studied and recombined during the "Special Virus Cancer Program"—are as follows:

Objection #1—The viruses discussed lack the "homology" needed to recombine.

I will grant you that some degree of homology is needed for recombination, and the more homology the more recombination. However, neither the whole genome needs to be homologous nor is there a requirement that the homologous regions be contiguous. Small stretches of even a few base pairs are all that is needed for recombination of type-C cancer viruses—the focus of substantial "Special Virus Cancer Program" research. HIV has been shown to evolve through type-C like morphogenesis. (Salakian, P et al. *J Virology* 70:3706-3715)

Moreover, random natural recombination is not the only issue. You may recall, given your first hand knowledge of bench level virology during the late 1960s and early 1970s, that people who were really up on molecular virology at the National Institutes of Health (NIH) including the late Dr. George Khoury, Ed Scolnic, and others, recombined such viruses in their labs. Documents show many government and industry researchers, known or unknown to you, were heavily involved in genetic engineering, in this time frame, preceding the discovery of HIV.

Additionally, some restriction enzymes were available before the discovery of HIV-1. Several enzymes were even publicly available to do gene cutting and pasting.

If you insist on homology of genomic organization, or nucleotide sequences, let me point out that the world of virology has known the lentiviruses for a long time. What about the bovine immunodeficiency virus? I do not need to tell you that there are a lot of organizational similarities between HIV and BIV.

You mentioned Ray Gilden during our interview. I am currently preparing a paper that discusses Gilden's warning in this regard. Following lengthy trials, concerning the homology of C-type cancer viruses, and the RD114 cat/human viral recombinant, Gilden stated: "[A] new virus with no growth restrictions may be accidentally introduced in a new species, perhaps by vaccine, and these become epigenetic as opposed to a rarely seen endogenous virus. Possibilities of recombinants are thus raised . . . , which could have an extended or newly acquired oncogenic potential." Gilden's warning obviously foreshadowed the AIDS pandemic. (See: *Viruses, Evolution, and Cancer: Basic Considerations—International Conference of Comparative Virology*, 2nd, Mont Gabriel, Can., 1973. New York: Academic Press, 1974, pp. 235-256.)

Regarding the little genetic similarity between the viruses used in your and Litton Bionetics's labs and HIV-1, this does not negate the probability that the SIVs and HIVs evolved from recombinant viral research. Having studied SV40, you may recall how this and another very dissimilar virus—the human adenovirus—were found to combine, creating a potentially deadly mutant—the ad-SV40 hybrid. In 1973, Andrew Lewis, at the NIAID (see: *Biohazards in Biological Research*, Cold Spring Harbor Laboratory, 1973, pp. 96-113) showed that following unexpected and unexplained recombination of these grossly different viruses, hybrids emerged that contained as little as 6% of the original SV40 genome.

P.O. Box 402. • Rockport, MA 01966 • Tele: 508-546-6586 • Fax: 508-546-9226 • E-mail: tetra@tetrahedron.org

Thus, few viral sequences resembling those of C-type cancer viruses may appear in HIV, yet this does not negate the possibility that some segments of the SIVs and HIVs may have come from NCI laboratory specimens.

Furthermore, molecular virology entails a lot more than homologous recombination. One could practically construct new viruses residue by residue using the general pattern of established viruses viz, the LTR, *gag, pol, env* and all the interesting genes sprinkled in. Though building and then testing the stability and function of new constructs is a painstaking and time consuming process, documented evidence shows this is precisely what was done during the 1960s and early 1970s by biological weapons contractors (see: Geissler E. *Biological and Toxin Weapons Today*. London: Oxford University Press, 1986 with contributions by David Baltimore and Raymond Zilinskas).

Additionally significant and suspicious is that HIV does not fit the mold for naturally evolved viruses. There is a lone~40 percent homologous virus—HIV-2—which may or may not have been a progenitor of HIV-1, and it may not have originated in monkeys. HIV-2 is definitely not endogenous to any of the species from which it has been isolated. The word "endogenous" is meant here in the classical sense. Which came first? The fact that we now find them in several monkeys and a group of individuals in one region of Africa (i.e., "high risk" Senegalese female prostitutes who, due to their "risk," and participation in public health/research programs, likely received the most suspected heptatitis B vaccine) makes one very suspicious. This is like the simian sarcoma virus complex (SSV, SSav and SiSV) which does not have any comparable viruses in the animal kingdom. There has not been a second isolation of that virus (HIV-2) yet.

Where did HIV-2 and other SIVs come from? The world of virology is still waiting for that answer. Max Essex informed me his isolation came from monkeys infected with human tissues during laboratory experiments. My theory of sloppy science (e.g., contaminated vaccines for HIV-1 and HIV-2, and contaminated monkeys being released back into the wild for the other SIVs) best explains the circumstantial and scientific evidence at hand. Do you have any better explanations? You indicated that you were able to provide a more "plausible" iatrogenic theory on the origin of AIDS but time did not permit you to explain. I await any additional insights you may be able to share.

Objection #2—Regarding the viruses I discussed as having been recombined by your colleagues at the NCI and Litton Bionetics, "not any one of them have any homology to what is HIV. Therefore, none of them could contribute to any part of HIV."

It is a matter of public record that once you firmly believed HIV was closely related to HTLV-1 and HTLV-II. Hence the name HTLV-III. As a matter of fact there was a publication in *Science* (see: Homology of AIDS-associated virus with genomes of human T-cell leukemia viruses, Arya SK, et al. *Science* 1984;225:927-930) showing molecular similarity. Did you ever withdraw that paper?

I agree that since there are no known viruses in the evolutionary scheme that look very similar to HIVs, HIV must be considered unique by design. However, you know that HIV is not totally unique. In very general terms, HIV is similar to both type C and type D viruses along with the inclusion of regulatory genes typical of lentiviruses.

Again, you may recall Ray Gilden's instruction on this subject in the "Comparison and Evolution of RNA Tumor Virus Components" (In: *Viruses, Evolution, and Cancer: Basic Considerations—International Conference of Comparative Virology*, 2nd, Mont Gabriel, Can., 1973. New York: Academic Press, 1974, pp. 235-256.):

> "The relationship of viruses such as Visna, Mason-Phizer, and mouse MTV (mammary tumor virus) to type C particles cannot be assessed in quantitative terms, yet the presence of reverse transcriptase and approximate morphologic similarity of virions present a strong case for common ancestry however remote. . . . We should stress here that *groupings such as "type C" are man-made abstractions*, and arguments of differences are only indicators of variability that are difficult for men to accommodate in simple classification schemes. . . . Once the ability to make comparisons is granted, a second major problem of critical significance to any attempt to discuss evolutionary relationships arises. Simply stated this is, *how do we know that the viruses chosen for analysis are representative of the species from which they were isolated?*"[emphasis added]

Though Gilden's conclusions were drawn long before the arrival of sophisticated DNA sequencing techniques, his point is still valid and particularly applicable to the question here: Did HIV evolve from laboratory experiments in which chance or intentional encounters occurred between different viruses of foreign species? The answer, as your comments suggest, is very plausibly "yes," despite the fact we may be unaware of the largest contributing virus(es).

Having studied SV40, you may again recall Andrew Lewis's conclusions at the NIAID (see: *Biohazards in Biological Research*, Cold Spring Harbor Laboratory, 1973, pp. 96-113.) Regarding the ad-SV40 hybrids, "Until satisfactory studies evaluate the long-term effects of SV40 infection in humans and clarify the relationship between SV40 and SV40-related agents to chronic degenerative central nervous system disease in humans, it appears to this reviewer that the laboratory manipulation of SV40 involves some risks."

Likewise, reflecting on your work with human white blood cells and type-C cancer viruses George Todaro (and Gallo), concluded:

> "Because viruses can alter their host range either by adaptation or selection, these human hybrid cells would appear to constitute a potential biohazard since, in this situation, one has an endogenous virus of a species being produced by cells which, at least in part, are human. These hybrid cells are being extensively explored by geneticists all over the world who do not realize that they contain high titers of potentially oncogenic [cancer causing] viruses. . . .What is not clear is the nature of the relationship between the acquisition of oncogenic potential by a cell and the expression of that cell's endogenous type C viral information. Type C viruses carry oncogenic information and can produce tumors (leukemias, lymphomas and sarcomas) by exogenous infection; whether horizontal spread (cell to cell and/or animal to animal) of exogenous type C virus is responsible for a significant portion of naturally occurring cancers in vertebrates is uncertain; that they can have oncogenic potential and can produce tumors in a variety of species is firmly established. It follows, then, that these viruses and the cells that produce them must be treated as potentially hazardous agents."

This is why I asked you in Vancouver whether you remain concerned that your early research with colleagues at Litton Bionetics might have given rise to AIDS virus progenitors.

A final point deserves mention here. HIV and other newly discovered viruses are still trying to stabilize themselves in their respective hosts. A similar situation was described by Todaro regarding "the feline leukemia and sarcoma viruses [that] might be derived from other species." (See Todaro's work "Endogenous type-C viruses in cell cultures. In: *Biohazards in Biological Research*. A Hellman, MN Oxman and R Pollack Eds. New York: CSHL, 1973, pp. 114-130.) Todaro, who cited additional examples of cross species laboratory transfers, noted that since these viruses grow so readily in cat cells, and spreads so "readily through the population, producing a high level of diseases, [their presence] represents an apparently unnatural situation among mammalian species." Likewise, Gerald Myers at Los Alamos recently shared with my colleague, author Ed Haslam, that HIV mutates faster than anything he has ever studied. In this manner, HIV stretches the bounds of nature. This, coupled with the fact that no close ancestors exist strongly suggests HIV is not natural but man-made.

Hopefully these extremely variable genomes may finally select a few stable versions, and like influenza, may settle down to be mildly harmful to its present hosts to mutual advantage.

In conclusion, in the absence of orderly evolution, uniquely high mutational tendencies, and its timely appearance the decade following recombinant biotechnology initiation, HIV was very possibly designed and put together along the lines of several well known agents with very adverse functional properties/consequences post infection in their present hosts.

Objection #3—"Obviously, you didn't say it was done intentionally, but just in case anybody ever said, it was impossible to do intentionally, because the viruses existed in human beings at least since the 1960s; and molecular techniques for gene cloning, doing these things in a laboratory, didn't evolve until the late '70s and early 1980s. So it's off by almost twenty years."

The earliest confirmed isolates of HIV go back only to 1976 (Myers and Pavlakis. *The Retroviridae*. New York: Plenum press. 1992, pg. 59). Regarding the reports claiming the earlier existence of HIV, I can only say—"What won't people do to get published?"

Recombinant DNA technology was beginning to unfold, even in the public domain, by the early 1970s. You even reported a cellular cloning operation involving SV40 in a 1972 publication (Gallagher R, Ting R, and Gallo, RC. *Biochemica et Biophysica Acta* 1972:272:570). Definitive experiments in phages and molecular biology using DNA manipulation goes back to 1952 (see: *Phage and the origin of Molecular Biology*, Eds. Cairas J, Stent GS, and Watson JD. Cold Springs Harbor Press, 1972).

Please allow me to refresh your memory that a 1969 *Congressional Record* cites Litton Bionetics as sixth largest U.S. Army biological weapons contractor. This is exactly the time when members of the National Academy of Sciences–National Research Council (NAS–NRC) informed

U.S. Department of Defense officials of their ability to produce, through genetic engineering, a "new infective microorganism" that may ravage the human immune system, and leave people susceptible to infectious diseases and cancers. Obviously then, by 1968, shortly after you began work at the NCI, the NAS–NRC was aware of genetic engineering capabilities, and offered to help develop "synthetic biological agents" for germ warfare. (See *Emerging Viruses: AIDS & Ebola*, pp. 6-7)

Objection #4—"Monkeys are infected with viruses . . . We know [HIV] came from monkeys. No rational informed person could argue otherwise."

The later is not true. I, like other researchers including Todaro (re: feline leukemia virus), Gerald Myers, and George Pavlakis, can argue otherwise.

Myers and Pavlakis, in "Evolutionary Potential of Complex Retroviruses (In: *The Retroviridae*, op cit.)" were unconvinced HIV evolved from either monkeys left alone in the wild or from monkeys at all! This was made clear when the authors discussed only the "possible simian origin of HIV." And though evidence, they said, was mounting HIV evolved from monkey virus relatives, they entertained the possibility ancestral viruses may have formed during the 1950s "as part of malaria experiments." (See page 59.)

I agree that HIV appears to have evolved substantially from monkeys and/or monkey virus parts. But as these scientists, as well as Ray Gilden (see Gilden, *op cit.*) indicated, we can't be sure. My investigation confirms that much was done to monkeys and monkey viruses that might have contributed to HIV's development.

Whereas I accept that SIV from the chimpanzee is the closest relative to HIV-1, and that HIV-2 is much like SIV present in wild sooty mangabeys, these viruses are all relatively recent isolates, and may themselves have evolved from laboratory experiments conducted during the 1950s, 1960s, or perhaps early 1970s when immune deficiency studies in New York City and Central Africa were in vogue.

Additional support for this iatrogenic theory comes from a series of letters/articles in the February 1988 issue of *Nature* wherein Essex and Kanki raised the "obvious possibility" that macaques "became infected with SIV from another primate species in captivity." Yet, Kestler, *et al.* concluded SIVmac, the laboratory contaminant identical to HIV-2, did not likely evolve from SIVagm or SIVmangabey. So if not from these primates, then where did SIVmac(HIV-2) come from?

"I am aware . . . of at least five instances in other laboratories in the United States and Europe where noninfected cell cultures became infected with HIV-1 in the same containment hood," wrote Carel Mulder in *Nature*. Thus, it remains highly plausible the original SIV evolved from laboratory outbreaks of HIV-1, or some related virus, carried by monkeys or vaccines into the wild. As John Martin reminded us in the foreword to *Emerging Viruses: AIDS & Ebola*, it was not uncommon to have experimental animals, particularly ailing ones, released back into the wild.

So, how did the infectious agent HIV enter humans around 1970? Well, documents show that in the late 1960s, and early 1970s, hepatitis B vaccine efforts concentrated in New York City and Central Africa. The virus was pooled from live, heavily infected, chimpanzees, Rhesus monkeys, and humans. Serum for the vaccine lots, containing 200,000 human doses, was obtained from the humans who received these viruses and, most assuredly, simian virus recombinants as well. By the way, these humans had received the earliest polio vaccines containing SV40, simian foamy retroviruses, and more. The primate resource for this effort was, as you mentioned, Litton Bionetics vis the U.S. Army.

In conclusion, I greatly appreciate this dialogue with you on a subject that has been kept in the closet for a variety of understandable reasons. Since I have your permission, I will incorporate your response in future work, and look forward to expanding common ground and reaching a scientific consensus regarding the origin of AIDS.

Yours in the Spirit of health,

Leonard G. Horowitz, D.M.D., M.A., M.P.H.

Now if you then say to me, 'Could it be an unidentified virus that mixed 'A' with 'B' with 'C', then I would say, 'Yeah that's possible. . . .'"

Further, Gallo stated my thesis was "not impossible. I can't even say it's improbable, that some viruses mixed could contribute to HIV. Because I told you that the closest we have to it is the chimp virus and HIV-2. The chimp virus is the closest we have to HIV-1, but there's something missing. That is, the chimp virus is about fifty/forty percent the same as HIV-1. We would have said it came from chimps into man, but we can't, because the virus in man is too different. We don't know where the rest came from."

"Okay," I interrupted, "I've got something for you. Did you know that in the 1974 subtype hepatitis B vaccine [trials], the viruses were prepared, were grown, in *chimps*?"

"No," he replied, "I did not know that."

"Don't you find that extraordinary?"

"Ahh. I did, I . . . I find it interesting. I don't find it extraordinary that they would grow in chimps. I mean people do grow things in monkeys. I did not know that, and that's interesting."

"And that's the subtypes," I offered, "that were used on Willowbrook State School mentally retarded children, and apparently [gay men and Blacks in Central Africa]. . . ."

"Ahh. Can I. . ." Gallo interrupted, "these are things, Leonard, I would never comment on, especially with a recorder, because I just don't know. I don't know the significance of that."

"I appreciate that. And your political position I can appreciate that [too]."

"Well, you know anything that I say, it's going to be in the newspapers."

"Right. And I don't want to put you in that position," unless I have to, I thought.

"No. I do want a discussion that's, ahh, honest, open, and frank. Ahh. But if I get into that, God knows how anybody could use it. . . ."

Our conversation ended shortly thereafter and, as agreed, I sent Gallo a copy of *Emerging Viruses: AIDS & Ebola*, along with an invitation to contribute any changes he felt were needed to improve the quality and accuracy of this work.

After transcribing his interview, and filing copies safely away with attorneys and colleagues, I ventured back to Harvard's Countway library to investigate Gallo's claims.

First, I was struck by the fact that he had attended the Gustav Stern Foundation virology symposium wherein Robert Purcell described his use of chimpanzees for pooling, that is growing, the hepatitis B viruses needed for the 1974 experiments that most plausibly brought AIDS to the world. Could Gallo's memory have conveniently lapsed, had he honestly forgotten, or had he simply been in the pissoir when Purcell presented this information?

Gallo's specific objections to my thesis were all unreasonable. As documented in a letter I subsequently sent to him (see figure 26.2), and a manuscript I prepared for scientific publication, all of his points were seriously weakened by the scientific facts.

Though my letter requested a response from him, four months later he still had not called or written. So I called him.

He took my call immediately, and with obvious jubilation he reported, "Have you heard the good news?"

"No. What's that?"

"You know the guy you implicate in your book? Maurice Hilleman?"

"Yes."

"President Clinton has announced he'll soon be awarding Hilleman a Presidential Medal of Honor for his service to American medicine and the military. What d'ya think of that?"

"I'm certain he'll be thrilled," I replied.

Not wanting to dwell on the "good news," I continued, "Bob, are you planning to respond to my letter of October 28, 1996, wherein I had requested some additional information?"

"You know, I do recall you sent me a letter, and that it contained some questions. I seem to have misplaced it."

"Would you like me to fax you a copy and then get back to me?"

"Yes. Please do."

"All right. I'll fax it at once."

That was on March 2, 1997. The transmittal was followed by a post script that said, "P.S. I have been asked to consent to debate the issues with you by several members of the media, including Michael Savage at KSFO in San Francisco, and Jane Freeman at Blackwell Television Corp. in Arlington, VA. I consented. If you are unwilling to do so, kindly specify your concerns so that when future requests of this nature are made, I can inform those requesting the interchange of your exact reason(s) for declining."

The answer came two days later from Mike Carrie who persisted in trying to schedule a debate.

"Gallo told his secretary to inform me," Mike said, "that he wouldn't dignify your comments with a response."

We both laughed, and that was our last attempt to gain a public discussion with Gallo that was, "ahh, honest, open, and frank."

Fulfilling a Prophecy

Late at night, on Friday, November 23, 1996, in Phoenix, Arizona, a middle-aged man named Jabril Muhammad slept soundly. The tall, good looking, articulate, man, of deep spiritual conviction, had retired earlier than usual that evening. Exhausted by the day's customary duties, this spiritual advisor to the highest leader of the Nation of Islam, Minister Louis Farrakhan, had the added burden of making several hospital visits that day to an ailing family member. Jabril was now recharging for what he hoped would be a more relaxed and focused weekend.

Suddenly, from the depths of his subconscious, a voice inside him shouted, "Jabril, wake up! Wake up and turn your radio on!"

"What?"

"Get up and turn on your radio," the inner messenger commanded.

Jabril complied instantly. He sat up, stripped the bedcovers from his chest, turned on his night light, and reached for the alarm radio on his night-table. He groped clumsily for the "on" switch, found it, and pushed it forward. An instant later the voice of Art Bell—latenight's leading radio talk show host filled Jabril's room.

"I'm interviewing Dr. Len Horowitz, the author of the book *Emerging Viruses: AIDS & Ebola—Nature, Accident or Intentional?*," Mr. Bell told his audience. For the next hour Jabril listened intently as I explained the work of Robert Gallo and Bionetics researchers, described the vaccines that most plausibly brought AIDS to the world, and implicated the Rockefeller-led military–medical–industrial complex whose plan for a New World Order called for massive depopulation at home and abroad. The spiritual advisor sat stunned.

In his transfixed state, Jabril could only listen. Writing down the book order line that the host liberally announced, along with my web site, and E-mail address, never entered Jabril's mind until the show ended. All at once, it seemed, his trance broke and he realized what had happened.

He reflected on the great prophecies of the Honorable Elijah Muhammad, the son of the Nation of Islam's Messiah, Master Fard Muhammad, responsible for bringing the Muslim faith to America for the liberation of enslaved Africans. The Honorable Elijah Muhammad was Jabril's teacher and Jabril was his favorite student. Elijah Muhammad dutifully prepared Jabril for his lifetime of human service. His instructions included ways of surviving the great tribulations he foresaw.

"Someday," the great prophet told Jabril, "a White man will come and explain why so many of our people are dying from plagues. When this man comes, reach out to him. Befriend him."

The next day Jabril phoned around feverishly to get a copy of this book. He called a dozen friends and bookstores countrywide but to no avail. Sunday passed likewise. Jabril retired Sunday night frustrated and disappointed. Not knowing where to turn next, he resigned his quest to a bedtime prayer.

"Jabril, wake up!"

The inner voice had returned. In fact, it was the same dream. "Wake up and turn your radio on!" the guide commanded.

Jabril was now familiar with the process. The outcome was identical.

Sunday night Art Bell always chose to rerun his best show of the week. He replayed our interview, and Jabril got my number.

The next morning my telephone rang. "Hello, my name is Jabril Muhammad," he announced. "I'm the spiritual advisor to Minister Louis Farrakhan. I heard you this weekend on the 'Art Bell Show.'"

Jabril then relayed to me the entire story described above. He ended by saying, "Minister Farrakhan would like to meet with you. Would you be willing to come to Chicago?"

Two days later I was honored to spend the evening with Minister Louis Farrakhan at his home in Chicago. The Nation of Islam's Health Minister, Dr. Abdul Alim Muhammad, from Washington, D.C., and Minister Farrakhan's AIDS czar, Dr. Barbara Justice Muhammad, from New York City, were also asked to attend and presented at the last minute.

The evening, and dinner, began with prayers and lessons for us from Minister Farrakhan. Acknowledging the unique assembly of a White Jewish man, with Christian beliefs, and Black brothers and sisters of the Muslim faith, we discussed the fears and concerns of people divided by the religious politics of a world gone mad.

Sure Jewish and Christian friends had advised me against accepting the risks of Minister Farrakhan's invitation. Forming an alliance with the leaders of The Nation of Islam for any reason seemed traitorous. The stereotyped Muslim is believed by the vast majority of Jews and Christians to be antisemitic and sexist. Likewise, Nation of Islam followers commonly view White Jews and Christians as racist and threatening.

Knowing, however, how the media, and the forces that wield it, are capable of distorting reality to divide and conquer, I remained open. I had also been primed for this meeting.

Months earlier I had witnessed a horrifying act of deception and treachery perpetrated by the major television networks against Louis Farrakhan and The Nation of Islam. During coverage of the "Million Man March" I noted a peculiar similarity in network coverage of the event. All networks portrayed the historic day of atonement, peacefully focused by the minister onto the fundamental need for building self-esteem, and spiritual devotion to God and family, as his ego trip.

"This march is about me," three of the four major networks broadcast Louis Farrakhan telling the masses with arms flailing. Reporters noted that the minister's speech lasted three-plus hours. What struck me odd was that all the networks, allegedly independent news sources, broadcast the same seconds of clip. How could this be? Only later, as I watched the entire speech on C-SPAN, did I realize the ruse.

What Minister Farrakhan had actually said was, "And *they* want you to believe that *this march is about me.*" The networks had purposely clipped his statement mid-sentence. They effectively distorted his meaning. I felt betrayed. Though I knew news organizations were capable of doing that, and that they routinely distorted the facts, witnessing the harsh reality left me feeling violated and cold.

So tempering my anxiety about messianic Jew meeting Islamic leader, and warming to the genuineness of the man and his message as we sat around the dinner table, was not difficult.

Indeed, Minister Farrakhan immediately hit a heartstring when, after praying for holy guidance, and a constructive outcome to our divinely inspired meeting, Minister Farrakhan turned to me and said, "You know, there's a lot more to this project than you might think. This is more than just an investigation into AIDS and Ebola viruses. I believe your greatest work is yet to come, and that you have been protected by the Lord and his angels to do this great work which involves extraordinary healing. Bridging the gap between people who have been, for so long, struggling against each other rather than against a common enemy. I see your greatest work is yet to come." Intuitively I knew this too.

A Political Time-bomb

Minister Farrakhan, and the others in the room, listened as I described my research and summarized this book. At the end of the meeting, he instructed his health advisors, Drs. Alim and Justice Muhammad, to study the book, decide their next steps, and report back. Health minister Alim Muhammad immediately suggested organizing a symposium to study the topic. It was later arranged to coincide with the Nation of Islam's "Saviour's Day" Convention in Chicago. Minister Farrakhan suggested that I might be invited to speak during the health ministry's session of the conference.

Three months later, in Chicago, before a "Saviour's Day" crowd of almost a thousand, the Minister of Health announced his recommendation for a moratorium on U.S. Government promulgated vaccines. He had studied the book and found it compelling enough to issue this warning. In essence, he lit the fuse on a political time-bomb. The blast would be determined by three months of deliberations by an official task force assembled by the health minister and the legislative committee of the National Medical Association—the American Black physician's counterpart to the American Medical Association. The task force proceedings were to be monitored, and resulting questions addressed, by top CDC and vaccine industry officials.

In fact, within days of Dr. Muhammad's controversial recommendation, CDC Director, David Satcher, M.D., Ph.D., a personal friend of the health minister, faxed Dr. Muhammad a letter expressing his views regarding my thesis on the man-made origin of HIV. He also voiced concern regarding the proposed moratorium on immunizations. In the letter Dr. Satcher invited Dr. Muhammad and I to "visit the Centers for Disease Control and Prevention to discuss these and other public health issues of mutual interest." The letter's content is reprinted in its entirety in figure 26.3.

In reply to Dr. Satcher's communication, Dr. Muhammad asked me to respond to the CDC Director's comments. The terms of my acceptance of Dr. Satcher's invitation, and rebuttal to his message regarding the iatrogenic theory of AIDS's origin through contaminated vaccines, is reprinted in figure 26.4.

The Health Minister's Concerns

The health minister's recommended moratorium on immunizations had been carefully considered. Dr. Muhammad's decision was based on previous research into the man-made theory of AIDS's origin, evidence that the pharmaceutical industry and FDA cooperatively allowed contaminated vaccines to be released, and ongoing concerns that the AIDS epidemic may be a genocidal effort to reduce Black populations. In addition, Dr. Muhammad was clearly impressed by the "smoking guns" delivered in this book.

The following is an interview with Dr. Muhammad. I began by asking the health minister to articulate his greatest concerns regarding the theory of AIDS as biological genocide:

Dr. Muhammad: I think that it is widely believed in the Black community that genocide is a very likely possibility. This is not only based on historical records which extend all the way back to the time of Columbus, wherein historians record that in the Caribbean Sea, on all of the islands, the Indian populations totaled approximately 15 million. But in one short generation, after Columbus's arrival, that population had been reduced to about 1,500 presumably due to the spread of epidemic diseases such as smallpox and measles to which the Indians had no natural immunity.

The same kind of thing happened in Mexico and South America. In fact, wherever the European "discoverers" ventured. They found that, amazingly, people seemed to die at their feet.

We know that Western science, at that time, had not yet developed a germ theory, so they substituted other theories to explain what was going on. Presumably it was the divine destiny of the European people to rule.

Now . . . in 1761 the British general Geoffrey Amhearst deliberately distributed smallpox infected blankets to some of the Indian tribes during the French–American War, and decimated entire villages and tribes. To my knowledge this was the first deliberate use of biological weapons even though, beginning with Columbus, that principle had been established as a way to depopulate and conquer territories so that they could be repopulated with another preferred group.

To bring this up to date, science today has reached a zenith. We live in a high-tech age when yesterday's works of science fiction are today's realities.

So when we look at Henry Kissinger's 1974 report—a study that was commissioned under Richard Nixon and completed during the Ford administration—the *National Security Memorandum 200*, some important concerns come to light. . . . One sees for the first time that Third World populations are specifically targeted by the United States as an enemy to the national security interests of America.[5]

It is not unimportant or coincidental, in my view, that starting in 1969, five years earlier, freshman Congressman George Bush from Texas, initiated a legislative investigating committee to look into the issue of planetary overpopulation.

So these forces were active at the time that people were being persuaded by propaganda to believe that population, in and of itself, was a problem. And that in the view of Henry Kissinger, the National Security Council, and the White House, it was their view that as a part of the national security interests, in order to safeguard America, you had to do something about population.

Fig. 26.3. Letter to Nation of Islam Health Minister Alim Muhammad From CDC Director David Satcher Expressing His Views on the Man-made Theory of AIDS's Origin and Vaccine Moratorium Recommendations

February 17,1997

Dear Dr. Muhammad:

This letter is in response to our conversation of February 13, 1997, regarding the safety of immunizations. We appreciate the opportunity to share detailed information with you regarding our efforts to protect our Nation's children against vaccine-preventable diseases. I am interested in discussing the safety of childhood vaccines further with you and Dr. Leonard G. Horowitz and invite you to visit the Centers for Disease Control and Prevention to discuss these and other public health issues of mutual interest.

Immunizations are among the most effective public health interventions in preventing illness and death throughout the world. Immunizations prevent an estimated 3 million deaths annually in children worldwide, and have resulted in more than 95 percent reduction in cases of all vaccine-preventable diseases in the U.S. compared to the pre-vaccine era. (See enclosed table.)

While routine childhood immunization has saved many lives and prevented disease epidemics both in the United States and elsewhere, it has paradoxically resulted in a decreased awareness by the public of the dangers of vaccine-preventable diseases. This decreased awareness can result in reduced vaccine coverage or delays in age-appropriate vaccination which frequently result in resurgent outbreaks of disease. The recent outbreak of diphtheria in Russia, pertussis in the United Kingdom in the 1970s, and, closer to home, the epidemic of measles in the United States in 1989-1991 illustrates this problem. Of particular note was the greatly increased burden of measles among unvaccinated preschool children in minority communities during the 1989-1991 measles epidemic. (See the enclosed article on "The Measles Epidemic.") This outbreak could have been prevented through use of the safe and effective measles vaccine, which is widely available through providers and public health clinics in the United States. We are, therefore, concerned that diseases like measles or whooping cough (pertussis) will continue to occur in young children in this country. Children who are not vaccinated will be at increase risk for disability and death associated with vaccine-preventable diseases. (See the enclosed issue of the *Morbidity and Mortality Weekly Report*, Vol. 44, No. 28.)

For several years, misinformation has circulated that vaccines are the source by which the human immunodeficiency virus (HIV) was introduced into the human population. One such misconception is based on an assumption that vaccines grown in monkey kidney cell cultures could have been infected with a monkey virus which eventually led to the spread of HIV infection and the resulting acquired immune deficiency syndrome (AIDS) epidemic. Though both are retroviruses, the simian virus is not the same as the human immunodeficiency virus. In fact, the genomic organization of the two viruses is very different.

Of the current universally recommended vaccines, only poliovirus vaccines are grown in monkey cells. The monkey kidney cell lines used in vaccines have been examined and demonstrated to be free of the simian virus and HIV. (See enclosed article by Khan et al.)

Use of these vaccines is critical to the worldwide polio eradication effort. The Western Hemisphere is now free of the wild polio virus, and worldwide, reported polio cases have been reduced by about 90 percent between 1988 and 1996--from 35,251 to 3,500, respectively. The goal is to eradicate polio worldwide by the year 2000, resulting in improvement in the health and well-being of all children as they no longer face the risk of death or paralysis from polio. Once polio is eradicated, the vaccination will eventually be stopped just as smallpox eradication led to cessation of that vaccination in the 1970s.

egarding the ebola outbreaks in Africa, concerns have been expressed that vaccines ould cause ebola or were contaminated with ebola virus. After the ebola virus was iscovered in 1976, testing to exclude its presence was incorporated into the mandatory rocedures for all tissues used in medical research or in the manufacture of other products, including vaccines. (These mandatory testing procedures are found in title 21 of te Code of Federal Regulations pertaining to the manufacturing and regulation of vaccines.)

ecause of economic constraints in Africa and other parts of the world, medical instruments designed for a single use are often reused. Under these circumstances, both the bola virus and HIV can, indeed, be spread; however, neither the ebola virus or HIV ave been spread through the use of a vaccine administered through properly sterilized ajection and other medical equipment.

accines have been and are made to protect the health and welfare of all persons and are ecommended by the Advisory Committee on Immunization Practices, the American cademy of Pediatrics, or the American Academy of Family Physicians for all children respective of race or ethnicity. The major threat to the health of African-American hildren comes not from vaccines, but from diseases that can occur if children are not ppropriately immunized.

hope this information and enclosed materials are helpful to you. I would also like to nvite you to our annual National Immunization Conference which will be held May 19-2 in Detroit. This conference is attended by medical and public health professionals rom the Federal, State, and local levels to discuss various topics related to vaccines. I tay be contacted at 404-639-7000. (FAX: 404-639-7111)

hank you for your interest in this very important health issue.

Sincerely,

David Satcher, M.D., Ph.D.
Director

nclosures

And in that *National Security Memorandum 200,* Kissinger goes on at length, not only ailing the populations that specifically he targeted, such as African nations, Black nations tside of Africa including Brazil, Iran, Iraq . . . and others. All tolled I think there were rteen. In fact, he detailed the kind of language that would have to be used in these proams to get around the political, cultural, and even religious objections that would be raised oopulation control efforts—whether it was through birth control programs or other means.

So, many years ago, we became aware of all of these policy objectives. And I think the auty of the book *Emerging Viruses: AIDS & Ebola* is that the documented proof was ught together in one place in a very powerful way."

Dr. Horowitz: That was my next question. What did you conclude after reading the ok?

Dr. Muhammad: Well Dr. Justice and I were convinced in 1991, that AIDS could not a naturally occurring virus. . . . From 1991 on, especially at important events like the ngressional Black Caucus weekends, where we were asked to present, we always raised the issue of genocide. And we called on Congressman Louis Stokes and others to convene investigatory hearings into the issue of whether or not AIDS was part of a genocidal policy of the United States government. . . .

Now *Emerging Viruses: AIDS & Ebola* basically begins where our efforts left off. It begins with that portion of the *Congressional Record* . . . dealing with the development of an artificial microorganism . . . and lays out in very precise detail how that work proceeded. So that by the end of the book, whether or not these are artificially created microoganisms is no longer a matter of mere speculation and circumstantial evidence, but I think it is conclusively proven.

I'm not in the legal profession, but I know in law there is a concept of "probable cause." I think certainly, the book provides probable cause to believe that Henry Kissinger and others were involved in the deliberate development of infective microorganisms for the purpose of genocide in Central Africa and other parts of the world. I think that the evidence is strong enough that were it to be reviewed by the appropriate legal authorities that it would serve to produce several indictments of those individuals that are involved. And it certainly is my hope that's exactly where this will lead. . . . To the same kinds of trials that were held in Nuremburg, and bring the accused before a bar of justice. And then let all the evidence contained in the book be heard and judged on its own merit.

I think that it is more than likely that we are in the midst of the worst genocide that has ever been carried out in the history of the world. It makes what Hitler did in Germany pale by comparison. It makes what Stalin did, and what Mao may have done, and others also pale by comparison.

Dr. Horowitz: All right then, Dr. Muhammad, how has this new knowledge, in relation to past knowledge, influenced your position regarding vaccines, number one, and what measures or political actions do you plan to now take?

Dr. Muhammad: Well, as discussed in the book, the role that vaccines played in the development of these artificial microorganisms is central. In fact, without the cancer virus and vaccine experiments, the knowledge of these microorganisms wouldn't have been gained, the cataloging of them wouldn't have taken place, and the ideas of recombining them in certain ways to produce cancer-causing microorganisms wouldn't have taken place. And so the problem of either accidental or deliberate biocontaminations of vaccines is just brought clearly to one's attention.

Along side of that you have to pay attention to epidemiological studies that seem to suggest that HIV is not primarily a sexually transmitted disease. . . .

One has to ask the question, 'If sexual transmission is not the primary means, what has been the primary means?' And I think the great thesis of the book is that it was through vaccine trials that this country was probably responsible for inoculating millions of people with HIV and perhaps other disease causing microorganisms.

And so that means that the distrust that already exists, especially in the Black communities, and in other communities as well, over public health measures such as vaccinations, is bolstered and substantiated. In fact, we have every reason to fear that the vaccines, that we are using, could be inadvertently, or deliberately, contaminated with viruses that could be part of the biological armamentarium that had been developed for cancer research, biological warfare, or genocide.

March 14, 1997

Dr. David Satcher, M.D., Ph.D.
Director
Centers for Disease Control and Prevention (CDC)
Atlanta, GA 30333

Dear Dr. Satcher:

Thank you for your invitation of Feb. 21, 1997 (that came by way of Minister of Health for the Nation of Islam, Dr. Abdul Alim Muhammad) to visit the Centers for Disease Control and Prevention to discuss the issue of vaccine contamination and "other public health issues of mutual interest," namely the origin of AIDS and Ebola viruses.

First, I greatly appreciate the opportunity to visit the CDC to present and discuss my investigation into the origin of AIDS and Ebola viruses. Last Fall, in the Bahamas, I met at length with your Associate Director for Minority Health, Reubin Warren, who likewise invited me to visit the CDC for this purpose. We have yet to set a date for this meeting.

Regarding your communication to Dr. Muhammad concerning the "misinformation . . . circulated that vaccines are the source by which the human immunodeficiency virus (HIV) was introduced into the human population, wherein you discuss "one such misconception," the polio vaccine theory, Dr. Muhammad asked me to reply to your comments.

For your information, you have apparently been misinformed. I challenge you, or any NIH investigator, to debate the scientific facts, the vast majority of which support the contention that contaminated vaccines have played a major role in the transmission of animal viruses to humans. A growing body of scientific evidence indicates vaccine contaminants are most plausibly related to certain types of cancers, and contemporary epidemics involving the human immune system including AIDS and chronic fatigue. Regarding AIDS, the evidence shows that the most supported theory on AIDS's origin, that is, the only theory that takes into account all of the confirmed scientific facts, as opposed to politically correct pseudo-scientific speculations, is the theory that I have advanced in *Emerging Viruses: AIDS & Ebola*.

I advance the theory that HIV, and simian immunodeficiency virus (SIV) relatives, evolved during the late 1960s to mid 1970s as a result of vaccine trials—including those conducted by Saul Krugman and later Maurice Hilleman at Merck pharmaceutical company (under NIH contract number 71-2059), along with coinvestigators at the CDC, FDA, and the National Institute for Allergies and Infectious Diseases (NIAID), as reported by Robert Purcell from NIAID. These investigators used heavily contaminated chimpanzees, and rhesus monkeys, supplied by the Army's sixth top biological weapons contractor—Litton Bionetics research lab (under NIH primate supply contracts including, but not limited to NIH 69-2160)—to "pool" hepatitis B viruses that were used to develop a reported 200,000 human doses of vaccine. Four subtypes of this hepatitis B vaccine were produced by these agencies and then simultaneously tested in New York City on gay men, Willowbrook State School mentally retarded children, on Staten Island, NY, and Blacks in Central Africa. The live hepatitis B viruses used to make these vaccines were extracted from the contaminated chimpanzees and rhesus monkeys, and then administered to these human subjects, along with all the other live viral contaminants these animals were infected with, including, but not limited to the herpes-type viruses, including simian cytomegalovirus, Epstein-Barr virus, and herpes B virus (all scientifically associated with chronic fatigue which, may I remand you, appeared on the planet at precisely the same time as the AIDS epidemic). Other viruses such as foamy retroviruses containing the AIDS-linked enzyme reverse transcriptase was also present in these animals. Additionally, most of the human subjects who received these infectious agents, and whose blood was later taken to make the suspected hepatitis B vaccines, had, approximately a decade earlier, received Salk or Sabin polio vaccines contaminated with SV40, and again, other common monkey kidney cell viral contaminants. This, of course, confounds my thesis, but significantly increased the likelihood that HIV progenitor viruses could have recombined to form HIV as well as SIV relatives—all a direct result of sloppy scientific methods and contaminated live viral vaccines.

My thesis explains the major scientific facts concerning the evolution of HIV including: 1) the earliest confirmed isolation of HIV, contrary to media headlines and popular belief, dates back only to 1976 as reported by Gerald Myers in Jay Levy's recently published textbook *The Retroviridae*; 2) by 1968 there were apparently HIV progenitors causing AIDS-like illnesses circulating in the U.S. as reported by Witte, et al.; 3) the closest relative to HIV-1 is the SIV from the chimpanzee; 4) the SIVs were discovered after HIV; 5) SIV from the macaque monkey, identical to HIV-2 found to be a laboratory contaminant, was not found in wild monkeys, only Senegalese female prostitutes, who because of their high risk trade, likely received contaminated hepatitis B vaccines during the 1970s. (How, other than through contaminated vaccines, could scores of these women have picked up a research laboratory monkey virus contaminant?); 6) the evolution of several subtypes of HIV around the planet by 1975, as detailed in Myers's "Big Bang" theory, coincides with the 1974 administration of the four subtypes of hepatitis B vaccine in various parts of the world including New York City and Central Africa by Hilleman's four teams; 7) the mutational frequency of HIV is consistent with that of a new virus; 8) the fact that HIV is associated with severe immunosuppression, and high mortality and morbidity, is also most consistent with a new virus requiring evolution to establish homeostasis in its new human host; 9) the mutational frequency range of HIV, again according to Myers (personal communication) exceeds that of anything natural, thus strongly suggesting an iatrogenic origin; 10) the unique epidemiology of AIDS in which the highest HIV seroprevalence rates exist in the exact regions of the world and populations wherein the hepatitis B vaccine was tested, namely New York City, Central Africa, and particularly in homosexual men, intravenous drug users, prisoners, and people of African decent, that is, people commonly used in vaccine trials; 11) Maurice Hilleman's 1986 admission that his team at Merck had brought the AIDS virus into North America in contaminated African green monkeys, again supplied by Litton; 12) that the epidemic broke out the decade following the 1960s wherein major advances in genetic biotechnology were made and wherein cell/virus cloning procedures exploded; 13) that contrary to popular belief and misinformation, sufficient homology exists between HIV and common polio vaccine viral contaminants, and viruses likely to have contaminated Litton laboratory animals and cell cultures at the time the earliest hepatitis B vaccines were produced, to advance this thesis, and last but not least,14) that scientists (including Dr. Robert Gallo and others) who advanced farfetched notions of the African green monkey theory of HTLV-1 and HIV, despite their sophisticated knowledge of the NCI's "Special Virus Cancer Program" in which viral recombinants and related vaccines were produced, have obviously incriminated themselves. A discussion of substantial self-incriminating evidence is provided on page 498 of *Emerging Viruses: AIDS & Ebola*. That virtually no attention has been paid by your organization, the NCI, as well as other AIDS investigators, to the iatrogenic theory of AIDS, is highly suspicious if not criminal.

On related notes, that leading AIDS investigators and public health officials have continued to downplay the need to determine HIV's origin, and possible continued spread through contaminated vaccines, flies in the face of ethical public health practice and preventative medicine. Moreover, you may not know that on February 18, 1997, Tammy Nunnally of your Office of Communications sent Gino Montesi and Mike Carrie from WXTK Radio on Cape Cod an official transmittal from your office that states, "the virus that causes AIDS, is not a man-made virus and did not originate in laboratories . . . It is a human virus that evolved naturally over time, as other viruses have." Who authorized her to communicate such misinformation? She references only the "World Book Encyclopedia which was written by one of our experts," as her definitive source. This is a sham—an absolute insult to medical intelligence. Why should I and the general public trust you, or the organization you represent, in light of such unfounded, biased, and misleading communications?

Finally, did I hear correctly that Dr. Gallo is, once again, under investigation for scientific misconduct or fraud? Having challenged Dr. Gallo at the XI International Conference on AIDS in Vancouver, regarding his role in the development of numerous immune system ravaging viruses while NCI project officer, overseeing Litton's NIH contract 71-2025—"Investigation of Viral Carcinogenesis in Primates"—I have reviewed his major objections to my thesis which, by the way, are discredited by his and his NIH mentors' earlier scientific contributions. I am enclosing a copy of a letter I sent to Dr. Gallo on October 28, 1996, wherein I refute his misleading claims. This transmittal followed a lengthy interview he provided me wherein he acknowledged my general thesis is plausible. Most importantly, he stated that he might be able to lend additional information in support of the accidental theory on the origin of AIDS. I still patiently await this information.

In conclusion, I gladly accept your invitation to discuss these mutual concerns, but I don't want to waste your time and mine playing lip service to the issues. If you or other CDC officials are willing to critically examine the facts, take a stand for common sense and scientific integrity, including a willingness to examine the CDC's apparent role in developing (along with Hilleman, Purcell et al.) the vaccine that most plausibly brought AIDS to the world, then I will be happy to schedule a visit to Atlanta to meet with you. If not, it's possible I'll see you in heaven or, with God's grace, and the support of the American people, before a Congressional investigating committee.

Sincerely yours,

Leonard G. Horowitz, D.M.D., M.A., M.P.H.
President, Tetrahedron Incorporated
a nonprofit educational corporation
Rockport, Massachusetts 01966
Telephone: 508-546-6586 • URL# http://www.Tetrahedron.org
E-mail: tetra@tetrahedron.org

So that forces us to the position of, at least, considering a moratorium on vaccines, and massive public education programs to inform people of this very real and probable risk. And it forces us to seek alternatives [to traditional public health practices]. . . .

The central points are clear. . . . There is, in the eyes of some, some potential public health risk in calling for a moratorium on vaccines. But our position really is that the policy of genocide is a real policy of the United States until proven and declared otherwise. And, therefore, the risk of that genocidal policy far outweighs any potential public health risk from a moratorium on vaccines.

Indeed, a basic tenant of prudent public health policy is that the benefits versus risks of that policy should be carefully weighed and prove positive. Regarding immunizations, the absence of such definitive analyses provides ample motive to pause and question both vaccination policy and its makers. By the CDC's own accounts more than 48,743 adverse vaccine reactions were reported between 1991 and 1996. During this time authorities acknowledged that more than 99 percent of the most severe cases were never reported.[10] Thus, annually, as many as 1 million Americans may have been harmed by vaccines, with, conservatively, tens of thousands seriously injured. In conclusion, the annual morbidity, if not mortality, from immunization practices in the United States approaches, and may even surpass, that of AIDS.

Fear's Call to Awareness and Action

People everywhere have wondered if I now fear for my life. A better question is, "Does the benefit of this work exceed the risk to a single life, mine or anyone's?"

During the past several months more than half of the audiences I polled knew friends or family members who, over the past few years, fell victim to bizarre immune-system-related disorders, or unique cancers, unrelated to family history.

My greatest fear is that the holocaust my mother survived in 1939, by coming to America, killed her—a victim of flu vaccine induced Guillain-Barré autoimmune disease and cancer—in 1994. We fought for years, she and I, over the likelihood of a contemporary holocaust. "It could never happen again," I blindly argued, "we have the media now." My mother was not like the rest of us who have been monumentally deceived.

Two years after my mother's death, I picked up a book entitled *The Secret War Against the Jews* (St. Martins, 1994) by John Loftus and Mark Aarons. The authors detailed the intricate deceptions carried out by international intelligence organizations as the forces of darkness moved to exterminate millions of Jews, Christians, homosexuals, Africans, Gypsies, and Indians. The world's masses knew nothing about the partnership, formed between John D. Rockefeller's Standard Oil Company, Germany's IG Farben, and Hitler's Third Reich. The "pirates of Wall Street," Allen and John Foster Dulles, of the law firm Sullivan & Cromwell, had secretly negotiated this alliance. It was not known to allied airmen, flying bombing missions over Germany, why the IG Farben plants, where Hitler's munitions were made, were exempted from attack. Likewise, when the IG Farben–Rockefeller consortium used concentration camp victims as slaves to build and run their factories it never made the news. Nor was it heralded that this same team patented and sold the gas that the Nazis used in the concentration camps to send millions to their graves. Recent headlines have asked to know where the Nazi gold went. Historians only recently recorded that the Rockefeller's Chase Bank was among the largest recipients.[10]

How could people have not known what was really going on? How could the Dulles brothers and Rockefeller-led military–medical–industrial complex have gotten away with committing treason against the United States? How could the Dulleses have, immediately following World War II, successfully engineered the next great conflict—the Cold War—behind the backs of Roosevelt and Truman? The common answer is: sophisticated intelligence and counterintelligence programs in support of covert operations.

In *Mein Kampf* Hitler wrote, "If you tell a lie long enough, eventually it will be believed as truth. . . . [and] the greater the lie, the more people will believe it." The phrase "vaccines are safe and effective" echoes in my mind as does the memory of those millions of holocaust victims who were marshalled into the gas chambers for "disinfection" as a "public health" measure. My greatest fear, given this history, is that today's public health clinics and physician's offices are like the concentration camps, and that our FDA approved vaccines are like the gas.

Health scientists, on whom we depend for miracle cures, have been lulled by the same siren's song of deception. Evidence, in Christopher Simpson's *The Science of Coercion*, shows the Rockefeller Foundation, in collusion with the CIA, largely controlled funding for scientific progress and academic research in the United States and elsewhere. "This was not a 'conspiracy,' in the hackneyed sense of that word. It was rather . . . informal authority" exercised by networks and projects that "advanced their conception of scientific progress and national security . . . to gain the financial support that is often a prerequisite to academic success." It is apparent that the "dominant paradigm" in health science is "in substantial part a *paradigm of dominance*" in which the inevitability of elite control is exercised.[11]

Thus, both of this century's worst genocides appear to have been determined by the same masterminds whose covert operations and deadly deceptions have beaten humanity by default. Sleeping sheeple fall prey to the forces of evil who divide the flock to conquer and wield ignorance to reign.

In this light, this work appears to be well timed as a call to action. Many people are poised to awaken and evolve beyond the disinformation and disturbing separation—rich from poor, Black from White, Jew from gentile, Christian from Muslim, New Ager from religious fundamentalist, Democrat from Republican, HIV-positive from HIV-negative, capitalist versus communist versus socialist—all conflicts championed by the dark forces of fascism.

The grave tribulations and plagues predicted in the *Book of Revelation* are here. Likewise, the challenges of a shifting paradigm to humanists, barriers to ascension into the light for New Agers, and atrocities of the New World Order for patriotic nationalists, all evolved from a common enemy. In this respect, Babylon is New York City. Those who "fornicated with the devil" and "deceived all the Kings" and the "wealthiest men of all the nations" are the Rockefellers *et al.* They have literally "stolen the blood of the prophets and saints" for their international blood trade. Contaminated vaccines and tainted bloods now flow, like Babylon's wine, full of impurities, into "rivers and streams" of people. Likewise, "beasts" deliver mad cow disease, leukemia and other plagues, arising from a similar source, to our world's population.[13]

Let it be known who wins in the end. "The meek shall inherit the Earth." For all of this, you see, I believe, was planned by God, and predicted by his prophets. They foretold that, indeed, someday soon, the "crystal clear waters" will once again flow through our rivers and streams. Trees bearing fruits will line their banks. And their leaves will bring forth "the healing of the nations."[13]

References and Notes

Prologue

1. Runnells RR. *AIDS in the Dental Office. The Story of Kimberly Bergalis and David Acer.* Fruit Heights, Utah: IC Publications, Inc., 1993, pp. 293-298; Johnson vs. Acer (Legal suit brought against dentist David Acer by Sherry Johnson). Deposition of Edward Parsons for Robert Montgomery, December 9, 1993. Visual Evidence, Inc., (407-655-2855).

2. United States General Accounting Office. AIDS-CDC's investigation of HIV transmission by a dentist. GAO/PEMD-92-31, Washington, D.C. September 29, 1992.

3. American Broadcasting Company. *20/20.* Interview with Edward Parson on the Florida dental AIDS tragedy. October 1, 1993.

4. Horowitz LG. *Deadly Innocence: Solving the greatest murder mystery in the history of American medicine.* Rockport, MA: Tetrahedron, Inc., 1994.

5. McLoed D. Did Dr. Acer intentionally kill patients? *Academy of General Dentistry Impact.* 1995;23;10:19.

6. Horowitz LG. Correlates and predictors of sexual homicide with HIV in the Florida dental AIDS tragedy. *AIDS Patient Care.* 1994;8;4:220-228.

7. Horowitz LG. Sexual homicide with HIV in a Florida dental office? *Journal of Clinical Pediatric Dentistry.* 1994;19;1:61-64.

8. Horowitz LG. Murder and cover-up may explain the Florida dental AIDS mystery. *British Dental Journal.* 1995;10;24:423-427.

9. Strecker R. *The Strecker Memorandum.* The Strecker Group, 1501 Colorado Boulevard, Los Angeles, CA 90041, 1988.

10. Edward Parsons personal communication.

11. Breo DL. The dental AIDS cases—Murder or an unsolvable mysery? *JAMA* 270:2732-2734, 1993.

12. CBS News—a *60-MINUTES* report. Kimberly's story. Produced by Josh Howard. June 19, 1994.

Chapter 1. Strecker's "World Health Organization Theory" of AIDS

1. Strecker R. *The Strecker Memorandum.* The Strecker Group, 1501 Colorado Boulevard, Los Angeles, CA 90041, 1988.

2. Gonda MA, Braun MJ, Carter SG, Kost TA, Bess Jr JW, Arthur LO and VanDer Maaten MJ. Characterization and molecular cloning of a bovine lentivirus related to human immunodeficiency virus. *Nature* 1987;330, 388-391; Mulder C. Human AIDS virus not from monkeys. *Nature* 1988;333:396; See also: Penny D. Origin of the AIDS virus. *Nature* 1988;333:494-495.

3. Collin J. They deployed the AIDS virus. *Townsend Letter for Doctors.* April, 1988 p.152.

4. Department of Defense Appropriations For 1970: Hearings Before A Subcommittee of the Committee on Appropriations House of Representatives, Ninety-first Congress, First Session, H.B. 15090, Part 5, Research, Development, Test and Evaluation, Dept. of the Army. U.S. Government Printing Office, Washington, D.C., 1969.

5. This text was typed at the top of page 129 in the document cited in reference #4 above. A portion of this DOD appropriations document was provided by The Strecker Group and published as document number RS-028. Los Angeles: The Strecker Group, 1988.

6. Szmuness W, Stevens CE, Harley EJ, Zang EA and Oleszko WR et al. Hepatitis B vaccine: Demonstration of efficacy in a controlled clinical trial in a high-risk population in the United States. *New England Journal of Medicine* 1980;303;15:833-841.

Chapter 2. WHO Plays in the Big Leagues

1. Horowitz LG. *Deadly Innocence: Solving the greatest murder mystery in the history of American medicine.* Rockport, MA: Tetrahedron, Inc., 1994. Includes a chapter titled "The Clinton–CIA Connection" which relays the story told by ex-intelligence asset Terry Reed. According to Reed's *Compromised* (S.P.I.Books, 1993), much of the Iran-Contra affair—the drugs for arms and hundreds of millions of dollars of laundered cash—was apparently handled by Clinton administration officials under a Banana Republic set up by the CIA and agents William Barr and Oliver North during the Reagan era.

2. Strecker RB. *The Strecker Memorandum: The cause, the effects and the possible cure for the pandemic AIDS.* Eagle Rock, CA: The Strecker Group, 1988.

3. Mathews AG. WHO's influence on the control of biologicals. *WHO Chronicle* 1968;23;1:3-15.

4. Glatt MM. The development of international control of drugs. *WHO Chronicle* 1970;24;5:189-197.

5. Payne AAM. Approaches to communicable disease control: Specialized and integrated services. *WHO Chronicle* 1968;22;1:3-7.

6. Tyrrell DAJ. The common cold research unit: WHO International Reference Centre for respiratory virus diseases. *WHO Chronicle* 1968;22;1:8-11.

7. WHO News and Notes. Genetic susceptibility to infection. *WHO Chronicle* 1968;22;4:162.

8. WHO News and Notes. Studies of the American Indian. *WHO Chronicle* 1968;22;10:459

9. Barrai I. Human genetics and public health. *WHO Chronicle* 1970;24;6:246-247.

10. WHO Report. Multipurpose serological surveys. *WHO Chronicle* 1971;25;3:99-101.

11. WHO News and Notes. Large-scale BCG trials. *WHO Chronicle* 1968;22;11:496.

12 WHO Current Research Projects. Live measles vaccines. *WHO Chronicle* 1968;22;12:534-5.

13. WHO Report (Based on a report presented to the Twenty-first World Health Assembly, and on discussions at the Assembly.) The smallpox eradication programme. *WHO Chronicle* 1968;22;8:354-362.

14. WHO Report (Based on a report presented to the Twenty-second World Health Assembly.) The smallpox eradication programme. *WHO Chronicle* 1969;23;10:465-476.

15. WHO News and Notes. Regional Committee for Africa. *WHO Chronicle* 1969;23;8:341-344.

16. Unfortunately, with the smallpox vaccination as with hepatitis B vaccination, the WHO reported that "in persons vaccinated only in infancy, the incidence of smallpox increases with age as immunity diminishes; the data indicate a high degree of protection for 4-5 years, followed by a slow decline, but even after a longer period, smallpox in vaccinated persons is usually milder than in unvaccinated persons and this appears to indicate some residual immunity. Similarly, the difficulty in producing a major reaction to revaccination lessens with time, but even after 10 or 20 years the vaccine required to produce a high percentage of takes must be at least 5-10 times more potent than vaccines that will produce the same percentage of takes in primary vaccinations. The duration of immunity after revaccination cannot be assessed accurately because not enough is known about the occurrence of smallpox in successfully revaccinated persons. . . ."
Quotation from: World Health Organization Report. Communicable diseases in 1970: Some aspects of the WHO programme. *WHO Chronicle* 1971;25;6:249-255.

17. Rowe DS. The WHO immunology laboratories at Lausanne. *WHO Chronicle* 1968;22;11:496.

18. WHO Report (Based on the 1969 report The medical research programme of the World health Organization, 1964-1968, Geneva.) Five years of research of virus diseases. *WHO Chronicle* 1969;23;12:564-572.

19. Kalter SS and Heberling. The study of simian viruses. *WHO Chronicle* 1969;23;3:112-117.

20. Siebert C. Smallpox is dead: Long live smallpox. *The New York Times Magazine*, Sunday, August 21, 1994, Section 6, pp. 31-55.

21. Walsh J. Civilian use for biological warfare facility under study. *Science* 1970;167;923:1359.

22 Henderson DA and Arita I. Monkeypox and its relevance to smallpox eradication *WHO Chronicle* 1973;27;4:145-148.

23. As defined in *Stedman's Medical Dictionary*, Kuru is a "highly localized, fatal disease found in New Guinea, resembling paralysis agitans; found among certain cannibalistic people who ingest raw brain of recently deceased victims of the disease. Also call laughing sickness."

24. Lederberg J. Biological warfare: a global threat. *American Scientist.* 1971 59;2:195-7.

25. *Department of Defense Appropriations For 1970: Hearings Before A Subcommittee of the Committee on Appropriations House of Representatives, Ninety-first Contress, First Session, H.B. 15090,*

Part 5, Research, Development, Test and Evaluation, Dept. of the Army. U.S. Government Printing Office, Washington, D.C., 1969.

26. Washington Correspondent. Gas and germ warfare renounced but lingers on. *Nature* 1970 228;273:707-8.

Chapter 3. Cold War, Biological Weapons, and World Health

1. Langer E. Chemical and biological weapons: Once over lightly on Capitol Hill. *Science* 1967 156;778:1073-5.

2. Anonymous. War on chemical and biological warfare. *Nature* 1968 218;145:905-6.

3. Lesse S. Editorial: Poison and the United States Public Health Service—a study of medical perversion. *American Journal of Psychotherapy* 1975;29;4:463-5.

4. Beckwith J. Science for the people. *Annals of the New York Academy of Sciences* 1972 196;4:236-40.

5. Anonymous. Can biological war be stopped? *Nature* 1968 219;155:665-6.

6. Crozier D. and Woodward TE. Report on research activities of the Commission on Epidemiological Survey. *Military Medicine* 1967 132;8:609-13.

7. Wallach DP. Deterrent value of CB research. *Science* 1968 161;842:631.

8. Lederberg J. Biological warfare: a global threat. *American Scientist* 1971 59;2:195-7.

9. Anonymous. The biological bomb. *Lancet* 1968;1;540:465.

10. Staff writer. War on chemical and biological warfare. *Nature* 1968;218:905-906.

11. The incomplete reference was given as "Hersh SM. Chemical and biological warfare. Indianapolis, N.Y., 1968.

12. Anonymous. Control of microbiological warfare. *The Lancet* 1968;2;564:391.

13. World Health Organization. Biomedical research: WHO's commitments examined. *WHO Chronicle* 1975;29:417-422.

14. McCrary DI. Letter to the Editor: Moral issues of CB warfare. *Science* 1967 156;780:1307-8.

15. WHO Group of Consultants. Chemical and biological weapons: The hazard to health. *WHO Chronicle* 1970 24;3:99-108.

16. Horowitz LG, Lewis PL, and Cohen P. AIDS-related fear: Beliefs, attitudes and behaviors. *Chicago Dental Society Review* 1993;86;2:18-23.

17. Horowitz LG and Kehoe L. Fear and AIDS: Educating the public about dental office infection control procedures. *Journal of the American Academy of General Dentistry* 1993;41;5:385-392.

18. Horowitz LG and Lipkowitz RD. Survey on AIDS, Fear and Infection Control: Attitudes affecting management decisions. *Journal of Clinical Preventive Dentistry* 1992;14;6:31-34.

19. Crozier D and Woodward TE. Report on research activities of the Commission on Epidemiological Survey, AFEB. *Military Medicine* 1967 132;8:609-13.

20. Covert NM. *Cutting Edge: A history of Fort Detrick, Maryland 1943-1993.* Fort Detrick: Headquarters U.S. Army Garrison Public Affairs Office (HSHD-PA), 1993.

21. Kalter SS and Heberling. The study of simian viruses. *WHO Chronicle* 1969;23;3:112-117.

22. World Health Organization Report. Communicable diseases in 1970: Some aspects of the WHO programme. *WHO Chronicle* 1971;25;6:249-255.

23. World Health Organization Report. Five years of research on virus diseases. *WHO Chronicle* 1969 23;12:564-572.

24. World Health Organization Report. Recent work on virus diseases. *WHO Chronicle* 1974;28:410-413.

25. World Health Organization Report. Communicable diseases in 1970: Some aspects of the WHO programme. *WHO Chronicle* 1971;25;6:249-255.

26. World Health Organization Report. The smallpox eradication programme. *WHO Chronicle* 1968 22;8:354-362.

27. World Health Organization Report. Smallpox eradication: the first significant results. *WHO Chronicle* 1969 23;10:465-476.

28. World Health Organization Report. The smallpox eradication programme. *WHO Chronicle* 1975 29:134-139.

29. World Health Organization Report. The eradication of smallpox. *WHO Chronicle* 1968. 22;12:523-527.

30. In other words, cancerous cells that have been presumably "transformed" by viral infections can be identified by specific foreign proteins (called antigens). Interestingly, The Group noted that these foreign proteins may enter a cell and thus be demonstrated regardless of the species or animal used as an infected host.

31. WHO Scientific Group on Viruses and Cancer (1965) Report, Geneva (Wld Hlth Org. techn. Rep. Ser., 1965, No. 295).

32. Mathews AG. WHO's influence on the control of biologicals. *WHO Chronicle* 1968;23;1:3-15.

33. WHO Scientific Group on Human Viral and Rickettsial Vaccines. *WHO Chronicle* 1966 20;7:255-261.

34. Gillette R. VEE Vaccine: Fortuitous Spin-off from BW Research. *Science* 1971;173;995:405-8.

35. WHO Respiratory and Enterovirus Centres. *WHO Chronicle.* 1974 28:410-413.

36. The Directors of WHO Respiratory and Enterovirus Centres. Recent work on virus diseases. *WHO Chronicle* 1974;28:410-413.

37. Tyrrell DAJ. The common cold research unit: WHO International Reference Centre for respiratory virus diseases. *WHO Chronicle* 1968;22;1:8-11.

38. Kalter SS and Heberling RL. The study of simian viruses—work of the WHO collaborating laboratory on comparative medicine: Simian viruses. *WHO Chronicle* 1969;23;3:112-117.

39. WHO Report (Based on the 1969 report The medical research programme of the World health Organization, 1964-1968, Geneva.) Five years of research of virus diseases. *WHO Chronicle* 1969;23;12:564-572.

Chapter 4. The Road to Fort Detrick Runs Through Bethesda

1. Washington Correspondent. Biological warfare: Detrick left hanging. *Nature* 1971;229:5279:8.

2. Washington Correspondent. Biological warfare: Relief of Fort Detrick. *Nature* November 28,1970;228:803.

3. Boffey PM. Fort Detrick: A top laboratory is threatened with extinction. *Science* January 22,1968;171:262-264.

4. Boffey PM. Detrick birthday: Dispute flares over biological warfare center. *Science* April 19,1968;171:285-288.

5. Allen JM, Emerson R, Grant P. Schneiderman HA and Siekevitz P. *Science* 1968;160;834:1287-8.

6. The incomplete reference was given as "Hersh SM. Chemical and biological warfare. Indianapolis, N.Y., 1968.

7. Anonymous. Control of microbiological warfare. *The Lancet* 1968;2;564:391.

8. World Health Organization. Biomedical research: WHO's commitments examined. *WHO Chronicle* 1975;29:417-422.

9. Covert NM. *Cutting Edge: A history of Fort Detrick, Maryland 1943-1993.* Fort Detrick, MD: Headquarters, U.S. Army Garrison, Public Affairs Office, 1993. [For copies call 301-619-2018]

10. Szmuness W, Stevens CE, Harley EJ, Zang EA and Oleszko WR et al. Hepatitis B vaccine: Demonstration of efficacy in a controlled clinical trial in a high-risk population in the United States. *New England Journal of Medicine* 1980;303;15:833-841.

11. Walgate R. Hepatitis B vaccine: Pasteur Institute in AIDS fracas. *Nature* 1983;304:104.

12. This knowledge also made me wonder whether Bethesda maintained any secret, highest biosafety level 4, BSL4, labs. Later I learned that, BSL 4 facilities were only available at Fort Detrick and at the CDC, they were not needed to produce or study the AIDS virus. This was confirmed during a telephone call to Bethesda's NCI AIDS research labs. The technician I spoke with there responded to my question, "Yes, we are handling the [AIDS] virus in level 3 labs as are numerous study groups around the country."

Despite the CDC labs ability to handle the AIDS-like viruses however, a review of the research literature from that period shows they were not active in such efforts. Only the NCI was conducting this kind of research and only in the Cell Tumor Biology Department at the NCI which was headed by Dr. Robert Gallo.

13. National Academy of Sciences. Symposium on chemical and biological warfare. *Proc. N.A.S.* 1970;65:250-279.

14. *Department of Defense Appropriations For 1970: Hearings Before A Subcommittee of the Committee on Appropriations House of Representatives, Ninety-first Contress, First Session, H.B. 15090,*

Part 5, Research, Development, Test and Evaluation, Dept. of the Army. U.S. Government Printing Office, Washington, D.C., 1969.

15. Staff writer. CBW: Geneva Protocol at last. *Nature* 1970;227;261:884.

16. Washington Correspondent. Gas and germ warfare renounced but lingers on. *Nature* 1970 228;273:707-8.

17. My hunch that the CIA might have been involved in viral research was based on my association with a Canadian colleague who relayed the story of Dr. Ewen Cameron. Cameron, the Chief of Psychiatry at McGill University's Allan Memorial Institute in Montreal, conducted LSD experiments for the CIA during a project code named MKULTRA. Victims of Cameron's brainwashing experiments were paid $7 million in settlements in a case which never went to court and was hushed up in the U.S. See: Bindman S. Ottawa has paid $7 million to brainwashing victims. *Montreal Gazette*, Wed. Jan. 19, 1994. p. B1.

18 The Rockefeller Commission. *Report to the President by the Commission on CIA Activities Within the United States.* Vice President Nelson A Rockefeller, Chairman. (Co-commissioners included Ronald Reagan). New York: The Rockefeller Foundation. 1975.

19. Moscow World Service in English. Belitskiy on How, Where AIDS Virus Originated. March 11, 1988. Published in *International Affairs.* FBIS-SOV-88-049, March 14, 1988, p. 24. Text discusses Seale's allegations, but does not furnish specifics.

20. *Havana International Service in Spanish.* German Claims AIDS Virus Created by Pentagon. FBIS-LAT 91-017. January 25, 1991. Caribbean, Cuba. Text discusses Dr. Jacobo Segal's allegations. Document PA 2401213091-0000 GMT 24, January 1991.

21. *Havana International Service in Spanish.* Commentary Accuses U.S. of Developing AIDS Virus. LAT 24, June 1987. Caribbean, Cuba "Viewpoint" commentary read by Angel Hernandez. Document PA 200342- 000GMT 19, June 1987. pp. A5-6.

22. McGinniss J. *The Last Brother: The Rise and Fall of Teddy Kennedy.* New York: Pocket Star Books, 1994.

23. World Health Organization. Biomedical research: WHO's commitments examined. *WHO Chronicle* 1975;29:417-422.32. Washington Correspondent. Relief of Fort Detrick. *Nature* 1970;228:803.

24. Brumter C. *The North Atlantic Assembly.* Dordrecht: Martinus Lijhoff Publishers, 1986, p. 215.

25. Washington Correspondent. Relief of Fort Detrick. *Nature* 1970;228:803.

26. Goldman BA and Chappelle M. Is HIV=AIDS wrong? *In These Times.* August 5-18, 1992, pp. 8-10.

27. Gallo R. RNA-dependent DNA polymerase in viruses and cells: Views on the current state. *Blood* 1972;39;1:117-137.

28. Shilts R. *And the Band Played On: Politics, People and the AIDS Epidemic.* New York: Penguin Books, 1987, pp. 450-453.

Chapter 5. The Emperor's New Virus

1. Shilts R. *And the Band Played On: Politics, People and the AIDS Epidemic.* New York: Penguin Books, 1987.

2. *Department of Defense Appropriations For 1970: Hearings Before A Subcommittee of the Committee on Appropriations House of Representatives, Ninety-first Contress, First Session, H.B. 15090, Part 5, Research, Development, Test and Evaluation, Dept. of the Army.* U.S. Government Printing Office, Washington, D.C., 1969.

3. Shilts R. *Op. cit.,* p. 269.

4. Shilts R. *Ibid.,* p. 270-271.

5. Shilts R. *Ibid.,* p. 151.

6. Shilts R. *Ibid.,* p. 163.

7. Shilts R. *Ibid.,* pp. 73-74.

8. Shilts R. *Ibid.,* p. 186.

9. Shilts R. *Ibid.,* p. 173.

10. Shilts R. *Ibid.,* p. 201-202.

11. Shilts R. *Ibid.,* p. 151.

12. Shilts R. *Ibid.,* p. 350.

13. Shilts R. *Ibid.,* pp. 366-367.

14. Walgate R. Hepatitis B vaccine: Pasteur Institute in AIDS fracas. *Nature* 1983;304:104.
15. Shilts R. *Ibid.*, p. 264.
16. Shilts R. *Ibid.*, p. 272.
17. Shilts R. *Ibid.*, p. 354.
18. Shilts R. *Ibid.*, p. 319
19. Shilts R. *Ibid.*, p. 444.
20. Shilts R. *Ibid.*, p. 451.
21. Shilts R. *Ibid.*, p. 528-29.
22. Shilts R. *Ibid.*, p. 452.
23. Gallo RC, Sarin PS, Allen PT, and Newton WA, et al. Reverse transcriptase in type C virus particles of human origin. *Nature New Biology* 1971;232:10-142.
24. Talal N and Gallo RC. Antibodies to a DNA:RNA Hybrid in systemic lupus erythematosus measured by a cellulose ester filter radioimmunoassay. *Nature New Biology* 1972;240:240-242.
25. Bobrow SN, Smith RG, Reitz MS and Gallo RC. Stimulated normal human lymphocytes contain a ribonuclease-sensitive DNA polymerase distinct from viral RNA-directed DNA polymerase. *Proc. Nat. Acad. Sci.* 1972;69;11:3228-3232.
26. Gallo RC. Reverse transcriptase, the DNA polymerase of oncogenic RNA viruses. *Nature* 1971;234:194-198.
27. Gallo RC and Whang-Peng JW. Enhanced transformation of human immunocompetant cells by dibutyryl adenosine cyclic 3'5' -monophosphate. *J. National Cancer Institute* 1971;47;1:91-94.
28. Gallo RC, Hecht SM, Whang-Peng J and O'Hopp S. N⁶-(²isopentenyl) adenosine: the regulatory effects of a cytokinin and modified nucleoside from tRNA on human lymphocytes. *Biochimica Et Biophysica Acta* 1982;281:488-500.
29. Herrera F, Adamson RH and Gallo RC. Uptake of transfer ribonucleic acid by normal and leukemic cells. *Proc. Nat. Acad. Sci.* 1970;67;4:1943-1950.
30. Among the human lymphocyte and RNA retrovirus reproductive stimulants Gallo and his co-workers studied were: phytohemagglutinin (a plant protein which makes red blood cells stick together)—see Riddick DH and Gallo RC. The Transfer RNA Methylases of Human Lymphocytes: Induction by PHA in Normal Lymphocytes. *Blood* 1971;37;3:282-292.; isopentenyladenosine (a plant hormone and component of yeast and mammalian tRNA)—see Gallo RC, Whang-Peng J and Perry S. Isopentenyladenosine Stimulates and Inhibits Mitosis in Human Lymphocytes Treated with Phytohemagglutinin. *Science*; 1969: 165:400-402; dibutyryl adenosine cyclic 3'5'-monophosphate (a chemical messenger and hormone stimulent in cells)—see Gallo RC, Whang-Peng J. Enhanced Transformation of Human Immunocompetent Cells by Dibutyryl Adenosine Cyclic 3',5'-Monophosphate. *Journal of the National Cancer Institute*. 1971;47;1:91-94; magnesium (an element and dietary component) see Gallo RC, Sarin PS, Allen, PT, Newton WA, Priori ES, Bowen JM and Dmochowski L. Reverse Transcriptase in Type C Virus Particles of Human Origin. *Nature New Biology* 1971;232;140-142; Epstein Barr virus (a virus strongly linked to Burkitt's-type lymphoma, cancer of the nasopharynx and infectious mononucleosis) see Fujioka S and Gallo RC. Aminoacyl Transfer RNA Profiles in Human Myeloma Cells. *Blood* 1971; 38;2:246-252; manganese (a metalic element)—see Smith RG and Gallo RC. DNA-Dependent DNA Polymerases I and II from Normal Human-Blood Lymphocytes. *Proceedings of the National Academy of Sciences* 1972; 69;10:2879-2884; adrenal corticosteroids and related steroid hormones including dexamethasone, prednisolone, fludrocortisone, hydrocortisone, corticosterone, cortisone, testosterone, progesterone, and insulin—see Paran M, Gallo RC, Richardson LS and Wu AM. Adrenal Corticosteroids Enhance Production of Type-C Virus Induced by 5-Iodo-2'-Deoxyuridine from Cultured Mouse Fibroblasts. *Proceedings of the National Academy of Sciences* 1973;70;8:2391-2395.

Chapter 6. Gallo's Research Anthology: The AIDS Buck and Virus Starts and Stops Here.

1. Germain RN. Antigen processing and CD4⁺ T cell depletion in AIDS. *Cell* 1988; 54:441-414.
2. Herrera F, Adamson RH and Gallo RC. Uptake of transfer ribonucleic acid by normal and leukemic cells. *Proc Nat Acad Sci* 1970;67;4:1943-1950. This paper was presented before the "International Symposium on Uptake of Informative Molecules by Living Cells, Mol, Belgium, 1970," the year in which $10 million in funds were appropriated by the Department of Defense for the development of AIDS-like viruses.
3. Gallo RC, Perry S and Breitman RT. The enzymatic mechanisms for deoxythymidine synthesis in human leukocytes. *Journal of Biological Chemistry* 1967;242;21:5059-5068.

4. Gallo RC and Perry S. Enzymatic abnormality in human leukaemia. *Nature* 1968;218:465-466.

5. Gallo RC and Breitman TR. The enzymatic mechanisms for deoxythymidine synthesis in human leukocytes: Inhibition of deoxythymidine phosphorylase by purines. *Journal of Biological Chemistry* 1968;243;19:4943-4951.

6. Gallo RC, Yang SS and Ting RC. RNA dependent DNA Polymerase of human acute leukaemic cells. *Nature* 1970;228:927-929.

7. Gallo RC and Longmore JL. Asparaginyl-tRNA and resistance of murine leukaemias to L-asparaginase. *Nature* 1970;227:1134-1136.

8. *Department of Defense Appropriations For 1970: Hearings Before A Subcommittee of the Committee on Appropriations House of Representatives, Ninety-first Contress, First Session, H.B. 15090, Part 5, Research, Development, Test and Evaluation, Dept. of the Army.* U.S. Government Printing Office, Washington, D.C., 1969.

9. Gallaher RE, Ting RC and Gallo RC. A common change aspartyl-tRNA in polyoma and SV transformed cells. *Biochimica Et Biophysica Acta* 1972;272:568-582.

10. Gallo RC, Sarin PS, Allen PT, Newton WA Priori ES, Bowen JM and Dmochowski L. Reverse transcriptase in type C virus particles of human origin. *Nature New Biology* 1971;232:140-142; see also Gallo RC. Transfer RNA and transfer RNA methylation in growing and "resting" adult and embryonic tissues and in various oncogenic systems. *Cancer Research* 1971;31:621-29.

11. Fujioka S and Gallo RC. Aminoacyl transfer RNA profiles in human myeloma cells. *Blood* 1971;38;2:246-252.

12. Smith RG and Gallo RC. DNA-dependent DNA polymerases I and II from normal human-blood lymphocytes. *Proceedings of the National Academy of Sciences* 1972;69;10:2879-2884.

13. Bobrow SN, Smith RG, Reitz MS and Gallo RC. Stimulated normal human lymphocytes contain a ribonuclease-sensitive DNA polymerase distinct from viral RNA-directed DNA polymerase. *Proceedings National Academy of Sciences* 1972;69;11:3228-3232.

14. Robert MS, Smith RG, Gallo RC, Sarin PS and Abrell JW. Viral and cellular DNA polymerase: Comparison of activities with synthetic and natural RNA templates. *Science* 1972;176:798-800.

15. Gallo RC, Abrell JW, Robert MS, Yang SS and Smith RG. Reverse transcriptase from Mason-Pfizer monkey tumor virus, avian myeloblastosis virus, and Rauscher leukemia virus and its response to rifamycin derivatives. *Journal of the National Cancer Institute* 1972;48;4:1185-1189.

16. NCI staff. *The Special Virus Cancer Program: Progress Report #8.* Office of the Associate Scientific Director for Viral Oncology (OASDVO). J. B. Moloney, Ed., Washington, DC.: U.S. Government Printing Office, 1971, p. 22.

17. Wu AM, Ting RC, Paran M and Gallo RC. Cordycepin inhibits induction of murine leukovirus production by 5-iodo-2'-deoxyuridine. *Proceedings of the National Academy of Sciences* 1972;69;12:3820-3824.

18. Gillespie D, Gillespie S, Gallo RC, East J and Dmochowski L. Genetic origin of RD114 and other RNA tumor viruses assayed by molecular hybridization. *Nature New Biology* 1973;224:52-54.

19. Gallo RC, Miller NR, Saxinger WC and Gillespie D. Primate RNA Tumor Virus-Like DNA Synthesized Endogenously by RNA-Dependent DNA Polymerase in Virus-like Particles from Fresh Human Acute Leukemic Blood Cells. *Proceedings National Academy of Sciences* 1973;70;11:3219-3224.

20. *Department of Defense Appropriations For 1970: Hearings Before A Subcommittee of the Committee on Appropriations House of Representatives, Ninety-first Contress, First Session, H.B. 15090, Part 5, Research, Development, Test and Evaluation, Dept. of the Army.* U.S. Government Printing Office, Washington, D.C., 1969, p. 689.

21. *Committee on Human Resources, United States Senate. Hearings before the Subcommittee on Health and Scientific Research, Biological Testing Involving Human Subjects by the Department of Defense, 1977: Examination of Serious Deficiencies in the Defense Departments Efforts to Protect the Human Subjects of Drug Research.* Washington, D.C.: U.S. Government Printing Office, May 8 and May 23, 1977, pp. 80-100.

Chapter 7. Interview with Robert Strecker

1. According to The Strecker Group, Dr. Strecker's brother, Ted Strecker, was found shot to death alone in his home in Springfield, Missouri, an apparent suicide, on August 11, 1988. In the past he suffered from depression and monumental frustration at the relative lack of interest in his findings. Ted had been working with Robert to uncover evidence linking the DOD to the development of HIV. Ted is

credited, along with Black military officer, Zears Miles, for having discovered and distributed fig. 1.1. However, Robert spoke with Ted the night before his death. He seemed cheerful—"in good spirits,"—looking forward to new developments that promised progress. The following day he was found dead. His 22-caliber rifle lay next to him. He left no note, no message, and he said no goodbyes. This was very untypical of him. Officially the death was ruled a suicide.

"Next," according to The Strecker Group, "Illinois State Representative Douglas Huff of Chicago was found alone in his home, dead from an apparent overdose of cocaine and heroin, on September 22, 1988. Representative Huff did everything in his power to make the Illinois State Legislature and the people of Chicago aware of Dr. Strecker's work. He was very vocal, gave many press interviews, was constantly on television and radio urging people to wake up to the coverup concerning AIDS. Did Representative Huff use drugs? Perhaps yes, but only occasionally and recreationally. Was he an addict? No. Would he have known how dangerous a massive overdose of cocaine and heroin was? Yes of course. Cause of death: officially a stroke. Dr. Strecker has serious doubts. . . ."

2. Strecker's comment came months prior to the first confirmed case of HIV transmission from a human bite. See: Singer G and Athans M. 91-year-old teaches world about AIDS: HIV contracted from prostitute's bite. *Sun-Sentinel* Saturday October 28, 1995 pp1A and 6A.

3. Several reports confirmed that The Wistar Institute is located at 36th and Spruce Sts. Philadelphia, PA 19104 (215-222-6700). See: *Science and Technology Division National Referral Center. Biological Sciences: A Director of Information Resources in the United States.* Washington, D. C.: Library of Congress, 1972, p. 493.

4. New Bolton Center is apparently now part of the University of Pennsylvania. One reference which appeared during my Medline search was: Bowman KF, Tate LP Jr., Evans LH and Donawick WJ. Complications of cleft palate repair in large animals. *Journal of the American Veterinary Medical Association* 1982;180;6:652-7.

5. Gonda MA, Braun MJ, Carter SG, Kost TA, Bess JW, Arthur LO and Van Der Maaten MJ. Characterization and molecular cloning of a bovine lentivirus related to human immunodeficiency virus. *Nature* 1987;330:388-391. This research group, which reported stark similarities between the bovine immunodeficiency-like virus (BIV) and HIV, interestingly enough was funded by the National Cancer Institute and based at the Frederick (Fort Detrick) Cancer Research Facility in Maryland.

6. *Stedman's Medical Dictionary*, Twenty-Second Edition. Baltimore Maryland: Williams & Wilkins Co., p. 1233.

7. Temin HM. The role of the DNA provirus in carcinogenesis by RNA tumor viruses. In: *The Biology of Oncogenic Viruses*, LG Silverster, Ed. New York: Elsevier, 1971, 176; Temin HM. The protovirus hypothesis. *J. National Cancer Institute* 1971;46:3. Also see: Temin HM. The participation of DNA in Rous sarcoma virus production. *Virology* 1964; 23:486; Temin HM and Mizutani S. *Nature* 1970; 226:1211.

8. Baltimore D. Viral RNA-dependent DNA polymerase. *Nature* 1970;226:1209.

9. Maruyama K and Dmochowski L. Cross-species transmission of mammalian RNA tumor viruses. *Texas Medicine* 1973;69:65-75. Regarding Hilary Koprowski serving at The Wistar Institute in Philadelphia, see: Silversti LG. *The Biology of Oncogenic Viruses.* New York: American Elsevier Publishing Company, Inc., 1971, p. 332; Huebner RJ, Todaro GJ, Sarma P, Hartley JW, Freeman AE, Peters RL, Whitmire CE, Meier H and Gilden RV. Switched Off" Vertically Transmitted C-type RNA Tumor Viruses as Determinants of Spontaneous and Induced Cancer: A New Hypothesis of Viral Carcinogenesis. In: *Defectiveness, Rescue and Stimulation of Oncogenic Viruses: Second International Symposium on Tumor Viruses*, Royaumont, France June 3-5, 1969. Paris: Centre National De La Recherche Scientifique, 1970, pp. 33-77; Montagnier L. Alterations de la surface des cellules BHK21 en rapport avec leur transformation par des virus ongogenes. *Ibid.*, p. 6; For more on ethnic cancer studies see: MacMahon B. The ethnic distribution of cancer mortality in New York City, 1955. *Acta Unio Internat. contra cancrum*, 1960 16;1716; Newill VA. Distribution of cancer mortality among ethnic subgroups of the white population of New York City, 1953-58. *J. National Cancer Institute* 1961 26:405.

10. Miller JM, Miller LD, Olsen C and Gillette KG. Virus-like particles in phytohemagglutinin-stimulated lymphocyte cultures with references to bovine lymphosarcoma. *Journal National Cancer Institute* 1969;43:1297-1305. See also: Miller JM and Van Der Maaten MJ. The biology of bovine leukemia virus infection in cattle. In: *Viruses in Naturally Occurring Cancers: Book B.* Essex M, Todaro G, and zur Hausen H, Eds. Cold Spring Harbor Conferences on Cell Proliferation, Vol. 7, New York: Cold Spring Harbor Laboratory, 1980, pp.901-909.

11. Burny A, Bex F, Chantrenne J, Cleuter Y, Dekegel D, Ghysdael J, Kettmann R, Leclercq M, Leunen J, Mammerickx M and Portetelle D. Bovine leukemia virus involvement in enzootic bovine leucosis [lymphosarcoma in cattle]. *Adv. Cancer Res.* 1978;28:251; See also: Burny A, Bruck G, Cleuter y et al. Bovine leukemia virus, a distinguished member of the human T-lymphotropic virus family. *Soc. Press.* Tokyo: VNU Science Press, Utrecht, pp. 219-227, 1983

12. Bobrow SN, Smith RG, Reitz MS and Gallo RC. Stimulated normal human lymphocytes contain a ribonuclease-sensitive DNA polymerase distinct from viral RNA-directed DNA polymerase. *Proc. Nat. Acad. Sci.* 1972;69;11:3228-3232; Gallo RC, Pestka S, Smith RG, Herrera, Ting RC, Bobrow SN, Davis C and Fujioka S. RNA-and DNA-dependent DNA polymerases of human normal and leukemic cells. *In* Silvestri, L. (Ed.): II. *Lepetit Colloquia on Biology and Medicine* "The Biology of Oncogenic Viruses." Amsterdam, North-Holland, 1971, p. 210.

13. Mussgay M, Dietzschold B, Lorenz R, Matheka HD, Matthaeus W, Straub OC, Weiland F, Wilesmith JW, Frenzel B and Kaaden O. Some properties of bovine leukemia virus, its use in seroepidemiological studies, and eradication of the disease from infected herds. In: *Viruses in Naturally Occurring Cancers: Book B.* M. Essex, G. Todaro and H zur Hausen, Eds. New York: Cold Spring Harbor Laboratory, 1980, pp. 911-925; Flensburg JC. Attempt to eradicate leukosis from a dairy herd by slaughter of cattle with lymphocytosis. Report over a ten-year period. *Vet. Microbiol.* 1976 1:301; Callahan R, Lieber MM, Todaro GJ, Graves DC and Ferrer FJ. Bovine leukemia virus genes in the DNA of leukemic cattle. 1976 *Science* 192:1005; Crespeau S, Sarsat FP, Vuillaume A, Levy D and Parodi AL. A two-year sero-epidemiological survey of bovine leukemia virus (BLV) infection in a high-incidence area of the southwest of France. *Ann. Rech. Vet.* 1978 9:747; Haase A. The slow infection caused by visna virus. *Curr. Top. Microbiol. Immunol.* 1975 72:101.; Narayan O, Griffin DE and Clements JE. Virus mutation during "slow infection"—Temporal development and characterization of mutants of visna virus recovered from sheep. *J. Gen. Virol.* 1978 41:343.

14. Though I was unable to locate the Montagnier publication re: placing EBV into infected T-cell culture to keep them alive, I did locate several articles published in the early 1970s that noted the presence EBV caused lymphocytes to proliferate. Several papers were presented during conferences attended by both Montagnier and Gallo that emphasized the role of EBV in molecular biology and tumor virology. Gallo wrote about the work of Pagano and the role of EBV in human cancer in his 1977 book, referred to EBV as a model oncogenic virus: "The evidence with EBV, although not definitive, has been extended from Burkitt's lymphoma to nasopharyngeal carcinomas." So he was certainly well aware of the ability of EBV to prompt lymphocytic proliferation. See: Gallo R. *Recent Advances in Cancer Research: Cell Biology, Molecular Biology, and Tumor Virology, Volume I.* Cleveland: CRC Press, Inc., 1977; In 1971 EBV was also studied by Gallo and co-workers. See Fujioka S and Gallo RC. Aminoacyl Transfer RNA Profiles in Human Myeloma Cells. *Blood* 1971; 38;2:246-252.

15. I was unable to find direct evidence that Montagnier had worked side-by-side with Gallo at the NCI. However, I located ample evidence that the two traveled in some of the same scientific circles, and attended many of the same cancer virus conferences. It is clear they were aware of each others' research from the late 1960s. Also, Montagnier published a report that suggested lings between LAV/HTLV-III and the bovine leukemia virus. See: Alizon M and Montagnier L. Relationship of AIDS to other retroviruses. *Nature* 1985;313:743.

16. Strecker's comments about the "famous cat house experiments," wherein Don Francis and Robert Gallo allegedly knew it was possible for mutant forms of feline leukemia virus (FeLV) to jump species to humans, are supported by parallel presentations made by the researchers during the same Cold Spring Harbor conference in 1980 See: Gutensohn N, Essex M, Francis DP and Hardy, Jr. WD. Risk to humans from exposure to feline leukemia virus: Epidemiological considerations; and Wong-Staal F, Koshy R and Gallo RC. Feline leukemia virus genomes associated with the domestic cat: A survey of normal and leukemic animals. In: *Viruses in Naturally Occurring Cancers: Book A.* Essex M, Todaro G, and zur Hausen H, Eds. Cold Spring Harbor Conferences on Cell Proliferation, Vol. 7, New York: Cold Spring Harbor Laboratory, 1980, pp. 699-706; 623-634.

17. World Health Organization Report. Five years of research on virus diseases. *WHO Chronicle* 1969 23;12:564-572; World Health Organization Report. Recent work on virus diseases. *WHO Chronicle* 1974;28:410-413; Kalter SS and Heberling RL. The study of simian viruses—work of the WHO collaborating laboratory on comparative medicine: Simian viruses. *WHO Chronicle* 1969;23;3:112-117.

18. Strecker was also accurate in reporting that Salk and colleagues at The Salk Institute had been researching RNA and DNA retroviruses including the simian monkey virus (SV40) with financial

support from the NCI and the West German Max-Planck Society. Thus, Salk quite plausibly participated, as Strecker alleged, in writing up the history of AIDS virus research, and in making "up a story." See: Tonegawa S, Walter G and Dulbecco R. Transcription of SV40 genome transformed and lytically infected cells; Eckhart W. Induction of cellular DNA synthesis after infection by polyoma virus: viral gene expression in the presence of hydroxyurea. (Both research teams from The Salk Institute) In: *The Biology of Oncogenic Viruses. Proceedings of the second Lepetit Colloquium, Paris France, November 1970.* LG Silvestri, Ed. New York: Elsevier, 1971, pp. 65-75;290-294.

19. Beardsley T. AIDS: Pasteur sues over patent. *Nature* 1985;318:595; Palca J. AIDS: US wins round in patent row. *Nature* 1986;322:200; Palca J. Franco—US agreement on AIDS test within sight: AIDS patent dispute near end? France and United States call truce. *Nature* 1987;326:115; See also: Staff writer. Settling the AIDS virus dispute. *Nature* 1987;326:425-426; Anderson C and Butler PD. US rejects French request to reopen AIDS patent deal. *Nature* 1987;326:425-426; Rensberger B. AIDS scientist Gallo, rival meet to discuss cooperation. *The Washington Post*, Saturday January 9, 1993, p. A2; Anderson C. Scientific misconduct: Popovic is cleared on all charges; Gallo case in doubt. *Science* 1993;262:981-983; Culliton BJ. Misconduct charges against Gallo withdrawn after Popovic decision. *Nature* 1993;366:191; Brown D and Schwartz J. Case against AIDS scientist dropped: Agency decides evidence insufficient to sustain Gallo charges. *The Washington Post* Saturday, November 13, 1993, pp A1;16; Greenberg DS. End of the Gallo case—maybe. *The Lancet* 1993;342:1289; Staff writer. What to do about scientific misconduct. *Nature* 194;369:261-262.

20. Gutensohn N, Essex M, Francis DP and Hardy, Jr. WD. Risk to humans from exposure to feline leukemia virus: Epidemiological considerations; and Wong-Staal F, Koshy R and Gallo RC. Feline leukemia virus genomes associated with the domestic cat: A survey of normal and leukemic animals. In: *Vruses in Naturally Occurring Cancers: Book A.* Essex M, Todaro G, and zur Hausen H, Eds. Cold Spring Harbor Conferences on Cell Proliferation, Vol. 7, New York: Cold Spring Harbor Laboratory, 1980, pp.699-706; 623-634.

21. Gold M. *Conspiracy of Cells* Albany, NY: State University of New York Press, 1986.

22. Szmuness W, Stevens CE, Harley EJ, Zang EA and Oleszko WR et al. Hepatitis B vaccine: Demonstration of efficacy in a controlled clinical trial in a high-risk population in the United States. *New England Journal of Medicine* 1980;303;15:833-841.

Regarding Szmuness, I later learned from AIDS researcher and physician Alan Cantwell, Jr. that Wolf Szmuness became a professor of epidemiology at Columbia University School of Public Health, and chief of epidemiology at the New York City Blood Center in Manhattan shortly after his arrival in the United States. According to Cantwell, who credits *Magic Shots* (1982) by Allan Chase, Szmuness was born in 1919 in Poland, and came to the United States in 1968 after being expelled from Poland "by the communist government in an anti-semitic purge." With no other history, it is interesting that Szmuness, so quickly, in 1969, became the chief epidemiologist at the New York City Blood Center. For more information see: Cantwell A. *AIDS and the Doctors of Death: An Inquiry into the Origin of the AIDS Epidemic.* Los Angeles: Aries Rising Press, 1988.

23. An *epitope* is a molecular region on the surface of an invading microorganism or infectious agent capable of eliciting an immune response and of combining with the specific antibody produced by such a response. It is also called a "determinant," or "antigenic determinant."

24. Gardner WU. International union against cancer: Brief history, organization, and program review of a nongovernmental voluntary organization. *National Cancer Institute Monograph* 1974 40:51-55; Higginson J and Muir CS. Epidemiologic program of the International Agency for Research on Cancer. *National Cancer Institute Monograph* 1974 40:63-70.

25. Koch's postulates were advanced as a scientific method to determine the cause and effect relationship between a germ and the disease it is believed to cause. It is based on three tests: 1) the microbe must be invariably found among organisms demonstrating the disease; 2) the microbe must not be present in disease-free organisms; and 3) the microorganisms must be effective in causing similar diseases among laboratory animals infected with the germ.

26. Strecker R. This is a bio-attack alert. The Strecker Group, 1501 Colorado Boulevard, Los Angeles, CA 90041. March 28, 1986, pp. 24-26.

27. Rowe DS. The WHO immunology laboratories at Lausanne. *WHO Chronicle* 1968;22;11:496.

28. WHO Report (Based on the 1969 report The medical research programme of the World health Organization, 1964-1968, Geneva.) Five years of research of virus diseases. *WHO Chronicle* 1969;23;12:564-572.

29. Kalter SS and Heberling. The study of simian viruses. *WHO Chronicle* 1969;23;3:112-117.

30. Three HIV genes—*gag*, *pol* and *env*—code for the structural parts of the AIDS virus envelope, or for the enzymes needed for gene transcription and insertion. According to authorities (Haseltine WA, Wong-Staal F. The molecular biology of the AIDS virus. *Scientific American* 1988;52-62; and Kieny MP. Structure and regulation of the human AIDS virus. *J AIDS* 1990;3:395-402), the *gag*, or group specific antigen, gene codes for the p24 proteins which form an "inner shell" within the virus. The *pol* gene codes for the reverse transcriptase enzyme which transcribes viral RNA to form a proviral form of DNA. The *pol* gene also codes for the endonuclease enzyme which transports the provirus into the host cell's nucleus and then deposits it into the host chromosome. The *env* gene codes for the "transmembrane protein" gp41 (glycosylated protein 41), which is incorporated into the envelope along with a closely associated gp120 protein which itself may have cell and nerve killing effects. The *tat* gene codes for a protein that enhances viral replication.

31. Moscow World Service in English. Belitskiy on How, Where AIDS Virus Originated. March 11, 1988. Published in *International Affairs*. FBIS-SOV-88-049, March 14, 1988, p. 24. Text discusses Seale's allegations, but does not furnish specifics.

32. Allison AC, Beveridge WIB, Cockburn WC, et al. Virus-associated immunopathology: Animal models and implications for human disease. *Bulletin WHO* 1972;47:257-263.

33. *Havana International Service in Spanish*. German Claims AIDS Virus Created by Pentagon. FBIS-LAT 91-017. January 25, 1991. Caribbean, Cuba. Text discusses Dr. Jacobo Segal's allegations. Document PA 2401213091-0000 GMT 24, January 1991.

34. Covert NM. *Cutting Edge: A history of Fort Detrick, Maryland 1943-1993*. Fort Detrick, MD: Headquarters, U. S. Army Garrison, Public Affairs Office, 1993. [For copies call 301-619-2018].

35. *Havana International Service in Spanish*. Commentary Accuses U.S. of Developing AIDS Virus. LAT 24, June 1987. Caribbean, Cuba "Viewpoint" commentary read by Angel Hernandez. Document PA 200342- 000GMT 19, June 1987. pp. A5-6.

Chapter 8. HIV-1, 2 and the "Big Bang"

1. Gonda MA, Braun MJ, Carter SG, Kost TA, Bess JW, Arthur LO and Van Der Maaten MJ. Characterization and molecular cloning of a bovine lentivirus related to human immunodeficiency virus. *Nature* 1987;330:388-391.

2. Maruyama K and Dmochowski L. Cross-species transmission of mammalian RNA tumor viruses. *Texas Medicine* 1973;69:65-75. Regarding Hilary Koprowski serving at The Wistar Institute in Philadelphia, see: Silversti LG. *The Biology of Oncogenic Viruses*. New York: American Elsevier Publishing Company, Inc., 1971, p. 332; Huebner RJ, Todaro GJ, Sarma P, Hartley JW, Freeman AE, Peters RL, Whitmire CE, Meier H and Gilden RV. Switched Off" Vertically Transmitted C-type RNA Tumor Viruses as Determinants of Spontaneous and Induced Cancer: A New Hypothesis of Viral Carcinogenesis. In: *Defectiveness, Rescue and Stimulation of Oncogenic Viruses: Second International Symposium on Tumor Viruses*, Royaumont, France June 3-5, 1969. Paris: Centre National De La Recherche Scientifique, 1970, pp. 33-77; Miller JM, Miller LD, Olsen C and Gillette KG. Virus-like particles in phytohemagglutinin-stimulated lymphocyte cultures with references to bovine lymphosarcoma. *Journal National Cancer Institute* 1969;43:1297-1305; Burny A, Bex F, Chantrenne J, Cleuter Y, Dekegel D, Ghysdael J, Kettmann R, Leclercq M, Leunen J, Mammerickx M and Portetelle D. Bovine leukemia virus involvement in enzootic bovine leucosis [lymphosarcoma in cattle]. *Adv. Cancer Res.* 1978;28:251; See also: Burny A, Bruck G, Cleuter y et al. Bovine leukemia virus, a distinguished member of the human T-lymphotropic virus family. *Soc. Press.* Tokyo: VNU Science Press, Utrecht, pp. 219-227, 1983.

3. McClure MA, Johnson MS, Feng DF and Doolittle RF. Sequence comparisons of retroviral proteins: Relative rates of change and general phylogeny. *Proceedings of the National Academy of Sciences* 1988;85:2469-73.

4. Devare SG. Bovine leukemia virus: an etiologic agent associated with lymphosarcoma of domestic cattle. In: *Viruses in Naturally Occurring Cancers: Book B*. Essex M, Todaro G, and zur Hausen H, Eds. Cold Spring Harbor Conferences on Cell Proliferation, Vol. 7, New York: Cold Spring Harbor Laboratory, 1980, pp. 943-952.

5. Gallo RC, Miller NR, Saxinger WC and Gillespie D. Primate RNA Tumor Virus-Like DNA Synthesized Endogenously by RNA-Dependent DN A Polymerase in Virus-like Particles from Fresh

Human Acute Leukemic Blood Cells. *Proceedings National Academy of Sciences* 1973;70;11:3219-3224.

6. Chopra H. Ebert P, Woodside N, Kvedar J, Albert S and Brennan M. Electron microscopic detection of simian-type virus particles in human milk. *Nature New Biology* 1973;243:159-160.

7.Gillespie D, Gillespie S, Gallo RC, East J and Dmochowski L. Genetic origin of RD114 and other RNA tumor viruses assayed by molecular hybridization. *Nature New Biology* 1973;224:52-54.

8. Gallo RC, Miller NR, Saxinger WC and Gillespie D. Primate RNA Tumor Virus-Like DNA Synthesized Endogenously by RNA-Dependent DN A Polymerase in Virus-like Particles from Fresh Human Acute Leukemic Blood Cells. *Proceedings National Academy of Sciences* 1973;70;11:3219-3224.

9. For documentation of Hilary Koprowski serving at The Wistar Institute in Philadelphia, see: Silversti LG. *The Biology of Oncogenic Viruses*. New York: American Elsevier Publishing Company, Inc., 1971, p. 332.

10. Montagnier L. Alterations de la surface des cellules BHK21 en rapport avec leur transformation par des virus ongogenes. In: *Defectiveness, Rescue and Stimulation of Oncogenic Viruses: Second International Symposium on Tumor Viruses*, Royaumont, France June 3-5, 1969. Paris: Centre National De La Recherche Scientifique, 1970, p. 6.

11. Huebner RJ, Todaro GJ, Sarma P, Hartley JW, Freeman AE, Peters RL, Whitmire CE, Meier H and Gilden RV. Switched Off" Vertically Transmitted C-type RNA Tumor Viruses as Determinants of Spontaneous and Induced Cancer: A New Hypothesis of Viral Carcinogenesis. In: *Defectiveness, Rescue and Stimulation of Oncogenic Viruses: Second International Symposium on Tumor Viruses*, Royaumont, France June 3-5, 1969. Paris: Centre National De La Recherche Scientifique, 1970, pp. 33-77

12. For more on ethnic cancer studies see: MacMahon B. The ethnic distribution of cancer mortality in New York City, 1955. *Acta Unio Internat. contra cancrum*, 1960 16;1716; Newill VA. Distribution of cancer mortality among ethnic subgroups of the white population of New York City, 1953-58. *J. National Cancer Institute* 1961 26:405.

It was also interesting to learn that the Public Health Research Institute of the City of New York, Inc.—a for-profit organization—promoted its "areas of interest" as "Virology, viral oncology; molecular biophysics; genetics; microbiology; and biochemistry." See: *Science and Technology Division National Referral Center. Biological Sciences: A Director of Information Resources in the United States*. Washington, D. C.: Library of Congress, 1972, p. 342.

13. Gardner WU. International union against cancer: Brief history, organization, and program reviwe of a nongovernmental voluntary organization. *National Cancer Institute Monograph* 1974 40:51-55.

14. Higginson J and Muir CS. Epidemiologic program of the International Agency for Research on Cancer. *National Cancer Institute Monograph* 1974 40:63-70.

15. Hilleman MR. Prospects for vaccines against cancer. In: *Viruses, Evolution and Cancer—Basic Considerations*. E. Kurstak and K. Maramorosch Eds. New York: Academic Press, 1974, pp. 549-560.

16. This expert comment raises the question as to whether genetic predisposition for at least some human cancers existed in nature prior to extensive viral experimentation beginning in the 1950s, as these experiments may have significantly altered gene pools and oncogenic susceptibility.

17. From: *American Men & Women of Science, 1995-96 • 19th Edition: A Biographical Directory of Today's Leaders in Physical, Biological and Related Sciences*, Volume 2, C-F. New Providence, NJ: R. R. Bowker, p. 1417.

18. Preston R. *The Hot Zone; A Terrifying True Story*. New York: Random House, 1994.

19. Gutensohn N, Essex M, Francis DP and Hardy, Jr. WD. Risk to humans from exposure to feline leukemia virus: Epidemiological considerations. In: *Vruses in Naturally Occurring Cancers: Book A*. Essex M, Todaro GJ, and zur Hausen H, Eds. Cold Spring Harbor Conferences on Cell Proliferation, Vol. 7, New York: Cold Spring Harbor Laboratory, 1980, pp.699-706; 623-634; Francis DP, Essex M and Hardy, Jr. WD. Excretion of feline leukaemia virus by naturally infected pet cats. *Nature* 269:252; Essex M and Francis DP. The risk to humans from malignant disease of their pets: An unsettled issue. *J. Am. Anim. Hosp. Assoc.* 1976 12:386.

20. Shilts R. *And the Band Played On: Politics, People, and the AIDS Epidemic*. New York: Penguin Books, 1987, p. 107;128-129.

21. Gallaher RE, Ting RC and Gallo RC. A common change aspartyl-tRNA in polyoma and SV transformed cells. *Biochimica Et Biophysica Acta* 1972;272:568-582.

22. Cold Spring Harbor Laboratory. *Viruses in Naturally Occurring Cancers: Book A. Cold Spring Harbor Conferences on Cell Proliferation Volume 7*, M. Essex, G. Todaro and H. zur Hausen Eds. New York: CHS Publications, 1980, pp. 589-708.

23. Shilts R. *Op. cit..*, p. 118.

24. Shilts R. *Ibid.*, p. 128.

25. Horowitz LG. *Deadly Innocence: Solving the Greatest Murder Mystery in the History of American Medicine*. Rockport, MA: Tetrahedron, Inc., 1994, p. 11.

26. Goldman BA and Chappelle M. Is HIV=AIDS wrong? *In These Times*. August 5-August 18, 1992. pp. 8-10; also see Duesberg's original arguments in: Duesberg P. HIV is not the cause of AIDS. *Science* 1988;241:514-515. Gallo's response to Duesberg's theory were also published during this policy forum. See: Blattner W, Gallo RC, and Temin HM. HIV causes AIDS. *Science* 1988;241:515-517.

27. Duesberg's study was revealed in: NCI staff. *The Special Virus Cancer Program: Progress Report #9* Office of the Associate Scientific Director for Viral Oncology (OASDVO). J. B. Moloney, Ed., Washington, D. C.: U. S. Government Printing Office, 1972, p. 233. Earlier studies at the University of California on sarcoma and leukemia viruses in cows and monkeys beginning in 1969 were revealed in: NCI staff. *The Special Virus Cancer Program: Progress Report #8*. Office of the Associate Scientific Director for Viral Oncology (OASDVO). J. B. Moloney, Ed., Washington, D. C.: U. S. Government Printing Office, 1971, pp. 257-258. Note: These reports are very hard to find. Few libraries hold them, including the NCI Library at Fort Detrick. It was available through Davies Library, The University of North Carolina, Chapel Hill, Government Documents Department Depository, Reference # HE 20.3152:V81.

28. Duesberg PH, Vogt PK and Canaani E. Structure and replication of avian tumor virus RNA. In: *The Biology of Oncogenic Viruses: Proceedings of the second Lepetit Colloquium*, Paris, November 1970. L. G. Silvestri, Ed., New York: Elsevier, 1971, pp. 154-166.

29. Duesberg PH and Robinson WS. Inhibition of mouse leukemia virus (MLV) replication by actinomycin D. *Virology* 1967 31:742-746.

30. Duesberg P, Beemon K, Lai M and Vogt PK. Recombinants of avian RNA tumor viruses: Characteristics of the virion RNA. In: *Viral Transformation and Endogenous Viruses*. A. S. Kaplan, Ed., New York: Academic Press, 1974, pp. 137-153.

31. Neth R, Gallo RC, Spiegelman S and Stohlman Jr. F. *Modern Trends in Human Leukemia: Biological, Biochemical and Virological Aspects*. New York: Grune & Stratton, Inc., 1974, pp. 348-349.

32. Wu AM and Gallo RC. Life cycle of RNA oncogenic viruses. *Ibid.*, p. 148; See also Wu A, Prival J, Paran M and Gallo RC. Hemopoietic stem cells and leukemia. *Ibid.*, p. 60.

33. Duesberg P. HIV is not the cause of AIDS. *Science* 1988;241:514-517; see also Blattner W, Gallo RC and Temin HM. HIV causes AIDS. *Science* 1988;241:515; see also: Duesberg P and Yiamouyiannis J. *AIDS*. Delaware, Ohio: Health Action Press, 1995; for discussion on virus/host protein complex interactions leading to autoimmune diseases see: World Health Organization. Memoranda: Virus-associated immunopathology: Animal models and implications for human disease—Effects of viruses on the immune system, immune-complex diseases, and antibody-mediated immunologic injury. *Bulletin of the WHO* 1972;47:2:257-263.

34. Corbitt G, Bailey AS and Williams G. HIV infection in Manchester, 1959. *The Lancet* 1990;336:51.

35. Zhu T and Ho D. Was HIV present in 1959? *Nature* 1995;374:503-504.

36. Garrett L. *The Coming Plague: Newly Emerging Diseases in a World Out of Balance*. New York: Penguin Books, 1994, p. 380.

37. Corbitt G and Bailey AS. AIDS in Manchester, 1959? *The Lancet* 1995;345:1058.

38. Nahmias AJ, Weiss J, Yao X, Lee F, Kodsi R, Schanfield M, Matthews T, Bologniesi D, Durack D, Motulsky A, Kanki P and Essex M. Evidence for human infection with an HTLV III/LAV-like virus in Central Africa, 1959. *The Lancet* May 31, 1986:1279-80.

39. Garrett, *Op. cit.*, pp. 371-81.

40. Saxinger WC, Levine PH, Deane AG, deThe, G, Lange-Wantzin, G, Moghissi, J, Mei Hoh, FL, Sarngadharan MH. and Gallo RC. Evidence for Exposure to HTLV-III in Uganda Before 1973. *Science* 1995;227:1036-1038.

41. Lyons SF, Schoub BD, McGillivray GM, Sher R, and Dos Santos, L. Lack of evidence of HTLV-III endemic in southern Africa. *New England Journal of Medicine* 1995;312:1257-1258.

42. Carswell JW, Sewankambo N, Lloyd G, and Downing RG., How long has the AIDS virus been in Uganda? *The Lancet* (May 24)1986;849:1217;

43. Levy J, Pan LZ, Beth-Giraldo E, Kaminsky LS, Henle G, Henle W, and Giraldo G. Absence of antibodies to the human immunodeficiency virus in sera from Africa prior to 1975. *Proc. Natl. Acad. Sci.* 1986;83:7935-7937;

44. Kuhls TL, Nishanian PG, Cherry JD, Shen JP, Neumann CG, Stiehm ER, Ettenger RB, Bwibo NO, and Koech D. Analysis of false positive HIV-1 serologic testing in Kenya. *Diagn. Microbiol. Infect. Dis.* 1988;9:179-185.

45. Szmuness W, Stevens CE, Harley EJ, Zang EA and Oleszko WR et al. Hepatitis B vaccine: Demonstration of efficacy in a controlled clinical trial in a high-risk population in the United States. *New England Journal of Medicine* 1980;303;15:833-841;

46. Shilts R. *And the Band Played On: Politics, People and the AIDS Epidemic.* New York: Penguin Books, 1987, p. 539.

47. Cantwell A. *Queer Blood: The secret AIDS genocide plot.* Los Angeles: Aries Rising Press, 1993, p. 27.

48. Krugman S, Overby LR, Mushahwar IK, Ling C-M, Forsner GG and Deinhardt F. Viral hepatitis, type B: Studies on natural history and prevention reexamined. *New England Journal of Medicine* 1979;200:101-6.

49. Witte MH, Witte CL, Minnich LL, et al., AIDS in 1968. *Journal of the American Medical Association* 1984;251:2657.

50. Garry RF, Witte MH, Gottlieb A, et al, Documentation of an AIDS Virus Infection in the United States in 1968. *Journal of the American Medical Association* 1988;260:2085-87.

51. Kyle WS. Simian retroviruses, poliovaccine, and origin of AIDS. *The Lancet* 1992;339:600-601.

52. Essex M, Kanki P. The origins of the AIDS virus. *Scientific American* 1988;259:64-71.

53. Stricker RB and Elswood BF. Origin of AIDS (letter to the editor). *The Lancet* 1992;339:867.

54. Schulz TF. Origin of AIDS (letter to the editor). *The Lancet* 1992;339:867.

55. Personal communication from Walter Kyle, May 19, 1996. Walter Kyle may be reached at his office at Sixty South Street, Hingham, MA 02043, telephone: 617-741-5953, fax: 617-741-5166.

56. Drew L, Lichtenstein, Issel CJ and Montelaro RC. Genomic quasispecies associated with the initiation of infection and disease in ponies experimentally infected with equine infectious anemia virus. *Journal of Virology* 1996;70;6:3346-3354.

57. Shaheen F, Duan L, Zhu M, Bagasra O and Pomerantz RJ. Targeting human immunodeficiency virus type 1 reverse transcriptase by intracellular expression of single-chain variable fragments to inhibit early stages of the viral life cycle *Journal of Virology* 1996;70;6:3392-3400.

58. Sakalian M, Parker SD, Weldon RA and Hunter E. Synthesis and assembly of retrovirus gag precursors into immature capsids in vitro. *Journal of Virology* 1996;70;6:3706-3715.

59. Gallo RC, Miller NR, Saxinger WC and Gillespie D. Primate RNA Tumor Virus-Like DNA Synthesized Endogenously by RNA-Dependent DNA Polymerase in Virus-like Particles from Fresh Human Acute Leukemic Blood Cells. *Proceedings National Academy of Sciences* 1973;70;11:3219-3224.

60. Chen Z, Telfer P, Gettie A, Reed P, Zhang L, Ho DD and Marx PA. Genetic characterization of New West African simian immunodeficiency virus SIVsm: Geographic clustering of household-derived SIV strains with human immunodeficiency virus type 2 subtypes and genetically diverse viruses from a single feral sooty mangabey troop. *Journal of Virology* 1996;70;6:3617-3627.

61. Kanki PJ, Barin S, M'B oup, et al., New human T-lymphotropic retrovirus (HTLV-IV) related to simian T-lymphotropicvirus Type III (STLV-IIIagm). *Science* 1986;232:238-43.

62. Kanki PJ, M'Boup S, Marlink R, et al., Sequence of simian immunodeficiency virus and its relationship to the human immunodeficiency viruses. *Nature* 1987;328:539-43.

63. Chakrabarti L, Guyader M, Alizon M, et al., Sequence of simian immunodeficiency virus from macaque and its relationship to other human simian retroviruses. *Nature* 1987;328:543-47.

64. Myers G, MacInnes K, and Myers L. "Phylogenetic Moments in the AIDS Epidemic," Chapter 12 in S. S. Morese, ed., *Emerging Viruses* (Oxford, Eng.: Oxford University Press, 1993).

65. Hope R. KU medical center virologist develops first model for testing HIV medications and vaccines. Univ. of Kansas Relations press release. October 10, 1995 (913-588-5240) and picked up by *AIDS Weekly* on October 23, 1995; see also Joag SV, Li Z, Foresman L, Stephens EB, Zhao LJ Pinson DM, McClure HM and Narayan O. SIV-HIV Chimeric virus that causes progressive loss of CD4+ T Cells and AIDS in pig-tailed macaques. Submitted to *J of Virology* in 1995.

Chapter 9. Early Targeting of Minority America

1. Dubos RJ. Environmental impact on health and disease. *Industrial Medicine and Surgery* 1961;30:369.

2. Von Hoffman N. *Citizen Cohn: The Life and Times of Roy Cohn.* New York: Doubleday, 1988, pp. 127-35; 284-87;331-41.

3. Powers RG. *Secrecy and Power: The Life of J. Edgar Hoover.* New York: The Free Press, 1987.

4. Strecker R. *The Strecker Memorandum.* The Strecker Group, 1501 Colorado Boulevard, Los Angeles, CA 90041, 1988.

5. Szmuness W, Stevens CE, Harley EJ, Zang EA and Oleszko WR et al. Hepatitis B vaccine: Demonstration of efficacy in a controlled clinical trial in a high-risk population in the United States. *New England Journal of Medicine* 1980;303;15:833-841.

6. Horowitz LG. *Deadly Innocence: Solving the greatest murder mystery in the history of American medicine.* Rockport, MA: Tetrahedron, Inc., 1994.

7. Lait J and Mortimer L. *Washington Confidential.* New York: Crown Publishers, 1953.

8. D'Emilio J. *Sexual Politics, Sexual Communities:* The Making of a Homosexual Minority in the United States, 1940-1970. Chicago: University of Chicago Press, 1983.

9. Newman DK. *Protest, Politics and Prosperity:* Black Americans and White Institutions, 1940-1975. New York: Pantheon Books, 1978.

10. Covert NM. *Cutting Edge: A history of Fort Detrick, Maryland 1943-1993.* Fort Detrick, MD: Headquarters, U. S. Army Garrison, Public Affairs Office, 1993, p. 39-40; Merriam Webster's Collegiate Dictionary. Tenth Edition. Springfield, MA 1994, pp. 710,924.

11. Buckley WF. Reeves' Kennedy. *National Review*, December 31, 1994 pp. 30-41.3. Hoover JE. "Turbulence on Campus," *PTA Magazine*, Feb. 1966, p. 4.

12. Hoover JE. "Turbulence on Campus," *PTA Magazine*, Feb. 1966, p. 4.

13. Goldstein RJ. *Political Repression in Modern America.* Cambridge, MA: Schenckmann/Two Continents, 1978, pp. 449-458.

14. Powers RG. *Op. cit*, p. 424-475.

15. Senate Select Committee. Final Report, Book III, pp. 179-189.

16. Hoover to SAC, Albany, Aug. 25, 1967, Senate Select Committee Hearings, Book, III, p. 180; Senate Select Committee, Hearings, Vol. 6, FBI, pp. 387-390.

17. See "King," Hoover O&C File 23, in which the Director attempted to persuade Senator Scott not to honor King, May 22, 1968; Hoover to Tolson and others, June 19, 1969, FBI File 67-9524, Tolson Personnel File. The Panther Directives were issued on November 25, 1968, and January 30, 1969 (See *Senate Select Committee, Final Report, Book III*, p. 22). Also see Sanford J. U. *FBI.* Boston: Atlantic Monthly Pres, 1975, p. 465; and Powers RG. *Op. cit.* p. 458.

18. Ungar SJ. *FBI.* Boston: Atlantic Monthly Pres, 1975, p. 466

19. Powers RG. *Op. cit*, p. 458.

20. Richards D. Played Out: The Jean Seberg Story. New York: Playboy, 1981, p. 237.

21. Powers RG. *Op. cit*, p. 460.

22. Bair D. *Simone de Beauvoir: a Biography.* New York: Summit Books, 1990, pp. 440-482.

23. Bair, *Ibid.* p. 518.

24. Bair, *Ibid.* p. 474.

25. Bair, *Ibid.* p. 480.

26. Goldstein RJ. *Op. cit.*, p. 458; *Senate Select Committee. Final Report, Book III*, p. 519; and for documentation on Dr. Henry Kissinger's powerful National Security Staff position, see: Isaacson W. *Kissinger: A Biography.* New York: Simon & Schuster, 1992, p. 135-672.

27. Rockefeller NA, Connor JT, Dillon CD, Griswold EN, Reagan R, and Kirkland, et al. *Report to the President by the Commission on CIA Activities Within the United States..* New York: The Rockefeller Commission, 1975, p. 211.

Chapter 10. African Foreign Policy and Population Control

1. Lambo TA. The African mind in contemporary conflict: The Jacques Parisot Foundation Lecture, 1971. *World Health Organization Chronicle* 1971;25;8:343-353.

2. Powers RG. *Secrecy and Power: The Life of J. Edgar Hoover.* New York: The Free Press, 1987, p. 469.

3. Kumar S. Cold war and covert action in Africa. In: *CIA and the Third World: A Study in Crypto-Diplomacy.* New Delhi: Vikas Publishing House Pvt. Ltd., 1981, pp. 65-92.

4. *Department of Defense Appropriations For 1970: Hearings Before A Subcommittee of the Committee on Appropriations House of Representatives, Ninety-first Contress, First Session, H.B. 15090, Part 5, Research, Development, Test and Evaluation, Dept. of the Army.* U.S. Government Printing Office, Washington, D.C., 1969—the text cited in previous chapters was discovered through the FOIA on page 129, but is missing from the public record.

5. House Republican Task Force Activities. Hon. George Bush of Texas in the House of Representatives. In: *Congressional Record: Proceedings and Debates of the 91st Congress First Session.* Volume 115-Part 16. July 29, 1969, p. 21304.

6. Rogers WP. *A report of the Secretary of State: United States Foreign Policy, 1971.* Washington, DC: U.S. Government Printing Office. Department of State Publication 8634, General Foreign Policy Series 260. Released March 1972. p. 328.

7. Nixon R. U. S. foreign policy for the 1970s: Shaping a durable peace. A report to the Congress by the President of the United States, May 3, 1973. *The Department of State Bulletin.* Volume LXVIII, No. 1771, June 4, 1973, pp. 794-798.

8. Williams MJ. Sahel African disaster relief and recovery assistance: Text of a Report for the President. *Department of State Bulletin*, November 26, 1973, pp. 669-673.

9. Newsom DD. African development and U. S. Foreign Policy. Speech made before the annual meeting of the African Studies Association at Syracuse, N.Y., on Nov. 2, 1997. *Department of State Bulletin*, December 31, 1973, p. 789.

10. Kissinger H. Foreign assistance and America's purposes in the world. Speech made before the House Committee on Foreign Affairs, June 4, 1974. *Department of State Bulletin*, June 24, 1974, pp. 710-715.

11. Kissinger H. Secretary Kissinger testifies on security assistance program. Statement made before the House Committee on International Relations. *Department of State Bulletin*, November 24, 1975, pp. 747-748.

12. Department of State. *Memorandum of Understanding Between ERTS-Zaire and the United States National Aeronautics and Space Administration (NASA). Diplomatic List.* Washington, D. C.: U. S. Government Printing Office, 1975, pp. 1700-1704.

13. Ranelagh J. *The Agency: The Rise and Decline of the CIA.* New York: Simon and Schuster, 1985, p. 732.

14. Department of State Staff. World Population: The Silent Explosion. *Department of State Bulletin.* November, 1978. pp. 1-8. The Series were available through the Correspondence Management Division, Bureau of Public Affairs, Depart of State, Washington, D.C. 20520

15. Fredericksen H. Feedbacks in economic and demographic transition. *Science* 1969;166:837.)

16. Ravenholt RT. Implications of mass immunization programs on the world population problem. In: *Pan American World Health Organization. Proceedings of the International Conference on the Application of Vaccines Against Viral, Rickettsial, and Bacterial Diseases in Man. December 14-18, 1970.* Scientific Publication No. 226. Washington, D.C.: Pan American Health Organization, 1971, pp. 527-528.

17. *Who's Who in America*, 49th Edition, Volume 1 A-K. New Providence, NJ: Marquis Who's Who, 1995, p. 552.

18. Califano, Jr. JA. Health: U. S. Initiatives in International Health. *Department of State Bulletin.* September, 1978, pp. 35-38.

19. Hartmann B. Population control as foreign policy. *Covert Action Information Bulletin.* Winter 1991-92;39:26-30.

20. Simons H. Repackaging population control. *Covert Action Quarterly* 1994;51:33-44.

21. Eberstadt N. *Foreign Aid and American Purpose.* Washington D.C.: American Enterprise Institute for Public Policy Research, 1988, p. 104.

22. Porrit J. Birth of brave New World Order. *Guardian Weekly* (London), September 11, 1994.

23. Gordon L. *Woman's Body, Woman's Rights: A Social History of Birth Control in America.* New York: Grossman, 1976. p. 400-401.

24. Foster G. quoted in "Global Demographic Trends to the Year 2010: Implications for U.S. Security," Washington Quarterly, Spring 1989, and *Information Project for Africa, Population Control and National Security.* Washington, D.C.: U. S. Government Printing Office, 1989, p. 54.)

25. *National Security Study Memorandum 200 (NSSM 200). "Implications of Worldwide Population Growth for US Security and Overseas Interests."* U.S National Security Council Report, December 10, 1974.

26. *Ibid.*, pp. 21-22;115.

27. Robinson, Jr LH. *Report to Africa Bureau, Office of Regional Affairs, Agency for International Development.* Battelle Human Affairs Research Centers, November 6, 1981, pp. 15-16; Also see *Ambassadors of Colonialism: the International Development Trap. An essay on the Benevolent Super-*

power, Sustainable Development, and Other Contemporary Myths, (Washington, D.C., Information Project for Africa, Inc., 1993.

28. Knowles JC. *"Tools for Population Policy Development OPTIONS for Population Policy Project"* (AID-funded project), 1988, p. 23.

29. In 1982 a U.S. General Accounting Office report cautioned that many NGOs in the U.S. were becoming overly dependent on USAID for financing their projects. See, "Voluntary Aid for Development: the Role of NGOs," OECD (Paris: OECD, 1988), p. 113.

30. NGO Review 1993. *The well-spent pound: an assessment of aid agencies's priorities for population activities.* London: House of Commons, March, 1994, p. 48. Author Helen Simmons reviewed this work and footnoted, "While UNICEF was set up by the U.N. and so is not strictly an NGO, it increasingly operates in and is treated as one in the development circles. Even relatively modest NGOs still have fantastic incomes in African terms. The Save the Children Fund's (SCF) income of over $149 million in 1991-92 outstrips that of the Eritrean government five times over."

31. Kaplan R. The coming anarchy. *Atlantic Monthly* February, 1994, p. 58.

32. Thoreau HD.*Journal [1906].* September 7, 1851

33. Sai FT and Chester LA. The role of the world bank in shaping Third World population policy. In: *Population Policy: Contemporary Issues*, G. Roberts, Ed., New York: Praeger, 1990, p. 183.

34. The Futures Group. The United Republic of Tanzania: Population and development. Washington, D.C., 1980, p. 45. For more information on the use of RAPID presentations, see Sai and Chester, *op. cit.*

35. Associated Press. HRS can't do everything for everybody, task group's chief says. *The Orlando Sentinel*, Tuesday, January 8, 1991. The position articulated here by Janet Reno, prior to becoming attorney general in the Clinton administration, was that social reforms were needed to respond to "the failed family institution." The breakdown of the family, she said was the chief cause of crime and drug use in the United States.

36. Ward SJ, Poernomo I, Sidi S, Simmons R and Simmons G. *Service Delivery Systems and Quality of Care in the Implementation of Norplant in Indonesia*. New York: Population Control Council, February, 1990, pp. 45, 50-51.

37. Allen C. Norplant—Birth control or coercion? *Wall Street Journal*, September 13, 1991, p. 10.

Chapter 11. Henry Kissinger's "New World Order"

1. Isaacson W. *Kissinger: A Biography.* New York: Simon & Schuster, 1992, pp. 26-28.

2. "America's Clausewitz was banned from Fürth's city schools," *Fürther Nachrichten*, Oct. 15, 1958; Collier BL. The Road to Peking. *NYT Magazine*, November 14, 1971. As noted in *Kissinger* by Kalb and Kalb, p. 35: "Almost word for word, he has relayed the same disclaimers to other interviewers."

3. Blumenfeld, R. *Henry Kissinger.* New York: New American Library, 1974, pp. 35-43.

4. Lina Rau Schubach, Dec. 8, 1988 quoted in Isaacson. *Op. cit.* p. 26.

5. Menachem Lion, May 10, 1988 quoted in Isaacson. *Op. cit.* p. 26.

6. Fritz Kraemer, May 14, 1988. quoted in Isaacson. *Op. cit.* p. 29. Kremer has reported essentially the same views over the years. See also the *New York Post*, June 3, 1974.

7. Ward D. "Kissinger: A psychohistory." In: *Henry Kissinger: His Personality and Policies*, Dan Caldwell, ed.: Durham, N.C.: Duke Univ. Press, 1983.

8. Dickson P. *Kissinger and the Meaning of History.* New York: Cambridge Press, 1979. p. 43.

9. Isaacson, *Op. cit.* p. 30-31.

10. Themes expressed in a letter from Kissinger to "My dear Mrs. Frank," April 21, 1946, courtesy of Paula Kissinger and Harold Reissner; *Ob. cit.* Issacson, p. 53.

11. Thimmesch N. The iron mentor of the Pentagon. *WP Magazine*, March 2, 1975; Fritz Kraemer, May 4 and May 14, 1988. See Isaacson, *Op. cit.*, p. 55.

12. "Memories of Mr. Henry," *Newsweek*, Oct. 8, 1973, p. 48; Henry Kissinger," December 19, 1988; Blumenfeld, *Op. cit.* pp. 68-80; Isaacson, *Op. cit.* pp. 53-55.

13. In 1945, the War Department set up a top-secret program initially named Project Overcast, and later renamed Project Paperclip which according to William Preston, a Professor of History at John Jay College of Criminal Justice of the City University of New York, was initiated to "locate, recruit, and exfiltrate to the United States hundreds of Nazi scientists, specialists in rocketry, biologi-

cal warfare, aviation medicine, wind tunnels, and the like." Quoting from a "Secret Security Information" memo on Paperclip, "The Department of Defense has two classified projects, deemed of utmost importance, that result in the employment and exploitation of foreign scientists by the Department: . . . PROJECT 63 is primarily a denial program with utilization as a desirable feature. The aim of this program is to secure employment in the United States of certain preeminent German and Austrian specialists, thus denying their services to potential enemies. Such specialists sign a six-month Department of Defense contract which guarantees them an income until permanent employment is arranged with Department of Defense agencies or industry within the United States." Please see: Preston W. The real treason. *Covert Action Information Bulletin* 1986;25:23-26.

14. Smith RN. *The Harvard Century*. New York: Simon & Schuster, 1986, p. 268-178; McGeorge Bundy, February 8, 1989.

15. Isaacson *Op. cit*, pp. 60-61.

16. Isaacson's interviews with: Henry Kissinger, March 8, 1989; Arthur Gilman, February 14, 1989; Herbert Engelhardt, February 27, 1989; and Kissinger transcripts, House file, Harvard Registrar's Office; *Ibid.*

17. Recommendation for Phi Beta Kappa, by Elliott, Kissinger House file; Isaacson *Op. cit*, p. 63.

18. Stoessinger J. *Henry Kissinger: The Anguish of Power*. New York: Norton, 1976, p. 4.

19. *Op. cit.* Isaacson, pp. 64-67.

20. Dickson P. *Kissinger and the Meaning of History*. New York: Cambridge, 1979.

21. Kissinger H. "The Meaning of History" Harvard University doctoral thesis. pp. 1-17.

22. Isaacson advises that Stanley Hoffmann, "a Harvard colleague, is the foremost analyst of the relationship between Kissinger's intellectual ideas and his policies. Particularly valuable are:" Hoffman S. *Dead Ends*. Cambridge: Ballinger, 1983, pp. 17-66; and Hoffman S. *Primacy or World Order*. New York: McGraw-Hill, 1978, pp. 33-97.

23. Dickson, *Op. cit.*, pp. 35, 47.

24. Graubard S. *Kissinger: Portrait of a Mind*. New York: Norton, 1973, p. 55.

25. Isaacson, *Op. cit.*, pp. 70-71.

26. Memo from the special agent in charge, Boston, to the Central Research Division of the FBI, July 15, 1953; see Diamond S. Kissinger and the FBI. *The Nation*, November 10, 1979; *Ibid.*

27. Henry Kissinger, March 8, 1989; letter from Kissinger to his parents, June 4, 1952; Isaacson, *Op. cit.*, pp. 80-81.

28. Kissinger H. *A World Restored: Metternich, Castlereagh, and the Problems of Peace, 1812-22*. Boston: Houghton Mifflin, 1957.; Kissinger, March 8, 1989; Hoffman, *Op. cit.*, p. 36; Isaacson, *Op. cit.*, pp. 75-76.

29. Stoessinger, *Op. cit.* p. 14.

30. Kissinger H. The limitations of diplomacy. *The New Republic*, May 9, 1955.

31. Isaacson, *Op. cit.*, pp. 82-86.

32. Graubard,*Op. cit.*, p. 104.

33. Isaacson, *Op. cit.*, 90-93

34. Starr P. *The Social Transformation of American Medicine: The rise of a sovereign profession and the making of a vast industry*: New York: Basic Books, Inc., 1982, pp. 338-341.

35. Strickland S. *Politics, Science and Dread Disease: A Short History of United States Medical Research Policy*. Cambridge: Harvard University Press, 1958, pp. 1-14.

36. Starr, *Op. cit.*, p. 340.

37. Brown RE. *Rockefeller Medicine Men: Capitalism and Medical Care in America*. Berkeley: University of California Press, 1979, pp. 3-4;119-30.

38. Kissinger, Reflections on American diplomacy. *Foreign Affairs*, October, 1956.

39. Isaacson, *Op. cit.*, 129-137.

40. *Department of Defense Appropriations For 1970: Hearings Before A Subcommittee of the Committee on Appropriations House of Representatives, Ninety-first Contress, First Session, H.B. 15090, Part 5, Research, Development, Test and Evaluation, Dept. of the Army*. U.S. Government Printing Office, Washington, D.C., July 1,1969, p. 129.

41. *Who's Who in America*, 49th Edition, Volume 1, A-K. New Providence, NJ., 1995, p. 123. Roy Ash's address for anyone wishing to write is: 1900 Avenue of the Stars, Suite 1600, Los Angeles, CA 90067-4407; Information on Alexander Meigs Haig, Jr. was found in the same publication on page,1002.

42. Isaacson, *Op. cit.*, 151-156.

43. Kissinger H. *The Necessity of Choice*. New York: Harper & Brothers, 1961, pp. 345-48.

44. Colodny L. *Silent Coup: The Removal of a President*. New York: St. Martin's Press., 199, p. 53; see also Isaacson, *Op. cit.* 186-188.

45. Hersh S. *The Price of Power: Kissinger in the Nixon White House*. New York: Summit, 1983, pp. 57-58; Morris R. *Haig: The General's Progress*. New York: Playboy, 1982, pp. 141-142.

46. Isaacson, *Op. cit.*, pp. 188-191.

47. Isaacson, *Op. cit.*, pp. 212-233; Morris R. *Uncertain Greatness*. New York: Harper & Row 1977, p. 159.

48. Summers A. *Official and Confidential: The Secret Life of J. Edgar Hoover*. New York: G.P. Putnam's Sons, 1993 p. 395.

49. Senate Foreign Relations Committee. *Dr. Kissinger's Role in Wiretapping*, 1974, p. 23.

50. Isaacson, *Op. cit.*, pp. 202-205.

51. Haldeman's handwritten meeting notes, June 4, 1969; *Ibid.*

52. Hersh S. *The Price of Power: Kissinger in the Nixon White House*. New York: Summit, 1983. p. 36.

53. *NYT*, February 5, 1969; *Time*, February 14, 1969.

54. *First Annual Report on U.S. Foreign Policy* ("State of the World" report, February 18, 1970, 124-25; Leacacos J. The Nixon NSC. *Foreign Policy*, Winter 1971-72, p. 7.

55. What's in a name? Coincidentally, the German word Zum-Walt, literally means "to the world."

56. Washington Correspondent. Gas and germ warfare renounced but lingers on. *Nature* 1970 228;273:707-8; National Academy of Sciences. Symposium on chemical and biological warfare. *Proc. Nat Acad Sci* 1970;65:250-279; *Department of Defense Appropriations For 1970: Hearings Before A Subcommittee of the Committee on Appropriations House of Representatives, Ninety-first Contress, First Session, H.B. 15090, Part 5, Research, Development, Test and Evaluation, Dept. of the Army*. U.S. Government Printing Office, Washington, D.C., 1969; WHO News and Notes. Regional Committee for Africa. *WHO Chronicle* 1969;23;8:341-344.

Chapter 12. Silent Coup in American Intelligence

1. Isaacson W. *Kissinger: A Biography*. New York: Simon & Schuster, 1992, p. 228.

2. Summers A. *Official and Confidential: The Secret Life of J. Edgar Hoover*. New York: G.P. Putnam's Sons, 1993 pp. 409-410.

3. Isaacson, *Op. cit.*, p. 148.

4. Summers, *Op. cit.*, p. 375-376.

5. U.S. House Resolution 262, 81st Cong., 1st sess., cited in Max Lowenthal, *The Federal Bureau of Investigation* (New York: William Sloan Associates, 1950), p. 546; Powers RG. *Secrecy and Power: The Life of J. Edgar Hoover*. New York: The Free Press, 1987, pp. 299;439-40.

6. Powers, *Op. cit*, p. 450.

7. Rockefeller NA, *et. al.*, *Op. cit.*, p. 233.

8. Summers, *Op. cit.*, p. 397-399.

9 *Ibid.*, p. 400-411.

10. William Preston, Jr. and Ellen Ray, chief administrators of the Fund for Open Information and Accountability, Inc. and frequent contributors to *Covert Action Information Bulletin*, published in Washington, D.C., cite many journalists who are "the disinformation peddlers—people who may, or may not at a given moment, be in the direct employ of the CIA or other intelligence agencies, but who can be counted on to report, embellish, or pass on whatever their disinformation masters in Washington decree.... In fact, coordination between the development of propaganda and disinformation themes by the covert media assets, the overt propaganda machine, and the bevy of puppet journalists is quite calculated. . . " Among this group's most common ploys is to publish politically correct exposés making the journalist an expert witness for interrogation by Congressional investigating committees. "After that," these authors note, "they are given credibility by the 'respectable' Cold War publications like the *National Review*, *Commentary*, and the *New Republic*. And finally, since they have repeated the theme so many times it must be true, they are given the opportunity to write Op Ed pieces for the *New York Times* or the *Washington Post*." Activities much like the one Summers chronicled regarding former Attorney General Ramsey Clark's editorial in *The Washington Post* which called for Hoover's resigna-

tion. For more information, please see: Preston W and Ray E. Disinformation and mass deception: Democracy as a cover story. *Covert Action Information Bulletin* 1983;19:7-8.

11. Rockefeller NA, Connor JT, Dillon CD, Griswold EN, Reagan R, and Kirkland, *et al. CIA's Relation to Events Preceding the Watergate Break-in. Report to the President by the Commission on CIA Activities Within the United States..* New York: The Rockefeller Commission, 1975, pp. 193-197.

12. Isaacson, *Op. cit.*, pp. 202-205.

13. *Ibid.* p.124-128.

14. Isaacson, *Op. cit.*, p. 134-139.

15. *Ibid.* 733-743; Boeing was apparently contracted to provide Henry Kissinger with his private 707 jet, see page 694.

16. Covert NM. *Cutting Edge: A history of Fort Detrick, Maryland 1943-1993.* Fort Detrick, MD: Headquarters, U. S. Army Garrison, Public Affairs Office, 1993. [For copies call 301-619-2018]

17. Szmuness W, Stevens CE, Harley EJ, Zang EA and Oleszko WR et al. Hepatitis B vaccine: Demonstration of efficacy in a controlled clinical trial in a high-risk population in the United States. *New England Journal of Medicine* 1980;303;15:833-841.

18. Summers, *Op. cit.*, p. 200; 414-416; Isaacson, *Op. cit.*, p. 222-229.

19. *Ibid.* 721; 606.

20. CBS News. Watergate: The secret story *CBS News* special program. June 17, 1992 (Burrelle's Information Services transcript) pg. 31 ; My statement that "it wouldn't be the first or last time CBS reported" falsehoods is based on my knowledge of what "60-Minutes" did with "Kimberly's story". Produced by Josh Howard on June 19, 1994, the program was largely about Kimberly Bergalis's allegedly withheld sexual practices. She along with Dr. David Acer's other victims, Mike Wallace claimed, had gotten AIDS from risky lifestyle practices in the Stuart, FL community. I thoroughly critiqued the segment in *Deadly Innocence* and concluded it was a "cruel hoax"—produced for chiefly political reasons. See Horowitz L. *Deadly Innocence: Solving the Greatest Murder Mystery in the History of American Medicine.* Rockport, MA: Tetrahedron, Inc., 1994; See also, Isaacson, *Op. cit.*, pg. 90-93.

21. *Who's Who in America*, 49th Edition, Volume 1, A-K. New Providence, NJ., 1995, p. 552. Joseph Califano's may be reached by contacting the Department of Public Health Policy, Columbia University Schools of Medicine and Public Health, New York City.

22. Colodny L. *Silent Coup: The Removal of a President.* New York: St. Martins Press, 1991.

23. Isaacson, *Op. cit.*, p. 143.

24. Summers, *Op. cit.*, p. 421-422.

25. Rockefeller NA, *et al., Op. cit.*, p. 451.

26. Isaacson, *Op. cit.*, p. 491-495

27. Schaap B. Administration stonewalls while covert operations escalate. *CovertAction Information Bulletin* 1982;16:31

28. Agee P. The range of covert intervention. In: *Dirty Work-2: The CIA in Africa.* Secaucus, Ray E, Schaap W, Van Meter K and Wolf L eds. Secaucus, NJ: Lyle Stewart, Inc., 1979, pp. 47-49.

29. Lederer R. Precedents for AIDS? Chemical-biological warfare, medical experiments, and population control. *overtAction Information Bulletin* 1987;28:33-42.

30. *U.S. House Committee on Foreign Affairs. Hearing on U.S. Chemical Warfare Policy. Cong. Sess. 93-2, May 1-14, 1974; U.S. Senate Committee on Foreign Relations. Prohibition of Chemical and Biological Weapons: Hearing to Consider Definition and Ratification of Geneva Protocol. December 10, 1974,* Cong. Sess. 93-2. The hearings indicated that two years after Nixon allegedly forbad the development of chemical and biological weapons arsenals, additional ones were being produced and stockpiles had not been destroyed.

31. *U.S. Select Senate Committee to Study Governmental Operations with Respect to Intelligence Activities. Intelligence Activities. Senate Resolution 21. Vol. 1: Unauthorized Storage of Toxic Agents. September 16-18, 1975.* Cong. Sess. 94-1, pp 22-23.

32. Isaacson, *Op. cit.*, pp. 530-531; 491-495; 389.

33. *Ibid.* pp. 699-701.

34. Jimmy Carter speech, the Foreign Policy Association, Oct. 3, 1976.

Chapter 13. USAID and New York Blood

1. Califano, Jr. JA. Health: U. S. Initiatives in International Health. *Department of State Bulletin.* September, 1978, pp. 35-38.

2. Stevenson RW. Glaxo offers $14 billion for Wellcome: A British drug alliance would be the world's largest. *New York Times*, Tuesday, January 24, 1995, p. D1. The report noted Merck's AIDS and herpes drug market share was the largest at 3.9 percent valued at close to $10 billion.

3. Covert NM. *Cutting Edge: A history of Fort Detrick, Maryland 1943-1993*. Fort Detrick, MD: Headquarters, U. S. Army Garrison, Public Affairs Office, 1993. [For copies call 301-619-2018].

4. Isaacson W. *Kissinger: A Biography*. New York: Simon & Schuster, 1992, pp. 186-188.

5. *Ibid.*, p. 734.

6. Hilleman MR. Whither immunization against viral infections? *Annals of Internal Medicine* 1984;101(6):852-8.

7. Ciesielski C, Marianos D, Ou CY, et al. Transmission of human immunodeficiency virus in a dental practice. *Annals of Internal Medicine* 1992;116:798-805.

8 Poiesz B, Tomar R, Lehr B and Moore J. (and anonymous CDC authors from division closely associated with Don Francis's work—Hepatitis Branch, Division of Viral Diseases, Center for Infectious Diseases, CDC.) Hepatitis B vaccine: Evidence confirming lack of AIDS transmission. *MMWR* 1984;33;49:685-687.)

9. Horowitz LG. *Deadly Innocence: Solving the greatest murder mystery in the history of American medicine*. Rockport, MA: Tetrahedron, Inc., 1994.

10. Szmuness W, Stevens CE, Harley EJ, Zang EA and Oleszko WR et al. Hepatitis B vaccine: Demonstration of efficacy in a controlled clinical trial in a high-risk population in the United States. *New England Journal of Medicine* 1980;303;15:833-841.

11. Lang WR, Snyder FR, Lozovsky D, Kaistha V, Kaczaniuk MA, Jaffe JH and the ARC Epidemiology Collaborating Group. Geographic distribution of human immunodeficiency virus markers in parenteral drug abusers. *American Journal of Public Health* 1988;78;4:443-446.

12. Shilts R. *And the Band Played On: Politics, People and the AIDS Epidemic*. New York: Penguin Books, 1987, p. 233.

13. Lederer R. Origin and spread of AIDS: Is the west responsible? *Covert Action Information Bulletin* 1988; 29:52-65; *JAMA*, February 7, 1986.

14. Hirsh R. *Hemophiliacs, blood transfusions and AIDS. In: Understanding AIDS*. V. Gong, ed., New Brunswick, NJ: Rutgers Univ. Press, 1985, p. 104.

15. Lehrman NS. Is AIDS Non-Infectious? The Possibility and its CBW Implications. *Covert Action Information Bulletin* 1987;28:55-62; Altman LK. AIDS development in infection: Data suggest AIDS rises yearly after infection. *New York Times*, March 3, 1987, p. C1.; Pugliese G and Lampinen T. *Am J Infection Control* 1989;17:1.

16. Shilts R. *Op. cit.*, p. 202-203.

17. *Ibid.*, pp. 371;409.

18. *Ibid.*, p. 553.

19. *Ibid.*, p. 458.

20. Physician and researcher Alan Cantwell, I later learned, likewise scrutinized the "Patient Zero" theory and came to the same conclusion. Cantwell observed that Shilts failed to mention "medical reports that indicate the AIDS virus was already 'introduced' into the New York City gay community, two years before Dugas was diagnosed! . . . In blood specimens dating back to 1980 (the year Gaetan Dugas was diagnosed)," Cantwell noted, that 20 percent of the men in Szmuness's hepatitis B vaccine experiment were already HIV-positive. Thus, by then, "it is inconceivable that Dugas could have flown in from Paris and infected such a large number of gays, some of whom were infected as early as 1978 to 1979. Furthermore, the 'source' of Dugas's own HIV infection was never ascertained." See: Cantwell A. *Queer Blood: The secret AIDS genocide plot*. Los Angeles: Aries Rising Press, 1993, p. 29; also see Shilts R. *Op. cit.*, pp. 23;460.

21. *Department of Defense Appropriations For 1970: Hearings Before A Subcommittee of the Committee on Appropriations House of Representatives, Ninety-first Contress, First Session, H.B. 15090, Part 5, Research, Development, Test and Evaluation, Dept. of the Army*. U.S. Government Printing Office, Washington, D.C., 1969, p. 689.

22. *Who's Who in America*, 49th Edition, Volume 1, A-K. New Providence, NJ., 1995, p.552.

23. The statement considers at least one year delay for the publication of Krugman's research results. See: Krugman S, Giles JP, Hammond J. Hepatitis virus: effect of health on the infectivity and antigenicity of the MS-1 and MS-2 strains. *J Infectious Disease*. 1970;122:432-6; Krugman S, Giles JP, Hammond J. Viral hepatitis, type B (MS-2 strain): Studies on active immunization. *JAMA* 1971;217:41-5; Krugman S, Giles JP. Viral hepatitis, type B (MS-2 strain); further observations on natural history

and prevention. *New England Journal of Medicine* 1973;288:755-60; and Krugman S, Overby LR, Mushahwar IK, Ling C-M, Forsner GG and Deinhardt F. Viral hepatitis, type B: Studies on natural history and prevention reexamined. *New England Journal of Medicine* 1979;200:101-6.

24. USDHEW. *Virology: Volume 4—Control of Viral Infections. NIAID Task Force Report.* Bethesda, MD: Public Health Service, National Institutes of Health (NIH) 79-1834, 1979, p. 20-65-78.

25. Centers for Disease Control. Guidelines for prevention of transmission of HIV and HBV to health-care and public safety workers. *MMWR* 1989;38:1-36; Seeff LB, Wright EC, Zimmerman HJ, Alter HJ, Dietz AA, Felsher BF, Finkelstein JD, Garcia-Pont P, Gerin JL, Greenlee HB, Hamilton J, Holland PV, Kaplan PM, Kiernan T, Koff RS, Leevy CM, McAuliffe VJ, Nath N, Purcell RH, Schiff ER, Schwartz CC, Tamburro CH, Vlahcevic Z, Zemel R and Zimmon DS. Type B hepatitis after needlestick exposure and its prevention with hepatitis B immune globulin. *Annals of Internal Medicine* 1978;88:285-293.

26. Poiesz BJ, Ruxcetti FW, Gazder AF, Bunn PA, Minna JD and Gallo RC. Detection and isolation of type C retrovirus particles from fresh and cultured lymphocytes of a patient with cutaneous T-cell lymphoma. *Medical Science* 1980;77:7415-9; Poiez BJ, Ruscetti FW, Reitz MS, Kalyanaraman VS and Gallo RC. (This reference appeared in Gallo's July 18, 1985 *Nature* article entitled "A molecular clone of HTLV-III with biological activity, Volume 316, pp. 262-265. It gave no title other than:) *Nature* 1981;294:268-271.

27. Ratner L, Haseltine W, Patarca R, Livak KJ, Starcich B, Josephs SF, Doran ER, Rafalski A, Whitehorn EA, Kaumeister K, Ivanoff L, Petteway SR, Pearson ML, Lautenberger JA, Papas RS, Ghrayeb J, Chang NT Gallo RC and Wong-Staal F. Complete nucleotide sequence of the AIDS virus, HTLV-III. *Nature* 1985; 313:277-284; Poiesz's citations included: Poiesz, B. J. *et al. Proc Nat Acad Sci* U.S.A. 77,7415-7419 (1980) and Robert-Guroff, M, Ruscetti FW, Posner LE, Poiesz BJ and Gallo RC. *J. Exp. Med.* 154, 1957-1964 (1981).

28. Wu AM, Ting RC, Paran M and Gallo RC. Cordycepin inhibits induction of murine leukovirus production by 5-iodo-2'-deoxyuridine. *Proc Nat Acad Sci* 1972;69;12:3820-3824;

29. Paran M, Gallo RC, Richardson LS and Wu AM. Adrenal Corticosteroids Enhance Production of Type-C Virus Induced by 5-Iodo-2'-Deoxyuridine from Cultured Mouse Fibroblasts. *Proc Nat Acad Sci* 1973;70;8:2391-2395.

30. NIAID Task Force Report. *Virology: Acute Viral Infections.* Bethesda, MD: U. S. Department of Health, Education and Welfare, Public Health Service, National Institute of Health [Volumes 1-5 (NIH) 79-1831-35]. 1979;20:65-69

31. Krugman S. Viral hepatitis type B: Prospects for active immunization. In: *International Symposium on Viral Hepatitis, Milan, Dec. 1974. Develop. biol. Standard. Vol. 30*, Munich: S. Karger Basel, 1975, pp. VI; 363-367; the General Discussion can be found on pp.375-379.

32. *Department of Defense Appropriations For 1970: Hearings Before A Subcommittee of the Committee on Appropriations House of Representatives, Ninety-first Contress, First Session, H.B. 15090, Part 5, Research, Development, Test and Evaluation, Dept. of the Army.* U.S. Government Printing Office, Washington, D.C., 1969, p. 689.

33. Other NYUMC biological weapons suppliers, Senate investigators learned within months following Krugman's presentation, included Dr. Alan W. Bernheimer, who supplied the Army's Special Operations Division with Staph bacteria and Botulinum toxin, and Dr. Arthur Eberstein, who manufactured or tested "shellfish poison" for the CIA. See: *U.S. Select Senate Committee to Study Governmental Operations with Respect to Intelligence Activities. Intelligence Activities. Senate Resolution 21. Vol. 1: Unauthorized Storage of Toxic Agents. September 16-18, 1975.* Cong. Sess. 94-1, pp. 216;221.

34. Szmuness W. Recent advances in the study of the epidemiology of hepatitis B. *American Journal of Pathology* 1975;81:629-49; Szmuness W, Harley EJ, Ikram H, Stevens CE, *et al.* Sociodemographic aspects of the epidemiology of hepatitis B. In: Vyas G, Cohen SN, Schmid R, eds. *Viral hepatitis.* Philadelphia: Franklin Institute Press, 1978:297-320.

35. Shilts, *Op. cit.*, p. 125.

36. Krugman S, Hoofnagle MD, Gerety RJ, Kaplan PM and Gerin JL. Viral hepatitis type B: DNA polymerase activity and antibody to hepatitis B core antigen. New Engl J Med 1994;290;24:1331-1335; see also: Reich WT. "Human research and the war against disease." In: *Encyclopedia of Bioethics: Revised Edition, Vol. 4.* New York: Simon & Schuster Macmillan, 1995, pg. 2253-2254; and Lederer R. Origin and spread of AIDS: Is the west responsible. *CovertAction Information Bulletin* 1988;29:52-66, and reference #42.

37. USPHS/NCI Staff. *Special Virus Cancer Program: Progress Report #8.* J. B. Moloney, ed., Bethesda: USPHS NCI, 1971. Univ. North Carolina, Davies Library call number #HE 20.3152:V81, pp. ;21-26;104.

38. Kalabus R, Sansarricq H, Lambin P, Proulx J and Hilleman MR. Standardization and mass application of combined live measles-smallpox vaccine in Upper Volta. *American Journal of Epidemiology* 1967;86:93-111.

39. Buynak EB, Weibel RE, Whitman, Jr, Stokes J and Hilleman MR. combined live measles, mumps, and rubella virus vaccines. *Journal American Medical Association* 1969;207;12:2259-2262.

40. Coursaget P, Deciron F, Tortey E, Barin F, Chiron JP, Yvonnet B, Diouf C, Denis F, Diop-Mar I, Correa P, et al. *IARC Scientific Publications* 1984;63:319-335.

41. Purcell RH. Current understanding of hepatitis B virus infection and its implications for immunoprophylaxis. In: *Antiviral Mechanisms: Perspectives in Virology IX, The Gustav Stern Symposium.* New York: Academic Press, 1975 pp. 49-76.

42. Krugman S, Giles JP and Hammond J. Infectious hepatitis: Evidence for two distinctive clinical, epidemiological, and immunological types of infection. *JAMA* 1967;200;5:366-373(96-103).

43. Moor-Jankowski J. Blood groups of apes and monkeys; Human and simian types. In: *Research Animals in Medicine: National Heart and Lung Institute National Institutes of Health,* Lowell T. Harmison, ed. Washington, DC: U. S. Department of Health, Education and Welfare, Public Health Service, National Institutes of Health, DHEW Publication No. (NIH) 72-333, October 2, 1973, pp. 483-488.

44. Schulz TF. Origin of AIDS (letter to the editor). *The Lancet* 1992;339:867.

45. Personal communication with Leonard Ciaccio, Staten Island Town Hall historian, 718-982-2000.

46. Epstein SS. *The Politics of Cancer*, Garden City, NY: Anchor Press/Doubleday, 1979, pp. 336-337.

Chapter 14. African Vaccination Programs

1. Coursaget P, Deciron F, Tortey E, Barin F, Chiron JP, Yvonnet B, Diouf C, Denis F, Diop-Mar I, Correa P, *et al. IARC Scientific Publications* 1984;63:319-335.

2. Perrin J, Ntareme F, Coursaget P and Chiron JP. Vaccination of the newborn against hepatitis B in Burundi. *IARC Scientific Publications* 1984;63:307-18.

3. Pan American/World Health Organization. *Proceedings of the International Conference on the Application of Vaccines Agasint Viral, Rickettsial, and Bacterial Diseases of Man.* December 14-18, 1970. Scientific Publication No. 226. Washington D.C.: World Health Organization, 1971.

4. Manaker, RA, Strother PC, Miller AA and Piczak CV. Behavior in vitro of a mouse lymphoid-leukemia virus. *J. Nat. Cancer Inst.* 1960;25:1411-1418.

5. *Hearings before the Subcommittee on Health and Scientific Research of the Committee on Human Resources, United States Senate, Ninety-fifth Congress, First Session, on Examination of Serious Deficiencies in the Defense Department's Efforts to Protect the Human Subjects of Drug Research, Biological Testing Involving Human Subjects by the Department of Defense.* Washington, D.C.: U.S. Government Printing Office, March 8 and May 23, 1977, pp. 147-148.

6. Pan American/World Health Organization, *Op. cit.*, pp. xi-xxiii.

7. Foege WH. Measles vaccination in Africa. In:*Ibid.*, pp. 207-213.

8. Millar JD and Goege WH. Status of eradication of smallpox (and control of measles) in West and Central Africa. *Journal of Infectious Diseases* 1969;120;6:725-732.

9. Shilts R. *And the Band Played On: Politics, People and the AIDS Epidemic.* New York: Penguin Books, 1987, pp. 500; 553.

10. Pan American/World Health Organization, *Op. cit.*, pp. 614-615.

11. Paran M, Gallo RC, Richardson LS and Wu AM. Adrenal corticosteroids enhance production of type-C virus induced by 5-iodo-2'-deoxyuridine from cultured mouse fibroblasts. *Proc Nat Acad of Sci* 1973;70;8:2391-2395.

12. Gonda MA, Wong-Staal F, Gallo RC et al. Sequence homology and morphologic similarity of HTLV-III and visna virus, pathogenic lentivirus. *Science* 1985;227:173-177;

13. Gonda MA, Braun MJ, Carter SG, Kost TA, Bess Jr JW, Arthur LO and VanDer Maaten MJ. Characterization and molecular cloning of a bovine lentivirus related to human immunodeficiency virus. *Nature* 1987;330, 388-391; Mulder C. Human AIDS virus not from monkeys. *Nature* 1988;333:396; See also: Penny D. Origin of the AIDS virus. *Nature* 1988;333:494-495; See also Dr. A.

F. Rasmussen, Jr.'s contribution in "The present and future of immunization: Discussion." In: Pan American/ World Health Organization., *Op. cit.*, p. 602.

14. Hilleman, during an open discussion, stated "following Dr. Krugman's work, we have prepared highly purified Australia antigen from hepatitis B antigenic plasma." He also credited Krugman's earlier work saying, "Dr. Krugman's demonstration of protective efficacy of . . . killed Australia antigen provided the sound basis and incentive to proceed with vaccine development. In the absence of such data, the activities in which we now engage [homosexual vaccine trials] might be regarded as foolhardy. His comments appear in: *International Symposium on Viral Hepatitis, Milan, Dec. 1974. Develop. biol. Standard. Vol. 30*, Munich: S. Karger Basel, 1975, p. 375.

15. *Department of Defense Appropriations For 1970: Hearings Before A Subcommittee of the Committee on Appropriations House of Representatives, Ninety-first Contress, First Session, H.B. 15090, Part 5, Research, Development, Test and Evaluation, Dept. of the Army.* U.S. Government Printing Office, Washington, D.C., 1969, p. 689.

16. Krugman S and Giles JP. Measles: The Problem. In: Pan American/ World Health Organization., *Op. cit.*, p. 195.

17. Gallo RC. The inhibitory effect of heme on heme formation In Vivo: Possible mechanism for the regulation of hemoglobin synthesis. *Journal of Clinical Investigation* 1967;46;1:124-132; Gallo RC, Whang-Peng J and Adamson RH. Studies on the antitumor activity, mechanisms of action, and cell cycle effects of camptothecin. *Journal of the National Cancer Institute* 1971;46;4:789-795; Wu AM and Gallo RC. Interaction between murine type-C virus RNA-directed DNA polymerases and rifamycin derivatives. *Biochimica et Biophysica Acta* 1974;340:419-436; Gallo RC, Sarin PS, Allen PT, Newton WA, Priori ES, Bowen JM and Dmochowski L. Reverse transciptase in Type-C virus particles of human origin. *Nature New Biology* 1971;232:140-142; and Gallo RC and Breitman TR. The enzymatic mechanisms for deoxythymidine synthesis in human leukocytes: II Comparison of deoxyribosyl donors. *Journal of Biological Chemistry* 1968;243;19:4936-4942.

18. Gallagher RE, Ting RC and Gallo RC. A common change of aspartyl-tRNA in Polyoma and SV40-transformed cells. *Biochimica et Biophysica Acta* 1972;272:568-582.

19. Ting RC, Yang SS and Gallo RC. Reverse transcriptase, RNA tumor virus transformation and derivatives of Rifamycin SV. *Nature New Biology* 1972;236:163-165. Dow Chemical provided a variety of Rifamycin derivatives used in this study of chemotherapeutic effects.

20. Pan American/World Health Organization, *Op. cit.*, pp. 602-604.

21. *Ibid.*, pp. 499-500.

22. *Ibid.*, pp. 490-491.

23. Wehrle PF. Need for international cooperation in immunization programs. In: Pan American/ World Health Organization, *Op. cit.*, pp. 518-521.

24. Bres P. The problem of yellow fever. *Ibid.*, pp. 25-28.

25. Taylor CE. Gaining public acceptance and maintaining regular programs in the developing countries. *Ibid.* pp. 511-517.

26. Pollock TM. *Trials of Prophylactic Agents for the Control of Communicable Diseases: A Guide to Their Organization and Evaluation.* Geneva: World Health Organization, 1966, pp. 73-74.

27. Pan American/World Health Organization, *Op. cit.*, p. 612.

28. Millar JD. Gaining public acceptance in maintaining regular programs in the developed countries. *Ibid.*, pp. 505-510.

29. Millar JD and Foege WH. Status of eradication of smallpox (and control of measles) in West and Central Africa. *J Infect. Disease* 1969;120;6:725-732; Kalabus FH, Sansarrico H, Lambin P, Proulx J and Hilleman MR. Standardization and mass application of combined live measles-smallpox vaccine in Upper Volta. Amer. *J. Epidemiology* 1967;86:93-111.

Chapter 15. The CIA/Detrick Operation

1. Rockefeller NA, Connor JT, Dillon CD, Griswold EN, Reagan R, and Kirkland, *et al. Report to the President by the Commission on CIA Activities Within the United States..* New York: The Rockefeller Commission, 1975.

2. *U. S. House of Representatives, Ninety-Third Congress. Second Session Hearings before the Committee on the Judiciary. Presidential Statements on the Watergate Break-In and its Investigation. A resolution . . . to investigate whether sufficient grounds exist for the House of Representatives to . . . Impeach Richard M. Nixon, President of the United States.* H. Res. 803. Washington, D.C.: U. S. Gov-

ernment Printing Office, May-June 1974; Isaacson W. *Kissinger: A Biography*. New York: Simon & Schuster, 1992, pp. 592-606.

3. U.S. *Select Senate Committee to Study Governmental Operations with Respect to Intelligence Activities. Intelligence Activities. Senate Resolution 21. Vol. 1: Unauthorized Storage of Toxic Agents. September 16-18, 1975.* Cong. Sess. 94-1.

4. U.S. Select Senate Committee *Op. cit.*, pp. 1-4.

5. *Ibid.* pp. 5-7.

6. *Ibid.* p. III-IV.

7. *Ibid.* pp. 200-203.

8. *Ibid.* pp. 207-209.

9. Though the SVCP was cited in numerous publications by dozens of authors as supplying the financial support for their cancer virus and vaccine research efforts, access to the program's protocol or related literature was very difficult. I happened to run across one of the most important documents by chance. The title: NCI Staff. *Special Virus Cancer Program: Progress Report #8*. Bethesda, MD: Office of the Associate Scientific Director for Viral Oncology, National Cancer Institute, National Institutes of Health, USPHS, August, 1971 is available through interlibrary loan from The University of North Carolina at Chapel Hill, Davies Library, Government Documents Department, Call number HE 20.3152:V81-1971

10. *Ibid.* pp. 216-239.

11. *Hearings before the Subcommittee on Health and Scientific Research of the Committee on Human Resources, United States Senate, Ninety-fifth Congress, First Session, on Examination of Serious Deficiencies in the Defense Department's Efforts to Protect the Human Subjects of Drug Research, Biological Testing Involving Human Subjects by the Department of Defense.* Washington, D.C.: U.S. Government Printing Office, March 8 and May 23, 1977, pp. 89-90.

12. Epstein SS. *The Politics of Cancer*, Garden City, NY: Anchor Press/Doubleday, 1979, pp. 306-307;333.

13. *Ibid.* pp. 240-243.

14. *Ibid.* pp. 8-9.

15. *Ibid.* pp. 13-14.

16. *Ibid.* pp. 15-16.

17. *Ibid.* pp. 17-20.

18. Kissinger, according to Isaacson's biography, often worked behind Melvin Laird's back when he desired to deal with the Navy. Then he sent orders directly through Admiral Elmo Zumwalt. Since the Navy maintained the most active viral research program at the time, it is possible Kissinger directed Zumwalt, and not Laird, to order the appropriations request for the development of AIDS-like viruses. However, according to Isaacson, who interviewed Zumwalt, the admiral always kept Laird informed regarding Kissinger's "out of channel" demands. See: Isaacson, *Op. cit.*, pp. 190; 202-205.

19. *Ibid.* pp. 20-21.

20. Mr. Sidney Gottlieb was the head of a special CIA covert operation called MKULTRA. The program, according to Irwin Block of the *Montreal Gazette*, was designed to "explore brainwashing techniques that the agency believed were being perfected by the Chinese and Soviet Communists. The goal was mind control," and some of the first known subjects were the psychiatric patients of the American psychiatrist Dr. Ewen Cameron who practiced at Montreal's Allan Memorial Institute. Later it was determined that the CIA gave "more than $60,000 to the institute between 1957 and 1961 for the research. (See: Block I. Agency spent millions studying mind control *Montreal Gazette*. Wednesday October 5, 1988)

In 1960, CIA MKULTRA director Gottlieb was sent to the Congo, the region that was later named Zaire. Gottliebs assignment was to help assassinate Prime Minister Patrice Lumumba, an anti-imperialist African leader. See: Lederer R. Precedents for AIDS? Chemical-biological warfare, medical experiments, and population control. *Covert Action Information Bulletin* 1987;28:33-42; U.S. Select Senate Committee *Ob cit*, pp. 22-25.

21. *Ibid.* pp. 26-28.

22. *Ibid.* p. 29.

23. *Ibid.* pp. 29-32; Colby may have perjured himself here as he acknowledged awareness of other biological weapons testing projects in which health effects were claimed by unsuspecting subjects. Investigative journalist Robert Lederer has written extensively on the subject of covert chemical and biological weapons testing by the American military. For more information, please see: Lederer R.

Precedents for AIDS? Chemical-biological warfare, medical experiments, and population control. *CovertAction Information Bulletin* 1987;28:33-42.

24. *Ibid.* pp. 32-35.
25. *Ibid.* p. 35.
26. *Ibid.* p. 38.
27. *Ibid.* p. 40.
28. *Ibid.* p. 41.

Chapter 16. PROJECT: MKNAOMI

1. *U.S. Select Senate Committee to Study Governmental Operations with Respect to Intelligence Activities. Intelligence Activities. Senate Resolution 21. Vol. 1: Unauthorized Storage of Toxic Agents. September 16-18, 1975.* Cong. Sess. 94-1, p. 44.

2. U.S. Select Senate Committee *Op. cit.*, pp. 45-46.

3. Classified PROJECT: MKNAOMI was a secret program of cooperation between the CIA and Army Special (meaning secret) Operations Division (SOD) at Fort Detrick to develop and covertly deploy a variety of biological weapons including natural toxins, lethal bacteria, and deadly viruses. Though the vast majority of text in this Congressional exhibit was illegible, the gist of the conversation suggests the principle purpose of MKNAOMI was to develop offensive biological weapons capabilities required to transmit lethal germs to mass populations. The Director of MKNAOMI is unknown but undoubtedly orders for its operation between 1969 through 1976 came from Dr. Henry Kissinger.

4. Isaacson W. *Kissinger: A Biography.* New York: Simon & Schuster, 1992, p. 667.

5. U.S. Select Senate Committee *Op. cit.*, pp. 52-61.

6. Herrera F, Adamson RH and Gallo RC. Uptake of transfer ribonucleic acid by normal and leukemic cells. *Proc Nat Acad Sci* 1970;67;4:1943-1950. This paper was presented before the "International Symposium on Uptake of Informative Molecules by Living Cells, Mol, Belgium, 1970," the year in which $10 million in funds were appropriated by the Department of Defense for the development of AIDS-like viruses.

7. Reference used: Rose LF and Kaye D. *Internal Medicine for Dentistry.* St. Louis: C. V. Mosby Company, 1983, p. 200.

8. U.S. Select Senate Committee *Op. cit.*, p. 66.

9. *Ibid.* p.p. 72-81.

10. Szmuness W, Stevens CE, Harley EJ, Zang EA and Oleszko WR et al. Hepatitis B vaccine: Demonstration of efficacy in a controlled clinical trial in a high-risk population in the United States. *New England Journal of Medicine* 1980;303;15:833-841.

11. Lederer R. Origin and spread of AIDS: Is the west responsible. *CovertAction Information Bulletin* 1988;29:52-66.

12. Krugman S, Giles JP, Hammond J. Hepatitis virus: effect of health on the infectivity and antigenicity of the MS-1 and MS-2 strains. *J Infectious Disease.* 1970;122:432-6; Krugman S, Giles JP, Hammond J. Viral hepatitis, type B (MS-2 strain): Studies on active immunization. *JAMA* 1971;217:41-5; Krugman S, Giles JP. Viral hepatitis, type B (MS-2 strain); further observations on natural history and prevention. *New England Journal of Medicine* 1973;288:755-60; and Krugman S, Overby LR, Mushahwar IK, Ling C-M, Forsner GG and Deinhardt F. Viral hepatitis, type B: Studies on natural history and prevention reexamined. *New England Journal of Medicine* 1979;200:101-6.

13. Szmuness W, Purcell RH, Dienstag JL and Stevens CE. Antibody to hepatitis A antigen in institutionalized mentally retarded patients. *JAMA* 1977;237:1702-1705.

14. Lederer provided an important reference linking Krugman, Hilleman from Merck, and Purcell, to the Army. See: "Current Investigation Studies Approved by the Army Investigational Drug Review Board." Investigator: S. Krugman, M.D., Biomedical and Behavioral Research, 1975, *Joint Hearings before the Subcommittee on Health of the Committee on Labor and Public Welfare and the Subcommittee on Administrative Practices of the Committee on the Judiciary, U.S. Senate, September 10, 12, and November 7, 1975*, p. 576.

15. Pollock TM. *Trials of Prophylactic Agents for the Control of Communicable Diseases: A Guide to Their Organization and Evaluation.* Geneva: World Health Organization, 1966, pp. 73-74.

16. Bres P. The problem of yellow fever. In: Pan American/World Health Organization. *Proceedings of the International Conference on the Application of Vaccines Agasint Viral, Rickettsial, and Bacterial*

Diseases of Man. December 14-18, 1970. Scientific Publication No. 226. Washington D.C.: World Health Organization, 1971, p. 25-28.

17. U.S. Select Senate Committee *Op. cit.*, p. 97-98.

Chapter 17. The CIA's Human Experiments

1. *U.S. Select Senate Committee to Study Governmental Operations with Respect to Intelligence Activities. Intelligence Activities. Senate Resolution 21. Vol. 1: Unauthorized Storage of Toxic Agents. September 16-18, 1975.* Cong. Sess. 94-1, pp. 93-125.

2. *House Committee on Appropriations. Department of Defense Appropriations for 1977, Part 1. Hearings before the Subcommittee on DOD Appropriations to consider DOD FY 77 budget request presented by CIA Director William E. Colby, January 22, 1976.*

3. *Ibid.*, see pp. 280-371 for appropriations for chemical and biological weapons, and page 406 for defense strategies against "Soviet and Cuban assistance in Africa."

4. *Senate Committee on Human Resources. Biological Testing Involving Human Subjects by the Department of Defense, 1977. Hearings before the Subcommittee on Health and Scientific Research to examine Army biological warfare research programs, March 8, 1977 and May 23, 1977.* Cong. Sess. 95-1, pp. 3; 22-234; 244-256.

5. Brumter C. *The North Atlantic Assemby.* Dordrecht: Martinus Nijhoff Publishers, 1986, p. 215.

6. Senate Committee on Human Resources. Biological Testing Involving Human Subjects by the Department of Defense, 1977., *Op. cit.*, p. 7-8.

7. *Department of Defense Appropriations For 1970: Hearings Before A Subcommittee of the Committee on Appropriations House of Representatives, Ninety-first Contress, First Session, H.B. 15090, Part 5, Research, Development, Test and Evaluation, Dept. of the Army.* U.S. Government Printing Office, Washington, D.C., 1969, see pp. 79 and then 129 of classified document obtainable through FOIA; See also: "Current Investigation Studies Approved by the Army Investigational Drug Review Board." Investigator: S. Krugman, M.D., Biomedical and Behavioral Research, 1975, *Joint Hearings before the Subcommittee on Health of the Committee on Labor and Public Welfare and the Subcommittee on Administrative Practices of the Committee on the Judiciary, U.S. Senate, September 10, 12, and November 7, 1975*, p. 576.

8. Senate Committee on Human Resources. *Op. cit.*, p. 9;11.

9. *Ibid.*, p. 79 (C-4 Addendum).

10. *Ibid.*, p. 14.

11. *Ibid.*, p. 265-267

12. *Ibid.*, pp. 91;125.

13. Rockefeller NA, Connor JT, Dillon CD, Griswold EN, Reagan R, and Kirkland, et al. *Report to the President by the Commission on CIA Activities Within the United States..* New York: The Rockefeller Commission, 1975, pp. 226-229. I thought it also interesting that the same year the Rockefeller commission reported its findings, Hoover's old friend and American counterintelligence asset Roy Cohn, made headlines for having engineered the resignation of President Jimmy Carter's chief of staff, Hamilton Jordan. Reportedly, Cohn leaked accusations to the *New York Times* that Jordan had been seen using cocaine in Manhattan's Studio 54. I noted that despite the changing of administrations, the old guard had remained intact and strong enough to undo what any President might. See: Von Hoffman N. *Citizen Cohn: The Life and Times of Roy Cohn.* New York: Doubleday, 1988, p. 405.

14. Lawrence Ken. The CIA and the mad scientist: Drugs, psychiatry, and mind control in Canada. *CovertAction Information Bulletin* 1987;28:29-32.

15. Commission of Inquiry Concerning Certain Activities of the Royal Canadian Mounted Police (McDonald Commission), *First Report: Security and Information* (Oct. 9, 1979; *Second Report: Freedom and Security Under the Law*, Volumes 1 and 2 (August 1981); and *Third Report: Certain R.C.M.P. Activities and the Question of Governmental Knowledge* (August 1981) Hull, Ont: Canadian Government Publishing Center, 1979-81.

16. Marks J. *The Search for the "Manchurian Candidate": The CIA and Mind Control.* New York: Time Books, 1979, pp. 134-135.

17. *Opinion of George Cooper, Q. C., Regarding Canadian Government Funding of the Allan Memorial Institute in the 1950s and 1960s.* Ottawa: Communications and Public Affairs, Department of Justice, 1986.

18. *Ibid.*, p. 20.

19. Untitled CIA memorandum from May 5, 1955. *Joint Hearing Before the Select Committee on Intelligence and the Subcommittee on Health and Scientific Research of the Committee on Human Resources, U. S. Senate, August 3, 1977, Project MKULTRA, the CIA's Program of Research in Behavioral Modification*. Washington, D.C.: U. S. Government Printing Office, 1977.

20. Marks, *Op. cit.*, p. 137-139.

21. Cooper, *Op. cit.*, p. 80.

22. Bulf E. Have mosquitoes been drafted in a secret war? *In These Times*, September 23-29, 1981, p. 22; and "U.S. Germ Warfare Tests Revealed—Target: Savannah, Georgia," *Revolutionary Worker*, November 21, 1980.

23. Lederer R. Precedents for AIDS? Chemical-biological warfare, medical experiments, and population control. *CovertAction Information Bulletin* 1987;28:33-42.

24. Senate Committee on Human Resources, *Op. cit.*, pp. 124-140.

25. Lederer refers interested readers to: "Guyana: The Faces Behind the Masks," *CovertAction Information Bulletin* 1980;10:21.

26. Shapo MS. *A Nation of Guinea Pigs: The Unknown Risks of Chemical Technology*. New York: Free Press, 1979, p. 91; Ana Maria Garcia, Study Guide for "La Operacion" (a documentary about sterilization of Puerto Rican women), 1986, available from Cinema Guild, New York City.

27. Mitford J. *Kind and Usual Punishment: The Prison Business*. New York: Knopf, 1976, pp. 138-67.

28. Lasagna L. Special subjects in human experimentation. In: Paul A. Fruend, ed., *Experimentation with Human Subjects*. New York: George Brazillier, 1969, p. 262.

29. Robbins W. "Dioxin Tests Conducted on 70 Philadelphia Inmates, Now Unknown, in 1960s," *New York Times*, July 17, 1983.

30. Mitford J. *Op. cit.*, pp. 157-167; Lastala J. "Atascadero: Dachau for Queers," *Advocate*, April 25, 1972, pp. 11-13.

31. Jones JH. *Bad Blood: The Tuskegee Syphilis Experiment*. New York: Free Press, 1981, p. 2.

32. Ortleb C. Bad Blood: The Health Commissioner, The Tuskegee Experiment, and AIDS Policy. *New York Native*, February 16, 1987, pp. 13-16; Ortleb C. Unpublished study suggests AIDS is caused by "virulent Immunosuppressant Spirochetes. *New York Native*, February 16,1987, p. 10.

33. CBS Television Network. Confirmation hearings of Dr. Henry Foster for U. S. Surgeon General. *CBS Evening News* with Dan Rather and Connie Chung. Tuesday May 2, 1995.

34. United States Senate. Proceeding and Debates of the 91st Congress, First Session. *Congressional Record*, Volume 115-Part 17, August 5, 1969, to August 12, 1969. Washington D.C.: U. S. Government Printing Office, 1969 p. 23075.

35. The statement considers at least one year delay for the publication of Krugman's research results. See: Krugman S, Giles JP, Hammond J. Hepatitis virus: effect of health on the infectivity and antigenicity of the MS-1 and MS-2 strains. *J Infectious Disease*. 1970;122:432-6; Krugman S, Giles JP, Hammond J. Viral hepatitis, type B (MS-2 strain): Studies on active immunization. *JAMA* 1971;217:41-5; Krugman S, Giles JP. Viral hepatitis, type B (MS-2 strain); further observations on natural history and prevention. *New England Journal of Medicine* 1973;288:755-60; and Krugman S, Overby LR, Mushahwar IK, Ling C-M, Forsner GG and Deinhardt F. Viral hepatitis, type B: Studies on natural history and prevention reexamined. *New England Journal of Medicine* 1979;200:101-6.

36. Shilts R. *And the Band Played On: Politics, People and the AIDS Epidemic*. New York: Penguin Books, 1987, p. 221-223.

37. Shilts, *Ibid.*, pp. 238-239.

38. *Ibid.*, p. 326.

39. Szmuness W, Stevens CE, Harley EJ, Zang EA and Oleszko WR et al. Hepatitis B vaccine: Demonstration of efficacy in a controlled clinical trial in a high-risk population in the United States. *New England Journal of Medicine* 1980;303;15:833-841.

40. Marennikova SS, Shelukhina EM, Mal 'tseva, Efremova EV and Matsevich GR. Data from the serological examination of the population of the Republic of Congo for the presence of antibodies to methods and general results. [Russian] *Zhurnal Mikrobiologii, Epidemiologii i Immunobiologii* 1984 (March) 3:95-100.

41. *International Symposium on Viral Hepatitis, Milan, Dec. 1974. Develop. biol. Standard. Vol. 30*, Munich: S. Karger Basel, 1975, pp. IV;480.

42. Krugman S, Overby LR, Mushahwar IK, Ling C-M, Forsner GG and Deinhardt F. Viral hepatitis, type B: Studies on natural history and prevention reexamined. *New England Journal of Medicine* 1979;200:101-6.

43. The 20 percent difference could be explained in two ways: It may have been due to the increased sexual exposures over time that the AIDS victims possibly received, that is, the gay men had developed natural immunity to hepatitis B viruses over the same period they were incubating AIDS viruses. Such a result could have occurred from simultaneous exposures to HIV and HBV during unprotected sex or through HIV tainted hepatitis B vaccines which contained either live hepatitis B viruses or HB core antigens. The Merck vaccines allegedly carried none of the above. Yet, with the large number of gay men in New York City who received the Merck vaccine, many of whom, shortly thereafter developed AIDS, it is questionable as to why so high a number as 88 percent would have developed immunity and therefore core HB blood markers against that which the vaccine allegedly reduced by 78.3 percent (according to Szmuness[37]), that is, HB virus infections.

44. Lederer's reference is "See, generally, Pedro I. Aponte Vázques, 'Yo Acuso! Tortura y Asesinato de Don Pedro Albizu Camp[os,' (Bayamon, Puerto Rico: Movimiento Ecuménico Nacional de Puerto Rico, 1985; and Pedro I Aponte Vászquez, 'Asesino Rhoads a Albizu?' pamphlet, no date or publisher listed."

Finally, Lederer noted it was common practice for branches of the American military to develop and test weapons and then contract with private firms to mass produce the final product for international sales. Such was the case in 1966 when the Army tested a new vaccine for Venezuelan equine encephalomyelitis (VVE).

In a most bizarre release—obviously designed to promote the Army's biological weapons development program—public relations offices reported,

> after animal tests were completed, the Army began controlled testing of the new vaccine among 40 young draftees at Fort Detrick in 1962 or 1963. All of these draftees were Seventh Day Adventists, and all were conscientious objectors who, at the behest of their national church organization, had volunteered as test subjects for experiments related to biological warfare. Of the 40, about 15 suffered feverish reactions similar to VEE. Nevertheless, the vaccine conferred a solid and long-lasting immunity. In 1966, the National Drug Company, a subsidiary of Richardson-Merrell, Inc., began producing the vaccine under an Army contract.

The National Drug Company and Richardson-Merrell, Inc. were no longer in business at the time of this writing. They had apparently merged with Dow Chemical. Narayan's study was funded by "Hoechst Marion Roussel, Inc., formally known as Marion Merrell Dow Inc." See reference #59 in Chapter 8.

45. NCI staff. *The Special Virus Cancer Program: Progress Report #8*. Office of the Associate Scientific Director for Viral Oncology (OASDVO). J. B. Moloney, Ed., Washington, D. C.: U. S. Government Printing Office, 1971, pp. 185-186.

46. NCI staff. *The Special Virus Cancer Program: Progress Report #9* Office of the Associate Scientific Director for Viral Oncology (OASDVO). J. B. Moloney, Ed., Washington, D. C.: U. S. Government Printing Office, 1972, pp. 175-176.

Chapter 18. Nazi Roots of American Central Intelligence: The Biological Warfare Industry

1. Scott PD. How Allen Dulles and the SS preserved each other. *Covert Action Information Bulletin* (Winter)1986;25:4-14.

2. Scott's references on Mengele's identification was.*Washington Post*, February 15, 1985, p. A4.

3. Scott's references on the Austrian arrest of Mengele was*The Nation*, March 2, 1985, p. 231; On U. S. response to Japanese CBW activities—*Le Monde Diplomatique*, July 1983, p. 24.

4. Isaacson W. *Kissinger: A Biography*. New York: Simon & Schuster, 1992, pp. 48-49.

5. Hunt L. *Secret Agenda: Nazi Scientists, The United States Government, and Project Paperclip, 1945 to 1990.* New York: St. Martin's Press, 1991, pp. 4;145-147 (for information on General Bolling); 186 (for Naval Medical Research Institute's employment of Paperclip Nazis for biological weapons testing); and 256 (for Dow Chemical employment of convicted Nazi Otto Ambros).

6. Barbie's service as a CDC informant against French communist intelligence was documented by Linklater M. et al., *The Nazi Legacy: Klaus Barbie and the International Fascist Connection*. New York: Holt, Reinhart and Winston, 1984, pp. 163,167

7. Scott reviewed the leaks from Army intelligence during the McCarthy era as detailed by Cook FJ. *The Nightmare Decade: The Life and Times of Senator Joe McCarthy*. New York: Random House, 1971, pp. 140, 411-424.

8. On Ryan's investigation of Barbie, see United States Department of Justice Criminal Division, *Klaus Barbie and the United States Government: A Report to the Attorney General of the United States by Allan A. Ryan* (Washington: Government Printing Office, 1983) p. 146, and Linklater, *op. cit.*, pp. 180-181, 192-193.

9. On name change from "Barbie" to "Barbier," and Lee "Henry" Oswald deception, Scott credits his book—*Crime and Cover-up*. Berkeley: Westworks, 1977, p. 12.

10. Scott's footnoted that "Ishii had embarked on his experiments after a visit to prewar Nazi Germany. " His references was Seiichi Morimura, *Akuma no Hoshaku*. Tokyo: 1981.

11. Linklater, *Op. cit.*, n. 4, pp. 228; 236-237.

12. Anne Burger biography and biological warfare job description: memo, C. R. Berrens, Naval Medical Research Institute, to Chief of Naval Operations, 27 November 1950, JIOA administrative files, Navy Escape Clause, RG 330, NARS. Erich Traub biography is in Traub's JIOA dossier, RG 330, NARS.

13. NCI staff. *The Special Virus Cancer Program: Progress Report #8*. Office of the Associate Scientific Director for Viral Oncology (OASDVO). J. B. Moloney, Ed., Washington, D. C.: U. S. Government Printing Office, 1971, pp. 224; 230-232.

14. Hervet F. Knights of darkness: The Sovereign Military Order of Malta. *Covert Action Information Bulletin* (Winter)1986;25:27-38.

15. Stevenson W. *The Bormann Brotherhood*. New York: Harcourt, Brace, Jovanovich, 1973, pp. 82-85.

16. *Ibid.*, p. 227.

17. Farago L. *Aftermath: Martin Bormann and the Fourth Reich*. New York: Avon, 1975, pp. 370 (Skorzeny);187 (Rudel); 305 (Rauff); 427 (Stangl); 289 (Eichmann).

18. *Ibid.*, pp. 204-213.

19. Bower T. *Klaus Barbie: The Butcher of Lyons*. London: Granada, 1984, p. 179.

20. Stevenson, *Op. cit.*, n. 11, p. 227.

21. Farago, *Op. cit.*, n. 13, p. 220.

22. Preston Jr. W. The real treason. *CovertAction Information Bulletin* (Winter) 1986;25:23-26.

23. Higham C. *Trading With the Enemy: An Exposure of the Nazi-American Money Plot, 1933-1949*. New York: Delacorte, 1983, pp. 20-31.

24. Hervet, *Op. cit.*, 27-38.

25. Chaitkin A. Population control, Nazis, and the U.N.: Rockefeller and mass murder. Internet: Sumeria, 1996, http://www.livelinks.com/sumeria/politics/eugenics.html; see also: Kuhl S. *The Nazi Connection: Eugenics, American Racism, and German National Socialism*. Oxford: Oxford University Press, 1994.

Chapter 19. The CIA in Africa

1. Stockwell J. *In Search of Enemies: A CIA Story*. New York: W.W. Norton & Company, Inc., 1978.

2. Ray E, Schaap W, Van Meter K and Wolf L, et al. *Dirty Work-2: The CIA in Africa*. Secaucus, NJ: Lyle Stewart, Inc., 1979.

3. Woodward B. *VEIL: the Secret Wars of the CIA 1981-1987*. New York: Simon and Schuster, 1987.

4. Stockwell J., *Op. cit.*, pp. 43-44; Colby W. *Honorable Men*. New York: Simon and Schuster, 1978, pp. 439-40.

5. U.S. Congress, Senate, Select Committee to Study Government Operations with Respect to Intelligence Activities, *Final Report*: Foreign and Military Intelligence, Book I, 94th Congress, 2nd Session, April 26, 1976, p. 131.

6. Agee P. The range of covert intervention. In: *Dirty Work-2: The CIA in Africa*. Secaucus, Ray E, Schaap W, Van Meter K and Wolf L eds. Secaucus, NJ: Lyle Stewart, Inc., 1979, pp. 47-49.

7. Rockefeller NA, Connor JT, Dillon CD, Griswold EN, Reagan R, and Kirkland, et al. *Report to the President by the Commission on CIA Activities Within the United States..* New York: The Rockefeller Commission, 1975, p. 211.

8. Schechter D, Ansara M and Kolodney D. The CIA as an equal opportunity employer. In: *Dirty Work-2: The CIA in Africa*. Secaucus, Ray E, Schaap W, Van Meter K and Wolf L eds. Secaucus, NJ: Lyle Stewart, Inc., 1979, p. 53.

9. Molteno R. Hidden sources of subversion. In: *Dirty Work-2: The CIA in Africa*. Secaucus, Ray E, Schaap W, Van Meter K and Wolf L eds. Secaucus, NJ: Lyle Stewart, Inc., 1979, pp. 100-101.

10. Center for National Security Studies. *The Consequences of "Pre-publication Review" A Case Study of CIA Censorship of The CIA and the Cult of Intelligence.*, CNSS Report No. 109. Washington, D. C.: Center for National Security Studies, September, 1983, p. ii.

11. Kissinger H. Congress and the U. S. Intelligence Community. Speech made before the Senate Committee on Government Operations on February 5, 1976. *Department of State Bulletin*, March 1, 1976, pp. 274-277

12. Nixon R. U. S. foreign policy for the 1970's: Shaping a durable peace. A report to the Congress by the President of the United States, May 3, 1973. *The Department of State Bulletin*. Volume LXVIII, No. 1771, June 4, 1973, pp. 794-798.

13. Williams MJ. Report to President Nixon by the Deputy Administrator of the Agency for International Development and the President's Special Coordinator for Emergency Relief to Sub-Sahara Africa. AID press release 73-76 dated October 23, 1973. *Department of State Bulletin*, November 26, 1973, pp. 669-671.)

14. Uganda Radio. CIA accused of plot to assassinate Amin. *Africa Diary* July 23-29,1978, p. 9103.

15. Bourderie J. A tough little monkey. In: *Dirty Work-2: The CIA in Africa.* Secaucus, Ray E, Schaap W, Van Meter K and Wolf L eds. Secaucus, NJ: Lyle Stewart, Inc., 1979, p. 211; Woodward, *Op. cit.*, pp. 139, 179;

16. Bourderie J. *Ibid.*, p. 213.

17. World Health Organization. Smallpox in 1974. *WHO Chronicle* 1975;29:134-139; Strecker R. The Strecker Memorandum: The Cause, The Effects and the Possible Cure for the Pandemic AIDS. Eagle Rock, CA: The Strecker Group, 1988.

18. Department of State. *Report on the Health, Population and Nutrition Activities of the Agency for International Development for Fiscal Years 1973 and 1974.* Washington, D.C., U. S. Government Printing Office, 1975.

19. According to Bob Woodward, "CIA ties with Mobutu dated back to 1960, the year the CIA [and Sidney Gottlieb] had planned the assassination of the Congolese nationalist leader Partice Lumumba. An August 25, 1960, cable to the CIA station chief from then DCI Allen Dulles stated that Lumumba's 'removal must be an urgent and prime objective and that under existing conditions this should be a high priority of our covert action.' Before the CIA plot could be effected, Lumumba was murdered by another group of Mobutu supporters. [CIA Director William] Casey had an important, personal relationship with Mobutu, and now [in 1983 during the Reagan Administration] they exchanged intelligence." Reference is Woodward, *Op. cit.*, pg. 268.

20. Staff reporter. Secretary Kissinger interviewed for *CBS-TV Evening News*. *Department of State Bulletin*, July 14, 1975, pp. 63-64.

21. Jeffreys-Jones R. *American Espionage: From Secret Service to CIA.* The Free Press, 1977, p. 5.

22. *U.S. Select Senate Committee to Study Governmental Operations with Respect to Intelligence Activities. Intelligence Activities. Senate Resolution 21. Vol. 1: Unauthorized Storage of Toxic Agents. September 16-18, 1975.* Cong. Sess. 94-1.

23. Kissinger H. Secretary Kissinger testifies on security assistance program. Statement Before House Committee on International Relations. *Department of State Bulletin*, November 24, 1975, pp. 742-748.

24. Goswami PK. CIA: *40 Inglorious Years (1947-1987)* Calcutta: Firma KLM Private Limited, 1989, pp 107-109.

25. Prados J. *President's Secret Wars: CIA and Pentagon Covert Operations From World War II Through IRANSCAM.* New York: Quill, William Morrow, 1986, pp. 339-340.

26. Kissinger H. Implications of Angola for future U. S. foreign policy. Speech made before the Subcommittee on African Affairs of the Senate Committee on Foreign Relations on January 29, 1976. *Department of State Bulletin*, February 16, 1976, pp. 174-182.

27. Weissman S. Zaire, OTRAG, and Angola: The CIA and U.S. Policy in Zaire and Angola. In: *Dirty Work-2: The CIA in Africa.* Secaucus, Ray E, Schaap W, Van Meter K and Wolf L eds. Secaucus, NJ: Lyle Stewart, Inc., 1979, pp. 183-207.

28. Stockwell, *Op. cit.*, letter is reproduced in appendix section of his book as it appeared in *The Washington Post*, April 10, 1977.

29. Weissman, *Op. cit.*, as referenced—*Times of Zambia*, March 21, 1977.

Chapter 20. OTRAG: Links to NATO, NASA, Nazis, the NCI and AIDS

1. Moscow World Service in English. Belitskiy on How, Where AIDS Virus Originated. March 11, 1988. Published in *International Affairs*. FBIS-SOV-88-049, March 14, 1988, p. 24.

2. Covert N. *Cutting Edge: A history of Fort Detrick, Maryland 1943-1993*. U.S. Army Garrison Public Affairs Office (HSHD-PA), Fort Detrick, MD., p. 54.

3. Informationsdienst Südliches Africa. OTRAG: Missiles against liberation in Africa. In: *Dirty Work-2: The CIA in Africa*. Secaucus, Ray E, Schaap W, Van Meter K and Wolf L eds. Secaucus, NJ: Lyle Stewart, Inc., 1979, pp. 215-219; Gesellschaft für Unternehmendberatung, Hamburg, 1976, Diagnosebericht OTRAG, p. 12.; *Der Spiegel*, August 4, 1978; The Evening Standard, February 13, 1978; Deutscher Bundestag, 8th Session, 98th Sitting, June 15, 1978, 11; *Aviation Week and Space Technology*, September 12, 1975.

4. Hussain F. Volksraketen for the Third World: A cheap rocket that could launch military reconnaissance satellites for developing countries has become involved in a tangled web of Nazi rocket scientists, *Penthouse* magazine, KGB disinformation, and a treaty reminiscent of the height of colonialism in Africa. *New Scientist* 1978 (March 23);77:802-803.

5. Brumter C. *The North Atlantic Assemby*. Dordrecth: Martinus Nijhoff Publishers, 1986, pp. 173-175.

6. Bennett, Jr. WT. U.S. reviews international cooperation in space activities and work of the U. N. Outer Space Committee in 1976. *Department of State Bulletin*, November 29, 1976, pp. 668-673.

7. *World Aviation Directory*. Germany: Messerschmitt-Bölkow-Blohm GmbH (MBB). Corporate listing under "Foreign Countries, Section, V-4400, Summer, 1979, pp. 1294-1295.

8. Preston Jr. W. The real treason. *Covert Action Information Bulletin* (Winter) 1986;25:23-26.

9. U. S. Government Press release 89 dated March 8, 1974. U. S. and Germany Discuss Cooperation in Science and Technology R. & D. *Department of State Bulletin*, March 25, 1974, pp. 300-301.

10. Hermann K. Klaus Barbie: A killer's career. *Covert Action Information Bulletin* (Winter) 1986;25:20.

11. Gallo RC, Sarin PS, Allen, PT, Newton WA, Priori ES, Bowen JM and Dmochowski L. Reverse Transcriptase in Type C Virus Particles of Human Origin. *Nature New Biology* 1971;232;140-142.

12. The *Who Chronicle* reported, "the present cooperation with investigators using primates in cancer studies is to be continued. . . . It should be reemphasized that there is a very practical, important side to this programme. Recent outbreaks of human and simian disease in several centres handling simians indicate that these animals are responsible for the transmission of the etiological agents. It is highly probable that more such incidents can be expected..." The reference is— Kalter SS and Heberling. The study of simian viruses. *WHO Chronicle* 1969;23;3:112-117.

13. *Department of Defense Appropriations For 1970: Hearings Before A Subcommittee of the Committee on Appropriations House of Representatives, Ninety-first Contress, First Session, H.B. 15090, Part 5, Research, Development, Test and Evaluation, Dept. of the Army*. U.S. Government Printing Office, Washington, D.C., 1969.

14. Litton Industries, Inc. Annual Report to the Securities and Exchange Commission for Fiscal Year Ended July 31, 1976. Commission file number 1-3998. Securities and Exchange Commission, Office of Reports, November 1, 1976.

15. Litton Industries, Inc. Annual Report to the Securities and Exchange Commission for Fiscal Year Ended July 31, 1977. Commission file number 1-3998. Securities and Exchange Commission, Office of Reports, October 31, 1977.

16. Litton Industries, Inc. Annual Report to the Securities and Exchange Commission for Fiscal Year Ended July 31, 1978. Commission file number 1-3998. Securities and Exchange Commission, Office of Reports, October 30, 1978.

17. Pan American/World Health Organization. *Proceedings of the International Conference on the Application of Vaccines Agasint Viral, Rickettsial, and Bacterial Diseases of Man*. December 14-18, 1970. Scientific Publication No. 226. Washington D.C.: World Health Organization, 1971, pp. 602-604; See also, USPHS/NCI Staff. *Special Virus Cancer Program: Progress Report #8*. J. B. Moloney, ed., Bethesda: USPHS NCI, 1971. Univ. North Carolina, Davies Library call number #HE 20.3152:V81, pp. ;21-26;104.

18. Rose LF and Kaye D. *Internal Medicine for Dentistry*. St. Louis: C. V. Mosby Company, 1983, pp. 131-132.

19. Kissinger H. Secretary Kissinger testifies on security assistance program. Statement Before House Committee on International Relations. *Department of State Bulletin*, November 24, 1975, pp. 742-748.; Kissinger H. Implications of Angola for future U.S. foreign policy. Speech made before the Subcommittee on African Affairs of the Senate Committee on Foreign Relations on January 29, 1976. *Department of State Bulletin*, February 16, 1976, pp. 174-182.; Kissinger H. Congress and the U. S. Intelligence Community. Speech made before the Senate Committee on Government Operations on February 5, 1976. *Department of State Bulletin*, March 1, 1976, pp. 274-277.

20. Williams MJ. Sahel African disaster relief and recovery assistance: Text of a Report for the President. *Department of State Bulletin*, November 26, 1973, pp. 669-673.; Nixon R. U.S. foreign policy for the 1970's: Shaping a durable peace. A report to the Congress by the President of the United States, May 3, 1973. *The Department of State Bulletin*. Volume LXVIII, No. 1771, June 4, 1973, pp. 794-798.; Newsom DD. African development and U. S. Foreign Policy. Speech made before the annual meeting of the African Studies Association at Syracuse, N.Y., on Nov. 2, 1997. *Department of State Bulletin*, December 31, 1973, p. 789.

21. State Department Staff. International cooperation in space. *Department of State Bulletin* August 26, 1974, pp. 326-329.

22. Litton Industries Press Release. Litton Industries Unit Gets Job. *Wall Street Journal*, Thursday, September 15, 1977, p. 4.

23. Litton Industries Press Release. Litton Industries awarded $19.8 million Army contract for missile fire-control equipment. *Wall Street Journal*, Monday, December 19, 1977, p. 21.

24. Litton Industries Press Release. Litton Industries awarded $32.9 million Air Force contract for electronic reconnaissance sensor equipment. *Wall Street Journal*, Friday, December 30, 1977, p. 6.

25. Litton Industries Press Release. Litton Industries Gets Order. *Wall Street Journal*, Tuesday, February 14, 1978, p. 33.

26. Staff Reporter. Litton Industries Gets $40 mil NATO Computerized Satcom Systems Order. *Wall Street Journal*. March 8, 1976, p. 12.; See also: Robertson J. Litton awarded 40m NATO contract. *Electron N*, March 8, 1976 Vol. 21, p. 42.*Iron Age*, May 10, 1976, p. 25.

27. Staff reporter. NATO seeks Phase 3 satellite proposals. *Aviation Weekly*, Vol. 95, August 23, 1971, p. 58; See also NATO modifies defense plans in S. Africa case. *Aviation Weekly*, Vol. 108, January 2, 1978, pp. 22-23.

28. Staff reporter. Siemens buys Boeing's 12% share in Messerschmitt-Boelkow. *Aviation Week*, July 17, 1978, p. 23.; See also, *Financial Times*, July 12, 1978, p. 22.

29. Staff reporter. Teledyne increases stake of Litton to about 20%; Teledyne boosts stake in Litton Industries from 22% to 27%. *Wall Street Journal*. May 12, 1977, p. 25., and December 11, 1978, p. 27.

30. Staff reporter. Grummann Aerospace subcontracts for Teledyne navigational computer and signal data converters. *Elec. News*, August 8, 1977, p. 24.

31. Staff reporter. Grumman Aerospace seeks $1 bil NATO radar-reconnaissance military aircraft deal. *Business Week*, April 18, 1977 p. 46.

32. Staff reporter. Court lets stand an indictment of Litton Unit. *Wall Street Journal*, Tuesday, October 3, 1978, p. 4.

33. Staff reporter. Suit against Litton may be renewed, says U. S. Appeals Court. *Wall Street Journal*, Friday, April 7, 1978, p. 12.

34. Staff reporter. Litton and Navy settle dispute over ship orders: Accord is to be reviewed by Congress; firm faces a loss of $200 million. *Wall Street Journal*, Wednesday, June 21, 1978, p. 4.

35. *Who's Who in America*, 49th Edition, Volume 1, A-K. New Providence, NJ., 1995, p.123.

36. For Nazis employed by the Navy to conduct cancer virus experiments, see: Hunt L. *Secret Agenda: Nazi Scientists, The United States Government, and Project Paperclip, 1945 to 1990*. New York: St. Martin's Press, 1991, pp. 186.

37. For U.S. Navy viral research program see: NCI staff. *The Special Virus Cancer Program: Progress Report #8*. Office of the Associate Scientific Director for Viral Oncology (OASDVO). J. B. Moloney, Ed., Washington, D. C.: U. S. Government Printing Office, 1971, p. 224.

38. For combined U.S. Navy and University of California program see: NCI staff. *The Special Virus Cancer Program: Progress Report #9* Office of the Associate Scientific Director for Viral Oncology (OASDVO). J. B. Moloney, Ed., Washington, D. C.: U. S. Government Printing Office, 1972, pp. 197-198.

Chapter 21. Marburg, Ebola and Chilling Propaganda in *The Hot Zone*

1. Johnson KM, Webb, PA, Lange JV and Murphy F. Isolation and partial characterization of a new virus causing acute hemorrhagic fever in Zaire. *Lancet*, 1977, March 12, 569-571. Summarized in: *Tropical Diseases Bulletin*, October, 1977, p. 900.

2. Herrera F, Adamson RH and Gallo RC. Uptake of transfer ribonucleic acid by normal and leukemic cells. *Proc Nat Acad Sci* 1970;67;4:1943-1950.

3. Siegert, R. *Marburg Virus*. New York: Springer-Verlag, 1972, pp. 98-100.

4. *Ibid.*, pp. 143-147.

5. Simpson DIH. *Marburg and Ebola Virus Infections: A Guide for their Diagnosis, Management, and Control.* Geneva: World Health Organization, Pub. No. 36.,1977, pp. 5-28.

6. NIAID Task Force. "The Evolution of Viruses". In: U. S. Department of Health, Education and Welfare. *Virology: NIAID Task Force Report*, Volume 2, Acute Viral Infections. Washington, D. C.: U. S. Government Printing Office, (NIH) 79-1832, 1979, pp. 155-160.

7. Gallo RC, Hecht SM, Whang-Peng J and O'Hopp S. N^6-(^{2}-Isopentenyl) Adenosine: The Regulatory Effects of a Cytokinin and Modified Nucleoside From tRNA on Human Lymphocytes. *Biochimica Et Biophysica Acta* 1972; 281:488-500.

8. NIAID Task Force, *Op. cit.*, p. 155.

9. *Ibid.*, p. 157

10. *Ibid.*, p. 159.

11. Preston R. *The Hot Zone*. New York: Random House, 1994, pp. 25-27.

12. Horowitz L. *Deadly Innocence: Solving The Greatest Murder Mystery in the History of American Medicine*. Rockport, MA: Tetrahedron, Inc., 1994,

13. Fine DL and Arthur LO. Prevalence of natural immunity to Type-D and Type-C Retroviruses in primates. In: *Viruses in Naturally Occurring Cancers: Book B*. Myron Essex, George Todaro and Harald zur Hausen, eds., Cold Spring Harbor, NY: Cold Spring Harbor Laboratory, 1980, Vol. 7, pp. 793-813; See also: Gallo RC, Wong-Staal F, Marhkam PD, Ruscetti R, Kalyanaraman VS, Ceccherini-Nelli L, Favera RD, Josephs S, Miller NR and Reitz, Jr MS. Recent studies with infectious primate retroviruses: Hybridization to primate DNA and some biological effects on fresh human blood leukocytes by simian sarcoma virus and Gibbon ape leukemia virus. *Ibid.*.

14. *Department of Defense Appropriations For 1970: Hearings Before A Subcommittee of the Committee on Appropriations House of Representatives, Ninety-first Contress, First Session, H.B. 15090, Part 5, Research, Development, Test and Evaluation, Dept. of the Army*. U.S. Government Printing Office, Washington, D.C., 1969.

15. Senate hearings on "Chemical and Biological Warfare." *Congressional Record*, Washington, D.C.: U. S. Government Printing Office. August 8, 1969, p. 23074.

16. Preston R. *Ob. cit.*, p. 31.

17. Cook R. *Outbreak*. New York: Berkeley Books, 1986.

18. Preston R. *Op. cit.*, p. 110; and Garrett L. *The Coming Plague* , New York: Penguin Books, 1994, pp. 598-599.

19. *Ibid.* p. 152.

20. Besides Litton Bionetics, another documented DOD biological weapons contractor, being cited as the major funding source for some of Gallo's experiments was Hazleton Laboratory in Vienna, Va. which participated in "The Special Virus Cancer Program" administered by the NCI. Hazleton supplied Rausher leukemia viruses for Gallo's studies. This is noteworthy as Hazleton's (Reston, Virginia) monkey facility was the site of the frightening Ebola-like virus outbreak in December, 1989. Nowhere in Richard Preston's best seller *The Hot Zone* was Hazleton mentioned as an actual supplier of RNA tumor viruses. In fact, Preston alleged the deadly viruses came from either the Philippines or Africa. See: Wu AM, Ting RCY and Gallo RC. RNA-Directed DNA Polymerase and Virus-Induced Leukemia in Mice. *Proceedings of the National Academy of Sciences* 1973;70;5:1298-1302.

21. Preston, *Op. cit.*, p. 44-46.

22. *Ibid.* p. 68-71.

23. Herrera F, Adamson RH and Gallo RC. Uptake of transfer ribonucleic acid by normal and leukemic cells. *Proc. Nat. Acad. Sci.* 1970;67;4:1943-1950.

24. *U.S. Select Senate Committee to Study Governmental Operations with Respect to Intelligence Activities. Intelligence Activities. Senate Resolution 21. Vol. 1: Unauthorized Storage of Toxic Agents. September 16-18, 1975.* Cong. Sess. 5-7; See also: Agee P. The range of covert intervention. In: *Dirty*

Work-2: The CIA in Africa. Secaucus, Ray E, Schaap W, Van Meter K and Wolf L eds. Secaucus, NJ: Lyle Stewart, Inc., 1979, pp. 47-49.

25. Preston, *Ob cit*, p. 78.

26. *Ibid.*, pp. 83-84.

27. Kissinger H. Secretary Kissinger testifies on security assistance program. Statement Before House Committee on International Relations. *Department of State Bulletin*, November 24, 1975, pp. 742-748; See also: Kissinger H. Implications of Angola for future U. S. foreign policy. Speech made before the Subcommittee on African Affairs of the Senate Committee on Foreign Relations on January 29, 1976. *Department of State Bulletin*, February 16, 1976, pp. 174-182; Goswami PK. CIA: *40 Inglorious Years (1947-1987)* Calcutta: Firma KLM Private Limited, 1989, pp 107-109; and Prados J. *President's Secret Wars: CIA and Pentagon Covert Operations From World War II Through IRANSCAM*. New York: Quill, William Morrow, 1986, pp. 339-340.

28. USAID. *A report on loans and grants from abroad for Congo (Kinshasa). June, 1969. Revision No. 256, April 1971*. Washington: U. S. Government Printing Office, 1971 p. 11(112).

29. Stockwell J. *In Search of Enemies: A CIA Story*. New York: W.W. Norton & Company, Inc., 1978, pp. 43-44; Colby W. *Honorable Men*. New York: Simon and Schuster, 1978, pp. 439-40.

30. *West Africa, London*. Zaire: Mobutu and the Americans. *Africa Diary* February 19-25, 1975 p. 7322.

31. *Daily News, Dar es Salaam; West Africa, London*. Zaire: Mobutu's Radicalism. *Africa Diary* February 12-18, 1975 p. 7310-11.

32. Staff reporter. Secretary Kissinger interviewed for *CBS-TV Evening News*. *Department of State Bulletin*, July 14, 1975, pp. 63-64.

Chapter 22. The Special Virus Cancer Program

1. NCI staff. *The Special Virus Cancer Program: Progress Report #8*. Office of the Associate Scientific Director for Viral Oncology (OASDVO). J. B. Moloney, Ed., Washington, D. C.: U. S. Government Printing Office, 1971. Note: This is a very hard publication to find. Few library data bases have it listed, including the NCI Library at Fort Detrick. It is available through the Davis Library, The University of North Carolina, Chapel Hill, Government Documents Department Depository, Reference # HE 20.3152:V81.

2. Bionetics Research Laboratories, Inc., A Division of Litton Industries. Progress report on investigation of carcinogenesis with selected virus preparations in the newborn monkey. *Ibid..*, pp. 273-278; See page 276 for *Cercopithecus aethiops* acknowledgment.

3. NCI staff. *The Special Virus Cancer Program: Progress Report #9* Office of the Associate Scientific Director for Viral Oncology (OASDVO). J. B. Moloney, Ed., Washington, D. C.: U. S. Government Printing Office, 1972.

4. NCI staff, 1971, *Op. cit.*, pp. 2-10.

5. *Ibid.*, 15-19; 20-26.

6. Goldman BA and Chappelle M. Is HIV=AIDS wrong? *In These Times*. August 5-18, 1992, pp. 8-10.

7. See the following Gallo *et al.*, publications: Gallaher RE, Ting RC and Gallo RC. A common change aspartyl-tRNA in polyoma and SV transformed cells. *Biochimica Et Biophysica Acta* 1972;272:568-582.; Bobrow SN, Smith RG, Reitz MS and Gallo RC. Stimulated normal human lymphocytes contain a ribonuclease-sensitive DNA polymerase distinct from viral RNA-directed DNA polymerase. *Proceedings National Academy of Sciences* 1972;69;11:3228-3232; Robert MS, Smith RG, Gallo RC, Sarin PS and Abrell JW. Viral and cellular DNA polymerase: Comparison of activities with synthetic and natural RNA templates. *Science* 1972;176:798-800.

8. NCI staff, 1971, *Op. cit.*, pp. 22-23.

9. Ting RC, Yang SS and Gallo RC. Reverse transcriptase, RNA tumor virus transformation and derivatives of Rifamycin SV. *Nature New Biology* 1972;236:163-165.

10. NCI staff, 1971, *Op. cit.*, pp. 24-26.

11. Litton Industries, Inc. Annual Report to the Securities and Exchange Commission for Fiscal Year Ended July 31, 1977. Commission file number 1-3998. Securities and Exchange Commission, Office of Reports, October 31, 1977.

12. Gallo R. *Recent Advances in Cancer Research: Cell Biology, Molecular Biology, and Tumor Virology, Volume I*. Cleveland: CRC Press, Inc., 1977; In 1971 EBV was also studied by Gallo and coworkers. See Fujioka S and Gallo RC. Aminoacyl Transfer RNA Profiles in Human Myeloma Cells. *Blood* 1971; 38;2:246-252.

13. Litton Industries, Inc. Annual Report to the Securities and Exchange Commission for Fiscal Year Ended July 31, 1978. Commission file number 1-3998. Securities and Exchange Commission, Office of Reports, October 30, 1978.

14. NCI staff, 1971, *Op. cit.*, pp. 27-31.

15. *Ibid.*, pp. 35-59.

16. Shilts R. *And the Band Played On: Politics, People and the AIDS Epidemic.* New York: Penguin Books, 1987, pp. 73-74.

17. NCI staff, 1971, *Op. cit.*, 63-271.

18. *Ibid.*, p. 104; 187 and NCI staff, 1972, *Op. cit.*, pp. 195-196;326. The complete title of the later study was "Investigation of the Carcinogenic Activity of Selected Virus Preparation in the Newborn Monkey."

19. NCI staff, 1971, *Op. cit.*, 111;139-141. The Merck and Company, Inc. study title: "Study of Viruses in Human and Animal Neoplasia," was actually an abridged title. The complete title was much more revealing. It was, "Research on Oncogenic and Potentially Oncogenic Viruses, Large-scale Virus Production and Vaccine Development." See also *Ibid.*, p. 373.

20. NCI staff, *Op. cit.*,1972, 324.

21. NCI staff, *Op. cit.*,1971, 257-258.

22. NCI staff, *Op. cit.*,1972, 130-131; spelled Hazleton on page 407 with the same grant number (69-2079).

23. NCI staff, *Op. cit.*,1971, p. 100.

24. *Ibid.*, p. 187; See also 68 and 362. The contract summary, produced by Robert Ting at Bionetics, and reviewed by NCI officers George Todaro, Paul Levine, and Robert Bassin—all Gallo co-authors—described their EBV studies conducted "under the supervision of Dr. Paul Levine." This contract, they said, provided "opportunity for systematic, large-scale effort to detect viruses or viral antigens in human or animal materials using tissue culture, immunological, biochemical and EM techniques."

Chapter 23. The Man-Made Origin of Marburg and Ebola

1. The practice of experimentally injecting monkey blood into humans initially carried out by Dr. Alexander S. Wiener at the Laboratory for Experimental Medicine and Surgery in Primates and simultaneously at the New York University Medical Center. See: Moor-Jankowski J. Blood groups of apes and monkeys; Human and simian types. In: *Research Animals in Medicine: National Heart and Lung Institute National Institutes of Health*, Lowell T. Harmison, ed. Washington, DC: U. S. Department of Health, Education and Welfare, Public Health Service, National Institutes of Health, DHEW Publication No. (NIH) 72-333, October 2, 1973, pp. 483-488.

2. NCI staff. *The Special Virus Cancer Program: Progress Report #8.* Office of the Associate Scientific Director for Viral Oncology (OASDVO). J. B. Moloney, Ed., Washington, D. C.: U. S. Government Printing Office, 1971. pp. 187; See also 68 and 362.

3. Higginson J and Muir CS. Epidemiologic Program of the International Agency for Research on Cancer (IARC). In: *The National Cancer Program and International Cancer Research.*, *National Cancer Institute Monograph* 1974; 40: 63-70.

4. Fine DL and Arthur LO. Prevalence of natural immunity to Type-D and Type-C Retroviruses in primates. In: *Viruses in Naturally Occurring Cancers: Book B.* Myron Essex, George Todaro and Harald zur Hausen, eds., Cold Spring Harbor, NY: Cold Spring Harbor Laboratory, 1980, Vol. 7, pp. 793-813; See also: Gallo RC, Wong-Staal F, Marhkam PD, Ruscetti R, Kalyanaraman VS, Ceccherini-Nelli L, Favera RD, Josephs S, Miller NR and Reitz, Jr MS. Recent studies with infectious primate retroviruses: Hybridization to primate DNA and some biological effects on fresh human blood leukocytes by simian sarcoma virus and Gibbon ape leukemia virus. *Ibid.*.

5. NCI staff, 1971, *Op. cit.*, pp. 104; 187. See also NCI staff. *The Special Virus Cancer Program: Progress Report #8.* Office of the Associate Scientific Director for Viral Oncology (OASDVO). J. B. Moloney, Ed., Washington, D. C.: U. S. Government Printing Office, 1972, pp. 195-196;326.

6. NCI staff, 1971, *Op. cit.*, 111;139-141.

7. Bionetics Research Laboratories, Inc., A Division of Litton Industries. Progress report on investigation of carcinogenesis with selected virus preparations in the newborn monkey. *Ibid.*, p. 273-278.

8. NCI staff, 1971, *Op. cit.*, pp. 224-225;376. Here an NCI contract given to the Naval Biological Laboratory in Oakland, California is described. The NCI project officer, and Chairman of Biohazards Control and Containment Segment of the SVCP, Dr. Alfred Hellman, had to have worked closely with Bionetics's NCI administrators. It is also very likely he held lengthy meetings with Robert Manaker

who was intimately connected to Gallo's group of Bionetics researchers as well as Hilleman's group at Merck. Hellman oversaw numerous co-carcinogen studies for the Navy and most plausibly the Army too.

9. Litton Industries, Inc. Annual Report to the Securities and Exchange Commission for Fiscal Year Ended July 31, 1978. Commission file number 1-3998. Securities and Exchange Commission, Office of Reports, October 30, 1978, p. 16.

10. According to physician author Samuel Epstein, Litton Bionetics was contracted by the NCI from 1963 to 1969 to conduct carcinogenicity tests on "approximately 140 industrial compounds and pesticides, selected because of strong suspicions of carcinogenicity. . . ." Bionetics tested the substances at "maximally tolerated doses in two strains of mice," and reported that less than 10 percent of test chemicals were carcinogenic. Epstein argued convincingly that Bionetics had been effectively lobbied and/or paid to produce or censor findings on behalf of numerous chemical firms including "Dow, Du Pont, Rohm and Haas, and Esso Research in addition to the Manufacturing Chemists Association and the Synthetic Organic Chemical Manufacturers Association," Shell Chemical Company, and Velsicol Chemical Company. See: Epstein SS. *The Politics of Cancer.* Garden City, NY: Anchor Books, 1979 pp. 306-307.

11. Preston R. *The Hot Zone.* New York: Random House, 1994.

12. Garrett L. *The Coming Plague: Newly Emerging Diseases in a World Out of Balance.* New York: Penguin Books, 1994, pp. 371-81.

13. Siegert, R. *Marburg Virus.* New York: Springer-Verlag, 1972, pp. 98-100.

14. Kotin P, Falk HL and McCammon CJ. The experimental induction of pulmonary tumors and changes in the respiratory epithelium in C57BL mice following their exposure to an atmosphere of ozonized gasoline. *Cancer* 1958;11:3:473-489.

15. Jurgelski Jr. W, Forsythe W, Dahl D, Thomas Ld, Moore JA, Kotin P, Falk HL and Vogel FS. The opossum as a biomedical model. II. Breeding the opossum in captivity: Facility design. *Laboratory Animal Science* 1974;24;2:404-411.

16. Kotin P. Standards in the workplace: Crisis, crusade or crucible? *Journal of Occupational Medicine* 1979;21;8:557-561.

17. Simmons ML. *Biohazards and Zoonotic Problems of Primate Procurement, Quarantine and Research: Proceedings of a Cancer Research Safety Symposium.* March 19, 1975, Conducted at the Frederick Cancer Research Center, Frederick, Maryland. DHEW Publication No. (NIH) 76-890, pp. 27; 50-52.

18. *Hearings before the Subcommittee on Health and Scientific Research of the Committee on Human Resources, United States Senate, Ninety-fifth Congress, First Session, on Examination of Serious Deficiencies in the Defense Department's Efforts to Protect the Human Subjects of Drug Research, Biological Testing Involving Human Subjects by the Department of Defense.* Washington, D.C.: U.S. Government Printing Office, March 8 and May 23, 1977, pp. 125-127.

Chapter 24. Ebola Kikwit and the Sloan/Hot Zone/Plague Connections

1. Altman L. Scientists investigate deadly viral outbreak in Zaire. *New York Times*, May 10, 1995, p. 1.

2. ABC News. Ebola. *Nightline* special report with Ted Kopel. Wednesday, May 10, 1995.

3. Arnot B. *CBS Evening News* with Dan Rather and Connie Chung. Ebola outbreak in Zaire. Thursday, May 11, 1995.

4. Ms. Garrett, telephoned at *Newsday* and in Manhattan for an interview, was unavailable for comment, and never returned my calls. Her book, *The Coming Plague* (Penguin Books, 1994), however, discusses these revelations on pages 33, 56, 595, 602 and 729.

5. Cowley G, Contreras J, Rogers A, Lach J, Dickey C and Raghavan S. Killer virus: Beyond the Ebola scare—What else is out there? *Newsweek* May 22, 1995, pp. 48-55.

6. Painter K. Trying to stop scariest microbes: But 'with an outbreak like (Ebola) they should have their own airplanes.' *USA Today* May 19-21, 1995, pp. A1-2.

7. Altman LK. Deadly virus still spreads in Zaire. *New York Times* May 11, 1995, p. A6.

8. O'Neill P. Dow Corning action riles women. *The Portland Oregonian* May 16, 1995, pp. A1;A5.

9. Hazleton RA. Junk science and the American economy. Speech before The Conference of The Manhattan Institute on Junk Science and the Courts, Washington, D.C., June 12, 1995. Reprint kindly provided by the media relations office of Dow Corning Corporation.

10. Personal communication with Dr. James Watson, Director of The Medical–Legal Foundation, 1564 A Fitzgerald Drive, Suite 240, Pinole, CA, 94564. Telephone: 510-222-9466; Fax: 510-222-0158.

11. *CBS Evening News* with Dan Rather and Connie Chung. "Reality Check: The Government's PR Machine.", September 7, 1993.

12. CBS News. Watergate: The secret story CBS News special program. June 17, 1992. Available through Burrelle's Information Services.

13. Editorial staff. Rather blunt. *The Spotlight*. December 6, 1993, p1.

14. Demac DD. *Keeping America Uninformed*. New York: The Pilgrim Press, 1984, pp. 91-92.

15. Covert Action Information Bulletin. Turner's "Born Again" CIA. In: *Dirty Work: The CIA in Western Europe*. P. Agee and L. Wolf, eds. Secaucus, NJ: Lyle Stuart Inc., 1977, pp. 313.

16. Gill K. Doctor ties gulf war illness to anti-chemical pills. *USA Today*. Thursday, March 28, 1996, p. 6A.

17. Fitz R. Gulf War G.I.s poisoned by American germ weapons: Scientist blows lid off huge govt. cover-up. *National Enquirer*, April 2, 1996, pp. 26-27.

18. Nicolson GL and Rosenberg-Nicolson NL. Doxycycline treatment and Desert Storm. (Letter to the editor) *JAMA* 1995;273;8:618-619.

19. Nicolson GL, Hyman E, Korenyi-Both A, Lopez DA, Nicolson N, Rea W, and Urnovitz H. Progress on Persian Gulf War illnesses—Reality and hypotheses. *International Journal of Occupational Medicine and Toxicology* 1995;4;3:1 In press galley copy

20. CBS News. Evening News with Dan Rather reporting on "Texas Southwest medical center studies on Gulf War chemical cocktail." Tuesday, April 16, 1996.

21. Schaap B. Deceit and secrecy: Cornerstones of U.S. Policy. *Covert Action Information Bulletin* 1982;16:24-31.

22. Arenson KW. Grants by foundations help technology books make it to the shelves. *New York Times*, Monday, August 21, 1995, p. D5.

23. Starr P. *The Social Transformation of American Medicine: The rise of a sovereign profession and the making of a vast industry*. New York: Basic Books, 1982, pp. 342-343.

24. Alfred P. Sloan Foundation: Report for 1967, pp. 2-6; for population control program see p. 79.

25. Keele HM and Kiger JC. *Foundations: The Greenwood Encyclopedia of American Institutions*. London: Greenwood Press, 1982, pp. 8-9; for early history of the Sloan Foundation see pp. 6-7.

26. A. P. Sloan Foundation, Op. cit., pp. 3;53-55; Alfred P. Sloan Foundation: Report for 1973, p. 46.

27. Alfred P. Sloan Foundation: Report for 1969, pp. 70-71; for Council on Foreign Relations funding see p. 57.; Alfred P. Sloan Foundation: Report for 1970, pp. 36;62-63.

28. A. P. Sloan Foundation Report for 1967, p. 79

29. Lawrence S. Rockefeller was cited in this manner in all annual Sloan Foundation reports reviewed.

30. *Who's Who in Finance and Industry, 17th edition, 1972-1973*. Chicago: Marquis Who's Who, Inc., 1973.

31. The Sloan Foundation's "Schedule of Marketable Securities" was listed in each annual report. References to Chase Manhattan Bank and Merck & Co., Inc. stocks are found as described in text.

Chapter 25. Smoking Guns and Conclusions

1. Walgate R. Hepatitis B vaccine: Pasteur Institute in AIDS fracas. *Nature* July 14,1983 Volume 304, pg. 104.

2. Guisnel J. Open Hunting Season on Intelligence at Bourget: Le Bourget, CIA, DGSE, Economic Spying Viewed published in Paris *Libération* in French on June 14, 1993, p. 10; and in English in *Government International News Reports*, FRANCE—FBIS-WEU-93-124, June 30, 1993, p. 19.

3. Javanovic P. Dassault and GIAT, Targets of the CIA. First published in Paris Le Quotidien De Paris in French on May 24, 1993, p. 7, and later in *Governments News Documents* FRANCE—FBIS-WEU-93-102, May 28, 1993, pg. 27.

4. Shorter E. *The Health Century: A companion to the PBS television series*. New York: Doubleday, 1987, pp. 67-69; 195-204, and acknowledgments page.

5. Dr. John Martin's address is: 1634 Spruce Street, South Pasadena, CA, 91030, Telephone: 818-799-4500; Fax: 818-799-1700. Dr. Martin requested credit for his copy of the Shorter/Hilleman tape be given to Dr. James Watson of The Medical–Legal Foundation in Pinole, CA.

6. Maurice Hilleman interview by Edward Shorter on February 6, 1987.

7. Sweet BH and Hilleman MR. "The Vacuolating Virus, S.V. $_{40}$," *Proceedings of the Society for Experimental Biology and Medicine* 105 (November 1960):420-27.

8. Shorter references Goffe AP, *et al*. Poliomyelitis vaccines. *Lancet* March 18, 1961:612.

9. An extensive literature review on the possible dangers of SV40's to public health was published by Fraumeni FJ, et al. "An evaluation of the carcinogenicity of simian virus 40 in man. *JAMA* 1963;185:713-18.

10. Schmeck HM. Studies identify virus in vaccine. *New York Times*, February 7, 1962, p. 27.

12. Paul JR. *History of Poliomyelitis*. New Haven, Conn.: Yale University Press, 1971, pp. 373-74.

13. *Congressional Record—Senate, Proceedings of October 15, 1971*, pp. S 16291-99; December 8, 1971, pp. S20902-14, and *Consumer Safety Act of 1972: Hearings before the Subcommittee on Executive Reorganization and Government Research of the Committee on Government Operations, United States, Senate, Ninety-Second Congress, Second Session on Titles I and II of S. 3419*. Washington, D.C.: Government Printing Office, 1972.

14. CovertAction Information Bulletin. Turners "Born Again" CIA. In: *Dirty Work: The CIA in Western Europe*. P. Agee and L Wolf, eds. Secaucus, NJ: Lyle Stuart Inc., 1977, pp. 313.

15. NCI staff. *The Special Virus Cancer Program: Progress Report #8*. Office of the Associate Scientific Director for Viral Oncology (OASDVO). J. B. Moloney, Ed., Washington, D. C.: U. S. Government Printing Office, 1971, pp. 63, 223-224.

16. Martin JW, Ahmed KN, Zeng LC, Olsen JC, Seward JG and Seehrai JS. African green monkey origin of the atypical cytopathic 'stealth virus' isolated from a patient with chronic fatigue syndrome. *Clinical and Diagnostic Virology* 1995;4:93-103.

17. Martin JW, Zeng LC, Ahmed K and Roy M. Cytomegalovirus-related sequence in an atypical cytopathic virus repeatedly isolated from a patient with chronic fatigue syndrome. *American Journal of Pathology* 1994;145;2:440-451.

18. Martin JW. "Stealth" Viruses. An oral presentation before the "Twentieth Century Plagues" symposia held at the Embassy Suites Hotel in Los Angeles on March 1, 1996, and at the San Francisco Airport Marriott Hotel on March 2, 1996. Text, slides and additional information is available at URL http://www.steathvirus.com.

19. Personal conversation with Dr. John Martin, Director of the Center for Complex Infectious Diseases, 3328 Stevens Avenue, Rosemead, California 91770, Telephone: 818-799-4500, and Walter Kyle, Attorney at law, Sixty South Street, Hingham, MA 02043, Telephone: 617-741-5953, Fax: 617-741-5166.

20. Staff writer. Porton opened to the public. *Nature* 1968 220(166):426. This article discussed state-of-the-art large-scale production facilities used for developing vaccines against a variety of viruses. Methods described included the use of "rolling bottles in a sealed unit—an apparatus only available at Porton (though one like it was known to also exist in Fort Detrick, MD[32])—it is possible to grow 2.1x10[11] (2,100,000,000,000) virus particles per batch."

21. Covert NM. *Cutting Edge: A history of Fort Detrick, Maryland 1943-1993*. Fort Detrick: Headquarters U.S. Army Garrison Public Affairs Office (HSHD-PA), 1993, pp. 85.

22. Strecker R. The Strecker Memorandum: The Cause, The Effects and the Possible Cure for the Pandemic AIDS. Eagle Rock, CA: The Strecker Group, 1988.

23. Walgate R. Hepatitis B vaccine: Pasteur Institute in AIDS fracas. *Nature* 1983;304:104.

24. *Hearings before the Subcommittee on Health and Scientific Research of the Committee on Human Resources, United States Senate, Ninety-fifth Congress, First Session, on Examination of Serious Deficiencies in the Defense Department's Efforts to Protect the Human Subjects of Drug Research, Biological Testing Involving Human Subjects by the Department of Defense*. Washington, D.C.: U.S. Government Printing Office, March 8 and May 23, 1977, p. 91.

25. *Department of Defense Appropriations For 1970: Hearings Before A Subcommittee of the Committee on Appropriations House of Representatives, Ninety-first Contress, First Session, H.B. 15090, Part 5, Research, Development, Test and Evaluation, Dept. of the Army*. U.S. Government Printing Office, Washington, D.C., 1969.

26. *Hearings before the Select Committee to Study Governmental Operations With Respect to Intelligence Activities of the United States Senate, Ninety-Fourth Congress, First Session, Vol. 1: Unauthorized Storage of Toxic Agents, Intelligence Activities Senate Resolution 21*, Washington, D.C.: U.S. Government Printing Office, September 16, 17, and 18, 1975 (pp. 97-98 for Kissinger's role in illegal stockpiling of biological weapons during the early to mid-1970s); for Kissinger's obvious directing of Zumwalt or Laird to obtain $10 million appropriated in 1970 for the development of AIDS-like viruses see also: Isaacson W. *Kissinger: A Biography*. New York: Simon & Schuster, 1992, p. 205.

27. NCI staff. *The Special Virus Cancer Program: Progress Report #8*. Office of the Associate Scientific Director for Viral Oncology (OASDVO). J. B. Moloney, Ed., Washington, D. C.: U. S. Government Printing Office, 1971

28. Bionetics Research Laboratories, Inc., A Division of Litton Industries. Progress report on investigation of carcinogenesis with selected virus preparations in the newborn monkey.*Ibid.*, pp. 273-278.

29. NCI staff. *The Special Virus Cancer Program: Progress Report #9* Office of the Associate Scientific Director for Viral Oncology (OASDVO). J. B. Moloney, Ed., Washington, D. C.: U. S. Government Printing Office, 1972.

30. See the following Gallo *et al.*, publications: Gallaher RE, Ting RC and Gallo RC. A common change aspartyl-tRNA in polyoma and SV transformed cells. *Biochimica Et Biophysica Acta* 1972;272:568-582.; Bobrow SN, Smith RG, Reitz MS and Gallo RC. Stimulated normal human lymphocytes contain a ribonuclease-sensitive DNA polymerase distinct from viral RNA-directed DNA polymerase. *Proceedings National Academy of Sciences* 1972;69;11:3228-3232; Robert MS, Smith RG, Gallo RC, Sarin PS and Abrell JW. Viral and cellular DNA polymerase: Comparison of activities with synthetic and natural RNA templates. *Science* 1972;176:798-800; Ting RC, Yang SS and Gallo RC. Reverse transcriptase, RNA tumor virus transformation and derivative of Rifamycin SV. *Nature New Biology* 1972;236:163-165.

31. Litton Industries, Inc. Annual Report to the Securities and Exchange Commission for Fiscal Year Ended July 31, 1977. Commission file number 1-3998. Securities and Exchange Commission, Office of Reports, October 31, 1977.

32. Negative Population Growth, Inc. Why we need a small U.S. population and how we can achieve it. *Foreign Affairs Magazine*. Council on Foreign Relations. March/April, 1996.

33. Urnovitz HB. Human ednogenous retroviruses: Nature, occurrence, and clinical implications in human disease. *Clinical Microbiology Reviews* January, 1996, pp. 72-99; see also: Fisher BL. Microbiologist issues a challenge to science: Did the first oral polio vaccine lots contaminated with monkey viruses create a monkey-human hybrid called HIV-1? *The Vaccine Reaction* 1996 (April);2;1:1-6.

34. Personal communication from Barbara Loe Fisher, May 20, 1996. To join the vaccine safety movement and work for social change, readers are encouraged to contact the NVIC at 512 W. Maple Avenue, Suite 206, Vienna, VA 22180 or call 1-800-909-SHOT. This charitable organization receives no government, foundation or corporate grants and exists entirely on memberships and donations from consumers for the information they make available, including a bimonthly newsletter *THE VACCINE REACTION* which keeps consumers updated on the latest political and scientific development in vaccine research and policymaking.

35. MacBride S. Preface. In: *Dirty Work-2: The CIA in Africa*. Secaucus, Ray E, Schaap W, Van Meter K and Wolf L eds. Secaucus, NJ: Lyle Stewart, Inc., 1979, pp. xiii-xiv.

36. Raeburn P. 1/3 of blacks asked in '90 said AIDS a form of genocide. Associated Press, Thursday, November 2, 1995; for primary reference, see Thomas SB and Quinn SC. Understanding the attitude of black Americans. In: *Dimensions of HIV Prevention: Needle Exchange*. J. Stryker and M. D. Smith, eds. Menlo Park, CA: Kenry J. Kaiser Family Foundation, 1993, pp. 99-128.

37. Henry P. Speech in Virginia convention. Richmond, VA. March 23, 1775. In: *Bartlett's Familiar Quotations*. E. M. Beck, ed. Boston: Little, Brown and Company, 1980, p. 383.

38. The harsh realities presented in this book could not be more painful. Seemingly unfortunate, is the fact that we depend on pain to be moved to change. Thus, this work holds great potential for changing the perception, and several widespread applications, of man's inhumanity toward man. In essence, now that we have diagnosed many gross injustices, perhaps now we can prevent some more.

Chapter 26. Epilogue

1. Horowitz LG, Strecker R, Cantwell A, Vid D, Grossman G, and Kyle W. The mysterious origin of HIV: Reviewing the natural, iatrogenic, and genocidal theories of AIDS. Abstract #: D3678. Paper presented during the social sciences section of the XI International Conference on AIDS, Vancouver, BC, Canada, July 10, 1996.

2. Herrera F, Adamson RH and Gallo RC. Uptake of transfer ribonucleic acid by normal and leukemic cells. *Proc Nat Acad Sci* 1970;67;4:1943-1950.

3. Gallo RC, Sarin PS, Allen PT, Newton WA Priori ES, Bowen JM and Dmochowski L. Reverse transcriptase in type C virus particles of human origin. *Nature New Biology* 1971;232:140-142.

4. It is now well established that the Bush administration supplied Sadam Hussein with military supplies, including chemical and biological weapons, as late as two weeks before Hussein's troops invaded Kuwait. Bush administration officials, including Secretary of State James Baker III, and Gen-

eral Norman Schwartzkopf, who knew of the biological and chemical perils facing troops headed for the gulf, have also been implicated in the ongoing cover-up of facts concerning Gulf War Syndrome. A class action suit filed on behalf of ailing veterans cites Tanox Biosystems, Inc., a Houston-based firm partly controlled by James Baker III and funded by George Bush, as partly responsible for developing and testing contaminated vaccines given to servicemen and women. One such vaccine appears to have been tested in Huntsville Prison (TX). Inmates, and later their guards and surrounding community members, developed GWS-like ailments before the Gulf War. The syndrome, it has been estimated, at the time of this writing, may be effecting as many as 200,000 veterans.

Following the war it was learned that Hill and Knowlton, Gallo's public relations firm, had fraudulently portrayed Hussein's elite guardsmen as having tortured and maimed babies. Infants thrown from windows, crashing to their graves, was the emotional bait that Hill and Knowlton cast through the press. The American public swallowed it hook, line, and sinker. The successful psychological warfare ploy was followed by George Bush's infamous call to arms— "This aggression will not stand."

See: McAlvany DS. Special report: Germ warfare against America—The desert storm plague and cover-up. *The McAlvany Intelligence Advisor*, August, 1996; Riegle DW, D'Amato AM. U.S. Chemical and biological warfare-related dueal use exports to Iraq and their possible impact on the health consequences of the Persian Gulf War. Committee on Banking, Housing and Urban Affairs with Respect to Export Administration. United States Senate, 103d Congress, 2d Session, May 25, 1994; Riley J. Contrary to what the Pentagon is telling you there is a deadly Gulf War biological disease ravaging our troops, and it is contagious! *The Washington Times*, November 3, 1996 p 5.

5. Garth Nicolson is respected as a hero to the masses of Gulf War syndrome veterans. Following the publication of several scientific reports indicating biological weapons and contaminated vaccines were associated with the veterans ailments, Dr. Nicolson's laboratory at M.D. Anderson Cancer Research Center in Houston was sabotaged. Refrigerators containing more than 5,000 study samples of sick veterans blood were unplugged. The tenured professor was thus compelled to seek a restraining order against the university. Later Dr. Nicolson, and his co-investigator/wife Nancy, were pressured to leave the University of Texas at Houston. He is currently in charge of the Institute for Molecular Medicine, Box 52470, Irvine, CA 92619, and he invites inquires from Gulf War veterans. For more on Persian Gulf War syndrome see: Nicolson GL, Hyman E, Korenyi-Both A, Lopex DA, Nicolson N, Rea W, Urnovitz H. Progress on Persian Gulf War illnesses—Reality and hypotheses. *Int J Occupational Medicine and Toxicology* 1995;4;3:1-6.

6. Names and specifics are withheld as requested by the research director as is customary prior to official scientific publication of data.

7. Geissler E. (with contributions by D. Baltimore)*Biological and Toxin Weapons Today*. Stockholm and London: Stockholm International Peace Research Institute; Oxford University Press, 1986. p. 31.

8. Personal communication from Tammy Nunnally, Office of Communications, Office of the Director, Centers for Disease Control and Prevention, February 18, 1997; Drotman DP. AIDS. *World Book Encyclopedia*, 1994 edition. World Book Publishing, Chicago; 1994:163-5.

9. In fact, direct quotes from Kissinger's *NSM200* document concerning Third World population control include: 1) "depopulation should be the highest priority of U.S. Foreign policy towards the Third World," 2) Reduction of the rate of population in these States is a matter of vital U.S. national security," 3) "The U.S. economy will require large and increasing amounts of minerals from abroad, especially from less-developed countries. That fact gives the U.S. enhanced interests in the political, economic and social stability of the supplying countries. Whereever a lessening of population can increase the prospects for such stability, population policy becomes relevant to resources, supplies and to the economic interest of the United States." See: National Security Council. *NSSM 200—Implications of Worldwide Population Growth for U.S. Security and Overseas Interests*. Washington, DC: The White House, December 10, 1974. Declassified, July 3, 1989, NSIAD-ROX-89-4. Also see: Rense J. *AIDS Exposed: Secrets, Lies, & Myths*. Goleta, CA: BioAlert Press, 1996, pp. 51 and 52.

10. Rock A. The lethal dangers of the billion-dollar vaccine business. *Money Magazine*, December 1996, p. 161.

11. Loftus J and Aarons M. *The Secret War Against the Jews: How Western Espionage Betrayed the Jewish People*. New York: St. Martin's Press, 1994.

12. Simpson C. *Science of Coercion: Communication Research & Psychological Warfare 1945-1960*. Oxford: Oxford University Press, 1994, pp. 60-62.

13. *The Holy Bible: Containing the Old and New Testaments* (translated from the original tongues being the [King James] version set forth A.D. 1611). London: Collins' Clear-Type Press, 1946, pp. 227-242.

Acknowledgments

I am deeply indebted to my wife Jackie for not only facilitating my research and writing, but also for her exceptional work in holding our family together during the two years this work drew on our attention and financial reserves.

My earliest AIDS investigation efforts began at the request of Stanley Bergman, the chief executive officer of Henry Schein, Inc. Thanks are given to him along with Jimmy Breslawski, both of whom were instrumental in financing my initial research on this topic.

There have been several very influential academicians who contributed greatly to my development as a researcher and educator who deserve my heart felt appreciation. The late James H. Leathem from Rutgers who taught me the meaning of inspired teaching. Joan and Myrin Borysenko for supporting me in reaching out for broader meanings in life and science. Helmut Zander who taught me to defend the knowledge we are privileged to hold. Jack Caton and Sean Meitner who made a surgeon out of me despite my initial distaste for the clinical art. Tony Adams for saving my life during a clinical emergency. Bill McHugh and Erling Johansen for validating my knowledge, writing, and researching skills. Chet Douglas for directing my post-doctoral research and studies at Harvard and for saying "If Horowitz says it, there's got to be something to it." Jack Dillenberg for being a model public health professional and human being. Al McAlister and Larry Green for many valuable lessons in public health education.

I also wish to thank my health care providers and friends for keeping me pain free during the countless hours I spent in front of a word processor. Tom Pearce for his medical expertise, Ivo Waerlop for keeping me aligned, Beth Goldberg for her spiritual guidance and inspired touch, Martha Woodworth for her reliable insights, Eli Jacob for hitting the right acupuncture points, and Rob Lipkowitz and Karen Cluett for my smile care.

Many people graciously assisted this effort by providing books, papers, and news clippings from which I drew. I would especially like to thank Charlotte Minisan, Hank and Marian Klein, Steven Bell, Virginia Moore-Barber, Bill Hershey, John Burgin, Gus Grossman, Harriet Wealth, Burton Linne, Pat Gross, Rick and Diane Balsara, Brian White, Rosemary

Lesch, Alan Cantwell, Walter Kyle, Dave Deeley, Ken and David Runkle, Abdul Alim Muhammad, Barbara Justice, and Captain Joyce Riley.

There are many other people who have supported or guided this work one way or another. Foremost I would like to thank Robert Strecker and The Strecker Group who's contributions led me and many others to consider the man-made origin of AIDS. Da Vid from the San Francisco Medical Research Foundation deserves special thanks for his practical and spiritual support along with his commitment to AIDS patient care. Barbara Loe-Fisher, for her research and recommendations and for guiding me to Rudy Shur who provided hours of thoughtful guidance. Nancy and Garth Nicolson for their constructive suggestions. Robert Fiske for his excellent editing services. In addition, I wish to thank Ian Shapolsky and Ann Cassouto, Roger Levin, John Seale, Eva Snead, and Vince Marshall, John Martin, and Jean-Pierre Eudier for their encouragement and advice. And special thanks to Larry Levin and Sam Fick for their financial support.

To my friends and family who tolerated my, at times, zealous recanting of my latest discoveries, and months of being incommunicado, including Barbara and Artie Heissenbottle, Nick and Martha Safford, Larry and Annette Knight, Tom and Lynn Bishop, cousins Danny and Shelly Horowitz, Vernon and Lenore Grubinger, Risa Gara, Lola Buchbinder, Beth Spittle, Michael Cook, Tarek and Georgie El Heneidy, John Cooney, Carra Hood, Jeanine Smith, George White, Duane Beers, Ralph Crapanzano, Bill Lewis, Peter Agnos, John McGannon, Keigm and Susan Crook, Steve and Sue Hamilton, and Rick Dolk.

Finally, I want to thank God for directing my work and my choice of parents, my father Sieg who instilled in me faith in myself when he professed "You can do anything you put your mind to," and my mother Lily, who I challenged incessantly, now in retrospect, blindly. Without your three way support, this book would not be.

574

Index

Aaron Diamond Research Center, 125
Abbott Laboratories, 126, 327
Acer, David, 139, 465, 540
Actinomycin-D, 123
Adams, James, 210
Adams, John, 294
Adenauer, Conrad, 338
aerosols (viral), 463
aflatoxin, 113
Africa, 18, 113, 115, 119, 151-154, 159, 161,
    174, 214, 233, 248, 250, 252, 255, 257,
    268, 269, 303, 305, 343, 347-361, 378,
    385, 388, 390, 393, 397, 399, 421, 422,
    461, 469, 483, 505, 514, 523, 524; AIDS
    case dating back to 1959 in, 126; AIDS
    belt in, 394; AIDS epidemic beginning in,
    130, 258; CIA covert operations in, 347-
    361, 523, 524; identified—T cell
    leukemia, 160; intelligence in, 309;
    measles vaccination in, 257; Kissinger's
    position on, 347-359; monkeys in, 3, 396,
    505; natives in, 12; vaccine trials in, 98,
African green monkey(s), 128, 130, 131, 364,
    389, 395, 420, 482-492, 505; immunode-
    ficiency viruses (SIV), 129
AFRICARE, 351
Agee, Philip, 352
Agency for International Development
    (USAID), 160, 172, 353
agent orange, 22, 323
AIDS, 4, 50, 100, 118, 129, 174, 180, 239, 240,
    249, 323, 324, 326, 328, 363, 394, 403,
    410, 450, 465, 483; belt in Africa, 394;
    "Big Bang" theory of, 131; case in 1968,
    127; cure for, 107; denial regarding
    intentional transmission, 485; discovery
    of the virus, 64; earliest cases, 125-128;
    epidemic, 32, 173, 240, 242; epidemic
    beginning in Africa, 130, 523, 524;
    French/American AIDS fracas(es), 57, 59,
    130, 414; GRID (Gay related immune

deficiency), 55, 62, 118, 123, 251; Haitian
origin theory of, 106; iatrogenic theory
on, 128-133, 496-498, 507; in Africa,
258; intentional transmission theory, 494-
496; pandemic, 295; poliovaccine theory
of, 128-130; related complex (ARC), 5;
related diseases, 32; related retrovirus
(ARV), 56, 63; striking Africans, 56;
striking Africans and homosexuals, 56,
137; tests, 379; transmission, 249, 541;
transmission for population control, 482;
transmission from the vaccine, 239, 524;
virus(es), 3, 4, 5, 39, 51, 55, 60, 87, 106,
154, 239, 242, 249, 255, 260, 363, 365,
541 (see also *HIV*) ; virus engineering, 87,
109
AIDS-like virus(es), 17, 32, 47, 49, 51, 70-76,
93, 125, 140, 203, 206, 212, 214, 305,
311, 384, 421, 422, 494, 497; experiments
to develop, 100, 485; evolution of, 130-
133; testing of, 40
Alessio, John, 230
Algren, Nelson, 151
Allan Memorial Institute (AMI), 319
Allen, John, 36
Allen, Richard, 205, 362
Alsop, Joseph, 195
Altman, Lawrence, 465, 470
Altmann, Klaus, 340
Ambros, Otto, 344
American Academy of Pediatrics, 499
American Cancer Society, 475
American Cyanimid, 492
American Enterprise Institute for Public Policy
    Research, 174
American Indians, 12
American Institute for Free Labor Development
    (AIFLD), 344
American Institute of Biological Sciences
    (AIBS), 36
American Liberty League, 342

About the Author

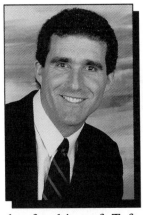

Leonard G. Horowitz, D.M.D., M.A., M.P.H., is a Harvard graduate, independent investigator, and an internationally known authority in behavioral science and public health education. He earned his doctorate in medical dentistry from Tufts University, a master of arts degree in health education from Beacon College, and a master of public health degree in behavioral science from Harvard University.

One of healthcare's most captivating motivational speakers, Dr. Horowitz has served on the faculties of Tufts University, Harvard University, and Leslie College's Institute for the Arts and Human Development. He has also served as a consultant to several leading healthcare corporations, national associations, and as a professional speaker, he travels to more than one-hundred locations a year to present keynote speeches, lectures, and seminars.

Dr. Horowitz has authored over eighty articles, ten audiocassettes, two videotapes and ten books including the critically acclaimed Florida dental AIDS tragedy exposé, *Deadly Innocence.* His other books include: *AIDS, Fear and Infection Control, Overcoming Your Fear of the Dentist, Choosing Health For Yourself: A Clear and Practical Guide to Motivating Self-Care, Freedom From Desk Job Stress and Computer Strain*, and his latest, *Taking Care of Yourself: An Audio Seminar and Workbook for Motivating Yourself to Optimal Health.*

Dr. Horowitz is also an avid fitness buff and spends his free time hiking, swimming, sailing, snorkeling, singing, and playing guitar with his wife and two daughters.